Restorative
Dental
Materials

Restorative Dental Materials

TENTH EDITION

Edited by
Robert G. Craig, Ph.D.
Marcus L. Ward Professor Emeritus
Department of Biologic and Materials Sciences
The University of Michigan School of Dentistry
Ann Arbor, Michigan

with 373 illustrations

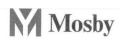 Mosby

St. Louis Baltimore Boston Carlsbad Chicago Naples New York Philadelphia Portland
London Madrid Mexico City Singapore Sydney Tokyo Toronto Wiesbaden

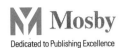

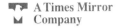

Vice President and Publisher: Don Ladig
Executive Editor: Linda L. Duncan
Developmental Editor: Jo Salway
Project Manager: Carol Sullivan Weis
Production: Shepherd, Inc.
Designer: Sheilah Barrett
Manufacturing Manager: Dave Graybill

TENTH EDITION

Copyright © 1997 by Mosby-Year Book, Inc.

Previous editions copyrighted 1960, 1964, 1968, 1971, 1975, 1980, 1985, 1989, 1993

Printed in the United States of America
Composition by Shepherd, Inc.
Printing/binding by Courier Westford, Inc.

Mosby-Year Book, Inc.
11830 Westline Industrial Drive
St. Louis, Missouri 63146

Library of Congress Cataloging in Publication Data

Restorative dental materials / edited by Robert G. Craig. – 10th ed.
    p. cm.
    Includes bibliographical references and index.
    ISBN 0-8151-1920-8
    1. Dental materials.   I. Craig, Robert G. (Robert George), 1923-

RK652.5.P47   1996
617.6'95–dc20
                                  96-28618
                                    CIP

98 99 00 / 9 8 7 6 5 4 3 2

Contributors

UNIVERSITY OF MICHIGAN
School of Dentistry
Ann Arbor, Michigan

Robert G. Craig, Ph.D.
Marcus L. Ward Professor Emeritus
Department of Biologic and Materials Sciences

Carl T. Hanks, D.D.S., Ph.D.
Professor
Department of Oral Medicine, Pathology, and Surgery

David H. Kohn, Ph.D.
Associate Professor
Department of Biologic and Materials Sciences

Andrew Koran, III, D.D.S., M.S.
Professor
Department of Prosthodontics

William J. O'Brien, Ph.D.
Professor
Department of Biologic and Materials Sciences

Warren C. Wagner, M.S.E., Ph.D.
Senior Research Associate
Department of Biologic and Materials Sciences

UNIVERSITY OF TEXAS HEALTH SCIENCES CENTER
Dental Branch
Houston, Texas

John M. Powers, Ph.D.
Professor
Department of Basic Sciences

MEDICAL COLLEGE OF GEORGIA
School of Dentistry
Augusta, Georgia

John C. Wataha, D.M.D., Ph.D.
Associate Professor
Department of Oral Rehabilitation

A Tribute to Floyd A. Peyton

D r. Floyd A. Peyton, the principal author of the first edition of *Restorative Dental Materials* published in 1960, died in July of 1994 at the age of 89 and a half, after a wonderfully long and productive career. It was my privilege to have been associated with him in a number of capacities. He was my mentor in the field of dental materials and was my department chairman, a research collaborator, a colleague, and a friend. His philosophy of instruction in dental materials was, "Keep it simple and make it fun," which I will paraphrase as, don't make it unnecessarily complicated and make it related to dentistry. That thought was the thrust of the writing of the first edition and continues to be our goal for the tenth edition.

Dr. Peyton's interest in disseminating information on dental materials was not limited only to students at The University of Michigan, but was nationwide and worldwide. This fact is evidenced by the number of leaders of dental materials programs at universities and industries in the United States and in countries such as Brazil, Argentina, Chile, Venezuela, Guatemala, New Zealand, Switzerland, Great Britain, Egypt, Japan, and Korea who received training at The University of Michigan. He also taught for extended periods at dental schools in Brazil, Uruguay, Egypt, Argentina, Chile, Venezuela, Guatemala, Colombia, New Zealand, and India. It

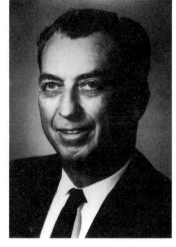

is not surprising, therefore, that various editions of *Restorative Dental Materials* have been translated into Spanish, Portuguese, Hindi, and Japanese, and about one third of the copies of the English editions are foreign sales.

Although Dr. Peyton's scientific contributions to the field of dental materials are impressive, his contributions of leadership because of his humanity are equally noteworthy. He consistently encouraged and was involved in the development of young teachers and investigators, and these efforts moved the field ahead by leaps and bounds. Thus his encouragement and insight will be missed, and we thank him for all his efforts on our behalf.

ROBERT G. CRAIG

Preface

The tenth edition of *Restorative Dental Materials* maintains its tradition of being a textbook for undergraduate dental students but would also be an excellent basic text for individuals in training to become dental technicians. Dental practitioners will find the text useful because it reviews important fundamental information on new classes of materials developed since their undergraduate degree.

The dramatic changes in restorative dental materials over the past 40 years have made frequent editions of the text essential. The development and introduction of zinc polyacrylate, glass ionomer, and resin cements; high copper amalgams; anterior and posterior composites; sealants; polyether and silicone impression materials; low gold alloys; silver-palladium alloys; titanium and its alloys; and metal ceramic systems occurred during this period. The use of high-speed cutting, visible light curing systems, automatic mixing systems, custom-made athletic mouth protectors, CAD-CAM processing of ceramics, disinfection of impression and model materials, and quantitative methods for evaluating cytotoxicity are further examples of changes in the biomaterials area during this period.

It is crucial that the basic sciences on which biomaterials is based be reviewed for dental students and examples of their application to biomaterials and clinical dentistry be presented. An understanding of the basic principles is important because of the rapid rate at which new materials and systems are being developed. An understanding of the fundamental and applied information about materials provides the background needed to correctly use current and future dental materials in the clinic and dental laboratory, as well as to intelligently select materials for a dental practice.

The text begins with a chapter describing the history of the development of restorative dental materials, which is followed by six chapters of basic science of special importance to dental materials. Although basic sciences are included in predental courses, the topics presented have probably not been emphasized and certainly few dental examples of their importance have been stressed. These chapters include a discussion of surface phenomena; optical, thermal, electrical, and mechanical properties of materials; the nature of metals and alloys; polymerization and polymers; and evaluation of the biocompatibility of dental materials. The remaining 12 chapters describe the properties of materials and the effect of manipulation on properties starting with direct restorative materials and followed by indirect restorative and laboratory materials.

Special features include review paragraphs at the end of major sections or chapters and problems and their solutions at the end of chapters to emphasize the problem-solving approach to the teaching of dental materials. Extensive use of figures and tables of data are made to complement the text. This edition uses metric units exclusively; however, an appendix at the end of the text provides conversion factors to English units. Each chapter has a list of references for further reading and is subdivided into topic sections. References to current reviews, as well as the most important research articles, are selected whenever possible.

All chapters have been revised, but major changes have been made in the following areas: (1) current review of the toxicity of mercury and its compounds; (2) new amalgams and amalgamators; (3) bonding of amalgam to tooth structure; (4) current review of adhesion of composites to tooth structure; (5) composition of composites, including filler types and levels and dual curing systems; (6) triple cure restorative composite-ionomer hybrids; (7) dual cure composite cements and triple cure composite-ionomer hybrid cements; (8) disinfection of impressions; (9) monophase impression materials; (10) automixing of very heavy consistency rubber impression materials; (11) major revision of gold, silver-palladium, and base metal casting alloys; (12) current review of titanium and its alloys; and (13) thorough review of biocompatibility testing of biomaterials and their interpretation.

I express my appreciation to Kitty Kahn for her diligent assistance in preparing the manuscript for the tenth edition. I especially thank L. Georgine Craig for her encouragement and forbearance during the revisions and proofreading.

ROBERT G. CRAIG

Contents

1   *Scope and History of Restorative Materials, 1*
Scope of Materials Covered in Restorative Dentistry, 1
     Basic sciences applied to restorative materials, 2
     Application of various sciences, 2
History, 3
     Early history, 4
     Medieval and early modern period, 5
       Some contemporary arts of the Middle Ages, 6
     Beginning of the dental science–1600 to 1840, 7
     The period of mechanical improvement–
       1840 to 1900, 9
     Advances since 1900, 11

2   *Applied Surface Phenomena, 16*
Characterization of Solid Surfaces, 17
The Colloidal State, 18
     Nature of colloids, 18
     Typical colloid systems, 19
     Gels, 19
     Syneresis, 20
     Emulsions, 20
Diffusion through Membranes and Osmotic
     Pressure, 20
Adsorption, Absorption, and Sorption, 20
Surface Tension and Wetting, 21
Capillary Rise, 24
     Penetration coefficient, 24
     Isolated capillaries, 24
Forces Involved in Denture Retention, 26
Adhesion, 27

3   *Optical, Thermal, and Electrical
Properties, 30*
Optical Properties, 30
     Color, 30
     Measurement of color, 31
       Instrumental technic, 31
       Visual technic, 32
       Surface finish and thickness, 34
     Pigmentation, 34
     Metamerism, 35
     Fluorescence, 35
     Opacity, translucency, and transparency, 35
       Measurement of contrast ratio, 36

     Index of refraction, 36
     Optical constants, 36
       Scattering coefficient, 37
       Absorption coefficient, 37
       Light reflectivity, 37
       Contrast ratio, 38
Thermal Properties, 38
     Temperature, 38
     Transition temperatures, 40
     Heat of fusion, 41
     Thermal conductivity, 42
     Specific heat, 42
     Thermal diffusivity, 44
     Coefficient of thermal expansion, 44
Electrical Properties, 45
     Electrical conductivity and resistivity, 45
     Dielectric constant, 47
     Electromotive force, 47
     Galvanism, 48
     Electrochemical corrosion, 49
     Zeta-potential, 50
Other Properties, 50
     Tarnish and discoloration, 51
     Water sorption, 51
     Solubility and disintegration, 51
     Setting time, 51
     Shelf life, 52

4   *Mechanical Properties, 56*
Force, 56
     Occlusal forces, 56
     Forces on restorations, 56
     Summary of occlusal forces, 57
Stress, 57
     Types of stress, 58
     Strain, 58
Stress-Strain Curves, 59
     Proportional and elastic limits, 61
     Yield strength, 62
     Ultimate strength, 63
     Fracture strength, 64
     Elongation, 64
     Elastic modulus, 65
     Poisson's ratio, 65

Ductility and malleability, 66
Resilience, 66
Toughness, 67
Fracture toughness, 67
Properties and stress-strain curves, 69
Other Mechanical Properties, 69
Tensile properties of brittle materials, 69
Compressive properties, 70
Shear strength, 71
Bond strengths, 72
Bending, 72
Transverse strength, 73
Permanent bending, 74
Torsion, 75
Fatigue strength, 76
Viscoelasticity, 77
Fluid behavior and viscosity, 77
Viscoelastic materials, 79
Mechanical models of viscoelasticity, 80
Creep compliance, 81
Dynamic Mechanical Properties, 83
Dynamic modulus, 83
Impact strength, 84
Tear Strength and Tear Energy, 84
Mechanical Properties of Composites, 85
Surface Mechanical Properties, 86
Indentation hardness, 86
Brinell hardness test, 87
Knoop hardness test, 88
Vickers hardness test, 89
Rockwell hardness test, 89
Shore A hardness, 90
Friction, 90
Wear, 91
Stress Analysis and Design of Dental Structures, 92
Two-dimensional photoelasticity, 92
Finite element analysis, 93
Summary, 93
Specifications for Restorative Materials, 94
American Dental Association specifications, 95
American Dental Association acceptance
program, 95
Index of Federal Specifications and Standards, 95

5   *Nature of Metals and Alloys, 104*
General Characteristics of Metals, 104
Metallic bonding and properties of alloys, 104
Crystal Structure of Metals, 104
Physical properties and crystal structure, 105
Deformation of metals, 106
Fracture of solids, 108

Nature of Alloys, 109
Classification of alloy systems, 110
Solid solution, 111
Intermetallic compounds, 111
Eutectic mixture, 111
Phase Diagrams, 112
Types of phase diagrams, 113
Solid solutions, 113
Eutectic alloy, 113
Intermetallic compounds, 115
Ternary phase diagrams, 115
Construction of phase diagrams, 116
Properties of Alloys, 117
Solid-solution alloys, 117
Eutectic alloys, 117
Intermetallic compounds, 117
Microstructure of Metals and Alloys, 118
Solidification of metals, 118
Solidification of alloys, 119
Cast microstructures, 120
Cold-worked microstructures, 121
Recrystallization and grain growth, 122
Techniques to Strengthen Metals
and Alloys, 124

6   *Polymers and Polymerization, 127*
Basic Nature of Polymers, 127
Chemical composition, 127
Molecular weight, 128
Spatial structure, 128
Preparation of Polymers, 130
Addition polymerization, 130
Free-radical polymerization, 130
Ring-opening polymerization, 132
Ionic polymerization, 133
Condensation polymerization, 133
Other polymers, 135

7   *Biocompatibility of Dental Materials, 137*
Biology and Inflammatory Response of Oral Tissue
to Injury, 140
The tooth, 140
Enamel, 140
Dentin and pulp, 140
Dentin permeability, 142
Bone, 143
Membranous bone formation, 143
Endochondral bone formation, 144
Periodontium, 144
Gingiva and mucosa, 145
Summary, 146

Types of Biocompatibility Tests, 146
 Initial tests, 147
  Cytotoxicity assays, 147
  Mutagenesis assays, 151
  Other assays, 152
 Secondary or intermediate tests, 153
 Usage tests in animals, 154
  Dental pulp irritation tests, 154
  Dental implants into bone, 154
  Mucosa and gingival usage tests, 155
 Correlation among screening and usage tests, 155
 Summary, 156
Biocompatibility of Various Dental Materials, 156
 Reactions of pulp, 156
  Microleakage, 156
  Dentin bonding, 157
  Dentin bonding agents, 158
  Resin-based materials, 159
  Amalgams and cast alloys, 159
  Glass ionomers, 161
  Liners, varnishes, and nonresin cements, 161
  Bleaching agents, 163
 Reaction of other oral soft tissues to restorative
  materials, 163
 Reaction of bone and soft tissues to implant
  materials, 165
  Reactions to ceramic implant materials, 165
  Reactions to pure metals and alloys, 166
  Reactions to other materials, 166
 Summary, 167

8 *Cements, 172*
Zinc Phosphate Cement, 173
 Composition, 173
  Powder, 173
  Liquid, 173
 Chemistry of the setting reaction, 174
 Manipulation, 174
  Mixing slab, 174
  Powder/liquid ratio, 174
  Care of the liquid, 174
  Mixing procedure, 174
  Frozen slab method, 175
 Characteristic properties, 175
  ANSI/ADA Specification No. 96 for dental
   water-based cements, 175
  Consistency and film thickness, 175
  Viscosity, 179
  Setting time, 179
  Strength, 181
  Solubility and disintegration, 181
  Dimensional stability, 182
  Acidity, 182
  Thermal and electrical conductivity, 182

Applications, 183
  Cementation of orthodontic bands, 183
Zinc Oxide–Eugenol and Non-Eugenol Cements, 183
 Composition, 183
 Chemistry of setting, 184
 Manipulation, 184
  Dispensing, 184
  Mixing procedures, 184
 Characteristic properties, 184
  Film thickness, 184
  Setting time, 184
  Compressive strength, 186
  Solubility, 186
 Applications, 186
  Base, 186
  Temporary cementation, 186
  Temporary restorations, 187
  Permanent cementation, 187
  Endodontic sealers, 187
  ANSI/ADA Specification No. 57 (ISO 6876), 187
  Tissue management, 189
Zinc Polyacrylate Cement, 189
 Composition and setting reaction, 189
 Manipulation, 190
 Properties, 190
  ANSI/ADA Specification No. 96, 190
  Viscosity, 190
  Setting time, 190
  Film thickness, 191
  Strength, 191
  Bond strength, 191
  Solubility and disintegration, 191
  Dimensional stability, 191
  Acidity, 191
 Applications, 191
Glass Ionomer Cement, 192
 Composition and setting reaction, 192
 Manipulation, 192
 Properties, 193
  Film thickness, 193
  Setting time, 193
  Strength, 193
  Bond strength, 193
  Solubility and disintegration, 193
  Biological properties, 193
 Applications, 194
Hybrid Ionomer Cement, 194
 Composition, 194
 Chemistry of setting, 194
 Manipulation, 194
 Characteristic properties, 194
 Applications, 194
Resin, Composite, and Adhesive Resin
  Cements, 195

Cementation of crowns, conventional bridges, resin-bonded bridges, and temporary restorations, 195
   Composition and setting, 195
   Properties, 195
   Applications, 196
Bonding of esthetic restorations, 196
   Composition, 196
   Manipulation, 196
   Properties, 196
Resin-metal bonding, 196
Bonding of orthodontic brackets, 196
   Composition and setting, 196
   Manipulation, 197
   Properties, 197
Cavity Varnishes, 198
  Composition, 198
  Manipulation, 198
  Properties, 199
  Applications, 199
Cavity Liners, 199
  Composition, 199
  Manipulation, 199
  Properties, 200
Low-Strength Bases, 200
  Composition and chemistry of setting, 200
   Calcium hydroxide bases, 200
   Zinc oxide–eugenol bases, 200
  Manipulation, 200
  Properties, 200
   Calcium hydroxide bases, 200
   Zinc oxide–eugenol bases, 201
High-Strength Bases, 202
  Properties, 202

9   *Amalgam, 209*
Dental Amalgam Alloys, 209
  Composition and morphology, 209
  Production, 211
   Irregular particles, 211
   Spherical particles, 212
  Silver-tin alloy, 212
Amalgamation Processes, 212
  Low-copper alloys, 212
  High-copper alloys, 213
   Reaction of mercury in an admixed high-copper alloy, 213
   Reaction of mercury in a unicompositional alloy, 214
  Microstructure of amalgam, 214
Properties of Amalgam, 214
  ANSI/ADA Specification No. 1 for amalgam alloy, 215

Physical and mechanical properties, 215
  Compressive strength, 215
  Tensile strength, 218
  Transverse strength, 218
  Strength of various phases, 218
  Elastic modulus, 219
  Creep, 219
  Dimensional change, 220
  Corrosion, 221
Properties of mercury, 222
Manipulation of Amalgam, 223
  Selection of alloy, 223
  Proportions of alloy to mercury, 224
   Size of mix, 224
  Mixing of amalgam, 224
   Undermix, normal mix, and overmix, 226
  Condensation of amalgam, 228
   Hand or mechanical condensation, 228
   Effect of delay in condensation, 228
   Mercury content of amalgam restorations, 229
   Moisture contamination during insertion, 229
  Factors related to finishing amalgam restorations, 230
  Bonding of amalgam, 231
Mercury Toxicity, 232
  Sources of mercury, 232
  Forms of mercury, 232
  Concentrations of mercury, 233
   Mercury in urine, 233
   Mercury in blood, 234
   Release of corrosion products, 234
  Are amalgams poisonous?, 234
   Local reactions, 235
   Systemic reactions, 235
  Risks to dentists and office personnel, 236

10   *Direct Esthetic Restorative Materials, 244*
Composite Restorative Resins, 244
  Composition and chemical reaction, 244
   Filler, 245
   Oligomers, 247
   Coupling agents, 247
   Initiators and accelerators, 248
   Pigments, 248
  Packaging of composites, 249
   Two-paste system, 249
   Single-paste systems for photoinitiation, 249
Properties of Direct Restorative Composites, 252
  Setting and working times, 252
  Polymerization shrinkage, 252
  Thermal properties, 253
  Water sorption, 254
  Solubility, 254
  Mechanical properties, 254

Radiopacity, 255
Depth of cure (photoinitiated resins), 255
Bond formation to tooth structure, 256
Enamel, 256
Dentin, 256
Biocompatibility, 260
Color, 260
Material selection, 261
Manipulation and Handling Characteristics, 262
Composites, 262
Two-paste system, 262
Insertion, 262
Single-paste system, 262
Finishing, 263
Effects of tooth bleaching agents, 264
Extended Applications for Composites, 264
Anterior veneers, 264
Porcelain bonding, 265
Core build-up, 265
Posterior restorations, 265
Orthodontics, 267
Pit and Fissure Sealants, 267
Composition and reactions, 268
Bis-GMA resins, 268
Properties, 269
Manipulation, 270
Enamel surface preparation, 270
Bis-GMA-amine–accelerated sealant, 271
Bis-GMA-light–accelerated sealant, 271
Clinical studies of sealants, 271
Glass Ionomers, 272
Composition and reaction, 272
Properties, 272
Clinical application, 272

11 *Impression Materials, 281*
Purpose of Impression Materials, 281
Desirable Qualities, 281
Types of Impression Materials, 283
Alginate Hydrocolloids, 283
Composition and chemistry, 283
Proportioning and mixing, 285
Properties, 285
Working time, 285
Setting time, 285
Permanent deformation, 286
Flexibility, 287
Strength, 287
Compatibility with gypsum, 287
Dimensional stability, 289
Disinfection, 289
Agar Hydrocolloids, 289
Chemical ingredients, 290
Critical factors of manipulation, 291

Properties, 292
Gelation temperature, 292
Permanent deformation, 292
Flexibility, 292
Strength, 292
Compatibility with gypsum, 292
Dimensional stability, 292
Agar-alginate combination impressions, 293
Duplicating impression materials, 295
Properties, 296
Rubber Impression Materials, 296
Composition and reactions, 300
Polysulfides, 300
Silicones, 302
Polyethers, 303
Setting properties, 303
Viscosity, 306
Working and setting times, 308
Dimensional change on setting, 308
Mechanical properties, 309
Permanent deformation, 310
Strain, 310
Flow, 310
Hardness, 311
Tear strength, 311
Detail reproduction, 311
Creep compliance, 311
Wettability of rubber impression materials, 312
Disinfection of rubber impressions, 312
Relationship of properties and clinical
application, 313
Rubber impression materials for bite
registrations, 314
Recent advances in rubber impression
materials, 314
Zinc Oxide–Eugenol Impression Pastes, 315
Nature and composition, 315
Setting reaction, 315
Characteristic properties, 316
Proportioning and mixing, 316
Effect of temperature and humidity on setting, 316
Modification of the setting time, 316
Dimensional changes of impressions, 316
Hardness, 317
Pouring and separating the cast, 317
ANSI/ADA Specification No. 16 for impression
paste–zinc oxide–eugenol type, 317
Dental Impression Plaster, 317
Composition and reactions, 317
Proportioning and mixing, 318
Storage problems, 318
Wax as an Impression Material, 318
Impression Compound, 318
Composition, 318
Thermal conductivity, 319

Softening and flow, 319
Cooling, 320
Effect of wet kneading, 320
Accuracy and dimensional stability, 320
Thermal contraction, 320
Tray compounds, 320
ANSI/ADA Specification No. 3 for dental
  modeling compound, 321
Die, Cast, and Model Materials, 321
Desirable Qualities of a Cast or Die Material, 321
Dental Plaster and Stone, 321
Dies Formed by the Electrodeposition of Metal, 322
  Electroforming impressions, 322
  Copper-formed dies, 323
  Silver-formed dies, 324
    Problems in metal-forming, 324
Epoxy Die Materials, 325
Comparison of Impression and Die Materials, 325

12 *Gypsum Products and Investments, 333*
Chemical and Physical Nature of Gypsum Products,
  333
  Manufacture of dental plaster, stone, and high-
    strength stones, 333
  Chemical reaction, 334
    Water/powder (W/P) ratio of dental stone
      and high-strength dental stone, 335
    Mechanism of setting, 335
    Volumetric contraction, 335
    Effect of spatulation, 336
    Effect of temperature, 336
    Effect of humidity, 337
    Effect of colloidal systems, 337
Properties, 337
  Setting time, 337
    Definition and importance, 337
    Measurement, 339
    Control of setting time, 339
  Consistency, 340
  Viscosity, 341
  Compressive strength, 341
  Surface hardness and abrasion resistance, 342
  Tensile strength, 343
  Reproduction of detail, 343
  Setting expansion, 344
Manipulation, 345
Casting Investments, 346
  Properties required of an investment, 346
  Composition, 347
    Refractory material, 347
    Binder material, 347
    Other chemicals, 347
  Calcium-sulfate–bonded investments, 347

Properties of calcium sulfate–bonded
  investments, 347
Effect of temperature on investment, 350
  Effect of temperature on silicon dioxide
    refractories, 350
  Effect of temperature on calcium sulfate binders, 351
  Cooling of the investment, 351
Setting and hygroscopic expansion of calcium
  sulfate–bonded investment, 351
  Water/powder ratio, 352
  Spatulation, 353
  Age of investment, 353
  Delay before immersion, 353
  Water bath temperature, 353
  Choice of binder material, 353
  Particle size of silica, 354
  Silica/binder ratio, 354
  Role of water, 354
Hygroscopic-thermal gold casting investment, 354
Investment for casting high-melting alloys, 354
  Phosphate-bonded investment, 354
  Silica-bonded investment, 356
Soldering investment, 357
Investments for all-ceramic restorations, 357

13 *Waxes, 361*
Waxes, Gums, Fats, and Resins, 361
  Natural waxes, 361
  Synthetic waxes, 364
  Gums, 364
  Fats, 364
  Resins, 365
Characteristic Properties of Waxes, 365
  Melting range, 365
  Thermal expansion, 366
  Mechanical properties, 367
  Flow, 368
  Residual stress, 370
  Ductility, 371
Dental Waxes, 371
  Inlay pattern wax, 371
    Composition, 372
    Properties, 372
    Flow, 373
    Thermal coefficient of expansion, 373
    Warpage of wax patterns, 373
  Casting wax, 374
    Physical characteristics, 375
  Resin modeling material, 376
  Baseplate wax, 376
    Composition, 376
    Physical characteristics, 377
  Boxing wax, 378
  Utility wax, 379

Sticky wax, 379
Corrective impression wax, 379
Bite registration wax, 380

14 *Noble Dental Alloys and Solders, 383*
Metallic Elements Used in Dental Alloys, 383
Noble metals, 383
Gold (Au), 383
Platinum (Pt), 385
Palladium (Pd), 385
Iridium (Ir), ruthenium (Ru), and
rhodium (Rh), 386
Base metals, 386
Silver (Ag), 386
Copper (Cu), 386
Zinc (Zn), 387
Indium (In), 387
Tin (Sn), 387
Gallium (Ga), 387
Nickel (Ni), 387
Binary combinations of metals, 387
Alloy composition and temperature, 387
Hardening of alloys, 389
Formulation of noble alloys, 390
Carat and fineness of gold-based alloys, 391
Casting Alloys, 391
Types and composition, 391
Grain size, 393
Properties, 394
Melting range, 394
Density, 394
Strength, 394
Hardness, 395
Elongation, 395
Gold-based alloys for porcelain-metal
restorations, 395
Wrought Alloys, 395
Microstructure, 396
Composition, 396
Properties, 396
Solders and Soldering Operations, 397
Types of solders, 397
Basis of selecting solders, 398
Composition, 398
Easy-flowing and free-flowing qualities, 399
Mechanical properties, 400
Color and tarnish resistance, 400
Pitted solder joints, 400
Microstructure of soldered joints, 400
Silver solder, 402
General suggestions for soldering, 402
Infrared soldering, 403
Casting to embedded metals or alloys, 404

15 *Cast and Wrought Base Metal Alloys, 408*
General Requirements of a Dental Alloy, 408
Cobalt-Chromium and Nickel-Chromium Casting
Alloys, 409
ANSI/ADA Specification No. 14, 409
Composition, 409
Function of various alloying elements, 409
Microstructure of cast base metal alloys, 410
Heat treatment of base metal alloys, 411
Physical properties, 412
Melting temperature, 412
Density, 412
Mechanical properties, 412
Yield strength, 412
Tensile strength, 412
Elongation, 413
Elastic modulus, 413
Hardness, 413
Corrosion, 414
Crown and bridge casting alloys, 414
Other applications of cast base metal
alloys, 414
Titanium and Titanium Alloys, 415
Commercially pure titanium, 415
Titanium alloys: general, 415
Ti-6Al-4V, 415
Cast titanium, 416
Dental implants, 418
Implant materials and processing, 419
Mechanisms of implant/tissue attachment, 419
Enhancing osseointegration, 419
Surface state and biocompatibility, 420
Summary, 421
Other applications of wrought titanium, 421
Wrought Stainless Steel Alloys, 421
Composition, 421
Function of alloying elements and chemical
resistance, 422
Stress-relieving treatments, 422
Stainless steel orthodontic wires, 423
Manipulation, 423
Properties, 423
Stainless steel endodontic instruments, 425
Properties, 426
Base metal prefabricated crowns, 427
Wrought Cobalt-Chromium-Nickel Alloy, 428
Composition, 428
Processing and manipulation, 428
Properties, 428
Wrought Nickel-Titanium Alloy, 430
Composition and shape-memory effect, 431
Properties and manipulation, 431

Wrought Beta-Titanium Alloy, 431
   Composition and microstructure, 431
   Manipulation, 431
   Properties, 431
New/Experimental Orthodontic Wires, 432
   Summary of orthodontic wires, 432
Some Other Alloys, 432

16 *Casting Procedures, 437*
Casting Practices for Low-Fusing Gold Alloys, 437
Dimensional Changes, 438
   Means of compensation, 438
Formation of Inlay Patterns, 439
   Direct wax patterns, 439
   Indirect wax patterns, 439
   Spruing the pattern, 440
   Wettability, 441
   Distortion, 442
Investing Procedure for Wax Patterns, 442
   Hand-investing procedure, 442
   Vacuum-investing procedure, 444
   Investing patterns for water-added technic, 445
   Heating the mold, 445
   Wax elimination, 446
   Oven temperature, 448
Practical Differences between Hygroscopic and
   High-Heat Technics, 448
Casting Facilities, 449
   Methods of melting alloys, 449
   Casting machines, 450
Some Common Casting Problems, 451
Casting and Soldering Fluxes, 453
Casting Porcelain Veneer Metal Structures, 454
Cleaning and "Pickling" Gold Alloys, 455
Casting of Cobalt-Chromium and Nickle-Chromium
   Alloys, 456
   Casting shrinkage compensation, 462
   Porosity in castings, 462
   Finishing of base metal partial denture castings, 463
Casting of Titanium, 463
Casting of Glass, 464

17 *Ceramics, 467*
Composition, 467
General Applications in Dentistry, 468
Porcelain as Tooth Restorative Material, 469
   Porcelain technic, 470
   Types of tooth restorative porcelain, 471
   Fusion of porcelain, 471
   Properties of fused porcelain, 472
   Porcelain crowns, 472
   Porcelain inlays, 473

   Machined restorations, 473
   Porcelain enamel-metal restorations, 474
   Core materials, 475
Cast Glass Ceramics, 476
   High-temperature injection molding, 477
Optical Properties, 477
Esthetic Porcelain Veneers, 479
Porcelain Artificial Teeth, 479
   Manufacture, 479
     Vacuum firing, 480
   Properties, 482

18 *Ceramic-Metal Systems, 485*
Ceramic-Metal Bonding, 485
   Evaluation of ceramic-metal bonding, 486
Ceramics for Porcelain-Fused-to-Metal Bonding, 488
Alloys for Porcelain-Fused-to-Metal Bonding, 490
   Composition of noble metal alloys, 490
   Composition of base metal alloys, 493
Properties of Alloys for Ceramic-Metal
   Restorations, 493
Preparation of Porcelain-Fused-to-Metal
   Restorations, 496

19 *Prosthetic Applications of Polymers, 500*
Properties of Denture Base Materials, 500
   Physical form and composition, 500
     Powder, 500
     Liquid, 502
     Gel types, 503
   Other denture materials, 503
     Pour type of denture resins, 503
     High-impact strength materials, 503
     Rapid heat-polymerized resins, 503
     Light-activated denture base resins, 503
   ANSI/ADA Specification No. 12 for denture base
     resins, 504
Properties of Dental Plastics, 504
   Strength properties, 504
     Tensile and compressive strength, 504
     Elongation, 504
     Elastic modulus, 504
     Proportional limit, 506
     Impact strength, 506
     Transverse strength and deflection, 508
     Fatigue strength, 508
     Fracture toughness, 509
     Compressive creep, 509
     Recovery after indentation, 509
     Hardness, 510
     Abrasion resistance, 510
   Thermal characteristics, 510
     Thermal conductivity, 510
     Specific heat, 510

Thermal coefficient of expansion, 510
Heat distortion temperature, 511
Other properties of denture plastics, 511
Density, 511
Polymerization shrinkage, 511
Dimensional stability and accuracy, 511
Water sorption and solubility, 513
Resistance to acids, bases, and organic solvents, 513
Processing ease, 513
Adhesion properties, 513
Esthetics, 513
Tissue compatibility, 514
Shelf life, 515
Summary, 515
Manipulation and Processing of Denture Base
Plastics, 515
Heat-accelerated acrylic denture plastics, 515
Proportioning, 516
Packing, 517
Processing, 518
Deflasking and finishing, 521
Residual monomer, 521
Dimensional changes, 522
Chemically accelerated acrylic denture
plastics–compression molding, 524
Manipulation and processing, 524
Properties, 524
Fluid resin acrylic denture plastics, 525
Light-cured denture plastic, 525
Forces involved in denture retention, 528
Effect of auxiliary materials on denture plastics, 528
Plaster and stone, 528
Impression materials, 528
Waxes, 528
Mold separators, 530
Characterization materials, 530
Denture cleansers, 530

Repair materials, 531
ANSI/ADA Specification No. 13 for denture self-
curing repair resins, 532
Relining and rebasing dentures, 532
Relining, 532
ANSI/ADA Specification No. 17 for denture base
temporary relining resin, 533
Rebasing, 533
Tissue conditioners, 533
Soft or resilient denture liners, 534
Mouth-cured soft liners, 534
Processed soft liners, 535
Denture Teeth, 537
ANSI/ADA Specification No. 15 for plastic teeth,
539
Maxillofacial Materials, 540
Poly(methyl methacrylate), 540
Plasticized polyvinylchloride, 540
Polyurethane, 541
Heat-vulcanized silicone, 541
Room temperature–vulcanized silicones, 541
Experimental elastomers, 541
Fabrication of the prostheses, 542
Physical properties, 542
Plastic Facings for Crown and Bridge Applications, 543
Temporary Crown and Bridge Restorations, 543
Occlusal Splints, 544
Athletic Mouth Protectors, 544
Inlay Patterns, 545
Impression Trays and Record Bases, 546

Appendix, 552

Index, 555

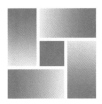

1 *Scope and History of Restorative Materials*

Humankind always has been plagued by the problem of restoring parts of the body lost as a result of accident or disease. Practitioners of dentistry have been confronted with this problem since the beginning of dental practice, and the means of replacing missing tooth structure by artificial materials continues to account for a large part of dental science. Modern dentistry recognizes preventive, corrective, and restorative types of practice, with the restorative types occupying the greatest amount of the time (variously estimated from 50% to 70%) of dentists in practice.

The replacement of lost teeth is desired for two primary reasons: esthetics and restoration of function (partial or complete). The ability of the dentist to accomplish the desired results has always been limited by certain basic factors. One is the availability of suitable materials for the construction of the restorative appliance; another is the development and control of suitable technical procedures for using the materials that are available. This search for the correct materials, with the aid of chemical, physical, and biological sciences, and for methods of manipulation or applied technics has continued from the beginning of dental art to the present. Throughout the ages dentistry has depended to a great degree on advances of the contemporary arts and sciences for improvements in materials and procedures. Although great improvements have been made recently in the restorative materials available to the dentist, this relationship to contemporary sciences still continues. The field of restorative materials is extensive with regard not only to the wide variety of materials and technics of manipulation but also to the related sciences that are employed.

■ SCOPE OF MATERIALS COVERED IN RESTORATIVE DENTISTRY

Restorative dental materials include such items as noble and base metals, amalgam alloys, cements, composites, ceramics, gypsum compounds, casting investments, dental waxes, impression-taking compounds, denture base resins, or any other such material used in restorative dental operations. In describing these materials, comparisons are usually made on the basis of typical physical and chemical characteristics. The line dividing restorative dental materials from therapeutic agents often is not clear. For example, the distinction is not pronounced in such cases as medicated cements, cavity liners, or root canal-filling materials. Usually in such borderline instances the materials are included in both fields of study, with emphasis placed on the properties related to the application involved.

This subject should be approached from the point of view of determining what the material is chemically, why it functions as it does physically and mechanically, and how it is manipulated technically to develop the most satisfactory properties. Emphasis should be placed on the manipulation and properties of the material as the basis for a practical interpretation of its fundamental physical and chemical characteristics.

The application of dental materials is not limited to any one branch of dentistry. There is scarcely a dental procedure that does not make use of dental materials in one or more forms. Some phases of restorative dentistry depend largely on various materials and their favorable properties for the existence of the practice. Other branches of dentistry, such as minor oral surgery and periodontics, require less use of materials, but even in these fields the physical characteristics of the equipment and the chemical characteristics of materials used are important. However, because most materials are used in restorations, either directly or indirectly, the subject is described as one dealing with restorative dental materials.

Most restorative materials are measured by a set of physical, chemical, or mechanical tests that lend themselves to duplication, and, as a result of these tests, a more uniform effort is being made to control the quality of and claims for the materials. This approach has led to a number of gradual improvements in the materials available to the profession. As refinement and improvement in properties have occurred, refinement in technic of application has become necessary.

Basic Sciences Applied to Restorative Materials

The scope of scientific principles applicable to dentistry is often not fully recognized. The sciences of primary interest to the dentist are all derived from the three basic scientific fields: biology, chemistry, and physics. No definite dividing lines regarding their importance to dentistry can be drawn among these three sciences for two reasons: (1) the mutual overlapping tends to produce a continuous field of knowledge and (2) investigations within each science are constantly encroaching on the area of the other. Most sciences can be traced to one or more of these basic fields, although an attempt to classify the fields of investigation into a single scheme often causes difficulties.

Fig. 1-1 indicates the relationship of the three basic fields to applied technics and clinical dentistry. The practice of clinical dentistry depends not only on a complete understanding of the various applied technics but also on an appreciation of the fundamental biological, chemical, and physical principles that underlie the applied technics. A failure to know the scientific principle on which a technic is established often leads to an incorrect conclusion for its application. On the other hand, an understanding of the well-balanced relationship that exists among the biological, chemical, and physical principles on which the various applied dental technics are established leads to a broader application of the clinical technics.

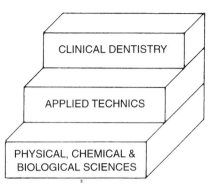

Fig. 1-1 Steps to understanding relations of materials science in dentistry.

It is evident that chemistry, physics, and related engineering sciences serve as the foundation for the science of restorative materials. In no way are the physiological and biological aspects of dentistry modified or subordinated by this physical science treatment of the materials, but rather the whole structure of restorative, corrective, and preventive dentistry is strengthened by its inclusion. Whereas the subject depends on one or more of these exact sciences, the chief problem in this field is to make the correct practical application and interpretation of information available from scientific studies. Most persons working with restorative materials believe that physical, chemical, and mechanical studies cannot be separated from physiological, pathological, or other biological studies of the tissue that support and tolerate the restorative structures. Certainly from the clinical standpoint it is desirable to keep the studies and interpretations as practical as possible. If practical clinical dentistry and the theoretical scientific aspects of restorative materials are allowed to develop without suitable correlation, neither is likely to progress as it should nor be useful to the other.

Application of Various Sciences

The fundamental principles of the physical sciences find application in the comparison of the physical characteristics with the structural applications of restorative materials. Often this situation is not fully appreciated because the application to dentistry of the various scientific principles has not been emphasized in undergraduate textbooks. In the chapters that follow, numerous practical examples of basic principles are presented, and throughout the discussions the fundamental characteristics are stressed, with a minimum of emphasis on test procedures and technics of manipulation.

Not all the theoretical aspects and applications of physical, chemical, and engineering principles can be described in detail in the limited space available. Such treatment should not be necessary because predental training includes an understanding of many of the basic principles, even though the practical applications may have been neglected. Therefore emphasis is placed on the application of significant fundamentals to dental operations.

A more complete understanding of these and other fundamental principles is important to the dentist as an aid in understanding such typical phenomena as the melting and freezing of casting alloys, the volatilization of liquids with the accompanying cooling action, or the crystal structure produced in solidified metals as compared with the essentially noncrystalline structure of hydrocolloid impression compounds and denture base materials. The branch of physical chemistry that considers the colloidal state of matter has for years been applied successfully to the sciences of medicine, physiology, botany, and engineering. Numerous illustrations of the application of colloid and surface chemistry to dentistry, oral conditions, and dental materials also are known.

To understand the complex nature of metals and alloys used for cast inlays or removable partial dentures, one should know something of the physical or chemical reactions that influence the combination of metals and alloys in the liquid and solid states. Alloys that demand heat treatment to produce the optimum properties offer an example of the application of such physicochemical principles. Using a knowledge of the physicochemical principles and numerous principles of good metallurgical casting practices and fabrication of structures through soldering and assembly, it is possible to design and construct remarkably effective dental structures and appliances.

Knowledge of organic and polymer chemistry, together with the mechanics of restorative structures and of mastication, and something of the biophysical principles involved in the complete denture restoration is desirable for designing and constructing complete dentures. Stress analysis of the various types of restorations involves physical principles that are closely related to successful design as well as the biophysical analysis of the support structures.

The toxicity of and tissue reactions to dental materials are receiving more attention as a wider variety of materials are being used and as federal agencies are demonstrating more concern in this area. A further indication of the importance of the interaction of materials and tissues is the development of recommended standard practices and tests for the biological interaction of materials through the auspices of the American Dental Association.

Throughout the study of biomaterials many examples will be observed in which these principles are found to apply. The characteristics of the restorative materials and the scientific principles on which the materials are used are intimately associated with the successful practice of restorative dentistry.

After many centuries, human beings continue to be confronted with the problem of replacing tooth tissue lost by either accident or disease. Until such time as there is no need for restorative materials and appliances, the dental profession will continue to draw from all the contemporary arts and sciences to further develop an improved and integrated science of dentistry.

■ HISTORY

An examination of the history of dentistry shows that the various materials available during any given period have always been important to contemporary restorative dental operations. The improvements continued to increase slowly and steadily over the centuries at about the same rate as related developments in other fields of science. It becomes evident therefore that many accepted technics, materials, and practices have resulted from systematic evaluation and development, so that now the branch of restorative materials has become an accepted part of the science of dentistry. The need for such materials has long been recognized, but only recently have the sciences of chemistry, physics, and engineering reached a stage where improved materials have become available to restorative dentistry.

More refinement and improvement of quality in restorative dental materials have taken place during the past generation than during any other period of dental history. An understanding of the factors that contributed to this progress enables us to appreciate better the limitations, developments, and future possibilities of this phase of dentistry. The problems of present-day dental materials cannot be fully evaluated without first having some knowledge of the past in this field.

Although no complete history of restorative materials has been written, it is possible to follow the general development of the subject by the progress that was made in the art and science of restorative dentistry throughout the centuries. Until recently this subject was not a distinct science but only a related phase of the art and science of dentistry. In the early development of dentistry the subject was sufficiently elementary that no separate study was devoted to materials. As dentistry developed and became more complex, so did the phase involving the restorative materials. Therefore the accumulated mass of information regarding the materials inevitably became so great as to be established as a separate science. As a science the subject is new, but as part of restorative practices it is as old as dentistry itself.

Early History   *700 hundred years ago gold structured from phoenicians.*

Among the earliest recorded examples of dental prostheses are the gold structures of the Phoenicians, the Etruscans, and, a little later, the Greeks and Romans. The earliest examples of dental prostheses are generally considered to be those found among the Phoenicians. All of the restorations date back to a period several hundred years before the beginning of Christianity, and for practical purposes it makes little difference which of the civilizations produced the first ones. It is much more interesting to observe that many of the materials and practices now in common use had a beginning application in dentistry hundreds of years ago.

Gold is one of the oldest materials used. It has been employed for prosthetic dental purposes for at least 2500 years. The ancient Babylonians, Assyrians, and Egyptians (4500 to 4000 BC), were familiar with gold, silver, copper, and lead. It remained for the Phoenicians (about 2700 BC), who were perhaps the

greatest commercial people of the ancient world, to spread the culture along the shores of the Mediterranean. They practically controlled the tin trade during the period 1000 to 300 BC, which was important for the bronze industry, and were considered the most skillful metallurgists of the ancient world. Iron was known to them as early as 990 BC.

Therefore a variety of metals was available for use by the ancient civilizations, and it seems reasonable to assume that the practice of using gold for dental appliances was common for centuries before the examples known to us were made. Evidence in favor of the antiquity of the art is found in the examination of the appliances. Many were prepared by soldering after reasonably careful assembly, and certainly this art was not developed for the convenience of only the few surviving examples.

It is not certain exactly how or by whom the appliances were constructed. Possibly they were made by skilled metalworkers and not by those who practiced the dental art. As pointed out by historians, the physicians and barber-surgeons probably performed the treatment and extractions, whereas goldsmiths and other artisans constructed the artificial restorations. The role played by the goldsmiths and other artisans is comparable to that of modern laboratory technicians. Persons qualified by practice and experience can often prepare a more artistic structure in less time than the one who visualized it, even though the functional design is the responsibility of the dentist.

The practice of using gold crowns and bridgework apparently flourished in Etruria and Rome as early as 700 to 500 BC. These people must have understood the arts of soldering and riveting to have prepared a restoration from pure gold rings soldered in correct relations, with the artificial tooth held in place by a pin that passed through both the artificial tooth and the gold ring. The extensive use of solder to prepare the appliance implies some knowledge of the simple alloying of gold and the preparation and use of fluxes and perhaps antifluxes. It seems incredible that the art of soldering dental appliances dates so far into the past, when so many other simple practices now considered commonplace were not known at that time.

The teeth used in the ancient appliances were either human or carved from the teeth of animals.

The early Phoenician restorations represent an interesting example of the use of wire to hold the teeth in a more or less fixed position. It appears therefore that the art of wire fabrication was known to this ancient civilization. Hippocrates, who was born in 460 BC, apparently used gold wire and linen thread for ligatures in the repair of bone fractures. He was likewise reported to be the inventor of a type of crude dental forceps and other dental instruments. In modern dentistry the oral surgeon is interested in the properties and behavior not only of ligature materials but also of hypodermic needles, cobalt-chromium and titanium alloy screws and appliances, tantalum or titanium plates, as well as various instruments. This interest started hundreds of years ago, before the introduction of the subject of dental materials.

Filling carious teeth for preservation apparently was not practiced extensively by ancient civilizations. Celsus (first century AD) recommended the filling of large cavities with lint, lead, and other substances before attempting extraction to prevent the tooth from breaking under the pressure of the instrument. This may have been the beginning of filling materials for carious teeth.

Restorative dental materials were relatively simple in character and few in number at the end of this ancient period; in general the structures were crude. However, a beginning had been made, and mankind was conscious of the desirability of replacement of lost tooth tissue. With all branches of civilization in an early state of development, the art of dentistry was equal to many others. Perhaps the need for better restorations was recognized but inasmuch as man had only recently emerged from the prehistoric ages, his tools and supplies were simple. Accordingly, persons who practiced the dental art depended on nature to provide the materials and on artisans to fashion the restorations.

Medieval and Early Modern Period

Dental historians describe little progress in the dental art from the beginning of the Christian era to about AD 1500. During this period little progress was made in any of the sciences. Historians doubt, however, that it was a period of retrogression or a "dark age" of physical inactivity. Probably there was much activity, creative thought, and invention, but

records were either not kept or else later destroyed through acts of superstition or religious fanaticism. The chief contribution to dentistry during this period appears to have been some shift in practice from prosthetic restorations to the restoration of carious teeth.

Some historians consider the sixteenth century to be the end of the Middle Ages. The invention of the printing press (1436), which aided in the dissemination of both cultural and technical knowledge, the emigration of Greek men of letters and science to Italy, and the discovery of America (1492) were all important events toward the close of this period. The end of the Middle Ages is generally considered to be a period of awakening of the common people. During the latter part of this period (between AD 1116 and 1289), universities with medical faculties were established at Bologna, Oxford, Paris, and Montpellier.

The development of books and writing on dental subjects was important to the progress of restorative dental materials. One of the first books to treat dentistry independently of medicine was written in German in 1548 by Walter Herman Ryff. This book, written in the language of the people, is significant because all previous works to describe the teeth were in Latin.

The use of gold leaf to fill cavities was perhaps the most significant development of the period from the standpoint of restorative materials. The first authentic record of the use of gold fillings in human teeth for purposes of their preservation appears to have been about 1480 by an Italian, Johannes Arculanus, who was at the University of Bologna and later at Padua. A description of the removal of carious matter from the teeth before filling them with gold leaf was given by Giovanni de Vigo (1460–1520). The practice of using gold leaf for fillings probably was not original with either of these writers because there is some indication that the custom may have dated back to the Middle East, several centuries before. It is certain, however, that gold leaf has been used for the past 500 years, or since about the time of Columbus.

Gold leaf was used for gilding and other commercial purposes in antiquity. The ancient Egyptians, Hebrews, and Greeks were familiar with the art, although the origin of gold leaf production was perhaps in the Far East. The early Greeks produced leaf of approximately 1/100,000-inch thickness, approaching the thickness of modern leaf or foil, which is approximately 1/300,000 inch. The methods for producing gold leaf have changed little throughout the ages, as is described in the discussion of gold foil as a restorative material.

Carious teeth were filled with ground mastic, alum, honey, or other substances during the period from about AD 1050 to 1122, according to the Arabian author Rhazes (al-Rāzi). Oil of cloves (eugenol) is mentioned by Riviére (1589) as being applicable to dental operations, but may have been used earlier (1562) by Ambroise Paré to alleviate toothache. Paré is also credited with having prepared artificial teeth from bone and ivory. Jacques Guillemeau, who was a pupil of Paré, prepared a substance by fusing together certain waxes, gums, ground mastic, powdered pearl, and white coral. This may have been the forerunner, in principle, of esthetic fused porcelain, which appeared many years later.

Some contemporary arts of the Middle Ages

The contemporary arts were also being developed during this period, the same as dentistry and medicine. The writings of Pliny (AD 23–79), Theophilus (eleventh century), and Cellini (1558) describe how painters, goldsmiths, ceramists, metalworkers, and others applied their art. None of the authors claim credit for complete originality of all their practices but rather indicate that they used them as routine methods.

In his *Natural History,* Pliny described bronze statuettes and other cast bronze or silver household articles such as candelabra and cups common to the period before AD 100. Pliny listed many dental practices that appear to be based on popular belief rather than on the practices of specialists, and in all his writings there is a sense of a certain amount of the impractical. Perhaps this tendency was characteristic of the age.

The priest and monk Theophilus in "An Essay upon Various Arts" shows certain improvements over the earlier writers. In preparing this essay, Theophilus has omitted certain erroneous practices of the previous period. In Book One he deals primarily with painting and the allied arts. Of considerable interest is his description of the method for forming gold leaf from gold of high purity by hammering, which is not unlike the recent practices of beating gold to form foil. Book Two deals predominantly with the ceramic art and gives a good description of early practices in glassworking.

In Book Three Theophilus describes metalworking and devotes considerable space to the work of the goldsmiths. There is a description of the casting of handles for a silver cup in which the "lost wax" method is given in detail. The casting practice was so clearly described by Theophilus that it is possible to follow him in practice as well as in principle. After fashioning the handle in wax, a wax "sprue," which was described as being round like a slender candle and half a finger in length, was attached. It was somewhat thicker at the top. This wax, called the funnel, was made fast with a hot iron. Well-beaten clay was used to cover the wax carefully, so that all details of the wax sculpture were filled. Afterward these molds were placed near warm coals, so that when the molds became warm it was possible to pour out the wax. After the clay mold was well baked and still hot, the molten metal was poured in through the funnel. When the mold and casting became cold, the clay mold was removed, and a metal replica of the wax model remained.

If a suitable dental casting investment, or mold material, had been used with an appropriate inlay wax, a balanced casting alloy, and a modern casting machine, the description might well apply to the dental casting process of today instead of to a practice in art used a thousand years ago.

A metal casting process very much like that of Theophilus is described by the Florentine artist Benvenuto Cellini in Chapter 41 of his *Memoires,* written in 1558. Cellini prepared a wax model and surrounded it with a plastic clay, which he allowed to dry and harden before attempting to melt the wax and pour the metal. He implies that he had frequently used wax patterns in previous castings. He claims no originality for the casting method, though he does indicate that the melting furnace that he used was original.

Cellini, like Pliny and Theophilus, also soldered gold by using copper acetate, nitre, and borax, which was considered very effective. Thus it is seen that certain metals and materials were available to the artisans for use in their trades. The secrets of these practices no doubt were often guarded so that they were not recognized outside the trade. Such dentistry was more of an art than a science, so that full use of existing skills and technics possibly was not made. Certainly the practice of casting restorations by the "lost wax" method was to wait several centuries before it was adopted by dentistry.

Beginning of the Dental Science—1600 to 1840

During the period from 1600 to 1840, the foundations for the science of dentistry were established. So little progress had been made up to that time that dentistry was merely an art practiced largely by the barber-surgeons or artisans as a part of their regular service. Few records of results were kept, and little thought was given to the improvement of methods before the beginning of the seventeenth century. Nevertheless, a special type of medical-dental practitioner was recognized by the medical profession.

By the end of the sixteenth century a limited knowledge of dentistry had spread to most of the countries in Europe. Carved bone and ivory teeth held to neighboring teeth with gold and silver wire were used in France, Germany, and Italy.

The contemporary sciences of chemistry and physics were being developed with the beginning of the seventeenth century. Galileo had stated his law of falling bodies and invented the telescope. The compound microscope and the printing press were in use. By the end of the century, chemical elements had been defined by Robert Boyle, and Sir Isaac Newton had demonstrated the law of gravitation. Similar developments were taking place in the biological sciences of bacteriology, anatomy, and physiology.

Wax models used in connection with prosthetic work are first mentioned by Matthaeus Gottfried Purmann in about 1700. It is supposed that the wax was carved to the desired shape, after which it was reproduced in bone or ivory by a craftsman.

Much progress in dentistry was made during the eighteenth century. Pierre Fauchard described the materials and practices of his time in his book published in 1728. He discussed many phases of dentistry, including operative and prosthetic procedures. He collected and catalogued much of the information about dentistry that was good during his time.

There were dental texts before the time of Fauchard, but they were considerably more limited in extent and application.

Fauchard mentioned lead, tin, and gold as filling materials. He preferred tin because of the ease with which it could be adapted to cavity walls. Separate ivory or natural teeth with wood pivots were fastened in position with a cement compound of sealing wax, turpentine, and white copal, or were set into low-melting alloy used to fill the canal. The use of the dental file had become common practice by the time of Fauchard, and emery wheels for grinding down teeth had been introduced by a Dutch physician, Kornelis van Soolingen, during the latter part of the seventeenth century. According to Vincenzo Guerini, it was Lorenz Heister (1683–1758) who first mentioned removable prosthetic appliances.

The early sixteenth century saw the beginning of useful dental literature, whereas the seventeenth century was a period of rapid development of the art of dental practice with a coordination of the scientific knowledge that had evolved during the past centuries. The introduction of fused porcelain for teeth in 1789 is regarded as one of the most important events in the history of dentistry. It represents the beginning of scientific improvements in the restorative art of dental practice.

The first book to describe mechanical dentistry was that of Claude Mouton in 1746. He mentioned gold shell crowns swaged from one piece of metal and the use of gold clasps instead of ligatures to retain artificial teeth. Clasps to retain partial dentures were in common use in 1796. Numerous other dental texts were written during the late eighteenth and early nineteenth centuries. Etienne Bourdet (1775) made the first reference to the use of a gold base to support artificial ivory teeth fixed with gold pins. Low-fusing metal alloy was introduced by Jean Darcet in 1770.

A complete baked porcelain denture made in a single block was first displayed by the French dentist Nicholas Dubois de Chemant in 1788. In 1797, he wrote a book in English describing porcelain. The Italian dentist Guiseppangelo Fonzi, who lived in Paris, is credited with preparing the first baked porcelain single tooth with attached platinum hooks about 1806 to 1808. He is credited also with preparing 26 shades of porcelain by use of metallic oxides.

It is claimed that the first American book on dentistry was written by R.C. Skinner (ca. 1801). By this time dentistry was no longer entirely in the hands of barbers or artisans but was practiced by professionally minded dentists or surgeons who warned the public against pretenders. There were 44 treatises on dentistry that appeared in the United States between 1800 and 1840. This is more than one each year, in addition to the numerous articles on dentistry that appeared in the medical journals.

The combination of silver and mercury to form amalgam "silver paste" was announced by O. Taveau of Paris in 1826. This was the beginning of dental amalgam, which is recognized as one of the outstanding developments in the field of restorative materials.

The French dentists may well be considered the leaders of this period, although the profession in other countries of Europe was quick to adopt the French practices or their equivalent, and in a few instances they made additional contributions. In Germany there was little progress until the sixteenth century. Mention of the use of gold foil in German writings during this century is common. Philip Pfaff (1756) is credited with being the first to use plaster models prepared from sectional wax impressions of the mouth. Other German contributions to prosthetic dentistry during this period do not appear to be well established in the literature.

In Great Britain, dentistry did not develop much until the eighteenth century. Even at that time the profession was not well established. The work of Fauchard was not generally known in Great Britain, and the first comprehensive textbook in English appeared in 1768, although in 1686 Charles Allen had written a book on teeth in which he described a method of transplantation. By the early part of the nineteenth century dental practice had apparently improved somewhat in Great Britain. Retentive cavities for gold fillings were prepared in Edinburgh in 1787.

James Snell (1832) wrote that he preferred forceps to the key for use in extractions. He chose gold for filling carious teeth, and he described two types of cement that might be used but without promise of much success. Zinc oxychloride cement did not come into use until 20 years later.

Considerable progress was made toward the perfection of porcelain teeth in France, England, and the United States before 1840. These teeth had been introduced in the United States from France in 1817. By 1825 porcelain teeth were being produced and improved in America. The replacement of carved bone and ivory or natural teeth by the fused mineral product was another step forward for the profession and represents one of the first great improvements in dental materials. The Ash tube tooth introduced in 1838 was produced until recent times with only slight modification in form.

In the United States, Wooffendale is said to have introduced gold foil after he settled in New York in 1767 to practice dentistry. Tin and lead also were used as filling materials at this time. Carved ivory and bone dentures, ivory or natural teeth with metal pivots, and silk and wire ligatures, as well as files for the removal of carious lesions, were in common use. Paul Revere is credited with being a skilled ivory turner and goldsmith who applied his skill to the production of artificial teeth. "Silver paste," the amalgam of silver with mercury, was introduced in the United States as a filling material by the Crawcour brothers in 1833. Gold points were used to fill root canals in 1805 by Edward Hudson in Philadelphia.

Dental materials were beginning to be produced in America during the early part of the nineteenth century. Before that time they were imported from Europe. Gold coins were rolled into a noncohesive gold filling material in 1800, and by 1812, gold foil was being produced by the beating method by Marcus Bull in Hartford, Connecticut. He founded a company that later became the J.M. Ney Company, which is still a leading dental gold alloy manufacturer. Thus the first American-made dental products were gold foil and dental porcelain.

By 1840 the practice of dentistry in America had reached a definite turning point. The first dental journal in the world, *The American Journal of Dental Science,* was established in 1839. The first national dental society, the American Society of Dental Surgeons, was established in 1840. The first dental school, the Baltimore College of Dental Surgery, was established the same year. H.H. Hayden and C.A. Harris were both active in these three institutions. This same year Charles Goodyear discovered the process of dry heat vulcanization of rubber that later made possible the introduction of a most useful dental material—vulcanite.

With the establishment of a dental society, a dental journal, and a dental school, the foundation was laid for the development of a dental science in the United States. The coordination and practical application of the knowledge and practice developed during the past centuries were begun, and uniform progress in all branches was seen. Dental materials in 1840 were still relatively simple, but such progress was being made in the industries that it could be expected that improvements would be forthcoming. Chemistry, physics, medicine, and the sciences generally were beginning to flourish in the schools. Inventions and the introduction of the railroad, the steamship, the postage stamp, improved highway systems, the Erie Canal, gas for illumination, phosphorous matches, and the telegraph all had their beginnings in the early nineteenth century. These improvements helped to promote dentistry and to create a turning point for civilization generally. Numerous respected men were in the practice of dentistry, both in the United States and in Europe. Through the efforts of these men improvements were made in the profession, and the barber-surgeon was forced to discontinue his trade.

Progress still was not rapid in the early part of the nineteenth century, but dentistry was becoming an improved and established science. It has been estimated that in 1830 the total number of dentists in the United States had increased to about 300, with an advancement in every department of dentistry as a science. The nineteenth century might be called a period of mechanical progress in contemporary fields and of the establishment of the dentist in society.

The Period of Mechanical Improvement–1840 to 1900

Dentistry, like the allied arts and sciences, took full advantage of the mechanical developments of the last half of the nineteenth and the early twentieth centuries. The application of chemical, physical, and engineering principles to dentistry was like a tonic for its improvement when combined with the improvements made available in the biological sciences. The developments in related arts and sciences stimulated further growth in the field of restorative materials. During this period applied mechanics was recognized as an essential supplement to the biological principles of dentistry. Apparently this was more quickly and completely recognized among U.S. dentists than among those of other countries, thereby advancing U.S. dentistry to the position it now holds. Few other nations had the early concept of coordination and balance between mechanical reconstruction and research and the biological fundamentals of dentistry.

Between 1839 and 1884 there were 44 dental journals established in the United States, and between 1842 and 1884 there were 103 dental societies organized. These assisted greatly in the dissemination of scientific dental information on practices and technics throughout the profession. At the beginning of this period dental materials were comparatively few in number, but this was the beginning of the application of physical principles to dental practices and processes, and the search had started for other and improved restorative materials.

By the end of the 60-year period from 1840 to 1900, many of the major present-day materials had been introduced to the profession along with a technic for their manipulation and use. After 1840 the United States began to acquire leadership in creating and producing restorative dental materials, and a substantial industry developed in this field. From this industry dentistry derived many valuable contributions, relationships, and benefits in the form of research and scientific development.

Because of the great number of improvements and developments introduced by dentistry during this period, it is possible here to enumerate in chronological order only a few of the most important. In 1844, S.S. White became interested in the production of porcelain teeth and their improvements in color and form. White was later to become a leading manufacturer and distributor of dental materials, establishing the S.S. White Dental Manufacturing Company. The records indicate, therefore, that the Ney and White Companies were among the oldest in the trade.

One of the early actions of the American Society of Dental Surgeons was to forbid its members to use silver amalgam for restoring lost tooth structure. Like many other acts of prohibition, this action of the society apparently served to stimulate thought on the use and study of the nature of amalgam. Years later, after much study, an improved amalgam was developed that eventually became one of the most popular and useful of all restorative materials.

About the time the society started the "war" against the use of silver amalgam, a companion material in the form of copper amalgam was introduced (1844). Mouth impressions were being taken in plaster about this same time. Gutta-percha was discovered in India in 1842, and by 1847 it was being used as a root canal filling material when mixed with chloroform. This material, chloropercha, remained in use until recent times as a cavity liner and varnish in deep cavities. Gutta-percha was mixed with zinc oxide for filling purposes by Asa Hill in 1848. In 1883, gutta-percha was dissolved in eucalyptol and used as a root canal filler. This was perhaps the beginning of the present-day gutta-percha points for root canals. Platinum-gold alloys, consisting of three-fourths gold and one-fourth platinum, were introduced in 1847.

In 1851, Nelson Goodyear announced the development of a method for producing vulcanite, or hard rubber, though about 10 years previously Charles Goodyear had discovered a method of dry-heat vulcanization of rubber in which he heated together caoutchouc, sulfur, and white lead. The discovery of vulcanite and its subsequent use for "dental plates," patented on March 5, 1855, was another outstanding advance in dental materials. Even though the material was not ideal as a denture base and its use was covered by restricting patents for many years, vulcanite served well as the first substitute for the carved ivory dentures. Not long afterward (1869) celluloid was introduced by J. Smith Hyatt, who was searching for a suitable material for billiard balls, and soon it was used as a denture base material. Thus a substitute for vulcanite was sought soon after its introduction. It was not until about 80 years later (1937), however, that the satisfactory substitute for vulcanite was obtained in a material known as acrylic resin.

The second dental school in the United States was established in Cincinnati in 1845. After this time, dental education was assured. By 1860 more than 200 dental books in German, Spanish, Italian, French, and English had appeared. The periodical literature had increased, with journals in the United States, Germany, England, and France, which assured a dissemination of knowledge.

The restrictions on the use of amalgam had not been completely successful. A silver-tin-mercury alloy, or amalgam, was introduced in 1855 by Elisha Townsend, followed by another formula by J.F. Flagg in 1860. Gold foil was becoming increasingly popular at the same time, with the introduction of cohesive annealed foil by Robert Arthur of Baltimore in 1855. Zinc oxychloride cement was in common use by this time as a filling and cementing medium. Low-melting point alloy baseplates were developed by Alfred A. Blandy in 1856, and a flexible dental engine cable was introduced by Charles Merry of St. Louis in 1858, followed by the angle handpiece in 1862. The rubber dam to isolate teeth from saliva was put into use by Phineas Taylor Barnum of Monticello in 1864, and four years later (1868) the profession was to benefit by the expiration of the patents controlling the use of vulcanite. About 1870 the zinc phosphate cements were first used, and they were introduced to the profession in 1879. Silicate cements were developed a few years later.

The practice of malleting for condensation of gold foil had been common since 1838, when it was introduced by E. Merrit of Pittsburgh. Since that practice started, numerous automatic mallets have been introduced, beginning with one developed by J.C. Dean in 1867. The introduction of automatic mechanical condensing devices has continued with varying degrees of success to the present time.

In 1850 the pivot crown was a crude structure with its wooden pin set into a tooth. The Richmond crown was introduced in 1878, followed by the Davis crown in 1885, and a modified form of the Davis crown in the same year by H.D. Justi, all making use of metal pins to replace the wood. These were only three of the many forms of porcelain pivot crowns common at that time. Much experimentation was being done during the same period with fused porcelain for inlays, jacket crowns, porcelain teeth set into vulcanite bases, and other modified porcelain structures. Some years later these ambitions were realized with the introduction of gas and gasoline furnaces for baking porcelain, porcelain jacket crowns, and high-fusing inlays by Charles Land (1889); an electric furnace for porcelain by Levitt Ellsworth Custer (1894); high-fusing porcelain inlays by W.E. Christensen (1895); the gingival shoulder for the porcelain jacket crown by E.B. Spalding (1903); and the summary of porcelain inlay construction in the technical publication of J.Q. Byram in 1905.

Circular inlays that were ground and fitted to position were in common use from 1858 to 1890. Aguilhon de Saran of Paris is credited with melting 24k gold in an investment mold to form inlays about 1884. J.R. Knapp in the United States invented a blowpipe in 1887, but not until 1907 did W.H. Taggart of Chicago succeed in introducing a practical casting method for the gold inlay. This was a long-sought-for invention, and although there is some question in the records about the authenticity of Taggart's invention and the ethics of its disposal, there can be no question about the merit of the practice and the advantages it has given to restorative dentistry. Solbrig in Paris, independent of Taggart, cast gold inlays by a similar method during the same year, and B.F. Philbrook had described in 1897 a method of casting metallic fillings. This indicates that much study was given to the problem throughout the profession and that its solution was a natural result of investigation. Why it was not done at an earlier date is now open to speculation, since it is known that Cellini and Theophilus used the same principles 1000 years before in their arts.

Continued progress was made in the work on amalgam alloy throughout the last of the nineteenth century. G.V. Black published the results of his studies in 1895, which marked the beginning of precision measurements on amalgam alloys. Black had previously published in 1891, his theories on cavity design and preparation, which are only remotely related to dental materials but include certain principles of mechanics that involve properties of materials used for restorations.

These are only a few examples of the many technics, practices, and principles that had their beginning in the late nineteenth century. This fact is often lost in the consideration of various materials and their use now in the latter half of the twentieth century. The fundamental principles underlying such operations as shaping cavities for various restorations; impression-taking; making wax patterns, models and indirect dies; the construction of complete and partial removable dentures; and creating many other types of structures were all recognized before the beginning of the twentieth century. Current developments and additional consideration of the historical background of individual materials will be considered in other discussions dealing with specific subjects.

Advances since 1900

With the beginning of the twentieth century came many refinements and improvements in the quality of various materials and processes used in restorative dentistry. Physical and mechanical tests combined with the fundamentals of engineering practice were applied to structural designs and restorative materials. From studies of physical and mechanical behavior, certain shortcomings of structures and materials were observed. When these shortcomings were detected, the process of improvement began with studies of methods of chemical combination or with physical improvement in fabrication. Thus for the first time, a concentrated effort was made to develop and improve products with specific properties designed for a definite purpose.

Before 1900 relatively few persons specialized in the improvement of dental materials or were able to verify the claims made for the materials that were available. Today more than 1500 persons who have a background of training and experience in physics, engineering, chemistry, and dentistry are engaged in research and development in this field and more than 65 universities offer graduate training in biomaterials. From 1900 to about 1925, frequent references to modifications, tests, and improvements of the materials and structures appeared in the literature. Unfortunately, a lack of uniformity of testing conditions prevailed, and it can be seen now that this often resulted in a failure to duplicate results and led to some misunderstanding of the science and studies as a whole. Since the early 1950s much has been done to clarify this situation, with cooperative effort among some of the dental schools; leaders in the profession; the American Dental Association Council on Dental Materials, Instruments, and Equipment, now the Council on Scientific Affairs; the National Bureau of Standards, now the National Institute for Standards and Technology; and the research departments of many reputable manufacturers.

Cooperative efforts among the workers in the field of restorative dentistry and materials appear to be stronger now than ever before. The researchers in this field, working in the profession, the schools, and the industries, are comparing results from tests and adopting a uniform method of testing. It is common practice now for the schools to exchange data with research departments of manufacturers and for each to supply information to the profession. This is a most constructive sign. It means that dentists in practice have an opportunity to compare results of different investigators more easily than in the past, and they probably will receive fewer conflicting statements of properties from research investigators.

During the early part of the present century, some of the persons engaged in improving the quality of restorative materials were associated with dental schools and others were in practice or engaged in research with manufacturers. At that time G.V. Black was still active both in the profession and at Northwestern University Dental School. The various editions of his textbook *Operative Dentistry* contained references to a variety of dental materials and in particular to the need for a balanced formula for an amalgam alloy. In addition, his rules on cavity design are still generally accepted, although there is a trend toward somewhat more conservative designs. In the related field of crown and bridge construction, F.A. Pesso was active in improving and modifying the technic and design of these restorations. At the University of Michigan School of Dentistry, M.L. Ward was active in the improvement of methods to measure dimensional change, flow, and other properties of amalgam. The development of the optical lever micrometer for measuring dimensional change in amalgam was one of the first refinements in dimensional change-measuring equipment for this and related materials. Ward also studied cements and improved designs in instruments and cavities, and made numerous contributions to the literature. Many of these are described in several editions of the *American Textbook of Operative Dentistry,* which he edited.

The term *dental metallurgy* was commonly used during the early part of the present century, and several books were written on the subject. The sixth edition of C.J. Essig and Augustus Koenig's book on dental metallurgy was published in 1909. This book fundamentally describes metallurgy of the various elements combined with procedures for melting and alloying. After a complete treatment of methods of extraction from the ore, together with methods of refinement of the various metals, there is a chapter on amalgam alloys with emphasis on their use in dentistry. The sixth edition of another popular book on dental metallurgy, written in 1924 by J.D.

Hodgen and G.S. Millberry, follows the same pattern of subject treatment. By that time considerable information had been accumulated on the various metals and particularly on amalgam and certain alloys used in dentistry, so that the book is somewhat more complete than previous editions. Dental metallurgy at that time, however, was not highly specialized, but perhaps that is to be expected because the subject was only beginning to take form and a limited amount of information was available on various materials and dental alloys. Books in this field written in later years adopted an entirely different style and included a different type of subject matter, as indicated by those of O.E. Harder, K.W. Ray, J.S. Shell, and E.W. Skinner.

Among the contributors to the periodical literature during the early part of the century were A.W. Gray, Paul Poetske, R.V. Williams, and W.S. Crowell. Gray reported numerous studies on amalgam alloy and its behavior when subjected to various practices of manipulation. He first offered a theory for the dimensional change resulting from the hardening of the amalgam mass. Poetske reported studies on both amalgam alloy and dental cement. Williams described methods of testing and improving dental gold alloys and Crowell contributed reports of investigations on cements and various other materials, as well as test practices.

At about this same time, James McBain and co-workers in England were studying the behavior of amalgam alloy subjected to different mixing procedures. At a later date M.L.V. Gaylor, working in the same laboratory, made significant observations about the way mercury and silver combine. Studies in Germany during this period dealt with the investigation of the theoretical behavior of metals and various alloys when combined under varying conditions. The theoretical behavior of structural designs was also being studied and reported from Germany. Significant studies on the method of combining gold and copper were reported from Russian laboratories in the early part of the twentieth century and were subsequently verified by studies in the United States and Great Britain. The discovery of copper-gold compound formation was most significant in the development and improvement of dental casting alloys.

In 1919 the National Bureau of Standards in Washington was requested by the United States government to formulate specifications for the selection of dental amalgam to be used in the federal services. Wilmer Souder directed this research and presented a report in 1920 that was well received and led to subsequent study of other materials. Shortly afterward the Weinstein Research Laboratories established a research associateship at the National Bureau of Standards, and studies were started on other materials. The first associates included R.L. Coleman, W.L. Swanger, and W.A. Poppe, who were under the direction of Dr. Souder. Their studies included investigations of the physical and mechanical properties of casting gold alloys, wrought gold alloys, and accessory casting materials. As a result of this investigation, research paper No. 32, which contained much fundamental information, was published in December 1928.

Since April 1928 the American Dental Association has maintained a research fellowship at the National Bureau of Standards. Numerous reports presented on the progress and investigations made under this fellowship have stimulated the advancement of information on many dental restorative materials. This research body has formulated a number of specifications, based on qualified investigations into the characteristic properties of each particular type of material. These specifications have been of great value to the profession in assuring greater uniformity and improved quality of restorative materials. The details of these specifications are described later in appropriate discussions.

Specifications have been developed in a number of countries but notably in Australia and the United States. Specifications for materials and devices are important in the practice of dentistry throughout the world, as evidenced by the establishment of international standards. The American Dental Association Specifications are submitted for approval to the American National Standards Institute and, if accepted, they become American National Standards. These standards may be submitted for acceptance by the International Organization for Standardization and, if approved, become an international standard. Of course, many countries contribute to the International Organization for Standardization, and specifications may be modified many times before they are finally accepted as international standards. The development of international standards will result in the improvement and reliability of materials and devices throughout the world and eliminates the need for each country to develop its own standards and specifications.

Because the development and acceptance of specifications frequently requires a number of years, the American Dental Association developed an Acceptance Program for dental materials in use but not covered by existing specifications. Manufacturers must submit test data that prove the materials function successfully for the specified application. Depending on the extensiveness of the laboratory and clinical results, products may be given provisional or complete acceptance. In 1993, the American Dental Association published a report, *Clinical Products in Dentistry—A Desktop Reference,* which lists accepted, certified, and recognized dental materials, instruments and equipment, and accepted therapeutic products. It is designed to be a quick reference for dentists concerning the status of new products and to assist them in the selection of products.

The Medical Devices Amendments, signed into law in 1976, were designed to protect the public from hazardous and ineffective devices. The responsibility for commercially available medical devices was divided among 19 panels, one of which was a dental panel. Each panel was to classify devices, identify known hazards, recommend characteristics for which standards should be developed, advise on the formulation of protocols and review premarket approval applications, recommend exemption for certain devices, and respond to requests from the FDA relating to the safety and effectiveness of devices. The Dental Device Classification Panel has classified life-sustaining and life-supporting devices, implants, and priority items for standards development. The list of dental devices includes 11 in the diagnostic area, 1 in monitoring, 51 in prosthetics, 82 in the surgical field, 2 in therapeutics, and 166 in the category of other devices.

If one were to list the major new materials, technics, or processes that have been developed or introduced since 1900, he or she would immediately realize that a continual search has been in progress for new and improved items and practices to replace those that have been accepted for 50 or more years. Dentistry as a whole, including the division of restorative materials, is continuing a vigorous, dynamic, and active search for items to replace those now in service. It seems unlikely that this branch of the profession will become dormant or static in the near future. The search continues throughout the contemporary arts and sciences, as well as within the dental profession, for ways to make restorative dentistry more acceptable and serviceable to the patient and convenient for the operator.

In the field of restorative materials and practices since 1900, several major items have been introduced, such as the casting process, the use of acrylic resins to replace vulcanized rubber in dentures, base metal casting alloys for partial dentures, and stainless steel for orthodontic and other appliances, as well as a variety of elastic impression materials. Each has made modern dental practice more acceptable to both the patient and the dentist. The development of carbide burs and diamond cutting instruments and the successful introduction of increased speeds for rotary instruments have aided materially in the operation of cutting tooth tissue. The development of resin composite and glass ionomer restorative materials, new and modified polymers for restorations and impressions, new phenolic cements, pit and fissure sealants, improved base metal alloys and amalgams, low- or no-gold casting alloys such as palladium-based alloys, ceramics fused to metal systems, and improved ceramics for single restorations have contributed to the service and function of restorative materials.

The extensively used acid etching of tooth structure and base metals to provide adhesion of resin composites has had a dramatic effect on restorative and orthodontic dental treatment. The recent improvements in bonding agents for composites and metals to enamel and dentin have provided the opportunity for major changes in cavity design. The improvements in composites have resulted in their extended application to the restoration of posterior teeth. The establishment of clinical and biological evidence of the success of titanium and titanium alloys for dental implants has made it possible to replace a tooth lost as a result of extraction.

Biophysical applications such as experimental stress analysis studies have resulted in better guidelines for the design of restorations in relation to the properties of particular materials. Materials used for maxillofacial applications or as dental implants have received increased attention; the urgent need for improvement has stimulated research in both of these areas.

The interaction of materials with the oral tissues has become increasingly important in the evaluation of these materials, as indicated by the interim acceptance by the Council on Dental Materials and Devices in November 1971 of recommended standard practices for the biological evaluation of dental materials. A series of handbooks has also been published reviewing the current knowledge about the biocompatibility of dental materials.

■ REFERENCES

American Dental Association: *Clinical products in dentistry—a desktop reference,* Chicago, 1993, American Dental Association.

American Dental Association: *Dentist's desk reference: materials, instruments and equipment,* ed 2, Chicago, 1983, American Dental Association.

American Dental Association: *Guide to dental materials and devices,* ed 8, Chicago, 1976, American Dental Association.

Coleman RL: Physical properties of dental materials, *J Res Nat Bur Stand* 1:868, 1928.

Council on Dental Materials and Devices, American Dental Association: Medical device legislation and the FDA Panel on Review of Dental Devices, *J Am Dent Assoc* 94:353, 1977.

Craig RG, Farah JW: Stress analysis and design of single restorations and fixed bridges, *Oral Sci Rev* 10:45, 1977.

Diefenbach VL: A national center for applied dental research, *J Am Dent Assoc* 73:587, 1966.

Docking AR: A critique of common materials used in dental practice, *Int Dent J* 12:382, 1962.

Essig CJ, Koenig A: *Dental metallurgy,* ed 6, Philadelphia, 1909, Lea & Febiger.

Gabel AB: The role of physics in dentistry, *J Appl Physics* 12:712, 1941.

Guerini V: *A history of dentistry,* Philadelphia, 1909, Lea & Febiger.

Harder OE: *Modern dental metallurgy,* Minneapolis, 1930, Burgess-Roseberry.

Hodgen JD, Millberry GS: *Practical dental metallurgy,* ed 6, St Louis, 1924, Mosby.

Lufkin AW: *A history of dentistry,* ed 3, Philadelphia, 1948, Lea & Febiger.

National Institute of Dental Research, National Institutes of Health: International state-of-the-art conference on restorative dental materials, Bethesda, Md, Sept 8–10, 1986.

Peyton FA: Significance of dental materials science to the practice of dentistry, *J Dent Educ* 30:268, 1966.

Ray KW: *Metallurgy for dental students,* Philadelphia, 1931, P Blakiston's Son.

Robinson JB: *The foundations of professional dentistry,* Baltimore, 1940, Waverly Press.

Shell JS: *Hodgen-Shell dental materials,* St Louis, 1938, Mosby.

Smyd ES: Bio-mechanics of prosthetic dentistry, *Ann Dent* 12:85, 1953.

Souder WH, Paffenbarger GC: Physical properties of dental materials, National Bureau of Standards Circular No C433, Washington, DC, 1942, US Government Printing Office.

Stanley HR: Biological testing and reaction of dental materials. In Craig RG, editor: *Dental materials review,* Ann Arbor, 1977, University of Michigan School of Dentistry.

Sturdevant CM, Roberson TM, Heyman HO, Sturdevant JR: *The art and science of operative dentistry,* ed 3, St Louis, 1995, Mosby.

Taylor JA: *History of dentistry,* Philadelphia, 1922, Lea & Febiger.

Townsend RB: Porcelain teeth and the Chevalier Dubois de Chemant, *Dent Mag & Oral Topics* 58:249, 1941.

Tylman SD, Malone P: *Theory and practice of crown and fixed partial prosthodontics (bridge),* ed 7, St Louis, 1978, Mosby.

Von Recum AF, editor: *Handbook of biomaterials evaluation,* New York, 1986, Macmillan.

Weinberger BW: *An introduction to the history of dentistry,* St Louis, 1948, Mosby.

Weinberger BW: The dental art in ancient Egypt, *J Am Dent Assoc* 34:170, 1947.

Weinberger BW: *Orthodontics, an historical review of its origin and evolution,* St Louis, 1926, Mosby.

Williams DF, editor: *Biocompatibility of dental materials,* vols 1–4, Boca Raton, Fla, 1982, CRC Press.

Williams DF, editor: *Concise encyclopedia of medical and dental materials,* New York, 1990, Pergamon Press.

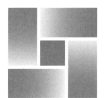

2 *Applied Surface Phenomena*

Atoms or molecules at the surfaces of solids or liquids differ greatly from those in the bulk of the solid or liquid, and neighboring atoms may be arranged anisotropically. Also, some atoms or molecules may accumulate at the surface and thus cause unusual physical and chemical properties. The surfaces of solids may contain 10^{15} atoms or molecules per square centimeter plus or minus a factor of three depending on the density. These solid surfaces have atoms of higher energy than bulk atoms because of the absence of some neighboring atoms and thus readily adsorb ambient atoms or molecules. It has been determined that to produce a clean solid surface, one with less than 1% of an adsorbed monolayer, a vacuum of 10^{-9} Torr or 1.33×10^{-7} Pa would be required to maintain that surface clean for about an hour. At a vacuum of about 3×10^{-6} Torr, a newly cleaned surface would be coated with ambient atoms or molecules in only a few seconds. Therefore all dental materials and dental surfaces would be covered with a layer of ambient atoms or molecules and thus adhesives would be bonding to these adsorbed monolayers.

The surface layer usually has a stronger bond to the substrate than to adjacent adsorbed molecules. Thus the surface can be described as two layers, the substrate layer and the adsorbed layer. The greatest interaction is between the substrate and the adsorbed layer, but interaction can involve several layers of adsorbed molecules. If the substrate is an insulator and an electrical charge exists at the interface between the solid and the liquid, the charge may extend a number of layers into the solid and several layers into the liquid.

The energy involved in the adsorption of atoms or molecules onto the substrate may be of the level of a chemical reaction (chemisorption) or may be of the level of van der Waal's reaction (physiosorption). The former is irreversible, whereas the latter is reversible.

Thus an important concept in surface chemistry is that critically important properties of a material may be more related to the chemistry of the surface layer and its composition than to the bulk properties. Such surface effects dominate the surface mechanical properties of adhesion and friction, the optical surface phenomena of the perception of color and texture, the tissue reaction to materials, the attachment of cells to materials, the wettability and capillarity of surfaces, the nucleation and growth of solids, and many other areas that are of crucial interest in biomaterials.

A few examples will convey the importance of surface chemistry to dentistry. Stainless steel used mainly in orthodontics is 72% to 74% iron but has acceptable corrosion resistance in the mouth because the 18% chromium present forms an adherent oxide layer on the surface, which provides corrosion resistance. Titanium, its alloys, and noble alloys containing small amounts of indium and tin have excellent biocompatibility properties as a result of oxides of titanium and of indium and tin on the surface.

Traditional methods and instrumentation allowed the measurement of adsorption and desorption of atoms or molecules to surfaces, the determination of thermodynamic properties of surfaces such as free energy and heats of adsorption and enthalpy, the evaluation of the contact angles of liquids on solid surfaces, and the study of adhesion, nucleation, friction, lubrication, and surface reactions.

New instrumentation and techniques developed during the past 20 years or so have permitted the study of surfaces on the atomic scale. The most common of these techniques involves scattering and absorption or emission of photons, electrons, atoms, or ions. Only three of the many methods that have been applied to the study of dental biomaterials will be described here. Other techniques are adequately described in textbooks on surface chemistry and catalysis.

■ CHARACTERIZATION OF SOLID SURFACES

Several methods have been developed that facilitate surface analysis on a routine basis. Because tissue reactions in contact with biomaterials have been found to be sensitive to cleanliness and contamination, as well as to surface composition, these approaches are used routinely in research.

Three widely used methods for surface analysis are x-ray photoemission spectroscopy, electron spectroscopy for chemical analysis, and Auger electron spectroscopy.

X-ray photoemission spectroscopy (XPS) is often used because it is highly sensitive to small amounts of surface contamination, since the x-ray beam does not penetrate deeply into the sample. The specimen to be studied with XPS is bombarded with x-ray photons, which results in the emission of electrons from the surface atoms. The electrons are then analyzed according to energy level and a spectrum is obtained, as shown in Fig. 2-1, for a titanium dental implant. The spectrum shows the presence of titanium and oxygen peaks, which indicates titanium oxide. Small peaks for carbon, nitrogen, calcium, and phosphorus are probably the result of contamination, which may or may not be significant in tissue attachment to the implant.

Electron spectroscopy for chemical analysis (ESCA) also employs a beam of x-rays that produce electron spectra characteristic of the atomic composition of the surface. The resolution of ESCA allows chemical analysis of areas as small as 200 μm diameter by focusing the x-ray beam on a small spot. Fig. 2-2 shows an ESCA spectrum of a hydroxyapatite surface after plasma cleaning. The spectrum shows the presence of fluorine, silica, and sodium contamination, as well as the expected C, P, and O peaks.

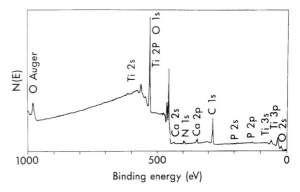

Fig. 2-1 XPS spectrum for Ti dental implant. The surface is dominated by TiO_2 peaks and smaller nitrogen, calcium, and phosphorous peaks resulting from surface contamination. (From Kasemo B, Lausmaa J: *Int J Oral and Maxillofac Implants* 3:253, 1988.)

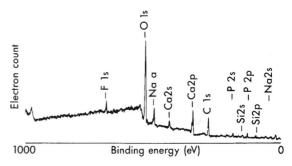

Fig. 2-2 ESCA spectrum from surface of hydroxyapatite after plasma cleaning. (From Smith DC, Pilliar RM, Metson JB, McIntyre NS: *J Biomat Res* 25:1080, 1991.)

Auger electron spectroscopy (AES) is another technic that can provide depth concentration profiles of elements. AES involves the bombardment of the specimen with electrons rather than x-ray beams and measurement of the secondary electrons emitted. At the same time, surface erosion is carried out by an ion bombardment process, called sputtering, to give the elemental analysis as a function of depth. Fig. 2-3 shows an AES spectrum from the surface of a titanium implant sample that shows the presence of Ti, O, and P as a function of sputter time and hence depth. The surface is dominated by TiO_2 with P contamination from treatment with H_3PO_4.

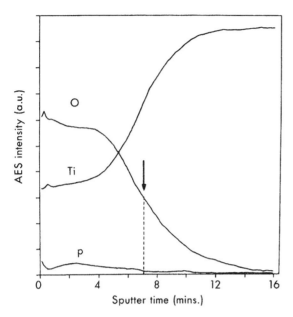

Fig. 2-3 AES depth profile for titanium implant surface as a function of depth removed by sputtering. (From Kasemo B, Lausmaa J: *Int Oral and Maxillofac Implants* 3:255, 1988.)

At deeper levels, sputtering uncovers the titanium under the oxide layer.

■ **THE COLLOIDAL STATE**

Colloids were first described by Thomas Graham (1861) as a result of his studies of diffusion in solutions. He observed that substances such as starch, albumin, and other gelatinous materials did not function in solution like acids, bases, and salts. Because these substances were all gluelike in nature, Graham described them as colloids, which was derived from the Greek word *kolla* for 'glue' and *-oid-* meaning 'like.' As studies continued to increase the understanding of the subject of colloids and their nature, the name came to include more than the original term implied. The term *colloid* now is used to describe a state of matter rather than a kind. The main characteristic of colloidal materials is their high degree of subdivision, although associated with these fine particles are certain physical properties such as electrical charges and surface energies that

control the characteristics of the colloids. It is not enough to confine the definition of colloids to particle size alone.

Nature of Colloids

Substances are called colloids when they consist of two or more phases, with the units of at least one of the phases having a dimension slightly greater than simple molecular size. Although the range of size is somewhat arbitrary, it is usually recognized as being approximately 1 to 500 nm in maximum dimension.* Thus colloidal systems can be fine dispersions, gels, films, emulsions, or foams.

Except for a dispersion of a gas in a gas, which is a true solution, each of the three forms of matter–gas, liquid, and solid–may be dispersed as colloidal particles in the others and in itself as well. Each type has numerous examples of industrial and commercial importance, and many are known to have applications to dentistry, oral conditions, and restorative materials. The dispersed phase, which may be in the form of a gas, liquid, or solid, may exist also in a variety of conditions. Some examples of these dispersed phases include: (1) colloidal silica as a filler in resin composites, (2) colloidal silica in water to be mixed with high-strength dental stone to improve abrasion resistance, (3) droplets of oil in a water base used to prevent rusting of dental instruments during steam sterilization, (4) fillers used in rubber impression materials to control properties such as viscosity, and (5) agglomerates of detergent molecules in water that serve as wetting agents for wax patterns.

The colloidal state represents a highly dispersed system of fine particles of one phase in another, and a characteristic property of the dispersed phase is an enormous surface area. This is true whether a dispersed phase of oil droplets in an emulsion or a finely divided solid suspended in a liquid is considered. To visualize the increase in surface area and its relation to particle size, consider a solid in the form of a 1 cm cube having a total surface area of 6 cm^2.

---

*A micrometer (μm) is equal to 0.001 mm (10^{-3} mm), and a nanometer (nm) is equivalent to 0.000001 mm (10^{-6} mm); 100 nm is equal to 0.0001 mm, or 0.1 μm.

When this mass is cut into 1000 cubes, each being 1 mm on an edge, the surface area is increased to 60 cm^2. The same material reduced to cubes of 1 μm on an edge, which still is not within the range of colloidal particles, has a surface area of 60,000 cm^2. A further reduction in size to 0.1 μm, which is the upper limit for colloids, develops the enormous surface area of 600,000 cm^2 from the same mass that originally had an area of 6 cm^2. If it is assumed that the particles were of uniform size, the 1 cm cube produced 10^{15} particles. This increase in surface area gives rise to a corresponding increase in surface energy and surface reactions. A study of colloids therefore is a study of small particles and the related surface effects in the form of surface electrical charge or surface adsorption. Not only is the surface energy important, but the interface between the two phases imparts important and characteristic properties to the system.

Suspended colloidal particles possess properties that permit the scattering of a beam of light or respond to superimposed electrostatic charges by being either attracted to or repelled by each other. Such a response is not characteristic of either true solutions or massive particles. Often it is difficult to distinguish the colloidal range of substances from true solutions or matter in the massive state. Often it is necessary to study not only the particle size but also the surface phenomena of the system. See also a discussion of the zeta-potential in Chapter 3.

Typical Colloid Systems

Some colloid systems are more important than others in relation to restorative materials. For example, the distinction between a sol and a gel is important because several of each find applications in dental operations. A sol resembles a solution, but it is made up of colloidal particles dispersed in a liquid. When a sol is chilled or caused to react by the addition of suitable chemicals, it may be transformed into a gel. In the gel form the system takes on a semisolid, or jellylike, quality.

The liquid phase of either a sol or a gel is usually water but may be some organic liquid such as alcohol. Systems having water as one component are described as hydrosols or hydrogels. A more general term might be hydrocolloid, which is often used in dentistry to describe the agar or alginate gels used as elastic impression materials. A general term to describe a system having an organic liquid as one component would be organosol or organogel.

Gels

Two examples of materials that involve gel structures are the agar and alginate hydrocolloid impression materials.

Gels possess an entangled framework of solid colloidal particles in which liquid is trapped in the interstices and held by capillarity. Such a gel has some degree of rigidity, depending on the extent of the structural solids present.

Gels that are formed with water are hydrophilic (water loving) in character and tend to imbibe large quantities of water if allowed to stand immersed. The imbibition is accompanied by swelling and a change in physical dimensions. When allowed to stand in dry air, the gel loses water to the atmosphere, with an accompanying shrinkage. Such changes may be observed readily in agar or alginate gels.

A very common method for forming a gel is to add water to gelatin, agar, starch, or another substance that develops a dispersed colloid of the sol type. Frequently such sols are heated to aid the dispersion. Simple cooling of this sol results in the gel formation. Such a gel may contain as little as 2% to 10% solid colloids as interlaced and entangled filaments of molecular aggregates. The remainder of the gel is water held by capillarity. Gels produced in this manner usually are reversible in nature because they can be reconverted to a sol by heating and again to a gel by cooling. A common example of such a gel is agar. Within limits, gels of this type can be dehydrated by being allowed to stand in air and be rehydrated by being reimmersed in water.

Another common method of forming gels is by a reaction of two chemicals. The best-known example in dentistry is alginate gel, which results from the reaction of soluble potassium alginate with calcium ions to form an insoluble calcium alginate gel. This gel is thermally nonreversible in contrast to the agar gel. Silicate-bonded dental investments set as a result of the formation of silica gel, which results from the reaction of sodium silicate and hydrochloric acid. This gel is an example of an inorganic nonreversible gel.

Syneresis

A characteristic of many gels is to contract on standing in closed containers and to exude or squeeze out some of the liquid phase. This process of accumulating an exudate on the surface is known as syneresis. The degree of attraction forces and the tenacity with which the filaments and fibers of the gel are held together have much to do with syneresis and the extent to which the exudate is formed. In dental impression-taking operations the formation of an exudate by syneresis is troublesome, as described in Chapter 11.   *Problematic*

Emulsions

A uniform dispersion of minute droplets of one liquid within another constitutes an emulsion. The two liquids are highly insoluble and immiscible, but by mechanical means a colloidal dispersion of one liquid is produced in the other. Mechanical blenders, homogenizers, or grinders are used for the purpose of preparation.

Normally, emulsions are of two types, an oil dispersion in water, and the reverse type of water in oil. Usually an emulsion developed by the mechanical dispersion of pure liquids is unstable, and the emulsion soon breaks, with the droplets coalescing and separating into layers. The emulsion may be stabilized by the addition of a small quantity of a third substance known as the emulsifier. The emulsifier enters into the interface between the droplet and the dispersing liquid to give stability to the system. The action of the emulsifier is to lower the interfacial tension between the two liquids. Generally it is necessary to employ only a small quantity of emulsifier to produce a stable emulsion.

The use of an emulsion to apply a protective film of oil to dental instruments during autoclave sterilization has been developed. By dipping the instruments into the emulsion, a thin coating of oil and protective chemicals is applied to the surface, which prevents corrosion and tarnish of the instruments during the process of steam autoclave sterilization. The emulsion in this case is composed of 2% oil dispersed in water, with less than 1% of sorbitan monooleate polyoxyethylene added as the emulsifier. Also dissolved in the water is 2% sodium benzoate, which aids in the reduction of corrosion.

■ DIFFUSION THROUGH MEMBRANES AND OSMOTIC PRESSURE

Osmotic pressure is the pressure developed by diffusion of a liquid or a solvent through a membrane. The solvent passes from the dilute to the more concentrated solution through the membrane separating the two solutions. The presence of dissolved material in a solvent lowers the escaping tendency of the solvent molecules, and the greater the concentration, the more the escaping tendency is lowered. Accordingly, the solvent will diffuse or pass through a membrane to a region of greater concentration, thus causing a dilution of the concentration of the solution.

The development of osmotic pressure has been used to explain the hypersensitivity of dentin. It has been considered that the change in pressure of solutions present in natural tooth dentin, in exposed carious teeth as the result of contact with saliva or concentrated solutions gives rise to diffusion throughout the structure to increase or decrease the pressure on the nerve system.

Not only the process of diffusion through membranes but also the diffusion from one substance of a given concentration to that of another concentration is important in many materials in dentistry. Studies have shown that salts and dyes will diffuse through human dentin. Stains and discoloring agents will diffuse through plastic restorative materials. Likewise, the diffusion of salts and acids through organic varnish-type cavity liners has been a problem.

■ ADSORPTION, ABSORPTION, AND SORPTION

It is common for both liquids and solids to adsorb gases or other liquids on their surfaces and the process is always exothermic. In the adsorption process a liquid or a gas adheres firmly to the surface by the attachment of molecules to the surface of the solid or liquid, thus reducing their surface free energy. In a physical sense, if the two substances were alike, as, for example, two pieces of the same metal in the solid state pressed closely together, the mass would be said to cohere. When a dissimilar substance, such as a gas or a liquid, is in intimate contact with the surface of the solid, it is said to adhere to the surface. The process of adsorption or adhesion to the surface of a substance is important in the wetting process, in which the substance is coated or wetted with a foreign substance such as a liquid. The degree to which saliva, for example, will wet or adhere to the surface of a resin denture depends on the tendency for surface adsorption. A substance that is readily wetted on the surface by water, as is glass or porcelain or the natural tooth surface, is considered to have adsorbed on its surface a layer of water molecules. High-energy surfaces such as metals will adsorb molecules more readily than low-energy surfaces such as waxes, whereas oxides have intermediate surface energies.

The process of adsorption differs somewhat from the process of absorption. In the process of absorption the substance absorbed diffuses into the solid material in a type of diffusion process and is not noted for concentration of molecules at the surface.

In instances in which both adsorption and absorption are known to exist and it is not clear which process predominates, the whole process is known as sorption. In measurement of the moisture content of dental resins the process is described as one of sorption of moisture by the resin.

Numerous examples of these processes are to be found in the use of various restorative dental materials. The process of absorption of water by the hydrocolloid impression materials is particularly important to the stability of this type of compound. When the quantity of liquid absorbed into a substance is relatively large, there is likely to be an accompanying change in the dimensions of the absorbent.

■ SURFACE TENSION AND WETTING

Surface tension is measured in terms of force per centimeter of the surface of liquid, and the units employed are dynes per centimeter. In the case of water at 20° C, the value is 72.8 dynes/cm. At the same temperature, benzene has a value of 29 dynes/cm; alcohol, 22 dynes/cm; and ether, 17 dynes/cm. By contrast, mercury at 20° C has a surface tension of 465 dynes/cm. The values for each of these substances are influenced by factors such as

temperature and purity. In general, there is a reduction in surface tension of all liquids as the temperature is increased. For example, the surface tension of water in dynes per centimeter is 76 at 0° C, 72 at 25° C, 68 at 50° C, and 59 at 100° C.

The surface tension of liquids is reduced also by the presence of impurities, some of which are exceedingly effective. Detergents such as sodium lauryl sulfate or the ingredients of soaps, including sodium stearate or sodium oleate, which have long hydrocarbon chains attached to hydrophilic groups such as $-COONa$, are particularly effective in reducing the surface tension of water. An example of the effectiveness of sodium oleate in minute concentrations is shown in Table 2-1; notice that the surface tension is reduced approximately one-half by the addition of only 0.02%, or 0.2 g/liter of solute in water.

These surface-active agents affect the surface tension by concentrating at the liquid-air or other interfaces or surfaces. As these molecules occupy surface positions in the water-air surface, they displace surface water molecules to reduce the cohesive force between water molecules over the surface area because the cohesion between water and surface active agent is less than that between water and water. This effect is demonstrated in Fig. 2-4, which represents two drops placed on wax, one of which is water and the other water with detergent. The presence of the surface-active agent molecules in the surface layer reduces the pull on the surface molecules toward the liquid mass. This reduces the surface tension to increase the wetting. The soap molecules are oriented so that the hydrophilic end is in the water and the hydrophobic (hydrocarbon) end is oriented toward the wax or air.

TABLE 2-1   Sodium Oleate in Water (Room Temperature, 22° C)

Solute Concentration	Concentration (%)	Surface Tension (dynes/cm)
Distilled water		72.8
1 part/500,000	0.0002	63.0
1 part/50,000	0.002	48.3
1 part/5000	0.02	35.3

WATER   SOAP – WATER

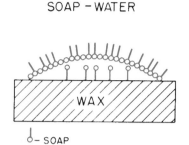

○– WATER   ↓– SOAP

Fig. 2-4 Spreading of pure water and water containing soap molecules on wax.

The increased wettability of solids with liquids of reduced surface tension is important in numerous dental applications. The wetting power of a liquid is represented by its tendency to spread on the surface of the solid. In restorative dental operations it often is necessary to form wax patterns that are to be wetted by water or water suspensions of such materials as plaster or casting investment. Wax is not well wetted by water, for which reason a dilute solution of some wetting agent (such as 0.01% aerosol) is first painted on the wax in small quantities to aid in the spreading of water mixtures in subsequent operations.

Much can be learned about the spreading of liquids on solids, or the tendency for wetting surfaces, by measurement of the angle of contact between the liquid and the solid surface. The angles of contact for different liquid droplets on a plane glass surface are illustrated in Fig. 2-5. The contact angle results from a balance of surface and interfacial energies. Notice that the surface energy of liquids is expressed as ergs per square centimeter, which is numerically equal to the surface tension in dynes per centimeter. The balance of these energies is shown in Fig. 2-6 for a solid and liquid where γ represents the surface energies and the subscripts sa, sl, and lv indicate solid-air, solid-liquid, and liquid-vapor interfaces. Notice that $\gamma_{sa} - \gamma_{sl}$ will be a maximum for a given liquid when the contact angle θ is 0 degree because the cosine has a maximum value of 1 for that value of θ.

The greater the tendency to wet the surface, the lower the contact angle until complete wetting occurs at an angle equal to zero.

Studies have been made to determine the contact angle of water and saliva on complete denture plas-

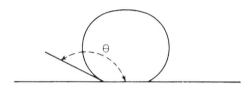

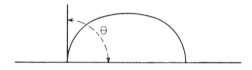

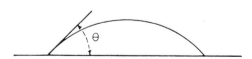

Fig. 2-5 Relation of contact angle to the spreading or wetting of a liquid on a solid.

tics because it relates to the retention of the denture (see Chapter 19). The contact angle and the tendency of a drop of water to spread on paraffin wax and dental methyl methacrylate plastic is shown for comparison in Fig. 2-7. The contact angle for water on wax is about 110 degrees and for water on the acrylic plastic is around 75 degrees. The contact angle for saliva freshly applied to the acrylic plastic surface is 75 degrees, which is the same as that for water. When saliva was allowed to stand overnight

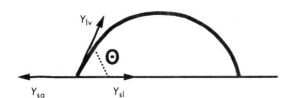

Fig. 2-6 Sketch of a contact angle formed by the balance of energies between the liquid and solid.

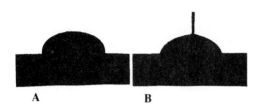

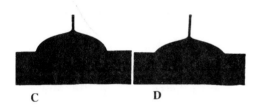

Fig. 2-7 Photographs to show the contact angle formed by a drop of water or saliva on wax and acrylic plastic. **A,** Water on wax. **B,** Water on plastic. **C,** Fresh saliva on plastic. **D,** Saliva after remaining in contact with plastic.

TABLE 2-2   Contact Angles of Water on Solids at 27° C

Solid	Advancing Angle (degrees)
Acrylic polymer	74
Teflon	110
Glass	14
Amalgam	77
Acrylic filling material	38
Composite filling material	51

Adapted from O'Brien WJ: Capillary penetration of liquids between dissimilar solids, doctoral thesis, Ann Arbor, 1967, University of Michigan, p 40.

TABLE 2-3   Surface Tension of Metals

Metal	Temperature (° C)	Surface Tension (dynes/cm)
Lead	327	452
Mercury	20	465
Zinc	419	758
Copper	1131	1103
Gold	1120	1128

in contact with the plastic material, the contact angle for saliva was reduced to approximately 68 degrees, which indicates that the surface wetting is somewhat improved after remaining in contact with the saliva. Table 2-2 gives contact angle values for water on selected materials.

Other examples of wetting of surfaces by liquids include the spreading of molten flux on hot metal during melting or soldering operations. The spreading of molten solder on the surface of the parts to be assembled is an example of liquid metal wetting the surface of a solid metal. If the wetting is not adequate, the operation may be unsuccessful, and if the contact angle of the solder is too great, it will not penetrate into the fine detail of the structures to be joined.

The surface tension of metals is relatively high compared with that of other liquids, an indication that greater cohesive forces exist between the liquid metal atoms in the liquid-air surface than between molecules of liquid compounds such as alcohol or water. The surface tension of most metals, except mercury, cannot be measured at room temperature because of the high melting points. Typical values of a few metals are included in Table 2-3, which shows that there is a difference in the surface tension of various metals and that the values are much greater than for other liquids.

The surface tension of molten metals, like that of other liquids, is reduced with an increase in temperature. This is fortunate for the operation of casting molten metal, since some increase in the temperature will aid in producing sharp detail in the casting. This assumes, however, that the metal is not oxidized excessively or otherwise damaged by heating to the elevated temperature. The presence of a suitable flux will aid in preventing damage during heating, as described in Chapter 16.

TABLE 2-4 Contact Angle of Mercury on Various Materials*

Material	Contact Angle (degrees)
γ (73.2% Ag/26.8% Sn)	145
Eutectic (71.9% Ag/28.1% Cu)	138
Mynol	150
Dispersalloy	145
AgO	130
Ag_2O	135
SnO	107
SnO_2	130

*From Baran G, O'Brien WJ: *J Am Dent Assoc* 94:898, 1977. Copyright by the American Dental Association. Reprinted by permission.

· Trituration of amalgam is important in amalgamation because of the degree of wetting of amalgam alloy by mercury. The contact angles of mercury on two common phases present in amalgam alloys, the silver-tin (γ) phase and the silver-copper eutectic phase, were found to be high and of the same order as those for commercial amalgam alloys. The high values are probably a result of the presence of silver and tin oxides on the surfaces of the alloys because the contact angle values for mercury on a set dental amalgam (Dispersalloy) is similar, as shown in Table 2-4. Trituration produces clean alloy surfaces that are readily wetted by mercury so amalgamation can occur.

■ CAPILLARY RISE

The penetration of liquids into narrow crevices is known as capillary action.

The following equation relates the differential capillary pressure developed when a small tube of radius *r* is inserted in a liquid of surface tension γ, usually expressed in dynes/cm, and with a contact angle θ:

$$\Delta P = \frac{2\gamma \cos \theta}{r}$$

It follows that if the contact angle of the liquid on the solid is less than 90 degrees as shown in Fig. 2-8, **A**, ΔP will be positive and the liquid will pene-

trate. If the contact angle is greater than 90 degrees (Fig. 2-8, **B**), ΔP will be negative and the liquid will be depressed.

Most restorative materials used at present in dentistry do not adhere strongly to tooth structure. As a result, a crevice usually exists between the restoration and the tooth tissue into which mouth fluids penetrate because of capillary action. The importance of gap or width has long been recognized as a factor influencing the degree of marginal leakage. However, wetting is also an important parameter in penetration. Fig. 2-9 describes the combined effects of gap width and contact angles on the capillary penetration of water between two plates. Two contact angles are involved, since one plate might be easily wetted, for example, glass, and the other might be a poorly wetted polymer.

Penetration Coefficient

Another aspect of capillary phenomena involves the rate of penetration of a liquid into a crevice. An example is the penetration of a liquid prepolymer sealant into a fissure and the fine microscopic spaces created by etching of an enamel surface. The properties of the liquid affecting the rate of penetration may be related to the penetration coefficient *(PC)* where γ is the surface tension, η is the viscosity, and θ is the contact angle of the sealant on the enamel:

$$PC = \frac{\gamma \cos \theta}{2\eta}$$

The penetration coefficients for sealants have been shown to vary from 0.6 to 12 cm/sec. Narrow occlusal fissures can be filled almost completely if the penetration coefficient value is at least 1.30 cm/sec when the sealant is applied at a proximal edge of the fissure on the occlusal surface and allowed to flow to the other edge. If the sealant is painted over the occlusal surface, air trapped in the fissure prevents penetration beyond a certain depth. The same analysis applies to the penetration of liquid sealants into the etched surface of enamel to form tags, as shown in Fig. 2-10.

Isolated Capillaries

Still another aspect of capillary phenomena is the adhesion of liquid bridges between solids. Liquid

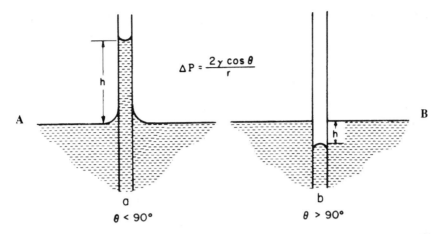

$$\Delta P = \frac{2\gamma \cos \theta}{r}$$

Fig. 2-8 Capillary penetration, **A,** and depression, **B.** (From O'Brien WJ, Craig RG, Peyton FA: *J Prosthet Dent* 19:400, 1968.)

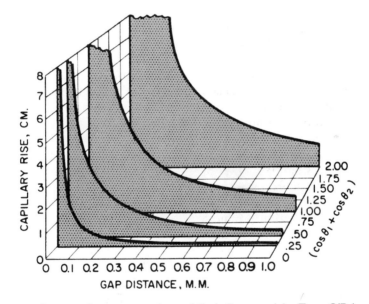

Fig. 2-9 Capillary rise curves for water between two plates of dissimilar materials. (From O'Brien WJ, Craig RG, Peyton FA: *J Colloid Interface Sci* 26:507, 1968.)

bridges were considered a contributing factor in denture retention (Fig. 2-11, **C**) when a thin film of saliva was present between the denture material and the mucosa. The source of capillary adhesion is the arrangement called an isolated capillary. As illustrated in Fig. 2-11, **A,** the differential pressure between a capillary and a connected reservoir is balanced by the hydrostatic pressure of capillary elevation. In capillaries isolated from a reservoir, as shown in Fig. 2-11, **B** and **C,** there is a negative dif-

ferential pressure that exerts an adhesive force. This force is partly responsible for denture retention but operates only if the film of saliva is isolated at the periphery of the denture. If the saliva film beneath the denture is connected to a reservoir of saliva beyond the borders of the denture, a negative differential pressure does not develop. Viscosity of the saliva film, however, offers some resistance to separation of the denture from the mucosa and thus contributes to retention.

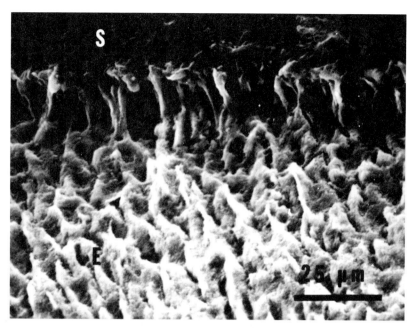

Fig. 2-10 Scanning electron micrograph of the interface of sealant *(S)* and enamel *(E)* showing sealant tags that had penetrated into the etched enamel surface. (From O'Brien WJ, Fan PL, Apostolidis A: *Oper Dent* 3:53, 1978.)

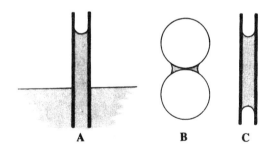

Fig. 2-11 Two classes of capillary systems. **A,** Connected capillary; **B** and **C,** Isolated capillaries (isocaps). (From O'Brien, WJ: *J Dent Res* 52:545, 1973.)

Isolated capillaries form around teeth when small quantities of saliva are trapped in interproximal spaces and occlusal fissures, as shown in Fig. 2-12. It is interesting that the growth rate of bacteria has been found to increase under these conditions of negative pressure.

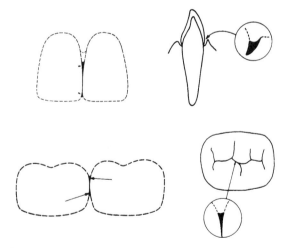

Fig. 2-12 Formation of isolated capillaries around teeth. (From O'Brien WJ: *J Dent Res* 52:547, 1973.)

■ FORCES INVOLVED IN DENTURE RETENTION

The accuracy of fit of a denture has been cited as an important factor in the retention of denture bases without any explanation as to why a better fit results in better retention. A technical discussion of all factors involved in the retention of dentures is not within the scope of this text, but a qualitative discussion is helpful in understanding the role of fit in denture retention. Factors include: (1) capillary forces involving the liquid film between the oral tissues and the denture base, (2) surface forces controlling the wetting of the plastic denture base by the saliva, (3) the seating force applied to the denture, which, for the most part, determines the thickness of the saliva film between the denture and the oral tissues, (4) the surface tension of the saliva, (5) the viscosity of the saliva, and (6) the atmospheric pressure.

The capillary force, F, responsible for retention of a denture can be expressed by the following equation:

$$F = \frac{\gamma A \left(\cos \theta_1 + \cos \theta_2 \right)}{dg}$$

in which γ is the surface tension of saliva, A is the surface area of the tissue surface of the denture, θ_1 and θ_2 are the contact angles of saliva against the plastic and the oral mucosa, d is the film thickness of the saliva between the denture and the tissue, and g is the gravitational constant.

Certain factors, such as wetting, are more important in the retention of a denture under static conditions, whereas other factors, such as capillarity and atmospheric pressure, are more effective when a force tends to dislodge the denture. The wetting of the plastic surface depends on the energy relationship between the solid and the liquid. If complete wetting occurs, the liquid will spread on the solid. If partial wetting occurs, the liquid will form droplets on the surface. The plastics used in dentistry are only partially wetted by saliva, but the wetting may improve after contact with oral fluids because of the adsorption of certain components of the saliva by the plastic surface.

The capillary force, which helps restrain any dislodging force on the denture, is increased by complete wetting of the denture surface, high surface-tension of the saliva, and large tissue-contact area of the denture. Patients with stringy (low surface tension) saliva experience difficulty with retention of dentures. The viscosity of saliva is low, and little difference in retention is observed regardless of whether the load is applied slowly or rapidly. The use of denture pastes, however, provides a film of increased thickness and viscosity, and if they are used, greater retention is observed when the load is applied rapidly. It has been shown that the use of adhesives has no detrimental effect on the health of the supporting tissues.

The viscosity of saliva from dentate and edentulous patients differs, with edentulous patients demonstrating a lower viscosity. The lower viscosity may be caused by stimulation of salivary flow with the denture acting as a foreign object, thereby producing a larger flow of saliva with a lower mucin content. Another possibility is that the mandibular denture may obstruct the ducts of the submandibular glands, which produce a greater proportion of mucous glycoprotein. Saliva also appears to act as a nonnewtonian fluid exhibiting lower viscosities at higher shear rates or shear thinning.

The capillary force is diminished when the distance between the denture and the oral tissues is increased. It is reduced to a very small value if the periphery of the denture is immersed in saliva or other fluids. This explains some of the difficulty patients may encounter when drinking fluids and the variation in retention of the maxillary compared with the mandibular denture. At best, the role of atmospheric pressure is that of a temporary restraining force because the pressure in the saliva film is only slightly less than atmospheric pressure. During the application of a dislodging force, however, a reduced pressure may occur under the denture, which may temporarily retard its movement.

The two factors just mentioned may explain in part the function of the peripheral seal. If all other factors are held constant for a particular patient, the fit of the denture controls the distance between it and the oral tissues, which in turn controls the force necessary to dislodge a denture. As a patient continues to wear a denture for a period of time, changes in the contour of the oral tissues and bone structure may eventually result in a poorer fit and decreased retention.

■ ADHESION

Adhesion is the bonding of dissimilar materials by the attraction of atoms or molecules. Because there is always some attraction between atoms, adhesive strength is a matter of magnitude. Stresses that weaken adhesive bonds are caused by differences in thermal expansion coefficients and dimensional changes during setting of the adhesive. In dental applications, moisture greatly weakens adhesion by hydrating the active groups of tooth structure.

Two mechanisms of adhesion may be distinguished: chemical and mechanical. Chemical adhesion involves bonding at the atomic or molecular level. Mechanical adhesion is based on retention by the interlocking of or the penetration of one phase into the surface of the other. In many cases chemical and mechanical adhesion occur together.

Adhesion with polymers has been achieved by etching tooth enamel with acids such as phosphoric acid. Adhesive bond strengths approaching the tensile strength of enamel have been found even after storage in water. Examination under high magnification shows the etched enamel to be greatly roughened. The adhesion of resins to etched enamel is a result of capillary penetration into surface irregularities. These polymer projections into enamel have been called tags. Enamel etching has been applied in the use of pit and fissure sealants to obtain adhesion and with composite filling materials to obtain adhesion to enamel margins. Some adhesion with polymers to dentin has been obtained using copolymer acids, acid-soluble glasses, and composites using treatment of the dentin with organic anhydrides, acids, or phosphates; however it is generally believed that the adhesion is primarily micromechanical in nature.

SELECTED PROBLEMS

Problem 1. Why is mercury difficult to handle without contamination of the operatory?

Solution. The high surface tension of mercury and high contact angles on most surfaces cause the mercury to cohere and roll off most surfaces. The vapor pressure of mercury at room temperature is high enough so that its concentration in air can be toxic. The solution is to handle free mercury over surfaces with lipped edges that can catch any spills or to use precapsulated amalgam systems.

Problem 2. Gold inlay castings made with the lost wax process were rough. What could have been the problem?

Solution. There could be several causes for the rough castings. A detergent or wetting agent may not have been used on the wax pattern before the investing procedure. Wax patterns are not readily wetted by the water-based gypsum investment unless a wetting agent is used; if one is not used, rough internal mold surfaces produce rough castings.

On the other hand, too much wetting agent placed on the wax will interfere with the setting of the investment and a rough surface will result. The wetting agent is painted on the wax pattern and the excess removed by painting with a dry brush. Very little wetting agent is needed (see Table 2-1).

Problem 3. The bond between a pit and fissure material that had just been removed from the refrigerator and etched enamel was found to be poor. Why?

Solution. The bonding of pit and fissure sealants to enamel depends on the capillary penetration of the sealant into the fine microscopic spaces produced by etching. The rate of capillary penetration is dependent upon the wetting and viscosity of the sealant. At lower temperatures, the viscosity of sealants is too high for rapid penetration. Therefore it is necessary to allow a refrigerated sealant to warm up to room temperature before application.

■ REFERENCES

Ackerman E: *Biophysical science,* Englewood Cliffs, NJ, 1962, Prentice Hall.

Baier RE, Meyer AE: Surface analysis. In von Recum, AF: *Handbook of biomaterials evaluation,* New York, 1986, Macmillan.

Baran G, O'Brien WJ: Wetting of amalgam alloys by mercury, *J Am Dent Assoc* 94:897, 1977.

Bonner FT, Phillips M: *Principles of physical science,* Reading, Mass, 1957, Addison-Wesley.

Bowen RL: A method for bonding to dentin and enamel, *J Am Dent Assoc* 107:734, 1983.

Craig RG, Berry GC, Peyton FA: Wetting of poly(methyl methacrylate) and polystyrene by water and saliva, *J Phys Chem* 64:541, 1960.

Dental composites and adhesives in the 21st century, The Gunnar Ryge Memorial Symposium, *Quintessence Internat* 24(9):605, 1993.

Fischer RB: *Applied electron microscopy,* Bloomington, Ind, 1953, Indiana University Press.

Flinn RA, Trojan PK: *Engineering materials and their applications,* ed 3, Boston, 1986, Houghton Mifflin.

Hildebrand JH, Powell RE: *Principles of chemistry,* ed 6, New York, 1952, Macmillan.

Iler RK: *The chemistry of silica-solubility, polymerization, colloid and surface properties, and biochemistry,* New York, 1979, John Wiley & Sons.

Masuhara E: Die neuentwickelten haftfuähigen Kunststoffe und ihre klinische Anwendung, *Dent Zahnüarztl Z* 37:155, 1982.

Moffatt WG, Pearsall GW, Wulff J: *The structure and properties of materials,* vol 1, *Structure,* New York, 1964, John Wiley & Sons.

Moskowitz HD, Ward GT, Wollridge ED, editors: *Dental adhesive materials,* symposium, New York University, New York, 1973, New York University Press.

Myers CL, Ryge G, Heyde JB, Glenn JA: *In vivo* test of bond strength, *J Dent Res* 42:907, 1963.

Norman AL: Frictional resistance and dental prosthetics, *J Prosthet Dent* 14:45, 1964.

O'Brien WJ: Capillary action around dental structures, *J Dent Res* 52:544, 1973.

O'Brien WJ: *Capillary effects in adhesion,* Proceedings of Conference on Dental Adhesive Materials, New York, 1973, New York University Press.

O'Brien WJ: Surface energy of liquids isolated in narrow capillaries, *J Surface Sci* 19:387, 1970.

O'Brien WJ, Craig RG, Peyton FA: Capillary penetration around a hydrophobic filling material, *J Prosthet Dent* 19:400, 1968.

O'Brien WJ, Craig RG, Peyton FA: Capillary penetration between dissimilar materials, *J Colloid Interface Sci* 26:500, 1968.

O'Brien WJ, Fan PL, Apostolidis A: Penetrativity of sealants and glazes, *Oper Dent* 3:51, 1978.

Shaw DJ: *Electrophoresis,* New York, 1969, Academic Press.

Siegel BM, editor: *Modern developments in electron microscopy,* New York, 1964, Academic Press.

Somorjai GA: *Introduction to surface chemistry and catalysis,* New York, 1994, John Wiley & Sons.

Sproell RL: *Modern physics,* New York, 1956, John Wiley & Sons.

van Pelt AWJ: *Adhesion of oral streptococci to solids,* Groningen, 1985, Drukkerij Van Denderen B.V.

Watt GW, Hatch LF: *The science of chemistry,* New York, 1949, McGraw-Hill.

Williams BF, von Fraunhofer JA, Winter GB: Tensile bond strength between fissure sealants and enamel, *J Dent Res* 53:23, 1974.

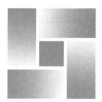

3 Optical, Thermal, and Electrical Properties

Restorative dental materials are developed by the producer and selected by the dentist on the basis of characteristic physical, chemical, and mechanical qualities of the materials, as well as their biological properties.

No single property can be used as a measure of quality of materials. Often several combined properties, determined from standardized laboratory and service tests, are employed to give a measure of quality. The information gained from an orderly laboratory investigation can assist greatly in the clinical evaluation of the particular product or technic by shortening the time required for service testing.

There are times when it is not possible to develop a test that is identical to practical conditions because of the nature of the material or the equipment involved. In such instances a systematic study is conducted with as practical an approach as possible, and then the results are interpreted on a comparative basis.

Standardization of test practices is essential, however, for control of quality or for duplication of results by other investigators. When possible, the test samples should approach the size and shape of the structure employed in practice, with mixing and manipulating procedures comparable with routine practical conditions.

Although it is important to know the comparative values of properties of different restorative materials, it is also essential to know the quality of the supporting tissue. Whereas many restorations fail in service because of fracture or deformation, it is not uncommon for a well-constructed restoration to be useless because the supporting tissue fails. Consequently, in designing restorations and interpreting test results, remember that the success of a restoration depends not only on its physical qualities but also on the biophysical or physiological qualities of the supporting tissues.

The physical properties described in this chapter include color and optical properties, thermal properties, and electrical and electrochemical properties. The color and optical properties are color and its measurement, pigmentation, metamerism, fluorescence, opacity, index of refraction, and optical constants. The thermal properties are temperature, heat of fusion, thermal conductivity, specific heat, thermal diffusivity, and coefficient of thermal expansion. The electrical and electrochemical properties are electrical conductivity, dielectric constant, electromotive force, galvanism, corrosion, and zeta-potential. Other, less specific properties are tarnish and discoloration, water sorption, solubility and disintegration, setting time, and shelf life. These properties generally are not concerned with the application of force to a body as mechanical properties are.

■ OPTICAL PROPERTIES

Color

The perception of the color of an object is the result of a physiological response to a physical stimulus. The sensation is a subjective experience, whereas the beam of light, which is the physical stimulus that produces the sensation, is entirely objective. The perceived color response results from either a reflected or a transmitted beam of white light or a portion of that beam. According to one of Grassmann's laws, the eye can distinguish differences in only three parameters of color. These parameters are dominant wavelength, luminous reflectance, and excitation purity.

The dominant wavelength (λ) of a color is the wavelength of a monochromatic light that, when

TABLE 3-1   Typical Quantities for Color Determined in Reflected Daylight (C.I.E. Source C)

Material	Dominant Wavelength (nm)	Luminous Reflectance	Excitation Purity
Denture resins	601–623	22.5–28.6	0.30–0.38
Denture resin (Meharry shade)	–493*	22.2	0.15
Composite resins	576–580	51.6–78.9	0.16–0.31
Glass ionomer (class V restorative)	577–579	55.2–67.7	0.19–0.27
Human teeth	566–586	35.8–44.8	0.34–0.40
Human facial skin			
Black	588–594	9.8–33.4	0.25–0.44
White	584–599	19.1–44.9	0.20–0.44
Oriental	588–593	22.4–37.4	0.27–0.38
Veneering resin	577–580	56.0–64.4	0.26–0.31

*The negative sign indicates a complementary wavelength and a dominant wavelength in the purple hue.

mixed in suitable proportions with an achromatic color (gray), will match the color perceived. Light having short wavelengths (350 nm) is violet in color, and light having long wavelengths (700 nm) is red. Between these two wavelengths are those corresponding to blue, green, yellow, and orange light. This attribute of color perception is also known as hue.

Of all the visible colors and shades, there are only three primary colors: red, green, and blue (or violet). Any other color may be produced by the proper combination of these colors. For example, yellow may be obtained by a correct mixture of green and red lights.

The luminous reflectance of a color permits an object to be classified as equivalent to a member of a series of achromatic objects ranging from black to white for light-diffusing objects and from black to perfectly clear and colorless for transmitting objects. A black standard is assigned a luminous reflectance of 0, whereas a white standard is assigned 100. This attribute of color perception is described as value in one visual system of color measurement.

The excitation purity or saturation of a color describes the degree of its difference from the achromatic color perception most resembling it. Numbers representing excitation purity range from 0 to 1. This attribute of color perception is also known as chroma.

Typical quantities for dominant wavelength, luminous reflectance, and excitation purity of mate-

rials and human tissues determined in reflected light are listed in Table 3-1.

Measurement of Color

The color of dental restorative materials is most commonly measured in reflected light by instrumental or visual technics.

Instrumental technic

Curves of spectral reflectance versus wavelength can be obtained over the visible range (405 to 700 nm) with a recording spectrophotometer and integrating sphere. Typical curves for a composite resin before and after 300 hours of accelerated aging in a weathering chamber are shown in Fig. 3-1. From the reflectance values and tabulated color-matching functions, the tristimulus values (X, Y, Z) can be computed relative to a particular light source. These tristimulus values are related to the amounts of the three primary colors required to give, by additive mixture, a match with the color being considered. Typically, the tristimulus values are computed relative to the Commission Internationale de l'Eclairage (C.I.E.) Source A (gas-filled incandescent lamp) or Source C (average daylight from overcast sky). The ratios of each tristimulus value of a color to their sum are called the chromaticity coordinates (x, y, z). Dominant wavelength and excitation purity of a color can be determined by referring its chromaticity coordinates to a chromaticity diagram such as the

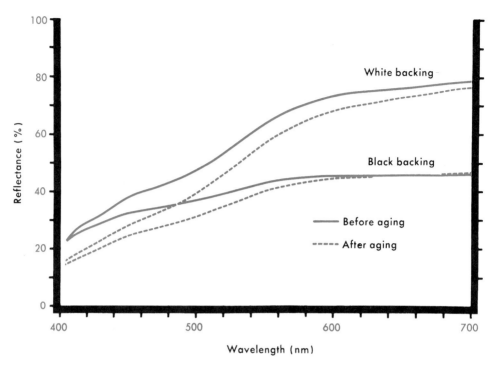

Fig. 3-1 Curves of spectral reflectance versus wavelength for a composite resin before and after exposure to conditions of accelerated aging. The specimen was exposed continuously for 300 hours to the radiation of a 2500-watt xenon lamp and intermittently sprayed with water. The aging chamber was held at 43° C and 90% relative humidity. Spectral reflectance curves for translucent specimens often are obtained with both black and white backings.

one shown in Fig. 3-2. The luminous reflectance is equal to the value of the second (Y) of the three tristimulus values. Some typical quantities for color of dental materials are listed in Table 3-1.

Differences between two colors can be determined from a color difference formula. One such formula has the form:

$$\Delta E(L^*a^*b) = [(\Delta L^*)^2 + (\Delta a^*)^2 + (\Delta b^*)^2]^{1/2}$$

where L^*, a^*, and b^* depend on the tristimulus values of the sample and of a perfectly white object. A value of ΔE^* of one can be observed visually by half of the observers under standardized conditions. A value of ΔE^* of 3.3 is considered perceivable clinically. A diagram of the C.I.E. $L^*a^*b^*$ color space is shown in Fig. 3-3. The $L^*a^*b^*$ color space is characterized by uniform chromaticities.

Visual technic

A popular system for the visual determination of color is the Munsell Color System, the parame-

ters of which are represented in three dimensions as shown in Fig. 3-4. The color considered is compared with a large set of color tabs. Value (lightness) is determined first by the selection of a tab that most nearly corresponds with the lightness or darkness of the color. Value ranges from white (10/) to black (0/). Chroma is determined next with tabs that are close to the measured value but are of increasing saturation of color. Chroma ranges from achromatic or gray (/0) to a highly saturated color (/18). The hue of the color is determined last by matching with color tabs of the value and chroma already determined. Hue is measured on a scale from 2.5 to 10 in increments of 2.5 for each of the 10 color families (red, R; yellow-red, YR; yellow, Y; green-yellow, GY; green, G; blue-green, BG; blue, B; purple-blue, PB; purple, P; red-purple, RP). For example, the color of the attached gingiva of a healthy patient has been measured as 5R 6/4 to indicate a hue of 5R, a value of 6, and a chroma of 4.

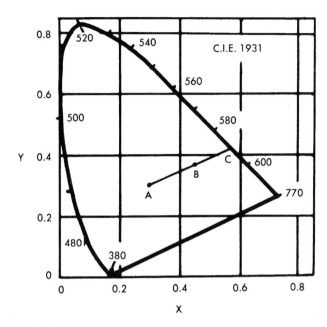

Fig. 3-2 Chromaticity diagram *(x, y)* according to the 1931 C.I.E. Standard Observer and coordinate system. Values of dominant wavelength determine the spectrum locus. The excitation purity is the ratio of two lengths *(AB/AC)* on the chromaticity diagram, where *A* refers to the standard light source and *B* refers to the color being considered. The point *C,* the intersection of line *AB* with the spectrum locus, is the dominant wavelength.

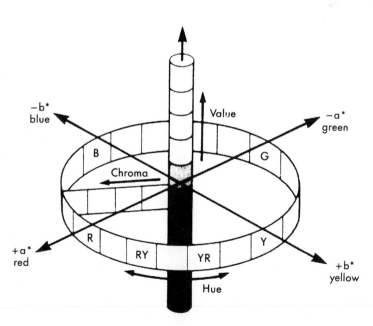

Fig. 3-3 C.I.E. *L*a*b** color arrangement. (From Seghi RR, Johnston WM, O'Brien WJ: *J Prosthet Dent* 56:35, 1986.)

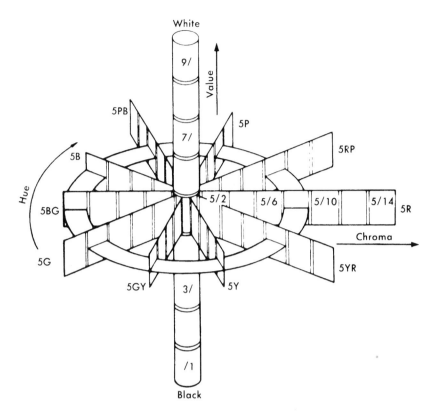

Fig. 3-4 Munsell scales of hue, value, and chroma in color space. (Adapted from Powers JM, Capp JA, Koran A: *J Dent Res* 56:112, 1977.)

Two similar colors can also be compared in the Munsell Color System by a color difference formula such as one derived by Nickerson:

$$I = (C/5)(2\Delta H) + 6\Delta V + 3\Delta C$$

where C is the average chroma and ΔH, ΔV, and ΔC are differences in hue, value, and chroma of the two colors. For example, if the color of attached gingiva of a patient with periodontal disease was 2.5R 5/6, the color difference, I, between the diseased tissue and the aforementioned healthy tissue (5R 6/4) would be:

$$I = (5/5)(2)(2.5) + (6)(1) + (3)(2) = 17$$

A trained observer can detect a color difference, I, equal to 5.

Surface finish and thickness

When white light shines on a solid, some of the light is directly reflected from the surface, and it remains white light. This light mixes with the light reflected from the body of the material and dilutes the color. As a result, an extremely rough surface appears lighter than a smooth surface of the same material. This problem is associated with unpolished or worn glass ionomer and composite restorations. For example, as the resin matrix of a composite material wears away, the restoration appears lighter and less chromatic (grayer).

The thickness of a restoration can affect its appearance. For example, as the thickness of a composite restoration placed against a white background increases, the lightness and the excitation purity decreases. The most dramatic change observed is the increase in opacity as the thickness increases. (See Fig. 10-13.)

Pigmentation

Esthetic effects are sometimes produced in a restoration by the incorporation of colored pigments in nonmetallic materials such as composite resins, dental acrylics, silicone maxillofacial materials, and dental porcelain. The color that is observed when pigments are mixed results from the selective absorption by the pigments and the reflection of certain colors. Mercuric sulfide, or vermilion, is a red pigment because it absorbs all colors except red. The mixing of pigments therefore involves the process of subtracting colors. For example, a green color may be obtained by mixing a pigment such as cadmium sulfide, which absorbs blue and violet, with ultramarine, which absorbs red, orange, and yellow. The only color reflected from such a mixture of pigments is green, which is the color observed.

Usually inorganic pigments rather than organic dyes are used because the pigments are more permanent and durable in their color qualities. When the colors are combined with the proper translucency, the restorative materials may be made to match closely the surrounding tooth structure or soft tissue. To match tooth tissue, various shades of yellow and gray are blended into the white base material, and occasionally some blue or green pigments are added. To match the pink soft tissues of the mouth, various blends of red and white are necessary, with occasional need for blue, brown, and black in small quantities. The color and translucency of human tissue shows a wide variation from patient to patient and from one tooth or area of the mouth to another.

Metamerism

Metameric colors are color stimuli of identical tristimulus values under a particular light source but different spectral energy distributions. The spectral reflectance curves of two such colors would be complicated, with perhaps three or more crossing points. Under some lights such colors would appear to match, but under other lights they would not match.

The quality and intensity of light are factors that must be controlled in matching colors in dental restorations. Because light from incandescent lamps, fluorescent lamps, and the sun differs, the match in color between a pigmented dental material and tooth structure may also vary. Whenever possible, colors should be matched in light corresponding to that of use.

Fluorescence

Fluorescence is the emission of luminous energy by a material when a beam of light is shone on it. The wavelength of the emitted light usually is longer than that of the exciting radiation. Typically, blue or ultraviolet light produces fluorescent light that is in the visible range. Light from most fluorescent substances is emitted in a single broad well-shaped curve, the width and peak depending on the fluorescing substance.

Sound human teeth emit fluorescent light when excited by ultraviolet radiation (365 nm), the fluorescence being polychromatic with the greatest intensity in the blue region (450 nm) of the spectrum. Some anterior restorative materials and dental porcelains are formulated with fluorescing agents (rare earths excluding uranium) to reproduce the natural appearance of tooth structure.

Opacity, Translucency, and Transparency

The color of an object is modified not only by the intensity and shade of the pigment or coloring agent but also by the translucency or opacity of the object. The body tissues vary in the degree of opacity that they exhibit. Most of them possess a degree of translucency. This is especially true of tooth enamel and the supporting soft tissues surrounding the teeth.

Opacity is a property of materials that prevents the passage of light. When all of the colors of the spectrum from a white light source such as sunlight are reflected from an object with the same intensity as received, the object appears white. When all the spectrum colors are absorbed equally, the object appears black. An opaque material may absorb some of the light and reflect the remainder. If, for example, red, orange, yellow, blue, and violet are absorbed, the material appears green in reflected white light.

Translucency is a property of substances that permits the passage of light but disperses the light so that objects cannot be seen through the material. Some translucent materials used in dentistry are porcelain, composite resins, and dental plastics.

Transparent materials allow the passage of light in such a manner that little distortion takes place and objects may be clearly seen through them. Transparent substances such as glass may be colored if they absorb certain wavelengths and transmit others. For example, if a piece of glass absorbed all wavelengths except red, it would appear red by transmitted light. If a light beam containing no red wavelengths were shone on the glass, it would appear opaque, since the remaining wavelengths would be absorbed.

Measurement of contrast ratio

The opacity of a dental material can be determined instrumentally or by visual comparison with opal glass standards. The opacity is represented by a contrast ratio, which is the ratio between the daylight apparent reflectance of a specimen (typically 1 mm thick) when backed by a black standard, and the daylight apparent reflectance of the specimen when backed by a white standard having a daylight apparent reflectance of 70% (or sometimes 100%) relative to magnesium oxide. The contrast ratio ($C_{0.70}$) for a composite resin should lie between the values of 0.55 and 0.70. The spectral reflectance curves of a composite resin backed by black and white standards are shown in Fig. 3-1. The contrast ratio also can be calculated from optical constants, as discussed later.

Index of Refraction

The index of refraction (ξ) for any substance is the ratio of the velocity of light in a vacuum (or air) to its velocity in the medium. When light enters a medium, it slows from its speed in air (300,000 km/sec) and may change direction. For example, when a beam of light traveling in air strikes a water surface at an oblique angle, the light rays are bent toward the normal. The normal is a line drawn perpendicular to the water surface at the point where the light contacts the water surface. If the light is traveling through water and contacts a water-air surface at an oblique angle, the beam of light is bent or refracted away from the normal. The index of refraction is a characteristic property of the substance (Table 3-2) and is used extensively for identification. One of the most important applications of refraction is the control of the refractive index of the dispersed and matrix phases in materials such as composite resins and dental porcelains, designed to have the translucent appearance of tooth tissue. A perfect match in the refractive indices results in a

TABLE 3-2   Index of Refraction of Various Materials

Material	Index of Refraction
Feldspathic porcelain	1.504
Quartz	1.544
Synthetic hydroxyapatite	1.649
Tooth structure, enamel	1.655
Water	1.333

transparent solid, whereas large differences result in opaque materials.

Optical Constants

Esthetic dental materials such as porcelain, composite resins, and human tooth structure are intensely light-scattering or turbid materials. In a turbid material the intensity of incident light is diminished considerably when light passes through the sample. The optical properties of these materials are described by the Kubelka-Munk equations, which develop relations for monochromatic light between the reflection of an infinitely thick layer of a material and its absorption and scattering coefficients. These equations can be solved algebraically by hyperbolic functions derived by Kubelka.

Secondary optical constants (*a* and *b*) can be calculated as follows:

$$a = [R(B) - R(W) - R_B + R_W - R(B)R(W)R_B \\ + R(B)R(W)R_W + R(B)R_B R_W \\ - R(W)R_B R_W] / 2[R(B)R_W - R(W)R_B]$$

and

$$b = (a^2 - 1)^{1/2}$$

where R_B is the reflectance of a dark backing (the black standard), R_W is reflectance of a light backing (the white standard), *R(B)* is the light reflectance of a sample with the dark backing, and *R(W)* is the light reflectance of the sample with the light backing.

These equations are used under the assumptions that (1) the material is turbid, dull, and of constant finite thickness; (2) the edges are neglected; (3) the optical inhomogeneities are much smaller than the thickness of the specimen and are distributed

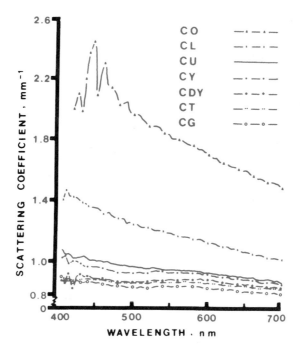

Fig. 3-5 Scattering coefficient versus wavelength for shades of a composite, *C*. Shades are *O,* opaque; *L,* light; *U,* universal; *Y,* yellow; *DY,* dark yellow; *T,* translucent; and *G,* gray. (From Yeh CL, Miyagawa Y, Powers JM: *J Dent Res* 61:797, 1982.)

uniformly; and (4) the illumination is homogeneous and diffused.

Scattering coefficient

The scattering coefficient is the fraction of incident light flux lost by reversal of direction in an elementary layer. The scattering coefficient, *S,* for a unit thickness of a material is defined as follows:

$$S = (1/bX) \text{ Ar ctgh } [1 - a(R + R_g) + RR_g/b(R - R_g)], \text{ mm}^{-1}$$

where *X* is the actual thickness of the sample, *Ar ctgh* is an inverse hyperbolic cotangent, and *R* is the light reflectance of the sample with the backing of reflectance, R_g.

The scattering coefficient varies with the wavelength of the incident light and the nature of the colorant layer as shown in Fig. 3-5 for several shades of a composite resin. Composites with larger values of the scattering coefficient are more opaque.

Absorption coefficient

The absorption coefficient is the fraction of incident light flux lost by absorption in an elementary layer. The absorption coefficient, *K,* for a unit thickness of a material is defined as follows:

$$K = S(a - 1), \text{ mm}^{-1}$$

The absorption coefficient also varies with the wavelength of the incident light and the nature of the colorant layer as shown in Fig. 3-6 for several shades of a composite resin. Composites with larger values of the absorption coefficient are more opaque and more intensely colored.

Light reflectivity

The light reflectivity, *RI,* is the light reflectance of a material of infinite thickness and is defined as follows:

$$RI = a - b$$

This property also varies with the wavelength of the incident light and the nature of the colorant layer.

The light reflectivity can be used to calculate a thickness, *XI,* at which the reflectance of a material with an ideal black background would attain 99.9%

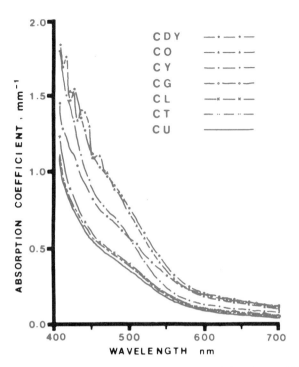

Fig. 3-6 Absorption coefficient versus wavelength for shades of a composite, *C*. Shades are *DY,* dark yellow; *O,* opaque; *Y,* yellow; *G,* gray; *L,* light; *T,* translucent; and *U,* universal. (From Yeh CL, Miyagawa Y, Powers JM: *J Dent Res* 61:797, 1982.)

of its light reflectivity. The infinite optical thickness, *XI,* is defined for monochromatic light as follows:

$$XI = (1/bS) \text{ Ar ctgh } [(1 - 0.999aRI)/0.999bRI], \text{ mm}$$

The variation of *XI* with wavelength is shown in Fig. 3-7 for a composite resin. It is interesting that composites are more opaque to blue than to red light, yet blue light is used to cure light-activated composites.

Contrast ratio

Once *a*, *b*, and *S* are obtained, the light reflectance *(R)* for a sample of any thickness *(X)* in contact with a backing of any reflectance *(R_g)* can be calculated by:

$$R = [1 - R_g(a - b \text{ ctgh } bSX)]/(a + b \text{ ctgh } bSX - R_g)$$

An estimate of the opacity of a 1 mm thick sample can then be calculated from the contrast ratio *(C)* as:

$$C = R_0/R$$

where R_o is the computed light reflectance of the sample with a black backing. If R_g is 0.70, then $C_{0.70}$ can be calculated (see Measurement of contrast ratio).

■ THERMAL PROPERTIES

Temperature

The temperature of a substance can be measured with a thermometer or a thermocouple. An important application of temperature measurement in dentistry is the measurement of heat during the shaping of cavities in teeth. Numerous studies have been made of the effect of speed and force on the rise of temperature in teeth. The increase in temperature during the cutting of tooth structure with various types of steel burs, carbide burs, and rotary diamond instruments also has been investigated. In addition, the rise in temperature in the tooth at various distances from the cutting instrument has been determined. A specific example of the effect of the speed of rotation and coolants on the increase in temperature in tooth structure is shown in Fig. 3-8. The temperature was measured by a thermocouple inserted into a small opening that extended into the dentoenamel junction. The tooth was then cut in the direction of the thermocouple and the maximum temperature recorded.

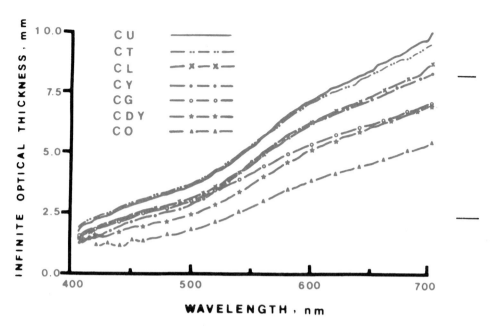

Fig. 3-7 Infinite optical thickness versus wavelength for shades of a composite, *C*. Shades are *U*, universal; *T*, translucent; *L*, light; *Y*, yellow; *G*, gray; *DY*, dark yellow; and *O*, opaque. (From Yeh, CL, Miyagawa Y, Powers JM: *J Dent Res* 61:797, 1982.)

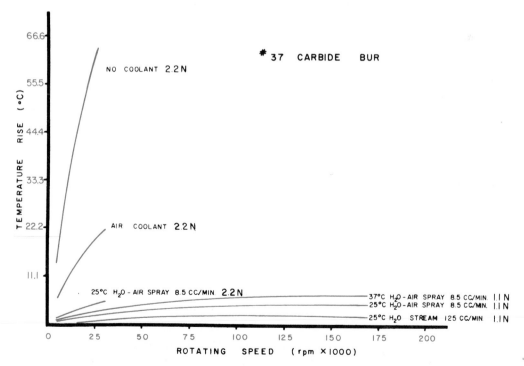

Fig. 3-8 Temperature rises developed by carbide burs during cutting of tooth tissue, operated at different speeds and with and without coolants. (Adapted from Peyton FA: *J Am Dent Assoc* 56:664, 1958.)

Transition Temperatures

The arrangement of atoms and molecules in materials is influenced by the temperature; as a result, thermal technics are important in understanding dental materials. The methods are differential thermal analysis, differential scanning calorimetry, thermogravimetric analysis, thermomechanical analysis, and dynamic mechanical analysis. Differential thermal analysis has been used to locate the temperature of transitions and to study the effect of variables such as composition and heat treatment on these transitions. Differential scanning calorimetry can determine the heats of transition and reaction. Thermogravimetric analysis measures the change in weight of materials as a function of temperature and environment and gives information related to the thermal decomposition of materials or their stability in various environments. Thermomechanical analysis measures the dimensional change with or without load as a function of temperature. Changes in the ease of deformation as the temperature increases indicate the presence of transitions. This method can also measure the

coefficient of thermal expansion as a function of temperature. Dynamic mechanical analysis measures the changes in modulus of elasticity and loss tangent as a function of temperature. This technic can be used to measure the glass transition temperature of polymers.

Differential thermal analysis (DTA) has been used to study waxes used in the compounding of dental waxes. The DTA curve of a mixture of paraffin and carnauba wax is shown in Fig. 3-9. The thermogram was obtained when the difference in temperature between the wax and a standard was recorded under the same heating conditions in which thermocouples were used. The difference in temperature was recorded as a function of the temperature of the surroundings. A decrease in the value of ΔT indicated an endothermic process in the sample. The endotherms at 31.5° and 35° C are solid-solid transitions occurring in the paraffin wax as the result of a change of crystal structure. The endotherm at 52° C represents the solid-liquid transition of paraffin wax, whereas the endotherms at 68.7° and 80.2° C result from the melting of carnauba wax. The heat of

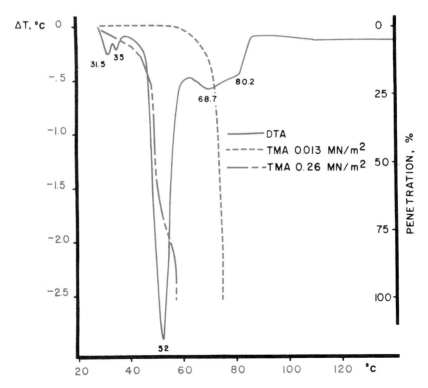

Fig. 3-9 Thermograms of a 75% paraffin-25% carnauba wax mixture.

transition of the two solid-solid transitions is about 8 cal/g, and the melting transition of paraffin and carnauba wax is approximately 39 and 11 cal/g, respectively. These and other thermograms show that 25% carnauba wax added to paraffin wax has no effect on the melting point of paraffin wax but increases the melting range by about 28° C.

Thermomechanical analysis (TMA) of the carnauba-paraffin wax mixture is also shown in Fig. 3-9. The percent penetration of the wax mixture by a cylindrical probe is shown for two stresses of 0.013 and 0.26 MPa. The penetration of the wax at the lower stress was controlled by the melting transition of the carnauba wax component, whereas the penetration at the higher stress was dominated by the solid-solid and solid-liquid transitions of the paraffin wax components. About 44% penetration, which is related to flow, occurred before the melting point of the paraffin wax was reached.

Other properties correlate with thermograms. The coefficient of thermal expansion of paraffin wax increases from about $300 \times 10^{-6}/°$ C to $1400 \times 10^{-6}/°$ C just before the solid-solid transition, and the flow also increases greatly in this temperature range.

Dynamic mechanical analysis (DMA) of a dimethacrylate copolymer is shown in Fig. 3-10. A thin film of the copolymer was subjected to a sinusoidal tensile strain at a frequency of 11 Hz. As temperature was increased, values of modulus of elasticity (E') and loss tangent (tan Δ) were obtained. The glass transition temperature (T_g) was determined from identification of the beginning of a rapid decrease in E' with temperature. The value of T_g identifies the temperature at which a glassy polymer goes to a softer, rubbery state upon heating. A lower value of T_g can result from a lower degree of conversion of double bonds or from saturation by water. As discussed later, the value of the coefficient of thermal expansion of a polymer changes at T_g.

Heat of Fusion

The heat of fusion, L, is the heat in calories, or joules, J, required to convert 1 g of a material from the solid to the liquid state at the melting temperature. The equation for the calculation of heat of fusion is $L = Q/m$, where Q is the total heat absorbed and m is the mass of the substance melted. Therefore in practical applications it is apparent that the larger the mass of material being melted, the more heat is required to change the total mass to liquid. The heat of fusion is closely related to the melting or freezing point of the substance because, when the change in state occurs, it is always necessary to apply the additional heat to the mass to cause liquefaction, and as long as the mass remains molten, the heat of fusion is retained by the liquid. When the mass is frozen, or solidified, the heat that was

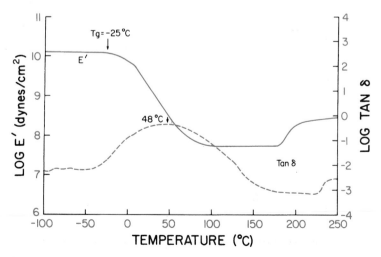

Fig. 3-10 Dynamic mechanical properties of a 75 wt % BIS–GMA/25 wt % TEGDM copolymer. (From Wilson TW, Turner DT: *J Dent Res* 66:1032, 1987.)

TABLE 3-3   Heat of Fusion of Some Materials

Materials	Temperature (° C)	Heat of Fusion (cal/g [J/g])
METALS		
Mercury	−39	3 [12]
Gold	1063	16 [67]
Silver	960	26 [109]
Platinum	1773	27 [113]
Copper	1083	49 [205]
Cobalt	1495	58 [242]
Chromium	1890	75 [314]
Aluminum	660	94 [393]
COMPOUNDS		
Alcohol	−114	25 [104]
Paraffin	52	35 [146]
Beeswax	62	42 [176]
Glycerin	18	47 [196]
Ice	0	80 [334]

retained in the liquid state is liberated. The difference in energy content is necessary to maintain the kinetic molecular motion, which is characteristic of the liquid state.

The values for heat of fusion of some common substances (given in round numbers) are listed in Table 3-3. It may be seen that the values for heat of fusion of gold and the metals used for dental gold alloys (silver and copper) are below those of many other metals and compounds. This is true also for the specific heat of gold and its alloys.

Thermal Conductivity

The thermal conductivity, K, of a substance is the quantity of heat in calories, or joules, per second passing through a body 1 cm thick with a cross section of 1 cm^2 when the temperature difference is 1° C. The units are cal/sec/cm^2/(° C/cm). The conductivity of a material changes slightly as the surrounding temperature is altered, but generally the difference resulting from temperature changes is much less than the difference that exists between different types of materials.

Common experience indicates that metals are better heat conductors than nonmetals. Several

important applications of thermal conductivity exist in dental materials. For example, a large gold or amalgam filling or crown that is in proximity to the pulp may cause the patient considerable discomfort as a result of temperature changes produced by hot or cold foods and beverages unless adequate tooth tissue remains or nonmetallic substances are placed between the tooth and filling for insulation. Such filling materials as cements are relatively poor conductors and insulate the pulp area.

The difference in thermal conductivity of denture base materials likewise may cause differences in soft-tissue response. A metal base, a good conductor, causes a prompt tissue response as shown in Fig. 3-11, whereas an acrylic denture base causes a more delayed response to thermal changes. Dental literature indicates that a good thermal conductor is preferred for denture bases to maintain good health in the supporting tissues by having the heat readily conducted to and from the tissue by the denture base. This concept has not been established on the basis of experimental data.

A better understanding of the conductivities of various restorative materials is desirable to develop an appropriate degree of insulation for the pulp tissue comparable with that in the natural tooth and to produce normal thermal stimulation in the supporting soft tissue under complete dentures. The conductivity of certain dental materials is listed in Table 3-4. Nonmetallic materials appear to be less effective as conductors than metals are, so they serve as good insulators. Dental cements seem to have a thermal conductivity similar to those of dentin and enamel. Note that the thickness of a cement base and its thermal conductivity are important in reducing the thermal transfer to the pulp and remember that the temperature difference across an insulator depends on the extent of the heating or cooling period and the magnitude of the temperature difference.

Specific Heat

The specific heat, Cp, of a substance is the quantity of heat needed to raise the temperature of one gram of the substance 1° C. Water is usually chosen as the standard substance and 1 g as the standard mass. The heat required to raise the temperature of 1 g of water from 15° to 16° C is 1 cal, which is

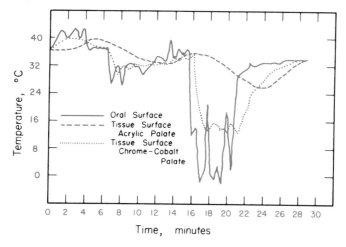

Fig. 3-11 Temperature on the oral surface and tissue surface of an acrylic and a cobalt-chromium palate while a subject was eating a meal. (Adapted from Wehner PJ: *Heat transfer properties of denture base materials,* master's thesis, Ann Arbor, Mich, 1959, University of Michigan School of Dentistry.)

used as the basis for the definition of the heat unit. Most substances are more readily heated, gram for gram, than water.

When the mass of a body is disregarded, the heat capacity of the substance is the quantity of heat needed to raise the temperature of the body 1° C and is controlled by the mass of the substance. Obviously the total heat required depends on the total mass and the specific heat of the substance. For example, 100 g of water requires more calories than 50 g of water to raise the temperature 1° C. Likewise, 100 g of water requires more heat than 100 g of alcohol to raise the temperature the same amount because of the difference in specific heat of water and alcohol. In general, the specific heat of liquids is higher than the specific heat of solids. Some metals have specific heat values of less than 10% of that of water.

During the melting and casting process the specific heat of the metal or alloy is important because of the total amount of heat that must be applied to the mass to raise the temperature to the melting point. Fortunately, the specific heat of gold and the metals used in gold alloys is low, and so prolonged heating is unnecessary. The specific heat of both enamel and dentin has been found to be higher than that of metals used for fillings, as is shown in Table 3-5.

TABLE 3-4   Thermal Conductivity of Various Materials

Material	Thermal Conductivity	
	cal/sec/cm^2/ (° C/cm)	J/sec/cm^2 (° C/cm)
METALS		
Silver	1.006	4.21
Copper	0.918	3.84
Gold	0.710	2.97
Platinum	0.167	0.698
Dental amalgam	0.055	0.23
Mercury	0.020	0.084
NONMETALS		
Gypsum	0.0031	0.013
Zinc phosphate cement	0.0028	0.012
Composite resin	0.0026	0.011
Porcelain	0.0025	0.010
Enamel	0.0022	0.0092
Dentin	0.0015	0.0063
Zinc oxide–eugenol cement	0.0011	0.0046
Acrylic resin	0.0005	0.0021
Beeswax	0.00009	0.0004

TABLE 3-5   Specific Heat of Various Materials

Material	Specific Heat (cal/g/° C [J/g/° C])
SOLIDS	
Gold	0.031 [0.13]
Platinum	0.032 [0.13]
Silver	0.056 [0.23]
Copper	0.092 [0.38]
Enamel	0.18 [0.75]
Quartz	0.19 [0.79]
Aluminum	0.21 [0.88]
Porcelain	0.26 [1.09]
Dentin	0.28 [1.17]
Acrylic resin	0.35 [1.46]
LIQUIDS	
Water	1.000 [4.18]
Paraffin	0.69 [2.88]
Glycerin	0.58 [2.42]
Alcohol (ethyl)	0.547 [2.29]
Mercury	0.033 [0.14]

TABLE 3-6   Thermal Diffusivity of Various Materials

Material	Thermal Diffusivity (mm^2/sec)
Pure gold (calculated)	119.0
Amalgam	9.6
Composite resin	0.675
Porcelain	0.64
Enamel	0.469
Zinc oxide–eugenol cement	0.389
Zinc phosphate cement	0.290
Dental compound	0.226
Zinc polyacrylate cement	0.223
Glass ionomer cement	0.198
Dentin	0.183
Acrylic resin	0.123

Thermal Diffusivity

The thermal diffusivity, Δ, is a measure of transient heat flow and is defined as the thermal conductivity, K, divided by the product of the specific heat, Cp, times the density, ρ:

$$\Delta = K/Cp \times \rho$$

The units of thermal diffusivity are mm^2/sec.

The thermal diffusivity describes the rate at which a body with a nonuniform temperature approaches equilibrium. For a gold inlay or crown or a dental amalgam, the low specific heat combined with the high thermal conductivity creates a thermal shock more readily than normal tooth structure does. Values of thermal diffusivity of some materials are listed in Table 3-6. These values of thermal diffusivity may vary somewhat with composition of the particular restorative material. For example, the thermal diffusivity of a zinc polyacrylate cement increases from 0.14 to 0.51 mm^2/sec as the powder/liquid ratio on a weight basis increases from 0.5 to 5.0.

As mentioned in the discussion of thermal conductivity, thickness of the material is important.

A parameter governing lining efficiency (Z) is related to thickness (T) and thermal diffusivity (Δ) as follows:

$$Z = \frac{T}{\sqrt{\Delta}}$$

Coefficient of Thermal Expansion

The change in length ($l_{final} - l_{original}$) per unit length of a material for a 1° C change in temperature is called the linear coefficient of thermal expansion, α, and is calculated as follows:

$$\frac{\left(l_{final} - l_{original}\right)}{l_{original} \times \left(° C_{final} - ° C_{original}\right)} = \alpha$$

The units are represented by the notation /° C, and because the values are usually small, they are expressed in exponential form such as 22×10^{-6}/° C. A less common practice is to report the change in parts per million (ppm) and the previous number would be expressed as 22 ppm.

The linear coefficients of thermal expansion for some materials important in restorative dentistry are given in Table 3-7. Although the coefficient is a material constant, it does not remain constant over wide temperature ranges. For example, the linear coefficient of thermal expansion of a dental wax

TABLE 3-7 Linear Coefficient of Thermal Expansion of Various Materials

Material	Coefficient $\times 10^{-6}/°$ C
Inlay waxes	350–450
Silicone impression material	210
Polysulfide impression material	140
Pit and fissure sealants	71–94
Acrylic resin	76.0
Mercury	60.6
Composite resins	
Anterior	17–50
Posterior	14–40
Zinc oxide–eugenol cement	35
Amalgam	22.1–28.0
Silver	19.2
Copper	16.8
Gold	14.4
Porcelain	12.0
Tooth (crown portion)	11.4
Glass ionomer (type 2)	10.2–11.4

may have an average value of $300 \times 10^{-6}/°$ C up to 40° C, whereas it may have an average value of $500 \times 10^{-6}/°$ C from 40° to 50° C. The coefficient of thermal expansion of a polymer changes as the polymer goes from a glassy state to a softer, rubbery material. This change in the coefficient corresponds to the glass transition temperature (T_g).

Either the linear or volumetric coefficient of thermal expansion may be measured, and for most materials that function as isotropic solids, the volumetric thermal coefficient may be considered to be three times the linear thermal coefficient.

Both linear expansion and volume expansion are important in restorative materials and processes. It is obvious that with a reduction of temperature, there is a contraction of the substance that is equal to the expansion that results from heating. Accordingly, tooth structure and restorative materials in the mouth will expand when warmed by hot foods and beverages but will contract when exposed to cold substances. Such expansions and contractions may break the marginal seal of an inlay or other filling in the tooth, particularly if the differ-

ence in coefficient of expansion is great between the tooth and the restorative material. The high coefficient of expansion of pattern waxes is an important factor in the construction of properly fitting restorations. The change in volume as a result of cooling is responsible for the shrinkage spots or surface cracks that often develop in gold alloy castings during solidification. Compensation for the contraction that occurs during the cooling of gold alloys must be made if accurate gold castings are to result. Therefore in some materials and in certain operations, the coefficient of thermal expansion may be equally as important as the strength, hardness, or esthetic appearance of the material. The values in Table 3-7 show that with comparable temperature changes, materials such as acrylic resin and amalgam expand more than tooth tissue, whereas porcelain expands less. The coefficient of inlay pattern wax is exceptionally high when compared with that of other materials.

Of particular importance in casting investments is the property of thermal expansion of three crystalline polymorphic forms of silica. As a principal ingredient in dental investments that are to be heated before a metal casting is made, the amount of expansion at various temperatures is critical and important. This quality of silica compounds in relation to use in casting investments was described in 1932. Curves in Fig. 3-12 illustrate the relative percentage of thermal expansion of the four forms of silica at different temperatures below about 800° C. Of the crystalline forms, cristobalite shows the greatest expansion at the lowest temperature and quartz requires a higher temperature to develop an equal amount of expansion as cristobalite. Fused silica has long been recognized as a material with an exceedingly low thermal expansion.

■ ELECTRICAL PROPERTIES

Electrical Conductivity and Resistivity

The ability of a material to conduct an electric current may be stated either as specific conductance or conductivity, or, conversely, as the specific resistance or resistivity. Resistivity is the more common term. The resistance of a homogeneous conductor of uniform cross section at a constant temperature varies directly with the length and inversely with the

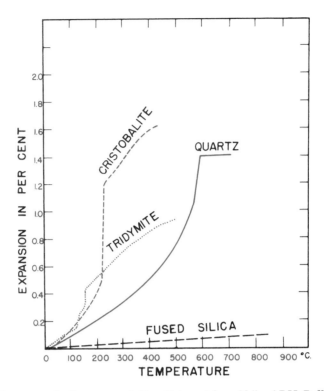

Fig. 3-12 Thermal expansion curves for four types of silica. (Adapted from Volland RH, Paffenbarger GC: *J Am Dent Assoc* 19:185, 1932.)

cross-sectional area of the sample, according to the following equation:

$$R = \rho \frac{l}{A}$$

in which R is the resistance in ohms, ρ (rho) is the resistivity, l is the length, and A is the section area. The resistivity depends on the nature of the material. If a unit cube of 1 cm edge length is employed, the l and A are equal to unity and in this case $R = \rho$. The resistivity is expressed as ohm-centimeters where R is in ohms, l is in centimeters, and A is in square centimeters.

The change in electrical resistance has been used to study the alteration in internal structure of various alloys as a result of heat treatment. An early investigation of the gold-copper alloy system by electrical conductivity methods revealed a change in internal crystal structure with an accompanying change in conductivity. The correlation of these conductivity studies with related changes in other prop-

erties established the fundamental basis of structural changes associated with heat-treatment operations on dental gold alloys.

Values for the resistivity of human tooth structure are shown in Table 3-8. The resistivity is important in the investigation of the pain perception threshold resulting from applied electrical stimuli, and of displacement of fluid in teeth caused by ionic movements. The electrical resistance of normal and carious teeth has been observed to differ, with less resistance offered by the carious tissue. Sound enamel is a relatively poor conductor of electricity, whereas dentin is somewhat better (Table 3-8).

The conductivity of materials used to replace tooth tissue is of concern in restorative dentistry. The effectiveness of insulating cement bases and other nonmetallic restorative materials is not yet established. Several studies have measured the resistivity of dental cements (Table 3-8). The zinc oxide–eugenol cements have the highest resistivity, followed by the zinc polyacrylate and zinc phosphate

TABLE 3-8 Values of Resistivity of Human Tooth Structure and Several Dental Cements

Material	Resistivity (ohm • cm)
Human enamel	
Bjorn (1946)	$2.9–3.6 \times 10^6$
Mumford (1967)	$2.6–6.9 \times 10^6$
Human dentin	
Bjorn (1946)	$0.7–6.0 \times 10^4$
Mumford (1967)	$1.1–5.2 \times 10^4$
Dental cement	
Glass ionomer	$0.8–2.5 \times 10^4$
Zinc oxide–eugenol	$10^9 – 10^{10}$
Zinc polyacrylate	$0.4–4 \times 10^5$
Zinc phosphate	2×10^5

TABLE 3-9 Dielectric Constant for Human Dentin and Several Dental Cements

Material	Dielectric Constant
Human dentin	8.6
Dental cements (set)	
Glass ionomer	$2–7 \times 10^5$
Zinc oxide–eugenol	10
Zinc polyacrylate	4×10^3 to 2×10^5

cements. The glass ionomer cements are the most conductive of the cements and have values most similar to dentin.

Dielectric Constant

A material that provides electrical insulation is known as a dielectric. The dielectric constant or relative permittivity, εr, compares the permittivity, ε, of the dielectric to the permittivity, ε_0, of empty space:

$$\varepsilon_r = \varepsilon/\varepsilon_0$$

where ε_0 of a vacuum is $8.854 \times 10{-12}$ farad/m. The dielectric constant varies with temperature, bonding, crystal structure, and structural defects of the dielectric.

Values of the dielectric constant for human dentin and several dental cements are listed in Table 3-9. The dielectric constant of a dental cement generally decreases as the material hardens. This decrease reflects a change from a paste that is relatively ionic and polar to one that is less so. As shown by the high values of permittivity of the glass ionomer and zinc polyacrylate cements in Table 3-9, these cements have a high ionic content and are quite polar compared with zinc oxide–eugenol cements and human dentin.

Dielectric measurements have been used to study polymer-filler interactions in dental composites with and without silane coupling agents, as well as the effect of moisture on these interactions. The measurements showed that increasing the filler content restricted the mobility of the main polymer chains and that compatible silanes did not form a separate interphase at the polymer-filler interface. It was also shown that bulk water could exist at the interface if the filler was not silanated. Therefore correct silanation of fillers used in dental composites is essential for their successful application.

The problem of electrical insulation is made more complex by the presence of galvanic currents in the mouth, resulting from cells formed from metallic restorations. Recent studies indicate that a cement base does not effectively insulate the pulp from the electric current developed in a metallic restoration in the mouth. How much insulation is essential or how to effectively restore the tooth to its original status of equilibrium is currently not known.

Electromotive Force

Working with metals and alloys for dental restorations or with instruments that are susceptible to corrosion necessitates some understanding of the relative position of the metal in the electromotive force series. The electromotive series is a listing of electrode potentials of metals according to the order of their decreasing tendency to oxidize in solution. This serves as the basis for comparison of the tendency of metals to oxidize in air. Those metals with a large negative electrode potential are more resistant to tarnish than those with a high positive electrode potential. In general, the metals above copper in the series, such as aluminum, zinc, and nickel, tend to oxidize relatively easily, whereas those below copper, such as silver, platinum, and gold, resist oxidation. A list of oxidation-reduction potentials for some common corrosion reactions in water and in

TABLE 3-10   Oxidation-Reduction Potentials for Corrosion Reactions in Water and Salt Water

Metal	Corrosion Reaction	In Water, Electrode Potential at 25° C, (Volts Versus Normal Hydrogen Electrode)	In Salt Water, Electrode Potential at 25° C, (Volts Versus 0.1 N Calomel Scale)
Aluminum	$Al \rightarrow Al^{3+} + 3e$	+1.662*	+0.83
Zinc	$Zn \rightarrow Zn^{2+} + 2e$	+0.763	+1.10
Chromium	$Cr \rightarrow Cr^{3+} + 3e$	+0.744	+0.4 to −0.18
Iron	$Fe \rightarrow Fe^{2+} + 2e$	+0.440	+0.58
Cobalt	$Co \rightarrow Co^{2+} + 2e$	+0.277	−
Nickel	$Ni \rightarrow Ni^{2+} + 2e$	+0.250	+0.07
Tin	$Sn \rightarrow Sn^{2+} + 2e$	+0.136	+0.49
Hydrogen	$H_2 \rightarrow 2H^+ + 2e$	0.000	−
Copper	$Cu \rightarrow Cu^{2+} + 2e$	−0.337	+0.20
	$4(OH^-) \rightarrow O_2 + 2H_2O + 4e$	−0.401	−
Mercury	$2Hg \rightarrow Hg_2^{2+} + 2e$	−0.788	−
Silver	$Ag \rightarrow Ag^+ + e$	−0.799	+0.08
Palladium	$Pd \rightarrow Pd^{2+} + 2e$	−0.987	−
Platinum	$Pt \rightarrow Pt^{2+} + 2e$	−1.200	−
	$2H_2O \rightarrow O_2 + 4H^+ + 4e$	−1.229	−
Gold	$Au \rightarrow Au^{3+} + 3e$	−1.498	−

Modified from Flinn RA, Trojan PK: *Engineering materials and their applications,* ed 3, Boston, 1986, Houghton Mifflin.
*A positive value indicates a strong tendency for the metal to go into solution. Higher positive values are more anodic, whereas higher negative values are more cathodic.

salt water is given in Table 3-10. The values of electrode potential and the order of the series change when measured in a saline solution rather than water. The electrode potentials of some dental alloys measured in artificial saliva at 35° C are listed in Table 3-11.

Likewise, it is possible to determine from the electromotive force series that the reduction of the oxides of gold, platinum, and silver to the pure metal can be accomplished more readily than with metals that have a higher electromotive force value.

Galvanism

The presence of metallic restorations in the mouth may cause a phenomenon called galvanic action, or galvanism. This results from a difference in potential between dissimilar fillings in opposing or adjacent teeth. These fillings, in conjunction with saliva or bone fluids as electrolytes, make up an electric cell. When two opposing fillings contact

TABLE 3-11   Galvanic Series of Some Dental Alloys in Artificial Saliva at 35° C

Material	Electrode Potential at 35° C (Volts)*
Tin crown form	+0.048
Hydrogen/H+	0.000
Amalgam	
Conventional spherical	−0.023
Dispersed high-copper	−0.108
Nickel-chromium alloy	−0.126 to −0.240
Cobalt-chromium alloy	−0.292
Gold alloy	
Au-Cu-Ag	−0.345
Au-Pt-Pd-Ag	−0.358 to −0.455

Modified from Arvidson K, Johansson EG: *Scand J Dent Res* 85:485, 1977.
*High positive sign indicates a strong tendency for the metal to go into solution.

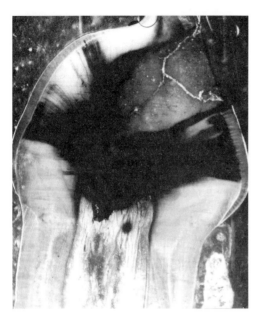

Fig. 3-13 Autoradiograph of a longitudinal section of a dog's permanent tooth in which the pulp has been capped with 45/20 Ca hydroxide. The dark areas in the tooth are evidence that migration of the Ca ions has occurred and that a circuit is possible. (Courtesy Avery JK, University of Michigan School of Dentistry, 1958.)

each other, the cell is short-circuited, and if the flow of current occurs through the pulp, the patient experiences pain, and the more anodic restoration may corrode. A single filling plus the saliva and bone fluid may also constitute a cell of liquid junction type. As shown in Fig. 3-13, ions capable of conducting electricity can easily migrate through dentin and around the margins of a restoration.

Studies have indicated that relatively large currents will flow through metallic fillings when they are brought into contact. The current rapidly falls off if the fillings are maintained in contact, probably as a result of polarization of the cell. The magnitude of the voltage, however, is not of primary importance, since indications support the fact that the sensitivity of the patient to the current has a greater influence on whether pain is felt. Some patients may feel pain at 10 μamp, whereas others do not experience it until 110 μamp are developed, although most patients feel pain at a value between 20 and 50 μamp. This may explain why some patients are bothered by galvanic action and others are not, despite similar conditions in the mouth.

The galvanic currents developed from the contact of two metallic restorations depend on their composition and surface area. An alloy of stainless steel develops a higher current density than either gold or cobalt-chromium alloys when in contact with an amalgam restoration. As the size of the cathode (such as a gold alloy) increases relative to that of the anode (such as an amalgam), the current density may increase. The larger cathode likewise can enhance the corrosion of the smaller anode. Current densities associated with non-γ_2-containing amalgams appear to be less than those associated with the γ_2-containing amalgams.

Electrochemical Corrosion

The corrosion and electrochemical behavior of restorative materials have received new interest with the study of multiphase systems such as gold alloys and amalgam. For example, the corrosion of γ, γ_1, and γ_2 phases in amalgam has been studied by electrochemical means. Anodic and cathodic polarization measurements indicated no strongly passive behavior of these phases in artificial saliva. The dental amalgam specimens became pitted at the boundaries between the phases or in γ_2 phase. Other studies, however, indicate that amalgam alloys exhibit decreasing electrochemical potentials, resulting in noble values when stored in neutral solutions. The addition of copper to amalgam alloys so that copper-tin compounds are formed during hardening has improved the resistance of amalgam to chloride and galvanic corrosion. As shown in Fig. 3-14 the anodic activity of AgSn amalgam is quite different from AgSn + AgCu amalgams. The AgSn + AgCu amalgam remains passive under the testing conditions, whereas the AgSn amalgam does not.

Studies of corrosion of surgical stainless steel, stainless steel orthodontic brackets, and endodontic silver cones also have been reported. Corrosion of these alloys and others can result in decreased mechanical properties and the formation of corrosion products, which in some instances accumulate in the human organs. As shown previously in Table 3-10, corrosion can be affected by the environment, and certain metals such as cobalt and copper corrode

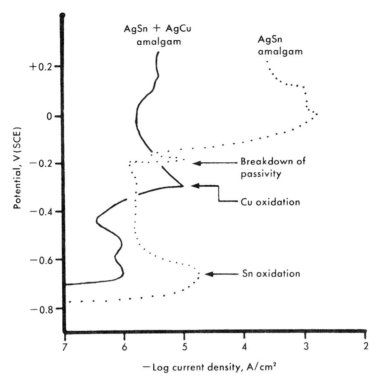

Fig. 3-14 Anodic polarization curves of two types of amalgam in synthetic saliva. (Adapted from Fairhurst CW, Marek M, Butts MB, Okabe T: *J Dent Res* 57:725, 1978.)

more rapidly in a saline solution containing serum albumin and fibrinogen proteins.

Zeta-Potential

A charged particle suspended in an electrolytic solution attracts ions of opposite charge to those at its surface. The layer formed by these ions is called the Stern layer. To maintain the electrical balance of the suspending fluid, ions of opposite charge are attracted to the Stern layer. The potential at the surface of that part of the diffuse double layer of ions is called the electrokinetic or zeta-potential.

The zeta-potential, ζ, of a solid as a porous plug can be determined by measurement of the streaming potential, E, which is the electric field caused when a liquid is made to flow along a stationary charged surface. The relation is as follows:

$$\xi = (8.47 \times 10^8)(\eta/\varepsilon)(\Delta E/\Delta P)(R_{0.1\ N\ KCl} \cdot k_{0.1\ N\ KCl}/R_p)$$

where η is viscosity in poises, E is in millivolts, R_p is resistance in ohms of the porous plug, k is in

ohm^{-1}cm^{-1}, and P is pressure in cm Hg. Rk is a cell constant for 0.1 N KCl. The term ε is the dielectric constant, which is 78.54 for water at 25° C.

The applications of electrophoresis include stability of colloids, adsorption of ions, and characterization of particle surfaces. Effects of pH, surface-active agents, and enzymes on zeta-potential are important. Zeta-potential may affect the near-surface mechanical properties (such as wear) of a material. The zeta-potentials of some materials are listed in Table 3-12.

■ OTHER PROPERTIES

Certain properties often are highly important in the selection and manipulation of materials for use either in the mouth or for laboratory applications. Five such properties are tarnish and discoloration, water sorption, solubility and disintegration, setting time, and shelf life.

TABLE 3-12   Zeta-Potential of Some Dental Materials

Material	Zeta-Potential (mV)
Hydroxyapatite	−9.0 to −10.9
Tooth structure*	
Calculus	−15.3
Cementum	
Exposed	−6.96
Unexposed	−9.34
Dentin	−6.23
Enamel	−9.04 to −10.3

Adapted from O'Brien WJ, Ryge G, editors: *An outline of dental materials and their selection,* Philadelphia, 1978, WB Saunders.
*Measured in Hanks' balanced salt solution at 30° C.

Tarnish and Discoloration

Discoloration of a restorative material from any cause is a very troublesome quality. The tarnish of metal restorations from oxide, sulfide, or any other surface reaction is a critical quality of metal restorations in the mouth or of instruments for either clinical or laboratory use. The process of steam sterilization of surgical instruments has long presented a serious problem of tarnish and corrosion. Many nonmetallic materials such as cements and composite restorations have displayed a tendency to discolor in service because colored substances penetrate the materials and continue chemical reactions in the composites.

Various in vitro tests have been proposed to study tarnish, particularly that of crown and bridge and partial denture alloys. Testing generally relies on controlled exposure of the alloy to a solution rich in sulfides, chlorides, and phosphates. Most recently the discoloration of alloys exposed to such solutions has been evaluated by spectrophotometric methods to determine a color-difference parameter discussed earlier in this chapter.

Water Sorption

Water sorption of a material represents the amount of water adsorbed on the surface and absorbed into the body of the material during fabrication or while the restoration is in service. The tendency of plastic denture base materials to have a high degree of water sorption is the reason this qual-ity was included in ANSI/ADA Specification No. 12 for this type of material. Usually a serious warpage and dimensional change in the material are associated with a high percentage of water sorption. The tendency of the hydrocolloid type of impression materials to imbibe water if allowed to remain immersed and then to change dimensions has been a serious problem associated with their use.

Solubility and Disintegration

Solubility and disintegration are measured gravimetrically by suspension of two disks 20 mm in diameter and 1.0 mm in thickness for 24 hours or longer in water at 37° C. The exposed surface area is about 13.8 cm^2. The units are percent mass loss or mg/cm^2. A conductimetric method for studying solubility and disintegration has the advantage of detecting the elution of volatile components and of using a smaller sample. Care should be taken in predicting in vivo properties from tests in water because abrasion and attack from other chemicals often occur intraorally.

The lack of correlation between in vivo testing of the degradation of cements and the aforementioned test of solubility and disintegration in water has led to the development of other in vitro tests. One test involves placement of cement between two round plane-parallel glass plates (16 mm in diameter) and exposure of this specimen to various acidic media. Changes in the cement are recorded photographically. Observations suggest that degradation may follow a sequence of absorption, disintegration, and solution. Variables such as cement composition, thickness, molarity, and pH of the medium are important.

Setting Time

Setting time characteristics are associated with the reaction rates and affect the practical applications of many materials in restorative dentistry. Materials such as cements, impression materials, dental plaster, stone, and casting investments depend on a critical reaction time and hardening rate for their successful application. From the practical standpoint of manipulation and successful application, the time required for a material to set or harden from a plastic or fluid state may be its most important quality. The setting time does not indicate the completion of the reaction, which may continue for a much longer time. The time varies for different materials, depending on the particular application, but duplication of results from one lot to another or from one trade brand of material to another is highly desirable. The influence of manipulative procedures on the setting time of various types of materials is important to the dentist and the assistant.

Shelf Life

Shelf life is a term applied to the general deterioration and change in quality of materials during shipment and storage. The temperature, humidity, and time of storage, as well as the bulk of material involved and the type of storage container, are all significant factors that vary greatly from one material to another. A material that has exceptionally good properties when first produced may be quite impractical if it deteriorates badly after a few days or weeks. These qualities are discussed particularly in chapters dealing with gypsum materials and impression materials. Some studies of these qualities of various materials have been made in recent years, and through the accelerated aging tests, improvements in quality can sometimes be made. X-ray film, anesthetics, and a few other products carry dates of expiration beyond which the product should not be expected to be serviceable. This practice assures the user that the material has not deteriorated because of age. Most materials that meet the requirements of the American Dental Association Specifications carry a date of production as a part of the serial number or as a separate notation.

SELECTED PROBLEMS

Problem 1. A hole was drilled in a gold crown to facilitate an endodontic procedure. Subsequently, the hole was filled with a dental amalgam. After several months the amalgam appeared discolored and corroded. What caused this problem, and how can it be avoided?

Solution. The dental amalgam is anodic to the gold alloy. Furthermore, the surface area of the gold restoration is much larger than that of the amalgam. Both of these factors will cause the amalgam to corrode by galvanic action. The hole should be filled with gold foil to minimize corrosion.

Problem 2. A porcelain veneer to be bonded on an anterior tooth matches the color of the shade guide but not the adjacent tooth. What most likely caused this problem, and how can it be avoided?

Solution a. If different light sources are used to match metameric shades, then the color could appear correct when observed under one light but not under the other. Be sure to match teeth and shade guides under appropriate lighting conditions.

Solution b. Porcelain is a translucent material, the color of which can be affected by the color of the cement retaining the restoration, particularly if the veneer lacks an opaque layer. Select a resin cement of an appropriate shade to bond the veneer.

Problem 3. A glaze applied to a porcelain restoration cracks on cooling. What caused the glaze to crack, and how can this problem be avoided?

Solution. Porcelain has a low thermal diffusivity and is subject to cracking as a result of thermal shock. Be sure to cool a porcelain restoration as recommended by the manufacturer to minimize larger thermal gradients.

Problem 4. A denture cleaned in hot water distorted and no longer fits the patient's mouth. Why?

Solution. If the temperature of the denture during cleaning exceeds the glass transition temperature of the resin, then distortion can occur readily. Be sure to use cool water to clean a denture.

■ REFERENCES

Color and Optical Properties

Asmussen E: Opacity of glass-ionomer cements, *Acta Odontol Scand* 41:155, 1983.

Baran GR, O'Brien WJ, Tien T-Y: Colored emission of rare earth ions in a potassium feldspar glass, *J Dent Res* 56:1323, 1977.

Colorimetry, official recommendations of the International Commission on Illumination (CIE), Publication CIE No 15 (E-1.3.1), 1971.

Crisp S, Abel G, Wilson AD: The quantitative measurement of the opacity of aesthetic dental filling materials, *J Dent Res* 58:1585, 1979.

Dennison JB, Powers JM, Koran A: Color of dental restorative resins, *J Dent Res* 57:557, 1978.

Groenhuis R: Scattering and absorption of light by turbid materials, especially dental enamel, doctoral dissertation, The Netherlands, 1981, Groningen State University.

Hall JB, Hefferren JJ, Olsen NH: Study of fluorescent characteristics of extracted human teeth by use of a clinical fluorometer, *J Dent Res* 49:1431, 1970.

Johnston WM, O'Brien WJ, Tien T-Y: The determination of optical absorption and scattering in translucent porcelain, *Color Res Appl* 11:125, 1986.

Johnston WM, O'Brien WJ, Tien T-Y: Concentration additivity of Kubelka-Munk optical coefficients of porcelain mixtures, *Color Res Appl* 11:131, 1986.

Jorgenson MW, Goodkind RJ: Spectrophotometric study of five porcelain shades relative to the dimensions of color, porcelain thickness, and repeated firings, *J Prosthet Dent* 42:96, 1979.

Judd DB: Optical specification of light-scattering materials, *J Res Nat Bur Standards* 19:287, 1937.

Judd DB, Wyszecki G: *Color in business, science, and industry,* ed 3, New York, 1975, John Wiley & Sons.

Koran A, Powers JM, Raptis CN, Yu R: Reflection spectrophotometry of facial skin, *J Dent Res* 60:979, 1981.

Kubelka P: New contributions to the optics of intensely light-scattering materials, part I, *Opt Soc Am J* 38:448, 1948.

Kubelka P, Munk F: Ein Beitrag zur Optik der Farbanstriche, *Z Tech Phys* 12:593, 1931.

Miyagawa Y, Powers JM: Prediction of color of an esthetic restorative material, *J Dent Res* 62:581, 1983.

Miyagawa Y, Powers JM, O'Brien WJ: Optical properties of direct restorative materials, *J Dent Res* 60:890, 1981.

Nickerson D: The specification of color tolerances, *Textile Res* 6:509, 1936.

Noie F, O'Keefe KL, Powers JM: Color stability of resin cements after accelerated aging, *Int J Prosthodont* 8:51, 1995.

O'Brien WJ, Johnston WM, Fanian F: Double-layer color effects in porcelain systems, *J Dent Res* 64:940, 1985.

O'Brien WJ, Johnston WM, Fanian F, Lambert S: The surface roughness and gloss of composites, *J Dent Res* 63:685, 1984.

O'Keefe KL, Powers JM, Noie F: Effect of dissolution on color of extrinsic porcelain colorants, *Int J Prosthodont* 6:558, 1993.

Panzeri H, Fernandes LT, Minelli CJ: Spectral fluorescence of direct anterior restorative materials, *Aust Dent J* 22:458, 1977.

Powers JM, Barakat MM, Ogura H: Color and optical properties of posterior composites under accelerated aging, *Dent Mater J* 4:62, 1985.

Powers JM, Capp JA, Koran A: Color of gingival tissues of blacks and whites, *J Dent Res* 56:112, 1977.

Powers JM, Dennison JB, Koran A: Color stability of restorative resins under accelerated aging, *J Dent Res* 57:964, 1978.

Powers JM, Dennison JB, Lepeak PJ: Parameters that affect the color of direct restorative resins, *J Dent Res* 57:876, 1978.

Powers JM, Koran A: Color of denture resins, *J Dent Res* 56:754, 1977.

Powers JM, Yeh CL, Miyagawa Y: Optical properties of composite of selected shades in white light, *J Oral Rehabil* 10:319, 1983.

Ruyter IE, Nilner K, Moller B: Color stability of dental composite resin material for crown and bridge veneers, *Dent Mater* 3:246, 1987.

Seghi RR, Johnston WM, O'Brien WJ: Spectrophotometric analysis of color differences between porcelain systems, *J Prosthet Dent* 56:35, 1986.

Specifying color by the Munsell system, D1535-68 (1974). In ASTM Standards, 1975, Part 20, Philadelphia, 1975, American Society for Testing and Materials.

Sproull RC: Color matching in dentistry, part III. Color control, *J Prosthet Dent* 31:146, 1974.

Van Oort RP: *Skin color and facial prosthetics—a colorimetric study,* doctoral dissertation, The Netherlands, 1982, Groningen State University.

Wyszecki G, Stiles WS: *Color science,* New York, 1967, John Wiley & Sons.

Yeh CL, Miyagawa Y, Powers JM: Optical properties of composites of selected shades, *J Dent Res* 61:797, 1982.

Yeh CL, Powers JM, Miyagawa Y: Color of selected shades of composites by reflection spectrophotometry, *J Dent Res* 61:1176, 1982.

Thermal Properties

Antonucci JM, Toth EE: Extent of polymerization of dental resins by differential scanning calorimetry, *J Dent Res* 62:121, 1983.

Brady AP, Lee H, Orlowski JA: Thermal conductivity studies of composite dental restorative materials, *J Biomed Mater Res* 8:471, 1974.

Brauer GM, Termini DJ, Burns CL: Characterization of components of dental materials and components of tooth structure by differential thermal analysis, *J Dent Res* 49:100, 1970.

Brown WS, Christiansen DO, Lloyd BA: Numerical and experimental evaluation of energy inputs, temperature gradients, and thermal stress during restorative procedures, *J Am Dent Assoc* 96:451, 1978.

Brown WS, Dewey WA, Jacobs HR: Thermal properties of teeth, *J Dent Res* 49:752, 1970.

Civjan S, Barone JJ, Reinke PE, Selting WJ: Thermal properties of nonmetallic restorative materials, *J Dent Res* 51:1030, 1972.

Craig RG, Eick JD, Peyton FA: Properties of natural waxes used in dentistry, *J Dent Res* 44:1308, 1965.

Craig RG, Peyton FA: Thermal conductivity of tooth structure, dental cements, and amalgam, *J Dent Res* 40:411, 1961.

Craig RG, Powers JM, Peyton FA: Differential thermal analysis of commercial and dental waxes, *J Dent Res* 46:1090, 1967.

Craig RG, Powers JM, Peyton FA: Thermogravimetric analysis of waxes, *J Dent Res* 50:450, 1971.

Dansgaard W, Jarby S: Measurement of nonstationary temperature in small bodies, *Odont Tskr* 66:474, 1958.

de Vree JH, Spierings TA, Plasschaert AJ: A simulation model for transient thermal analysis of restored teeth, *J Dent Res* 62:756, 1983.

Fairhurst CW, Anusavice KJ, Hashinger DT, Ringle RD, Twiggs SW: Thermal expansion of dental alloys and porcelains, *J Biomed Mater Res* 14:435, 1980.

Henschel CJ: Pain control through heat control, *Dent Dig* 47:294, 444, 1941.

Lisanti VF, Zander HA: Thermal conductivity of dentin, *J Dent Res* 29:493, 1950.

Lloyd CH: The determination of the specific heats of dental materials by differential thermal analysis, *Biomaterials* 2:179, 1981.

Lloyd CH: A differential thermal analysis (DTA) for the heats of reaction and temperature rises produced during the setting of tooth coloured restorative materials, *J Oral Rehabil* 11:111, 1984.

McCabe JF, Wilson HJ: The use of differential scanning calorimetry for the evaluation of dental materials. I. Cements, cavity lining materials and anterior restorative materials, *J Oral Rehabil* 7:103, 1980.

McCabe JF, Wilson HJ: The use of differential scanning calorimetry for the evaluation of dental materials. II. Denture base materials, *J Oral* 7:235, 1980.

McLean JW: Physical properties influencing the accuracy of silicone and thiokol impression materials, *Br Dent J* 110:85, 1961.

Murayama T: *Dynamic mechanical analysis of polymeric materials,* New York, 1978, Elsevier Science.

Pearson GJ, Wills DJ, Braden M, McCabe JF: The relationship between the thermal properties of composite filling materials, *J Dent* 8:178, 1980.

Peyton FA: Effectiveness of water coolants with rotary cutting instruments, *J Am Dent Assoc* 56:664, 1958.

Peyton FA: Temperature rise and cutting efficiency of rotating instruments, *NY J Dent* 18:439, 1952.

Peyton FA, Morrant GA: High speed and other instruments for cavity preparation, *Int Dent J* 9:309, 1959.

Peyton FA, Simeral WG: The specific heat of tooth structure, *Alum Bull U Mich School Dent* 56:33, 1954.

Powers JM, Craig RG: Penetration of commercial and dental waxes, *J Dent Res* 53:402, 1974.

Powers JM, Fan PL, Hostetler RW: Properties of class V restorative materials, *Mich Dent Assoc J* 63:275, 1981.

Powers JM, Hostetler RW, Dennison JB: Thermal expansion of composite resins and sealants, *J Dent Res* 58:584, 1979.

Rootare HM, Powers JM: Determination of phase transitions in gutta-percha by differential thermal analysis, *J Dent Res* 56:1453, 1977.

Soderholm KJ: Influence of silane treatment and filler fraction on thermal expansion of composite resins, *J Dent Res* 63:1321, 1984.

Souder WH, Paffenbarger GC: *Physical properties of dental materials,* National Bureau of Standards Circular No C433, Washington, DC, 1942, US Government Printing Office.

Soyenkoff BC, Okun JH: Thermal conductivity measurements of dental tissues with the aid of thermistors, *J Am Dent Assoc* 57:23, 1958.

Tay WM, Braden M: Thermal diffusivity of glass-ionomer cements, *J Dent Res* 66:1040, 1987.

Walsh JP, Symmons HF: A comparison of the heat conduction and mechanical efficiency of diamond instruments, stones, and burs at 3,000 and 60,000 rpm, *NZ Dent J* 45:28, 1949.

Watts DC, Smith R: Thermal diffusion in some polyelectrolyte dental cements: the effect of powder/liquid ratio, *J Oral Rehabil* 11:285, 1984.

Watts DC, Smith R: Thermal diffusivity in finite cylindrical specimens of dental cements, *J Dent Res* 60:1972, 1981.

Wilson TW, Turner DT: Characterization of polydimethacrylates and their composites by dynamic mechanical analysis, *J Dent Res* 66:1032, 1987.

Electrical and Electrochemical Properties

Arvidson K, Johansson EG: Galvanic series of some dental alloys, *Scand J Dent Res* 85:485, 1977.

Bergman M, Ginstrup O, Nilner K: Potential and polarization measurements in vivo of oral galvanism, *Scand J Dent Res* 86:135, 1978.

Bjorn H: Electrical excitation of teeth, *Svensk Tandlak T* 39(Suppl):1946.

Braden M, Clarke RL: Dielectric properties of polycarboxylate cements, *J Dent Res* 54:7, 1975.

Braden M, Clarke RL: Dielectric properties of zinc oxide–eugenol type cements, *J Dent Res* 53:1263, 1974.

Cahoon JR, Holte RN: Corrosion fatigue of surgical stainless steel in synthetic physiological solution, *J Biomed Mater Res* 15:137, 1981.

Clark GCF, Williams DF: The effects of proteins on metallic corrosion, *J Biomed Mater Res* 16:125, 1982.

Fairhurst CW, Marek M, Butts MB, Okabe T: New information on high copper amalgam corrosion, *J Dent Res* 57:725, 1978.

Gjerdet NR, Brune D: Measurements of currents between dissimilar alloys in the oral cavity, *Scand J Dent Res* 85:500, 1977.

Holland RI: Galvanic currents between gold and amalgam, *Scand J Dent Res* 88:269, 1980.

Maijer R, Smith DC: Corrosion of orthodontic bracket bases, *Am J Orthodont* 81:43, 1982.

Marek M, Hochman R: *The corrosion behavior of dental amalgam phases as a function of tin content.* Microfilmed paper no 192, delivered at the Annual Meeting of the International Association for Dental Research, Dental Materials Group, Washington, DC, April 12–15, 1973.

Mohsen NM: *Physical, chemical and biological characterizations of urethane dimethacrylate biomaterial composite,* doctoral dissertation, Ann Arbor, Mich: 1995, University of Michigan School of Dentistry.

Mumford JM: Direct-current electrodes for pulp testing, *Dent Pract* 6:236, 1956.

Mumford JM: Direct-current paths through human teeth, master's thesis, Ann Arbor, Mich, 1957, University of Michigan School of Dentistry.

Mumford JM: Electrolytic action in the mouth and its relationship to pain, *J Dent Res* 36:632, 1957.

Mumford JM: Path of direct current in electric pulp-testing, *Br Dent J* 106:23, 1959.

Mumford JM: Resistivity of human enamel and dentin, *Arch Oral Biol* 12:925, 1957.

O'Brien WJ: Electrochemical corrosion of dental gold castings, *Dent Abstracts* 7:46, 1962.

Phillips LJ, Schnell RJ, Phillips RW: Measurement of the electric conductivity of dental cement. III. Effect of increased contact area and thickness: values for resin, calcium hydroxide, zinc oxide–eugenol, *J Dent Res* 34:597, 1955.

Phillips LJ, Schnell RJ, Phillips RW: Measurement of the electric conductivity of dental cement. IV. Extracted human teeth; in vivo tests; summary, *J Dent Res* 34:839, 1955.

Rootare HM, Powers JM: Comparison of zeta-potential of synthetic fluorapatite obtained by stepwise and continuous methods of streaming, *J Electrochem Soc* 126:1905, 1979.

Schreiver W, Diamond LE: Electromotive forces and electric currents caused by metallic dental fillings, *J Dent Res* 31:205, 1952.

Shaw DJ: *Electrophoresis,* New York, 1969, Academic Press.

Tay WM, Braden M: Dielectric properties of glass ionomer cements, *J Dent Res* 47:463, 1968.

Wilson AD, Kent BE: Dental silicate cements. V. Electrical conductivity, *J Dent Res* 47:463, 1968.

Zitter H, Plenk H, Jr: The electrochemical behavior of metallic implant materials as an indicator of their biocompatibility, *J Biomed Mater Res* 21:881, 1987.

Other Properties

German RM, Wright DC, Gallant RF: In vitro tarnish measurements on fixed prosthodontic alloys, *J Prosthet Dent* 47:399, 1982.

Koran A, Powers JM, Lepeak PJ, Craig RG: Stain resistance of maxillofacial materials, *J Dent Res* 58:1455, 1979.

Mesu FP: Degradation of luting cements measured in vitro, *J Dent Res* 61:655, 1982.

Raptis CM, Powers JM, Fan PL, Yu R: Staining of composite resins by cigarette smoke, *J Oral Rehabil* 9:367, 1982.

Solovan DF, Powers JM: Effect of denture cleansers on partial denture alloys and resilient liners, *Mich Dent Assoc J* 60:135, 1978.

Walls AW, McCabe JF, Murray JJ: An erosion test for dental cements, *J Dent Res* 64:1100, 1985.

Wilson AD, Merson SA, Prosser HJ: A sensitive conductimetric method for measuring the material initially water-leached from dental cements. I. Zinc polycarboxylate cements, *J Dent* 8:263, 1980.

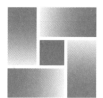

4 *Mechanical Properties*

M ost restorative materials must withstand forces, during either fabrication or mastication. Mechanical properties are therefore important in understanding and predicting a material's behavior under load. Because no single mechanical property can give a true measure of quality, understanding the principles involved in a variety of mechanical properties is essential to obtain the maximum service. Quantities of force, stress, strain, strength, hardness, friction, and wear can help identify the properties of a material. In general, the stability of a solid under applied load is determined by the nature and strength of atomic binding forces. In this chapter, the concepts of elastic, viscoelastic, and surface mechanical properties are introduced, and the importance of these concepts in dentistry is emphasized.

■ FORCE

In general, force is gained through one body pushing or pulling on another. Forces may be applied through actual contact of the bodies or at a distance. The result of an applied force on a body is a change in position of rest or motion of the body. If the body to which the force is applied remains at rest, the force causes the body to deform. A force is defined by three characteristics: the point of application, the magnitude, and the direction of application. The direction of a force is characteristic of the type of force. The unit of force is the newton, N.

Occlusal Forces

One of the most important applications of physics in dentistry is the study of forces applied to teeth and dental restorations. There are numerous reports in the dental literature that describe the measurement of biting forces on teeth. The maximum reported forces, measured by strain gages and telemetric devices, have ranged from 200 to 3500 N.

Biting forces on adult teeth decrease from the molar region to the incisors, with forces on the first and second molars varying from 400 to 800 N. The average force on the bicuspids, cuspids, and incisors has been reported to be approximately 300, 200, and 150 N, respectively. A somewhat irregular but definite increase in force from 235 to 494 N occurs in growing children, with an average yearly increase of 22 N.

Forces on Restorations

Equally important to the study of forces on natural dentition is the measurement of forces and stresses on restorations such as inlays, fixed bridges, removable partial dentures, and complete dentures. One of the first investigations of occlusal forces showed that the average biting force for patients who had a fixed bridge replacing a first molar was 250 N on the restored side and 300 N on the opposite side where natural dentition occurred. For comparison, the average biting forces on permanent teeth were 665, 450, and 220 N on molars, bicuspids, and incisors, respectively.

In another study, force measurements of patients with removable partial dentures ranged from 67 to 235 N. For patients with complete dentures, the average force on the molars and bicuspids was about 100 N, whereas the forces on the incisors averaged 40 N. These spreads in results were possibly caused by the age and gender variations of the patient populations. In general, the biting force applied by women is 90 N less than that applied by men.

These studies and others indicate that the chewing force on the first molars of patients with a fixed bridge is about 40% of the force exerted by patients with natural dentition. A further decrease in force is obtained in patients with complete or removable partial dentures. Patients who wear such appliances exert only about 15% of the force applied by persons with normal dentition.

Recent measurements made with the smaller strain gage devices have been more precise than those made with the early equipment, but in general, the conclusions are similar. The distribution of force between the first bicuspid, second bicuspid, and the first molar of a complete denture has been established as approximately 15%, 30%, and 55% of normal. The average force on the first bicuspid, second bicuspid, and first molar while the patient chewed peanuts, coconut, or raisins was 6.6, 12.0, and 22.6 N, respectively. These values are low because they are forces required to chew the food rather than average maximum forces. Therefore patients wearing a complete denture may facilitate the chewing of tough foods by increasing the force or number of chewing thrusts or by shifting the food to the small bicuspids where the stress is greater. Because the range of force application is small, shifting the food forward would be the better solution.

Summary of Occlusal Forces

In general, the studies cited above were for small patient populations and/or patients of different ages and, based on the range of data reported, research on forces of mastication should be conducted on a large number of controlled patient groups for more accurate quantification. However, we may surmise that the forces of occlusion and the response of the underlying tissue change with anatomical location, age, malocclusion, and placement of a restorative appliance. Therefore a material or design sufficient to withstand the forces of occlusion on the incisor of a child may not be sufficient for the first molar of an adult who has a malocclusion or bridge.

■ STRESS

When a force acts on a body, tending to produce deformation, a resistance is developed to this external force application. The internal reaction is equal in intensity and opposite in direction to the applied external force, and is called stress. Both the applied force and internal resistance (stress) are distributed over a given area of the body, and so the stress in a structure is designated as the force per unit area. In this respect, stress resembles pressure, because both stress and pressure are represented by the following equation:

$$\text{Stress} = \frac{\text{Force}}{\text{Area}}$$

Technically, stress is the internal resistance of the body in terms of force per unit area. Because the internal resistance to force applications is impractical to measure, the more convenient procedure is to measure the external force (F) applied to the cross-sectional area (A), which can be described as the stress, typically denoted as S or σ. The unit of stress, therefore, is the unit of force (N) divided by a unit of area or length squared and is commonly expressed as Pascal (1 Pa = 1 N/m^2 = 1 MN/mm^2). It is common to report stress in units of megapascals (MPa), where 1 MPa = 10^6 Pa.

Because the stress in a structure varies directly with the force and inversely with area, it is necessary to determine the area over which the force acts. This is particularly true in dental restorations because the areas over which the forces are applied often are extremely small. For example, the clasps on removable partial dentures, orthodontic wire structures, or small occlusal restorations may have cross-sectional areas of only 0.16 to 0.016 cm^2.

As a numerical example, a 20-gage orthodontic wire has a diameter of 0.8 mm and a cross-sectional area of 0.5 mm^2. If a 220 N force is applied to a wire of this diameter, the stress developed is equivalent to 220 N/0.5 mm^2, or 440 N/mm^2 (MPa).

Stress is always stated as though the force were equivalent to that applied to a 1 m^2 section, but a dental restoration obviously does not have a square meter of exposed occlusal surface area. A small occlusal pit restoration may have no more than 4 mm^2 of surface area if it were assumed that the restoration were 2 mm on a side. If a biting force of 440 N should be concentrated on this area, the stress developed would be 100 MPa. Therefore stresses equivalent to several hundreds of MPa occur in many types of restorations.

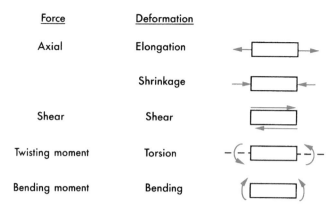

Fig. 4-1 Schematic of the different types of stresses and their corresponding deformation.

Types of Stress

A force can be directed to a body from any angle or direction, and many times several forces are combined to develop complex stresses in a structure. In general, individually applied forces may be axial (tensile or compressive), shear, bending, or torsional. These directional forces are illustrated in a simplified manner in Fig. 4-1. All stresses, however, can be resolved into combinations of two basic types—axial and shear.

Tension results when a body is subjected to two sets of forces that are directed away from each other in the same straight line. Compression results when the body is subjected to two sets of forces in the same straight line and directed toward each other. Shear is the result of two sets of forces directed parallel to each other. Torsion results from the twisting of a body, and bending results from an applied bending moment. When tension is applied, the molecules in the body must resist being pulled apart. When compression is applied, they resist being forced more closely together. As a result of a shear stress application, one portion of the body must resist sliding past another. These resistances of a material to deformation represent the basic qualities of elasticity of solid bodies.

An example of the complexity and varying direction and magnitude of the stresses in the oral cavity is shown in Fig. 4-2, in which a photoelastic model of a three-unit bridge has been loaded in compression by the opposing occlusion. The arrows in Fig. 4-2, A, indicate locations of contact that are under

compressive stress. Fig. 4-2, B, shows the type of stress at the periphery of the model and illustrates that the occlusal surface of the bridge is subjected alternately to areas of compression and tension, whereas the gingival portion of the pontic is under tensile stress. The soldered joints, however, are under both tensile and shear stress.

Strain

In the discussion of force, it was pointed out that a body undergoes deformation when a force is applied to it. It is important to recognize that each type of stress is capable of producing a corresponding deformation in a body. The deformation resulting from a tensile or pulling force is an elongation of a body in the direction of applied force, whereas a compressive or pushing force causes compression or shortening of the body in the direction of loading. Strain, ε, is described as the change in length ($\Delta L = L - L_o$) per unit length (L_o) of the body when it is subjected to a stress. Strain has no unit of measurement but is represented as a pure number obtained from the following equation:

$$\text{Strain } (\epsilon) = \frac{\text{Deformation}}{\text{Original length}} = \frac{(L - L_o)}{L_o} = \frac{\Delta L}{L_o}$$

Thus if a sample with an original length of 2 mm is pulled to a new length of 2.02 mm, it has deformed 0.02 mm and the strain is 0.02/2 = 0.01 or 1%. Strain is therefore reported as an absolute value or as a percentage. The amount of strain will differ with each type of material subjected to stress and

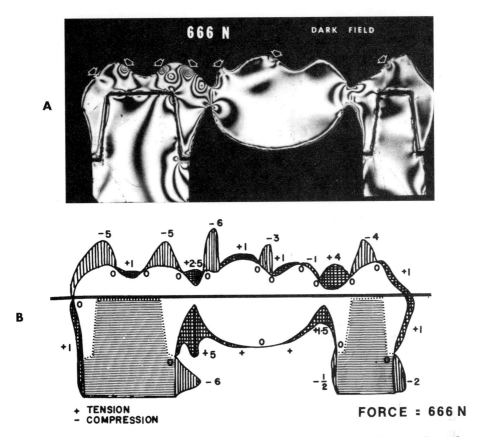

Fig. 4-2 Stress distribution in a model of a dental bridge showing **A**, the isochromatic fringes or lines of constant stress when loaded in compression, and **B**, the fringe order or a measure of the magnitude of the stress at the periphery. (From El-Ebrashi MK, Craig RG, Peyton FA: *J Prosthet Dent* 23:177, 1970.)

with the magnitude of the stress applied. Note that regardless of the composition or nature of the material and regardless of the magnitude and type of stress applied to the material, deformation and strain result with each stress application. The importance of strain in dentistry is that a restorative material, such as a clasp or an orthodontic wire, which can withstand a large amount of strain before failure, can be bent and adjusted with less chance of fracturing.

■ STRESS-STRAIN CURVES

Consider a bar of material subjected to an applied force. We can measure the magnitude of the force and the resulting deformation (Δ). If we next take another bar of the same material, but different

dimensions, the force-deformation characteristics change (Fig. 4-3, *A*). However, if we normalize the applied force by the cross-sectional area (stress) of the bar and normalize the deformation by the original length (strain) of the bar, the resultant curve now becomes independent of the geometry of the bar (Fig. 4-3, *B*). It is therefore preferential to report the stress-strain relations of a material rather than the force-deformation characteristics. The stress-strain relationship of a dental material is studied by measuring the load and deformation and then calculating the corresponding stress and strain.

The testing of many materials necessitates loads of 2220 N or more and the measurement of deformations of 0.02 mm or less. Another requirement may be that the load should be applied at a uniform rate or that the deformation should occur at a uniform

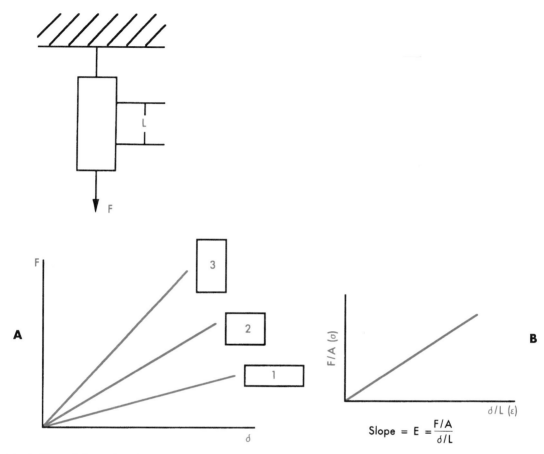

Fig. 4-3 A, Force-deformation characteristics for the same material but having different dimensions. **B,** Stress-strain characteristics of the same group of bars. The stress-strain curve is independent of the geometry of the bar.

rate. A typical machine that permits testing in tension, compression, or shear is shown in Fig. 4-4. In the figure a stainless steel rod is clamped between two jaws, and the tensile properties are measured by pulling the specimen. The load is measured electronically with a strain-gage transducer and recorded on the vertical axis of a strip-chart recorder. The deformation is measured with an extensometer clamped over a given length of the sample, and is recorded on the horizontal axis of the recorder. One therefore obtains a plot of load versus deformation, which can be converted to a plot of stress versus strain (Fig. 4-5) by the simple calculations described previously.

In the calculation of stress, it is assumed that the cross-sectional area of the specimen remains constant during the test. The resulting stress-strain curve is called an engineering stress-strain curve, and stresses are calculated based on the original cross-sectional area. For many materials, significant changes in the area of the specimen may occur as it is being deformed. A stress-strain curve based on stresses calculated from a nonconstant cross-sectional area is called a true stress-strain curve. At high loads a true stress-strain curve may be quite different from an engineering stress-strain curve because significant changes in the area of the specimen may occur. For example, if a sample is being tested in tension and the area decreases, the engineering stress will be lower than the true stress. The engineering stress-strain curve is used throughout the remaining chapters.

A stress-strain curve for a hypothetical material that was subjected to increasing tensile stress until

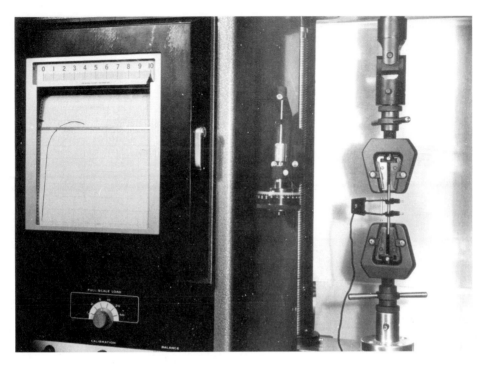

Fig. 4-4 Mechanical testing instrument.

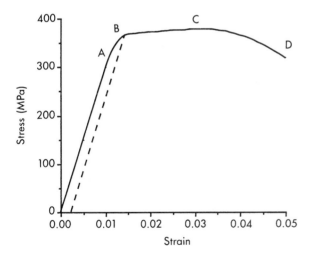

Fig. 4-5 Stress-strain curve for a material subjected to a tensile stress.

fracture is shown in Fig. 4-5. The stress is plotted vertically, and the strain is plotted horizontally. As the stress is increased, the strain is increased. In fact, in the initial portion of the curve, from 0 to *A*, the strain is proportional to the stress, and as the stress

is doubled, the amount of strain also is doubled. When a stress that is higher than the value registered at *A* is achieved, the strain changes are no longer linearly proportional to the stress changes. Hence the value of the stress at *A* is known as the proportional limit.

Proportional and Elastic Limits

The proportional limit is defined as the greatest stress that a material will sustain without a deviation from the proportionality of stress to strain. Below the proportional limit, no permanent deformation occurs in a structure. When the stress is removed, the structure will return to its original dimensions. Within this range of stress application, the material is elastic in nature, and if the material is stressed to a value below the proportional limit, an elastic or reversible strain will occur. The region of the stress-strain curve below the proportional limit is called the elastic region. The application of a stress greater than the proportional limit results in a permanent or irreversible strain in the sample, and the region of the stress-strain curve beyond the proportional limit is called the plastic region.

The elastic limit is defined as the maximum stress that a material will withstand without permanent deformation. For all practical purposes, therefore, the proportional limit and elastic limit represent the same stress within the structure, and the terms are often used interchangeably in referring to the stress involved. Keep in mind, however, that they differ in fundamental concept, in that one deals with the proportionality of strain to stress in the structure, whereas the other describes the elastic behavior of the material. The proportional limit of the material in Fig. 4-5 is approximately 330 MPa. Both the proportional and elastic limits are quite different in values for different materials. Values for proportional or elastic limits in either tension or compression can be determined, but the values obtained in tension and compression will differ for the same material.

The concepts of elastic and plastic behavior can be realized with a schematic model of the deformation of atoms in a solid under stress (Fig. 4-6). The atoms are shown in Fig. 4-6, *A*, with no stress applied, and in Fig. 4-6, *B*, with an applied stress that is below the value of the proportional limit. When the stress shown in *B* is removed, the atoms return to their positions shown in *A*. When a stress

is applied that is greater than the proportional limit, the atoms move to a position as shown in Fig. 4-6, *C*, and, after removal of the stress, the atoms remain in this new position. The application of a stress less than the proportional or elastic limit therefore results in a reversible strain, whereas a stress greater than the proportional or elastic limit results in an irreversible or permanent strain in the sample.

The model described in Fig. 4-6 is considerably oversimplified, and a more realistic but more complicated model of plastic deformation is shown in Fig. 4-7. In this schematic the atoms move to new stable positions, resulting in plastic deformation due to the movement of dislocations or imperfections in the structure of the solid. These imperfections allow the consecutive movement of atoms without the need for an entire row or plane of atoms to move.

Yield Strength

Stress-strain curves determined in the laboratory are rarely as ideal as the curve shown in Fig. 4-5. Therefore it is not always feasible to explicitly measure the proportional and elastic limits. The yield

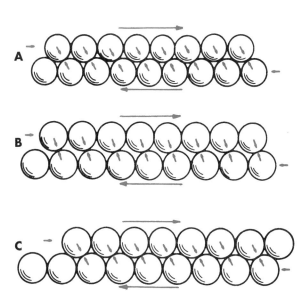

Fig. 4-6 Sketch of an atomic model showing atoms in **A**, original position; **B**, after elastic deformation; and **C**, after plastic deformation. (Adapted from Cottrell AH: *Sci Am* 217(3):90, 1967.)

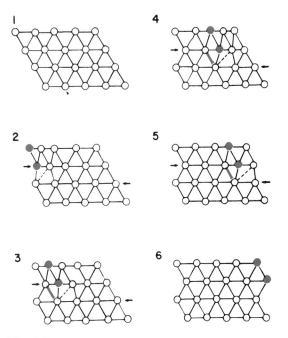

Fig. 4-7 Sketch of an atomic model showing plastic deformation taking place due to the movement of dislocations. (Adapted from Cottrell AH: *Sci Am* 217(3):90, 1967.)

strength or yield stress (*YS*) of a material is a property that can be determined readily and is often used to describe the stress at which the material begins to function in a plastic manner. At this stress, a limited permanent strain has occurred in the material. The yield strength is defined as the stress at which a material exhibits a specified limiting deviation from proportionality of stress to strain. The amount of permanent strain is arbitrarily selected for the material being examined and may be indicated as 0.1%, 0.2%, or 0.5% (0.001, 0.002, 0.005) permanent strain. The amount of permanent strain may be referred to as the percent offset. Many specifications use 0.2% as a convention.

The yield stress is determined by selecting the desired offset and drawing a line parallel to the linear region of the stress-strain curve. The point at which the parallel line intersects the curve is the yield stress. On the stress-strain curve shown in Fig. 4-5, for example, the yield strength is represented by the value B. This represents a stress of about 360 MPa at a 0.25% offset. This yield stress is slightly higher than that for the proportional limit and also indicates a specified amount of deformation. Note that when a structure is permanently deformed, even a small amount (such as the amount of deformation at the yield strength), it does not completely return to its original dimensions when the stress is removed. For this reason, the proportional limit, elastic limit, and yield strength of a material are among its most important properties.

Any dental structure that is permanently deformed in service, due to the forces of mastication and use, is usually a functional failure to some degree. For example, a bridge that is permanently deformed in service due to excessive biting forces is shifted out of the proper occlusal relation to which it was originally designed. The prosthesis is permanently deformed because a stress equal to or greater than the yield strength and greater than the elastic limit was developed in the structure. Recall also that malocclusion changes the stresses placed on a restoration, and therefore a deformed prosthesis may be subjected to greater stresses than originally intended. Usually a fracture does not occur under such conditions but rather only a permanent deformation results, which represents a destructive example of deformation. A constructive example of permanent deformation and stresses in excess of the elastic limit is observed when an appliance or dental structure is adapted or adjusted for purposes of design. In the process of shaping an orthodontic appliance or adjusting a clasp on a cast removable partial denture, it is necessary to introduce a stress into the structure that is greater than the yield strength if the material is to be permanently bent or adapted. Values of yield strength for some partial denture alloys are listed in Table 4-1.

Ultimate Strength

In Fig. 4-5, the test sample is subjected to its greatest stress at point *C*. The ultimate tensile strength or stress (UTS) is defined as the maximum stress that a material can withstand before failure in tension, whereas the ultimate compressive strength or stress (UCS) is the maximum stress a material can withstand in compression. If the direction of loading has previously been specified, then the term *ultimate strength* (stress) is often used. The ultimate stress is determined by dividing the maximum load in tension or compression by the original cross-sectional area of the test sample. The ultimate tensile strength of the material in Fig. 4-5 is about 380 MPa.

The ultimate strength of an alloy is used in dentistry to give an indication of the size or cross section required for a given restoration. It should be noted that an alloy that has been stressed to near the ultimate strength will be permanently deformed, and so a restoration receiving that amount of stress during function would be useless. Therefore although data on materials used in dentistry usually specify values for ultimate strength, the use of ultimate strength as a criterion for evaluating the relative merits of various materials should not be

TABLE 4-1   Values of Yield Strength for Some Partial Denture Alloys

Material	Yield Strength, 0.2% Offset MPa
Nickel-chromium alloy	690
Cobalt-chromium alloy	572
Gold (type IV) alloy	621*

*0.1% offset.

overemphasized. The yield strength is of greater importance than ultimate strength because it is a gage of when a material will start to deform.

Fracture Strength

In Fig. 4-5 the test sample fractured at point *D*, at the end of the curve. The stress at which a material fractures is called the fracture strength or fracture stress. Note that a material does not necessarily fracture at the point at which the maximum stress occurs. Some materials begin to elongate excessively, and the stress calculated from the force and the original cross-sectional area may drop before final fracture occurs. Accordingly, the stress at the end of the curve is less than at some intermediate point on the curve. Therefore in the most general case, the ultimate and fracture strengths are different. However, for the specific cases of many dental alloys subjected to tension, the ultimate and fracture strengths are the same, as is seen later.

Elongation

The deformation that results from the application of a tensile force is elongation. Elongation is extremely important because it gives an indication of the workability of an alloy. As may be observed from Fig. 4-5, the elongation of a material during a tensile test can be divided conveniently into two parts: (1) the increase in length of the specimen below the proportional limit (from 0 to *A*), which is not permanent and is proportional to the stress applied; and (2) the elongation beyond the proportional limit and up to the fracture strength (from *A* to *D*), which is permanent. The permanent deformation may be determined after the test is completed by measuring the increase in the distance between two fixed points on the sample when the fractured ends are placed together or, more accurately, it may be measured with an extensometer while the material is being tested and calculated from the stress-strain curve. A common method to express total elongation is in percentage, such as 20% elongation for a 5-cm test specimen. The percent elongation (% EL) would be calculated as follows:

$$\% \text{ Elongation} = \frac{\text{Increase in length}}{\text{Original length}} \times 100\%$$

We see that elongation and axial strain are similar.

TABLE 4-2 Values of Percent Elongation of Some Crown and Bridge and Partial Denture Alloys

Alloy	% Elongation
Crown and bridge	
Gold (type III)	34.0
40% Au-Ag-Cu	2.0
Nickel-chromium	1.1
Partial denture	
Gold (type IV)	6.5
Nickel-chromium	2.4
Cobalt-chromium	1.5
Iron-chromium	9.0
Cobalt-nickel-chromium	8-10

The total percent elongation includes both the elastic elongation and the plastic elongation. The plastic elongation usually is the greater of the two, except in materials that are quite brittle or that have very low elastic moduli. A material that exhibits a 20% total elongation at the time of fracture has increased in length a total of one-fifth more than its original length. Such a material, as many dental gold alloys, has a high value for plastic or permanent elongation and, in general, is a ductile type of alloy, whereas a material with only 1% elongation would possess little permanent elongation and would be considered brittle.

Values of percent elongation of some crown and bridge and partial denture alloys are compared in Table 4-2. An alloy that has a high value for total elongation can be bent permanently without danger of fracture. Clasps can be adjusted, orthodontic appliances can be prepared, and crowns or inlays can be burnished if they are prepared from alloys with high values for elongation. Therefore in the selection of alloys for specific purposes, it is necessary to recognize that they may be subjected to permanent deformation and adaptation during the construction or assembly of the restoration, and so it is necessary to have an acceptable amount of elongation. In other restorations in which permanent deformation is not anticipated, materials can be employed that have a lower value for elongation. A relationship exists between elongation and yield strength for many materials, including dental gold alloys, where, generally, the higher the yield strength, the less the elongation.

Elastic Modulus

The measure of elasticity of a material is described by the term *elastic modulus*, also referred to as modulus of elasticity or Young's modulus, and denoted by the variable *E*. The elastic modulus represents the stiffness of a material within the elastic range. The elastic modulus can be determined from a stress-strain curve (see Fig. 4-5) by calculating the ratio of stress to strain or the slope of the linear region of the curve. The modulus is calculated from the equation

$$\text{Elastic modulus} = \frac{\text{Stress}}{\text{Strain}} \text{ or } E = \frac{\sigma}{\in}$$

Because strain is dimensionless, the modulus has the same units as stress, and is usually reported in MPa or GPa.

The elastic qualities of a material represent a fundamental property of the material. The interatomic or intermolecular forces of the material are responsible for the property of elasticity (Fig. 4-6). The stronger the basic attraction forces, the greater the values of the elastic modulus and the more rigid the material. Because this property is related to the attraction forces within the material, it usually is the same when the material is subjected to either tension or compression. The property generally is independent of any heat treatment or mechanical treatment that a metal or alloy has received, but is quite dependent on the composition of the material.

The elastic modulus represents the slope of the elastic portion of the stress-strain curve. The slope is calculated by choosing any two stress and strain coordinates in the elastic or linear range. As an example, for the curve in Fig. 4-5, the slope can be calculated by choosing the following two coordinates:

$\sigma_1 = 150$ MPa, $\in_1 = 0.005$; and $\sigma_2 = 300$ MPa, $\in_2 = 0.010$

The slope is therefore

$(\sigma_2 - \sigma_1)/(\in_2 - \in_1) = (300-150)/(0.010 - 0.005) = 30,000$
MPa $= 30$ GPa

Stress-strain curves for two hypothetical materials, *A* and *B*, of different composition are shown in Fig. 4-8. Inspection of the curves shows that for a given stress, *A* is less elastically deformed than *B*, with the result that the elastic modulus for *A* is greater than for *B*. This difference can be demonstrated, numerically, by a calculation of the elastic moduli for the

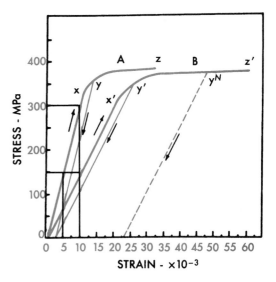

Fig. 4-8 Stress-strain curves of two hypothetical materials subjected to tensile stress.

two materials subjected to the same stress of 300 MPa. At a stress of 300 MPa, material *A* is strained to 0.010 (1%) and the elastic modulus is

$$E = \frac{300 \text{ MPa}}{0.010} = 30,000 \text{ MPa} = 30 \text{ GPa}$$

On the other hand, material *B* is strained to 0.02 (2%), or twice as much as material *A* for the same stress application. The equation for the elastic modulus for *B* is

$$E = \frac{300 \text{ MPa}}{0.020} = 15,000 \text{ MPa} = 15 \text{ GPa}$$

The fact that material *A* has a steeper slope in the elastic range than material *B* means that a greater stress application is required to deform material *A* a given amount than for material *B*. From the curves shown in Fig. 4-8, it can be seen that a stress of 300 MPa is required to deform *A* the same amount elastically that *B* is deformed by a stress of 150 MPa. Materials such as rubber and plastics have low values for the elastic modulus, whereas many metals and alloys have much higher values, as shown in Table 4-3.

Poisson's Ratio

During axial loading in tension or compression there is a simultaneous axial and lateral strain.

TABLE 4-3 Values of Elastic Modulus of Some Restorative Dental Materials

Material	Elastic Modulus GPa*
Cobalt-chromium partial denture alloy	218.0
Gold (type IV) alloy	99.3
Enamel	84.1
Feldspathic porcelain	69.0
Zinc phosphate cement (base)	22.4
Amalgam	27.6
Dentin	18.3
Composite resin	16.6
Zinc phosphate cement (luting)	13.7
Acrylic denture resin	2.65
Silicone rubber (maxillofacial)	0.002

*1 gigapascal (GPa) = 103 MPa.

TABLE 4-4 Values of Poisson's Ratio of Some Restorative Dental Materials

Material	Poisson's Ratio
Acrylic restorative resin	0.35
Amalgam	0.35
Zinc phosphate cement	0.35
Enamel	0.30
Composite resin	0.24

Under tensile loading, as a material elongates in the direction of load, there is a reduction in cross section. Under compressive loading, there is an increase in the cross section. Within the elastic range, the ratio of the lateral to the axial strain is called Poisson's ratio (ν). In tensile loading, the Poisson's ratio indicates that the reduction in cross section is proportional to the elongation during the elastic deformation. The reduction in cross section continues until the material is fractured.

Poisson's ratios of some dental materials measured by an ultrasonic technic are listed in Table 4-4. Brittle substances, such as hard gold alloys and dental amalgam, show little permanent reduction in cross section during a tensile test. More ductile materials such as soft gold alloys, which are high in gold content, show a high degree of reduction in cross-sectional area.

Ductility and Malleability

Two significant properties of metals and alloys are ductility and malleability. These properties cannot always be determined with certainty from a stress-strain curve. In general, ductility is the ability of a material to be plastically deformed, and it is indicated by the plastic strain.

In general, a high degree of compression or elongation indicates good malleability and ductility, although certain metals show some exception to this rule. The reduction in area in a specimen, combined with the elongation at the breaking point, is, however, a good indication of the relative ductility of a metal of alloy.

The ductility of a material represents its ability to be drawn into wire under a force of tension. The material is subjected to a permanent deformation while being subjected to these tensile forces. The malleability of a substance represents its ability to be hammered or rolled into thin sheets without fracturing.

Ductility is a property that has been related to the workability of a material in the mouth. Ductility has also been related to burnishability of the margins of a casting. Although ductility is important, the amount of force necessary to cause permanent deformation during the burnishing operation also must be considered. A burnishing index has been used to rank the ease of burnishing alloys and is equal to the ductility (elongation) divided by the yield strength.

The relative malleability and ductility of 10 metals used in dentistry and industry are given in Table 4-5. It is interesting that gold and silver, used extensively in dentistry, are the most malleable and ductile of the metals, but other metals do not follow the same order for both malleability and ductility. In general, metals tend to be ductile, whereas ceramics tend to be brittle.

Resilience

Resilience is the resistance of a material to permanent deformation. It indicates the amount of energy necessary to deform the material to the proportional limit. Resilience is measured by the area under the

TABLE 4-5   Relative Ductility and Malleability
of Metals in Decreasing Order

Ductility	Malleability
Gold	Gold
Silver	Silver
Platinum	Aluminum
Iron	Copper
Nickel	Tin
Copper	Platinum
Aluminum	Lead
Zinc	Zinc
Tin	Iron
Lead	Nickel

Note: Some authorities consider tungsten to be the most ductile
metal.

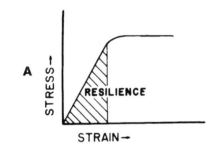

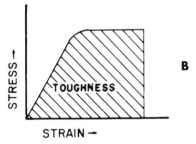

Fig. 4-9 Stress-strain curves showing **A**, the area
indicating the resilience, and **B**, the area representing
the toughness of a material.

elastic portion of the stress-strain curve, as illustrated in
Fig. 4-9, *A*. The resilience can be measured by idealiz-
ing the area of interest as a triangle and calculating the
area of the triangle, ½bh. The resilience of the material
in Fig. 4-5, for example, would be $\frac{1}{2} \times 0.011 \times 330$
$= 1.82$ m MN/m^3. The units are m MN/m^3
(meter · meganewtons per cubic meter), which represents an energy per unit volume of material.

Resilience has particular importance in the evaluation of orthodontic wires because the amount of
work expected from a particular spring in moving a
tooth is of interest. There is also interest in the
amount of stress and strain at the proportional limit
because these factors determine the magnitude of
the force that can be applied to the tooth and how
far the tooth will need to move before the spring is
no longer effective.

Toughness

Toughness is the resistance of a material to fracture and it is an indication of the amount of energy
necessary to cause fracture. The area under the elastic and plastic portions of a stress-strain curve, as
shown in Fig. 4-9, *B*, represents the toughness of a
material. Toughness is not as easy to calculate as
resilience, and the integration is usually done numerically. The units of toughness are the same as the
units of resilience—m MN/m^3 or MPa/m. Toughness
therefore represents the energy required to stress the
material to the point of fracture. A material can be
tough by having a combination of high yield and
ultimate strength and moderately high strain at rupture, or by having moderately high yield and ultimate strengths and a large strain at rupture.

Fracture Toughness

Recently the concepts of fracture mechanics have
been applied to a number of problems in dental
materials. Fracture mechanics characterizes the
behavior of materials with cracks or flaws, which
may arise naturally in a material or nucleate after a
time in service. In either case, any defect generally
weakens a material, and sudden fractures can arise at
stresses below the yield stress. Sudden, catastrophic
fractures typically occur in brittle materials that don't
have the ability to plastically deform and redistribute
stresses. The field of fracture mechanics provides an
analysis of and design basis against these types of
failures.

Two simple examples illustrate the significance of
defects on the fracture of materials. If one takes a
piece of paper and tries to tear it, greater effort is
needed than if a tiny cut is made in the paper.
Analogously, it takes a considerable force to break a
glass bar; however, if a small notch is placed on the
surface of the glass bar, less force is needed to cause

fracture. If the same experiment is performed on a ductile material, we find that a small surface notch has no effect on the force required to break the bar, and the ductile bar can be bent without fracturing (Fig. 4-10). For a brittle material, such as glass, no local plastic deformation is associated with fracture, whereas for a ductile material, plastic deformation, such as the ability to bend, occurs without fracture. The ability to be plastically deformed without fracture, or the amount of energy required for fracture, is the fracture toughness.

In general, the larger a flaw, the lower the stress needed to cause fracture. This is because the stresses, which would normally be supported by material, are now concentrated at the edge of the flaw. The ability of a flaw to cause fracture depends on the fracture toughness of the material. Fracture toughness is a material property and is proportional to the energy consumed in plastic deformation.

A material is characterized by the energy release rate, G, and the stress intensity factor, K. The energy release rate is a function of the energy involved in crack propagation, whereas the stress intensity factor describes the stresses at the tip of a crack. The stress intensity factor changes with crack length and stress according to

$$K = Y\sigma a^{1/2}$$

where Y is a function that is dependent on crack size and geometry. A material fractures when the stress intensity reaches a critical value, K_c. This value of the stress intensity at fracture is called the fracture toughness, which gives a relative value of a material's ability to resist crack propagation. The units of K_c are units of stress (force/length^2) × units of length$^{1/2}$, or force × length$^{-3/2}$, and are typically reported as MN m$^{-3/2}$ or MPa-m$^{1/2}$.

Fracture toughness has been measured for amalgams, acrylic denture base materials, posterior composites, porcelain, dental ceramics, ceramic crowns and orthodontic brackets, cements, calcium hydroxide, and human enamel and dentin. Typical values are in the range of 0.75-2.2, 2.6, 1.5-2.1, 0.61-1.8, and 3.08 MN m$^{-3/2}$ for composites, porcelain, other ceramics, enamel, and dentin, respectively.

Low-copper amalgam is usually of higher toughness than high-copper amalgam, and fracture toughness progressively decreases with increasing copper

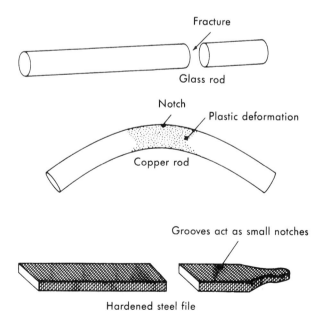

Fig. 4-10 Schematic of different types of deformation in brittle (glass, steel file) and ductile (copper) materials of the same diameter and having a notch of the same dimensions. (From Flinn RA, Trojan PK: *Engineering materials and their applications,* Boston, 1981, Houghton Mifflin, p 535.)

content. The presence of fillers in polymers substantially increases the fracture toughness. The mechanisms of toughening are presumed to be matrix/filler interactions, but are not yet established. Similarly, the addition of up to 50 wt% zirconia to porcelain increases the fracture toughness. As with other mechanical properties, aging or storage in a simulated oral environment or at elevated temperatures can decrease the fracture toughness, but there is no uniform agreement in the literature. Attempts to correlate fracture toughness with wear resistance have been mixed, and therefore it is not an unequivocal predictor of the wear of restorative materials. Also, numerical analysis technics have been applied to composites and the tooth-denture base joint to determine energy release rates in the presence of cracks.

Properties and Stress-Strain Curves

The shape of a stress-strain curve and the magnitudes of the stress and strain allow classification of materials with respect to their general properties. The idealized stress-strain curves in Fig. 4-11 represent materials with various combinations of physical properties. For example, materials *1* to *4* all have high stiffness; materials *1, 2, 5,* and *6* all have high strength; and materials *1, 3, 5,* and *7* have high ductility. If the only requirement for an application is stiffness, materials *1* to *4* would all be satisfactory. However, if the requirements are both stiffness and strength, only materials *1* and *2* would

now be acceptable. If the requirements were to also include ductility, the choice would be limited to material *1*. Therefore it is clear that the properties of stiffness, strength, and ductility are independent, and materials may exhibit various combinations of these three properties.

■ OTHER MECHANICAL PROPERTIES

Tensile Properties of Brittle Materials

A variety of brittle restorative materials, including dental amalgam, cements, ceramic materials, plaster and stone, and some impression materials, is important to dental practice. In many instances the material is much weaker in tension than in compression, which may contribute to failure of the material in service. Such material should therefore only be used in areas subjected to compressive stresses.

Previously, test methods were described for the development of stress-strain curves resulting from tensile measurements on ductile materials such as metals, alloys, and some types of plastics. Similar test methods have been applied to brittle materials. However, brittle materials must be gripped with caution, and any stress concentrations at the grips or anywhere else in the sample can lead to premature fracture. As a result there has been large variability in tensile data on brittle materials. Although special grips have been used to permit axial tensile loading

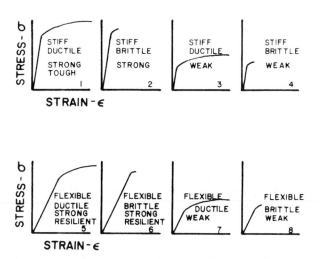

Fig. 4-11 Stress-strain curves for materials with various combinations of properties.

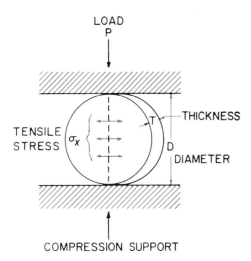

Fig. 4-12 Drawing to illustrate how compression force develops tensile stress in brittle materials.

TABLE 4-6 Values of Tensile Strength for Some Restorative Dental Materials

Material	Diametral Tensile Strength MPa	Ultimate Tensile Strength MPa
Gold alloy	–	448
Amalgam	65.7	–
Dentin	–	98.7
Composite resin	45.5	–
Feldspathic porcelain	–	24.8
Enamel	–	10.3
Zinc phosphate cement	8.1	–
High-strength stone	7.66	–
Calcium hydroxide liner	0.96	–

with a minimum of localized stress concentrations, obtaining uniform results is still difficult, and such testing is relatively slow and time consuming.

An alternative method of testing brittle materials, in which the ultimate tensile strength of a brittle material is determined through compressive testing, has become popular because of its relative simplicity and reproducibility of results. The method is described in the literature as the diametral compression test for tension, the Brazilian test, or the indirect tensile test. In this test method, a disk of the brittle material is compressed diametrically in a testing machine until fracture occurs, as shown in Fig. 4-12. The compressive stress applied to the specimen introduces a tensile stress in the material in the plane of the force application of the test machine. The tensile stress is directly proportional to the load applied in compression through the following formula:

$$(\text{Tensile stress}) \; \sigma_x = \frac{2P}{\pi \times D \times T} \; \frac{(\text{Load})}{(\text{Diameter} \times \text{Thickness})}$$

Note that if the specimen deforms significantly before failure or fractures into more than two equal pieces, the data may not be valid. Some materials yield different diametral tensile strengths when tested at different rates of loading and are described as being strain-rate sensitive. (Strain-rate dependence is discussed later in the chapter.) The diametral tensile test is not valid for these materials, and

thus the strain-rate sensitivity of a material should be determined before this test is used to evaluate the tensile strength. Values of diametral and ultimate tensile strength for some dental materials are listed in Table 4-6.

Compressive Properties

Compressive strength is important in many restorative dental materials and accessory items used in dental technics and operations. This property is particularly important in the process of mastication because many of the forces of mastication are compressive. Compressive strength is most useful for comparing materials that are brittle and generally weak in tension and that as a result are not employed where tensile forces predominate. It is somewhat less useful to determine the compressive properties of ductile materials such as gold alloys. Compressive strength is therefore a useful property for the comparison of dental amalgam and cements and for determining the qualities of other materials such as plaster, investments, and some impression materials. Typical values of compressive strength of some restorative dental materials are given in Table 4-7.

Certain characteristics observed in materials subjected to tension are also observed when a material is in compression. For example, a stress-strain curve can be recorded for a material in compression similar to that obtained in tension. Such a curve represents a

TABLE 4-7 Compressive Strength of Some Restorative Dental Materials

Material	Compressive Strength MPa
Enamel	384
Amalgam	388
Dentin	297
Composite resin	277
Feldspathic porcelain	149
Zinc phosphate cement	117
High-strength stone	81
Calcium hydroxide liner	8

material that has both elastic and plastic characteristics when subjected to compressive stress although the plastic region is generally small. The modulus of elasticity of a material in compression can be determined from the ratio of the stress to the strain in the elastic region. Such a modulus value is usually similar for a material whether tested in compression or tension. A proportional limit or yield strength in compression can also be observed. The ultimate compressive strength is calculated from the original cross-sectional area of the sample and the maximum applied force in a similar manner to the ultimate tensile strength.

When a structure is subjected to compression, note that the failure of the body may occur as a result of complex stress formations in the body. This is illustrated by a cross-sectional view of a right cylinder subjected to compression as shown in Fig. 4-13. It is apparent from Fig. 4-13 that the forces of compression applied to each end of the sample are resolved into forces of shear along a cone-shaped area at each end and into tensile forces in the central portion of the mass as a result of the action of the two cones on the cylinder. Because of this resolution of forces in the body, it has become necessary to adopt standard sizes and dimensions to obtain reproducible test results. Fig. 4-13 shows that if a test sample is too short, the force distributions become more complicated as a result of the cone formations overlapping in the ends of the cylinder. If the sample is too long, buckling may occur. Therefore for the most satisfactory results, the cylinder should have a length approximately twice that of the diameter.

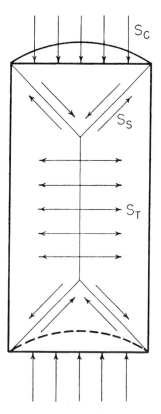

Fig. 4-13 Drawing of complex stress pattern developed in cylinder subjected to compressive stress.

Shear Strength

The shear strength is the maximum stress that a material can withstand before failure in a shear mode of loading. It is particularly important in the study of interfaces between two materials, such as a porcelain fused to metal restoration or an implant/tissue interface. One method of testing the shear strength of dental materials is the punch or push-out method, in which an axial load is applied to push one material through another. The shear strength (τ) is calculated by

$$\text{Shear strength}(\tau) = F/\pi dh$$

where F is the compressive force applied to the specimen, d is the diameter of the punch, and h is the thickness of the specimen. Note that the stress distribution caused by this method is not "pure" shear and that results often differ because of differences in specimen dimensions, surface geometry, composi-

TABLE 4-8 Values of Shear Strength Tested by the Punch Method for Some Restorative Dental Materials

Material	Shear Strength MPa
Amalgam	188
Dentin	138
Acrylic denture resin	122
Porcelain	111
Enamel	90
Zinc phosphate cement	13

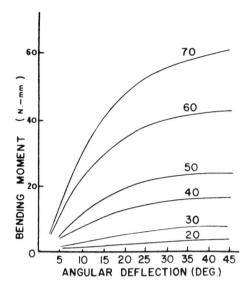

Fig. 4-14 Bending moment-angular deflection curves for endodontic reamers sizes 20 through 70.

tion and preparation, and mechanical testing procedure. However, it is a simple test to perform and has been used extensively. Alternatively, shear properties may be determined by subjecting a sample to torsional loading. Shear strengths of some dental materials are listed in Table 4-8.

Bond Strengths

A variety of tests have been developed to measure the bond strength between two materials such as porcelains to metal; cements to metal; and polymers, ceramics, resin composites, and adhesives to human enamel and dentin. Most of the tests are designed to place the bond in tension, although a few, especially for ceramics to metals, place the bond in shear. To simulate oral conditions, many of the test samples are subjected to numerous temperature cycles in water, ranging from 5° to 50° C, before measurement of the bond strength. These bond strength values may not simulate the clinical situation because of differences between the geometry of the test samples and the clinical application. Bond strength values typically overestimate the bond strength obtained in clinical usage and should therefore be viewed with caution.

Bending

The bending properties of many materials are equally as or more important than their tensile or compressive properties. The bending properties of stainless steel wires, endodontic files and reamers, and hypodermic needles are especially important. For example, both ANSI/ADA Specification No. 28 for endodontic files and reamers and No. 32 for orthodontic wires not containing precious metals require bending tests.

Bending properties are usually measured by clamping a sample at one end and applying a force at a fixed distance from the face of the clamp. Samples are subjected to conditions that resemble pure bending, and the cantilever beam theory has been used to analyze the data. As the force is increased and the sample is bent, corresponding values for the angle of bending and the bending moment (force × distance) are recorded. Graphic plots of the bending moment versus the angle of bending are similar in appearance to stress-strain curves. As an example, a series of plots for various sizes of endodontic reamers is shown in Fig. 4-14. An instrument will be permanently bent if the bending angle exceeds the value at the end of the linear portion of the curve. The larger instruments are stiffer, as shown by the initial steeper slope. The initial linear portion of the curve is shorter for the larger instruments and thus the deviation from linearity occurred at lower angular bends.

The maximum bending stress σ in a wire is

$$\sigma = My/I$$

where M is the bending moment, y is the distance from the neutral axis (plane of the sample, which is stress free) to the outer surface of sample, and I is

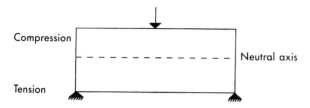

Fig. 4-15 Schematic of a three-point bending (transverse strength, flexural strength, modulus of rupture) test.

TABLE 4-9 Values of Transverse Strength for Some Restorative Dental Materials

Material	Transverse Strength MPa
Gold foil	292
Composite resin	139
Lathe-cut amalgam	124
Feldspathic porcelain	65
High-strength stone	17

the moment of inertia, which indicates the distribution of forces relative to the sample geometry.

The maximum angle of bending, θ_{max}, of a wire fixed at one end may be determined by the following formula:

$$\theta_{max} = Ml/EI$$

where l is the distance from the point of force application to the fixed end, and E is the modulus. For round wires with $l/d \sim 15$ and $l = 25$ mm, the elastic modulus in bending (also called modulus of stiffness) approximates the elastic modulus in tension. The equation is

$$E = (32\ l/\pi d^4)M/\theta$$

where l is the span length of the wire, d is the diameter of the wire, and M/θ is the slope of a plot of bending moment versus angular deflection in radians. The use of cantilever beam theory to calculate E results in values about two-thirds those determined in tension.

Transverse Strength

The transverse strength of a material is obtained when a load is applied in the middle of a simple beam, which is supported at each end (Fig. 4-15). Such a test is called a three-point bending (3PB) test, and transverse strength is often described in technical, dental, and engineering literature as the modulus of rupture (MOR) or flexure strength. The transverse strengths for several dental materials are shown in Table 4-9. The transverse strength test is especially useful in comparing denture base materials in which a stress of this type is applied to the denture during mastication. This test determines not only the strength of the material indicated, but also the amount of distortion expected. The transverse deflection test is a part of ANSI/ADA Specification No. 12 for denture base resins. The transverse

strength and accompanying deformation are important also in long bridge spans in which the biting stress may be severe.

The stresses and deflections in three-point bending can be determined as specific cases of the more general formulae presented in the last section. A beam having a rectangular cross section of width, b, and height, d, has a moment of inertia of

$$I = bd^3/12$$

For a load, P, applied in the center, the bending moment is

$$M = \frac{1}{4}Pl$$

Substituting these relations for I and M into the general equation $\sigma = My/I$, the equation for the maximum stress developed in a rectangular beam loaded in the center of the span becomes

$$\text{Stress} = \frac{3 \times \text{Load} \times \text{Length}}{2 \times \text{Width} \times \text{Thickness}^2}$$

or

$$\sigma = \frac{3Pl}{2bd^2}$$

The resulting deformation or displacement in such a beam or bridge can be calculated from

$$\text{Deformation} = \frac{\text{Load} \times \text{Length}^3}{4 \times \text{Elastic modulus} \times \text{Width} \times \text{Thickness}^3}$$

or

$$\delta = \frac{Pl^3}{4Ebd^3}$$

The significance of length, thickness, and width of the restoration in relation to the strength and deformation is evident from these formulae. Both the length and the thickness of the span are critical because the deformation varies as the cube of these two dimensions.

As a numerical example, consider a simple beam, such as the one shown in Fig. 4-15, with a rectangular cross section of 6.4 mm in thickness and 25.4 mm in height and a concentrated load of 666 N applied in the center. The total length of the beam is 102 mm, and the distance between the supports is 89 mm. Because this is a static situation (i.e., the beam does not move), the reactant forces at the supports in this symmetrical loading are 333 N each. The solution for this beam may be calculated as follows:

$$M = \frac{1}{4}\,Pl = \frac{1}{4} \times 666\ \text{N} \times 89\ \text{mm} = 14,800\ \text{mmN}$$

The moment of inertia is determined by

$$I = (6.4)(25.4)^3/12 = 8740\ \text{mm}^4$$

Thus at the lower surface of the beam, $y = 12.7$ mm and

$$\sigma = \frac{14,800\ \text{mmN} \times 12.7\ \text{mm}}{8740\ \text{mm}^4}$$

or 21.5 MPa. The lower surface of the beam is under a tensile stress of 21.5 MPa, and the upper surface is under a compressive stress of 21.5 MPa. The maximum deflection is

$$\frac{-PL^3}{48EI} = -0.36\ \text{mm}$$

The transverse strength of a beam can also be determined by the photoelastic method of analysis. A model of the simple beam used in this example is shown in Fig. 4-16, *A*. The isochromatic fringes, or lines of constant principle stress, are shown in Fig. 4-16, *A*, with the neutral axis, *NA*. The fringe order of the isochromatics is shown in Fig. 4-16, *B*, and the isotropic point can be seen in the center. Below the loading point and above the support points, the beam is in compression; in the center of the lower portion, the beam is in tension. Along any isochromatic fringe the difference in the principal stresses is constant, and the difference in the state of stress between fringes is 0.41 MPa/fringe.

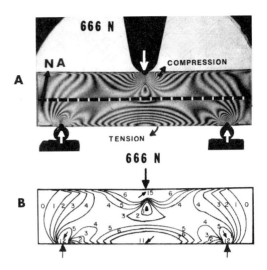

Fig. 4-16 Analysis of transverse bending. **A,** Photoelastic model with isochromatic fringes. **B,** Drawing to illustrate isochromatic fringe order.

Permanent Bending

During fabrication many dental restorations are subjected to permanent bending. The adjustment of removable partial denture clasps and the shaping of orthodontic appliances are two examples of such bending operations. Also bends are often introduced into hypodermic needles or root canal files in service. Comparisons of wires and needles of different compositions and diameters subjected to repeated 90-degree bends are often made. The number of bends a sample will withstand is influenced by its composition and dimensions, as well as its treatment in fabrication. Such tests are important because this information is not readily related to standard mechanical test data such as tensile properties or hardness.

Severe tensile and compressive stresses can be introduced into a material subjected to permanent bending. It is partly for this reason that tensile and compressive test data on a material are so important. Fig. 4-17 shows the internal structure of a segment of gold wire that was bent severely for purposes of adaptation. The outer portion of the bend was subjected to tensile stresses to the point of rupture. In the center of the wire, probably little or no stress developed during the bending, but the inner portion of the bend shows evidence of severe compression.

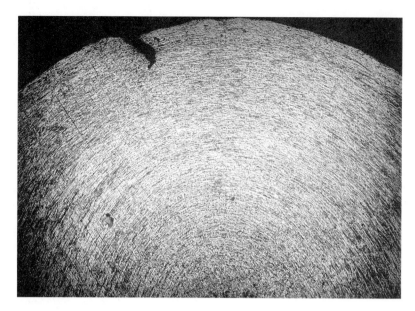

Fig. 4-17 Severe bend of gold wire showing evidence of tensile and compressive stress.

Torsion

Another mode of loading important to dentistry is torsion or twisting. When an endodontic file is clamped at the tip and the handle is rotated, the instrument is subjected to torsion. Because most endodontic files and reamers are rotated in the root canal during endodontic treatment, their properties in torsion are of particular interest. ANSI/ADA Specification No. 28 for endodontic files and reamers describes a test that uses a torque meter to measure resistance to fracture by twisting. Torsion results in a shear stress and a rotation of the sample. In these types of applications, we are interested in the relation between torsional moment (M_t = shear force × distance) and angular rotation π. A series of graphs in which torsional moment was measured as a function of the angular rotation is shown in Fig. 4-18. In this example, the instruments were twisted clockwise, which results in an untwisting of the instrument. As was the case with bending, the curves appear similar to stress-strain curves, with an initial linear portion followed by a nonlinear portion. The instruments should be used clinically so that they are not subjected to permanent angular rotation; thus the degrees of rotation should be limited to values within the linear portion of the torsional moment–angular rotation curves. The larger instruments are stiffer in torsion than the smaller sizes, but their linear portion is less. The irregular shape of

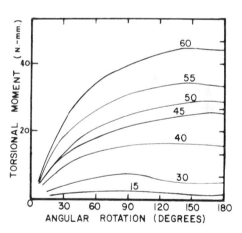

Fig. 4-18 Torsional moment-angular rotation curves for endodontic files sizes 15 through 60.

the curves at high angular rotation results from the untwisting of the instruments.

The resultant shear stress in a wire of radius r may be calculated from

$$\tau = M_t \times r/I_z$$

where I_z is the polar moment of inertia. The angular rotation may be calculated from

$$\phi = \frac{M_t L}{G I_z}$$

where L is the length of the shaft, and G is the shear modulus.

Fatigue Strength

Based on the previous discussions, a structure that has been subjected to a stress below the yield stress and subsequently relieved of this stress should return to its original form without any change in its internal structure or properties. It has been found that a few such applications of stress do not appreciably affect a material. However, when this stress is frequently repeated, the strength of the material may be drastically reduced and ultimately cause failure. Fatigue is defined as a progressive fracture under repeated loading. Fatigue tests are performed by subjecting a specimen to alternating stress applications below the yield stress until fracture occurs. Tensile, compressive, shear, bending, and torsional fatigue tests can all be performed.

The fatigue strength is the stress at which a material fails under repeated loading. Failure under repeated or cyclic loading is therefore dependent on the magnitude of the load and the number of loading repetitions. Fatigue data are often represented by an S-N curve, a curve depicting the stress (or strain) at which a material will fail as a function of the number of loading cycles. An example of such a curve is shown in Fig. 4-19. From this curve we see that when the stress is sufficiently high, the specimen will fracture at a relatively low number of cycles. As the stress is reduced, the number of cycles required to

cause failure increases. Therefore when specifying a fatigue strength, the number of cycles must also be specified. For some materials, a stress at which the sample can be loaded an infinite number of times without failing is eventually approached. This stress is called the endurance limit.

The determination of fatigue properties is of considerable importance for certain types of dental restorations subjected to alternating forces during mastication. Structures such as complete dentures, implants, and metal clasps of removable partial dentures, which are placed in the mouth by forcing the clasps over the teeth, are examples of restorations that undergo repeated loading. It has been estimated that alternate stress applications of the fatigue type occurring during mastication may amount to approximately 300,000 flexures per year, whereas the greater stress necessitated in removing restorations from the mouth or placing them in position probably amounts to less than 1500 per year. Because dental materials can be subjected to moderate stresses repeated a large number of times, it is important in the design of a restoration to know what stress it can withstand for a predetermined number of cycles. Restorations should be designed so that the in-service cyclic stresses are below the fatigue limit. Many gold cast alloys, for example, can withstand from 1 million to 25 million flexures without fracture when a stress below the yield stress is applied.

Fatigue fractures develop from small cracks and propagate through the grains of a material. In general, the causes of cyclic failure in a material are inhomogeneities and anisotropy of the material. These imperfections lead first to the development of microcracks, which coalesce, and ultimately lead to a macroscopic crack and failure. Areas of stress concentration, such as surface defects and notches, are particularly dangerous and can lead to catastrophic failure.

Fatigue properties do not always relate closely to other mechanical properties. Some parameters that influence fatigue are grain size and shape, composition, texture, surface chemistry and roughness, material history (i.e., fabrication and heat treatment), and environment. For example, in dental appliances made of resin, the internal stresses developed during the molding and processing tend to subject the structure to fatigue failure.

Note that the environment a material is subjected to is a critical factor in determining the fatigue proper-

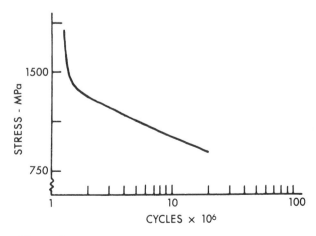

Fig. 4-19 Flexural fatigue curve for a cobalt-chromium-nickel alloy used for partial dentures.

ties. Any environmental agent that can degrade a material will reduce fatigue strength. Therefore elevated temperatures, humidity, aqueous media, biological substances, and pH deviations away from neutral can reduce fatigue properties. As a result, fatigue data, which are typically presented based on tests in laboratory air at room temperature, are not always relevant to the service conditions in the oral cavity. The higher temperature, humidity, saline environment with proteins, and fluctuating pH all tend to reduce fatigue strength from its level in the laboratory.

■ VISCOELASTICITY

In the previous discussions of the relationship between stress and strain, the effect of load application rate was not considered. In many brittle materials the effect is rather small. However, the rate of loading is important in many materials, particularly polymers and soft tissues. The mechanical properties of many dental materials, such as agar, alginate, and rubber impression materials, as well as amalgam, plastics, waxes, and dentin, oral mucosa, and periodontal ligaments, are dependent on how fast they are stressed. For these materials, increasing the loading (strain) rate produces a different stress-strain curve with higher rates giving higher values for the elastic modulus, proportional limit, and ultimate strength. Materials that have mechanical properties independent of loading rate are termed *elastic*. Materials that have mechanical properties dependent on loading rate are termed *viscoelastic*. In other words, these materials have characteristics of an elastic solid and a (viscous) fluid. The properties of an elastic solid were previously discussed in detail. Before viscoelastic materials and properties are presented, fluid behavior and viscosity are reviewed.

Fluid Behavior and Viscosity

In addition to the many solid dental materials that exhibit some fluid characteristics, many dental materials such as cements and impression materials are in the fluid state when formed. Therefore (viscous) fluid phenomena are important. Viscosity (η) is the resistance of a fluid to flow and is equal to the shear stress divided by the shear strain rate, or

$$\eta = \tau/[d\epsilon/dt]$$

When a cement or impression material sets, the viscosity increases, making it less viscous and more solid-like. The units of viscosity are poise, p, (1p = 1Pa-s = 1N-s/m), but often data are reported in centipoise, cp, (1cp = 100p). Some typical values of viscosity for dental materials are listed in Table 4-10. As a basis for comparison, the viscosity of water at 20° C is 1 cp.

Rearranging the equation for viscosity, we see that fluid behavior can be described in terms of stress and strain, just like elastic solids.

$$\tau = \eta[d\epsilon/dt]$$

In the case of an elastic solid, stress (σ) is proportional to strain (ϵ), with the constant of proportionality being the modulus of elasticity (E). The above equation indicates an analogous situation for a viscous fluid, where the (shear) stress is proportional to the strain rate, and the constant of proportionality is the viscosity. The stress is therefore time dependent, because it is a function of the strain rate, or rate of loading. To better comprehend the concept of strain rate dependence, consider two limiting cases—rapid and slow deformation. A material pulled extremely fast (dt→0) results in an infinitely high stress,

TABLE 4-10   Viscosity of Some Dental Materials Soon after Mixing

Material	Temperature (° C)	Viscosity (cp)
Cements		
Zinc phosphate	18	43,200
	25	94,700
Zinc polyacrylate	18	101,000
	25	109,800
Endodontic sealers	37	7000-678,000
Fluid denture resins	23	67-575
Impression materials		
Agar	45	281,000
Alginate	37	252,000
Impression plaster	37	23,800
Polysulfide, light	37	57,200
Polysulfide, heavy	36	1,360,000
Silicone, syringe	37	95,000
Silicone, regular	36	420,000
Zinc oxide–eugenol	37	99,600

whereas a material pulled infinitesimally slow results in a stress of zero.

The behavior of elastic solids and viscous fluids can be understood from simple mechanical models. An elastic solid can be viewed as a spring (Fig. 4-20). When the spring is stretched by a force, F, it displaces a distance, x. The applied force and resultant displacement are proportional, and the constant of proportionality is the spring constant, k. Therefore

$$F = k \times x$$

Note that this relation is equivalent to

$$\sigma = E \times \in$$

Also note that the model of an elastic element does not involve time. The spring acts instantaneously when stretched. In other words, an elastic solid is independent of loading rate.

A viscous fluid can be viewed as a dashpot, or a shock absorber with a damping fluid (Fig. 4-21). When the fluid-filled cylinder is pulled, the rate of straining ($d\in/dt$) is proportional to the stress (τ), and the constant of proportionality is the viscosity of the fluid (η).

Although the viscosity of a fluid is proportional to the shear rate, the proportionality differs for different fluids. Fluids may be classified as newtonian, pseudoplastic, or dilatant depending on how their viscosity varies with shear rate, as shown in Fig. 4-22. The viscosity of a newtonian liquid is constant and independent of shear rate. Certain dental cements and impression materials are newtonian. The viscosity of a pseudoplastic liquid decreases with increasing shear rate. Several endodontic cements are pseudoplastic, as are "single-mix" rubber impression materials. When subjected to low shear rates during spatulation or while an impression is made in a tray, these impression materials have a high viscosity and possess "body" in the tray. These materials, however, can also be used in a syringe, because at the higher shear rates encountered as they pass through the syringe tip, the viscosity decreases by as much as

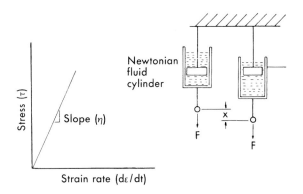

Fig. 4-21 Stress versus strain rate for a dashpot, which can be used to model the response of a viscous fluid. (From Park JB: *Biomaterials science and engineering,* New York, 1984, Plenum Press, p 26.)

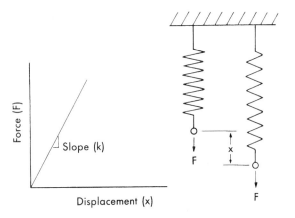

Fig. 4-20 Force versus displacement of a spring, which can be used to model the elastic response of a solid. (From Park JB: *Biomaterials science and engineering,* New York, 1984, Plenum Press, p 26.)

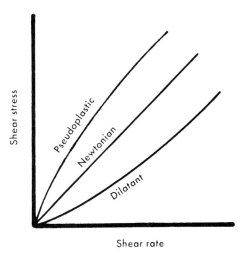

Fig. 4-22 Shear diagrams of newtonian, pseudoplastic, and dilatant liquids. The viscosity is shown by the slope of the curve at a given shear rate.

tenfold. The viscosity of a dilatant liquid increases with increasing shear rate. Examples of dilatant liquids in dentistry include the fluid denture-base resins.

Two additional factors that influence the viscosity of a material are time and temperature. The viscosity of a nonsetting liquid typically is independent of time and decreases with increasing temperature. Most dental materials, however, begin to set after the components have been mixed and their viscosity increases with time, as evidenced by most dental cements and impression materials. A notable exception is a zinc oxide–eugenol material that requires moisture to set. On the mixing pad these materials maintain a constant viscosity that is described clinically as a long working time. Once placed in the mouth, however, the zinc oxide–eugenol materials show rapid increases in viscosity because exposure to heat and humidity accelerates the setting reaction.

In general, for a material that sets, viscosity increases with increasing temperature. However, the effect of heat on the viscosity of a material that sets depends on the nature of the setting reaction. For example, the initial viscosities of a zinc phosphate cement (material *A*) and a zinc polycarboxylate cement (material *B*) are compared at three temperatures in Fig. 4-23. The setting reaction of *A* is highly exothermic, and mixing at reduced temperatures results in a lower viscosity than when mixed at higher temperatures. The setting reaction of *B* is less affected by temperature. Clinically, additional working time is achieved for these cements by the use of cool- or frozen-slab mixing technics.

Viscoelastic Materials

For viscoelastic materials, altering the strain rate alters the stress-strain properties. The tear strength of alginate impression material, for example, is increased about four times when the rate of loading is increased from 2.5 to 25 cm/min. Another example of strain rate dependence is the elastic modulus of dental amalgam, which is 21 GPa at slow rates of loading and 62 GPa at high rates of loading. A viscoelastic material, therefore, may have widely different mechanical properties depending on the rate of load application, and for these materials it is particularly important to specify the loading rate with the test results.

Materials that have properties that are dependent on the strain rate are better characterized by relating stress or strain as a function of time. Two properties of importance to viscoelastic materials are stress

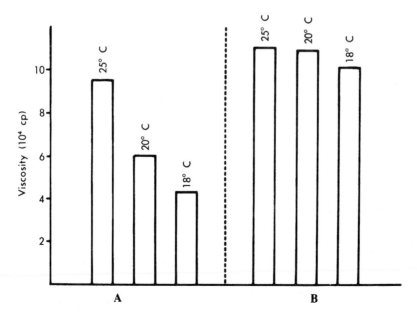

Fig. 4-23 Changes in initial viscosity with temperature of **A,** a zinc phosphate cement, and **B,** a zinc polycarboxylate cement. (Adapted from Vermilyea S, Powers JM, Craig RG: *J Dent Res* 56:762, 1977.)

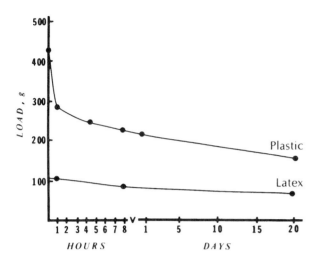

Fig. 4-24 Decrease in load of latex rubber and plastic bands as a function of time at a constant extension of 95 mm. (From Craig RG, ed: *Dental materials: a problem-oriented approach,* St Louis, 1978, Mosby.)

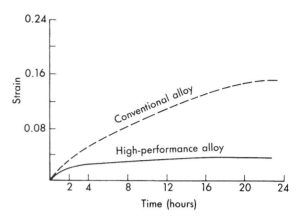

Fig. 4-25 Creep curves for conventional (low copper) and high-performance (high copper) amalgams. (From O'Brien WJ: *Dental materials properties and selection,* Chicago, 1989, Quintessence, p 25.)

relaxation and creep. Stress relaxation is the reduction in stress in a material subjected to constant strain, whereas creep is the increase in strain in a material under constant stress.

As an example of stress relaxation, consider how the load-time curves at constant deformation are important in the evaluation of orthodontic elastic bands. The decrease in load (or force) with time for a latex and a plastic band of the same size at a constant extension of 95 mm is shown in Fig. 4-24. The initial force was much greater with the plastic band, but the decrease in force with time was much less for the latex band. Therefore plastic bands are useful for applying high forces, although the force decreases rapidly with time; latex bands apply lower forces, but the force decreases slowly with time in the mouth, and these bands are useful for applying more sustained loads.

The importance of creep can be seen by interpreting the data in Fig. 4-25. In the figure, creep curves for low- and high-copper amalgam are shown. For a given load, at a given time, the low-copper amalgam has a greater strain. The implications and clinical importance of this are that the greater creep in the low-copper amalgam makes it more susceptible to strain accumulation and fracture, and also marginal breakdown, which can lead to secondary decay.

Mechanical Models of Viscoelasticity

Because a viscoelastic material may be viewed as a material exhibiting behavior characteristic of both a solid and a fluid, we may also understand the behavior of a viscoelastic material in terms of combinations of the simple mechanical models of a spring and dashpot, introduced previously. Strain as a function of time for the various combinations is shown in Fig. 4-26. When a constant load is applied (at time t_0) to a spring (an ideal elastic element), an instantaneous strain occurs and the strain remains constant with time; when the load is removed (at time t_1), the strain instantaneously decreases to zero. When a constant load is applied to an ideal viscous element, the strain increases linearly with time, and when the load is removed, no further increase or decrease in strain is observed. The elastic element reacts instantaneously (changes strain) to a change in load, and the viscous element reacts after a finite time.

The relative time-course of spring and dashpot reactions is observed when the two ideal elements are combined. When a spring and viscous element are in series (a Maxwell model), and a fixed load is applied, a rapid increase in strain occurs and is followed by a linear increase in strain with time. The resultant strain, frequently referred to as the viscoelastic strain, represents a combination of elastic and viscous responses. The rapid increase in strain represents the elastic portion of the strain (i.e., response of the

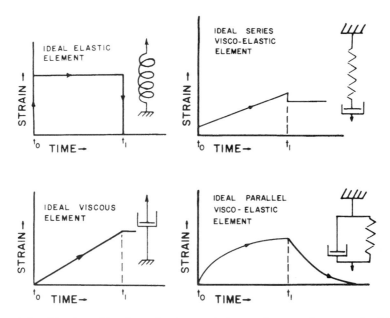

Fig. 4-26 Strain-time relationship of combinations of springs and viscous elements. A constant load is applied at time t_0 and removed at time t_1.

elastic spring), whereas the linear increase represents the viscous portion of the strain (i.e., response of the viscous component). When the load is removed an instantaneous recovery of the elastic strain occurs, but the viscous strain remains.

A constant load applied to a spring and viscous element in parallel (a Kelvin or Voigt model) causes a nonlinear increase in strain with time as a result of the viscous element and reaches a constant value as a result of the spring. On removal of the load, the spring acts to decrease the strain to zero. However, the strain does not instantaneously diminish to zero because of the action of the dashpot. Note, also, that real materials exhibit more complex behavior than these simple models predict, and modeling the strain-time properties requires a combination of the elements described. Impression materials such as agar, alginate, polysulfide, and silicone have been modeled by a Maxwell model in series with a Kelvin model.

An example of the importance of viscoelasticity lies with impression materials. Because these materials are viscoelastic, they do not immediately lose their strain when a load is removed. Therefore on removal from the mouth, these materials remain stressed, and thus time is required for the material to recover before a die can be poured.

The viscoelasticity of the oral tissues also has important clinical implications. Experiments on monkeys have shown that the palatal mucosa has little resistance to loading compared with the periodontal ligament. Thus denture baseplates supported by palatal mucosa show substantially more displacement as a function of load than those supported by teeth (Fig. 4-27). The creep of the palatal mucosa under load is sustained and recovery is prolonged and variable because the mechanism of deformation and recovery is controlled by physiological and physical factors. Making an impression of the mucosal tissues in their resting state therefore requires that the tissues be allowed to recover free of the denture for several hours. Teeth, on the other hand, will recover from load within minutes. Recording the mucosal tissues under load will result in recoil of these tissues, initially displacing the denture base and artificial teeth to a position superior to the natural teeth. However, the tissues will return to their displaced state on loading of the denture.

Creep Compliance

A creep curve yields insight into the relative elastic, viscous, and anelastic response of a viscoelastic material, and such curves can be interpreted in terms

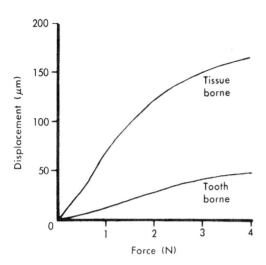

Fig. 4-27 Displacement versus force for denture baseplates supported by six teeth and by mucosa alone. Loading rate was 4 N/sec. (Adapted from Wills DJ, Manderson RD: *J Dent* 5:310, 1977.)

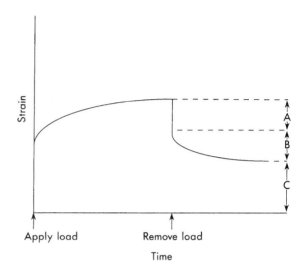

Fig. 4-28 Creep recovery curve, showing *A,* elastic, *B,* anelastic, and *C,* viscous strain.

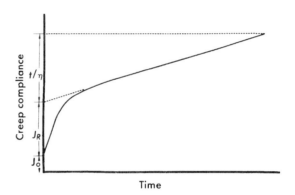

Fig. 4-29 Creep compliance versus time for a viscoelastic material. (Adapted from Duran RL, Powers JM, Craig RG: *J Dent Res* 58:1801, 1979.)

of the molecular structure of the associated materials, which have structures that function as elastic, viscous, and anelastic elements. On removal of a load a creep recovery curve can be obtained (Fig. 4-28). In such a curve, after the load is removed, there is an instantaneous drop in strain and a slower strain decay to some steady state strain value, which may be nonzero. The instantaneous drop in strain represents the recovery of elastic strain. The slower recovery represents the anelastic strain, and the remaining, permanent strain represents the viscous strain. A family of creep curves can be determined by using different loads. A more useful way of presenting these data is by calculating the creep compliance. Creep compliance (J_t) is defined as the strain divided by the stress at a given time. Once a creep curve is obtained, a corresponding creep compliance curve can be calculated. The creep compliance curve shown in Fig. 4-29 is characterized by the equation

$$J_t = J_0 + J_R + (t/\eta)$$

where J_0 is the instantaneous elastic compliance, J_R is the retarded elastic (anelastic) compliance, and t/η represents the viscous response at time t for a viscosity η. The strain associated with J_0 and J_R is completely recoverable after the load is removed; how-

ever, the strain associated with J_R is not recovered immediately but requires some finite time. The strain associated with t/η is not recovered and represents a permanent deformation. If a single creep compliance curve is calculated from a family of creep curves determined at different loads, the material is said to be linearly viscoelastic. The viscoelastic qualities can be described concisely by a single curve.

The creep compliance curve therefore permits an estimate of the relative amount of elastic, anelastic and viscous behavior of a material. J_0 indicates the flexibility and initial recovery after deformation, J_R the amount of delayed recovery that can be

TABLE 4-11   Values of Dynamic Modulus and Dynamic Resilience as a Function of Temperature for Some Dental Elastomers

Material	Temperature (° C)	Dynamic Modulus MPa	Dynamic Resilience (%)
Maxillofacial materials			
Polyurethane	−15	5.98	15.0
	37	3.06	19.9
Polyvinylchloride	−15	12.2	6.0
	37	2.51	19.6
Silicone	−15	2.84	16.0
	37	2.36	23.2
Polyvinylacetate-polyethylene mouth protectors			
New	37	9.39	23.4
Worn	37	7.23	20.2

expected, and t/η the magnitude of permanent deformation to be expected. Creep compliance curves for rubber impression materials are shown in Chapter 11.

■ DYNAMIC MECHANICAL PROPERTIES

Although static properties frequently can be related to the function of a material under dynamic conditions, there are limitations to using the static properties to estimate the properties of materials subjected to dynamic loading. Static testing refers to continuous application of force at slow rates of loading, whereas dynamic testing involves cyclic loading or loading at high rates (commonly referred to as impact). Dynamic methods including a forced oscillation technic, used for determining dynamic modulus, and a torsion pendulum, used for impact testing, have been used to study viscoelastic materials such as dental polymers. Ultrasonic technics have been used to determine elastic constants of viscoelastic materials such as dental amalgam and dentin. Impact testing has been applied primarily to brittle dental materials.

Dynamic Modulus

The dynamic modulus (E_D) is defined as the ratio of stress to strain for small cyclical deformations at a given frequency and at a particular point on the stress-strain curve. When measured in a forced oscillation instrument, the dynamic modulus is computed by

$$E_D = mqp^2$$

where m is the mass of the vibrating yoke, q is the height divided by twice the area of the cylindrical specimen, and p is the angular frequency of the vibrations.

In conjunction with the dynamic modulus, values of the internal friction and dynamic resilience can be determined. Cyclical stretching or compression of an elastomer results in irreversibly lost energy that manifests itself as heat. The internal friction of an elastomer is comparable with the viscosity of a liquid. The value of internal friction is necessary to calculate the dynamic resilience, which is the ratio of energy lost to energy expended.

The dynamic modulus and dynamic resilience of some dental elastomers are listed in Table 4-11. These properties are affected by temperature (−15° to 37° C) for some maxillofacial elastomers, such as plasticized polyvinylchloride and polyurethane, but not so much for silicones. As shown in Table 4-11 the dynamic modulus decreases and the dynamic resilience increases as the temperature increases. As a tangible example, the dynamic resilience of a polymer used for an athletic mouth protector is a measure of the ability of the material to absorb energy from a blow and thereby protect the oral structure. Once the mouth protector has been worn, however, a deterioration in properties is observed compared with the properties before the material was exposed to the oral environment.

Impact Strength

A material may have reasonably high static strength values, such as compressive, tensile, and shear strengths, and even reasonable elongation, but may fail when loaded under impact. Materials such as fused glasses, cements, amalgam, and some plastics have low resistance to breakage when a load is applied by an impact. Such a sudden blow might correspond to the energy of impact resulting from an accident to a person wearing a restoration or from dropping the restoration on a floor.

The impact resistance of materials is determined from the total energy absorbed before fracture when struck by a sudden blow. Often a bar of material is supported as a beam and struck either at one end or in the middle with a weighted pendulum. A test sample in an impact instrument is shown in Fig. 4-30. The energy absorbed by the blow can be determined by measuring of the reduction in swing of the pendulum compared with the swing with no sample present. The values are usually reported in joules, J (1J = 1Nm) for a sample of a specific shape. Some substances offer relatively little resistance to the shock, whereas others of different composition may not fracture under the same impact. For example, the Charpy impact strength of unnotched specimens of denture resins ranges from 0.26 J for a conventional denture acrylic to 0.58 J for a rubber-modified acrylic resin.

■ TEAR STRENGTH AND TEAR ENERGY

Tear strength is a measure of the resistance of a material to tearing forces. Tear strength is an important property of dental polymers used in thin sections, such as flexible impression materials in interproximal areas, maxillofacial materials, and soft liners for dentures. Specimens are usually crescent shaped and notched. The tear strength of the notched specimen is calculated when the maximum load is divided by the thickness of the specimen and the unit of tear strength is N/m.

Tear strength depends on the rate of loading because of the viscoelastic nature of the materials tested. More rapid loading rates result in higher values of tear strength. Clinically, the rapid (or snap) removal of an alginate impression is recommended to maximize the tear strength and also to minimize permanent deformation. Typical values of tear strength are listed in Table 4-12 for some dental materials. The table indicates that the rubber impression materials have superior values of tear strength compared with agar and alginate hydrocolloids.

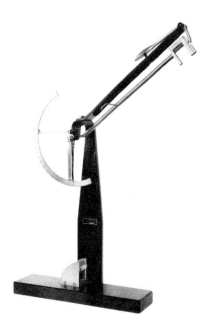

Fig. 4-30 Impact-testing instrument.

TABLE 4-12   Tear Strength of Some Dental Materials

Material	Tear Strength* kN/m
Agar duplicating material	0.22
Denture liners	2.6-45
Impression materials	
Agar	0.99
Alginate	0.47
Polysulfide	4.0
Polyvinylacetate-polyethylene mouth protectors	114

*Crosshead speed, 25 cm/min.

The tear energy (T) is a measure of the energy per unit area of newly torn surface and is determined from the load (F) required to propagate a tear in a trouser-shaped specimen by

$$T = (F/t)(\lambda + 1)$$

where t is the sample thickness and λ is an extension ratio. Typical values of tear energy determined for some dental impression materials and maxillofacial materials are listed in Table 4-13.

■ MECHANICAL PROPERTIES OF COMPOSITES

Many materials used in dentistry are not homogeneous solids but consist of two or more essentially insoluble phases. There may be one continuous phase and one or more dispersed phases, or there may be two or more continuous phases, with each of these phases containing one or more dispersed phases. These materials are called composites. A composite can be generally defined as a combination of two or more different materials, still present as separate entities in the final material. The materials are combined to take advantage of selected properties of each individual material in the final material, and the physical and mechanical properties of the composites are different from those of the separate phases. The trend in the development of materials for various applications is toward composites rather than completely new classes of materials. There can be metal, ceramic, and polymer-based

TABLE 4-13 Tear Energy of Some Dental Materials

Material	Tear Energy* (J/m^2 [Mergs/cm^2])	
Impression materials		
Alginate	66	[0.066]
Polyether	640	[0.64]
Polysulfide	1100-3000	[1.1-3.0]
Silicone	390-1150	[0.39-1.15]
Maxillofacial materials		
Polyurethane	1800	[1.8]
Polyvinylchloride	11,000	[11]
Silicone rubber	660	[0.66]

*Crosshead speed, 2 cm/min.

composites. Important examples of dental composites include posterior composite resins used as direct esthetic restorative materials. Such composites are made from an organic polymer matrix (usually a diacrylate) filled with an inorganic phase, such as quartz, borosilicate or strontium glass, lithium or barium, aluminum silicate, or colloidal silica.

Factors that affect the properties of composites include: (1) the state of matter of the second (dispersed) phase; (2) the geometry of the second phase; (3) the orientation of the second phase; (4) the composition of the dispersed and continuous phases; (5) the ratio of the phases; and (6) bonding of the phases. Examples of properties that can be changed (improved if the composites are judiciously developed) are (1) modulus, (2) strength, (3) fracture toughness, (4) abrasion resistance, (5) thermal expansion, and (6) chemical and corrosion resistance.

A simple example of how adding a second phase affects properties is now illustrated. Consider a series of continuous parallel glass fibers all oriented in the same direction in a plastic matrix. If a tensile load is applied to the sample in the direction of the fibers, the elastic modulus of the composite E_c is

$$E_c = E_f V_f + E_m V_m \text{ or } E_f V_f + E_m (1 - V_f)$$

where E_f, E_m, V_f, and V_m represent the elastic modulus and volume fraction of the fiber and matrix. If, on the other hand, the tensile load is applied in the direction transverse to the fibers, the composite elastic modulus would be

$$E_c = \frac{E_f E_m}{E_m E_f + E_f V_m}$$

If the volume fraction of fibers is zero (i.e., the material is strictly a polymer), the modulus is that of the polymer, and if the volume fraction is 100%, the material is a glass and has the modulus of glass. Thus, the moduli of the polymer and glass serve as lower and upper bounds on the composite modulus. Furthermore, from the above two equations, we see that in addition to the ratio of the two phases, the orientation of the second phase also plays an important role in the composite properties.

The basis for the function of a dispersed phase in a matrix is shown in Fig. 4-31. A single fiber is shown surrounded by a matrix, and the tensile stress in the fiber is plotted versus the distance along the fiber. The load is applied to the matrix and is

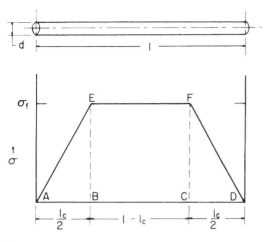

Fig. 4-31 Stress on a glass fiber in a plastic matrix. (Adapted from Titelman AS, McEvily AJ, Jr: *Fracture of structural materials,* New York, 1967, John Wiley & Sons, pp 635-661.)

transferred to the fiber by shear at the interface. The elastic and plastic deformation in the matrix can be transferred to the fiber if the modulus of the matrix is less than that of the fiber. Also, the bond between the matrix and the fiber must be maintained or the stress will drop to the frictional force. As the load is increased, the tensile stress in the fiber may reach the ultimate shear stress and the fiber will fail.

Continually increasing the volume fraction of the fibers should continue to increase the strength of the composite. However, as the concentration of fibers increases, more and more contact of the fibers with each other occurs, and premature rupture results. Therefore for many composites the maximum strength occurs at a volume fraction of 60% for the dispersed phase.

As a further illustration of the factors that effect the properties of a composite, consider the filled polymer resins used in dentistry. For many of these dental composites a random arrangement of the dispersed phase is used, even though a random orientation results in about a sixfold lower strength compared to an oriented dispersed phase. However, the resultant lower strength due to random second phase orientation can be counteracted in several ways. The use of a fine (e.g., < 3 μm) dispersed phase increases strength. Also, the selection of the shape of the dispersed particles is important, with rods and plates being more effective than spheres in improving the strength. The principal factors needed are (1) a high-

strength dispersed phase; (2) a more ductile matrix phase; (3) fine dispersed particles at the optimum volume fraction; and (4) adhesion between the dispersed and matrix phases. The last requirement is usually accomplished by treating the dispersed phase with an organosilane. The silanes, often called coupling agents, react with the glass or water adsorbed on the glass and form a bond with the resin.

■ SURFACE MECHANICAL PROPERTIES

In our discussion so far, we have discussed mechanical properties that are mainly dependent on the bulk characteristics of a material. In this section, mechanical properties that are more a function of the surface condition of a material are presented. In particular, the concepts of hardness, friction, and wear are summarized.

Indentation Hardness

The property of hardness is of major importance in the comparison of restorative materials. Hardness may be broadly defined as the resistance to permanent surface indentation or penetration. Formulating a more rigorous definition of hardness is difficult because any test method will, at a microscopic level, involve complex surface morphologies and stresses in the test material, thereby involving a variety of qualities in any single hardness test. Despite this condition, the most common concept of hard and soft substances is their relative resistance to indentation. Hardness is therefore a measure of the resistance to plastic deformation and is measured as a force per unit area of indentation (Fig. 4-32).

Based on this definition of hardness, it is clear why this property is so important to dentistry. Hardness is indicative of the ease of finishing of a structure and its resistance to in-service scratching. Finishing or polishing a structure is important for esthetic purposes and, as discussed previously, scratches can compromise fatigue strength and lead to premature failure.

Some of the most common methods of testing the hardness of restorative materials are the Brinell, Knoop, Vickers, Rockwell, and Shore A hardness tests. Each of these tests differs slightly from the others, and each presents certain advantages and disadvantages. They have a common quality, however, in

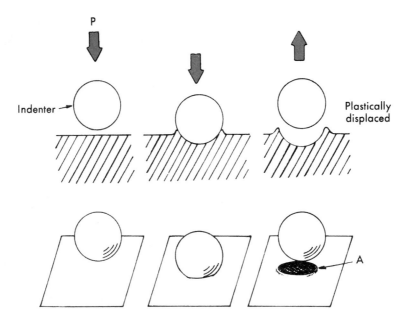

Fig. 4-32 Schematic representation of a hardness test. (From Park JB: *Biomaterials science and engineering,* New York, 1984, Plenum Press, p 18.)

that each depends on the penetration of some small, symmetrically shaped indenter into the surface of the material being tested. The various hardness tests differ in the indenter material, geometry, and load. The indenter may be made of steel, tungsten carbide, or diamond and be shaped as a sphere, cone, or pyramid. Loads typically range from 1 to 3000 kg. The choice of a hardness test depends on the material of interest, the expected hardness range and the desired degree of localization.

The general procedure for testing hardness, independent of the specific test, is as follows. A standardized force or weight is applied to the penetrating point. Such a force application to the indenter produces a symmetrically shaped indentation, which can be measured under a microscope for depth, area, or width of the indentation produced. The indentation dimensions are then related to tabulated hardness values. With a fixed load applied to a standardized indenter, the dimensions of the indentation vary inversely with the resistance to penetration of the material tested. Thus lighter loads are needed for softer materials.

Brinell hardness test

The Brinell hardness test is among the oldest methods used to test metals and alloys used in den-

tistry. The method depends on the resistance to the penetration of a small steel or tungsten carbide ball, typically 1.6 mm in diameter, when subjected to a weight of 123 N. In testing the Brinell hardness of a material, the penetrator remains in contact with the sample tested for a fixed time of 30 seconds, after which it is removed and the indentation diameter is carefully measured. A diagram showing the principle of Brinell hardness testing, together with a microscopic view of the indentations into a gold alloy, is shown in Fig. 4-33. The resulting hardness value, known as the Brinell hardness number (BHN), is computed as a ratio of the load applied to the area of the indentation produced. The formula for computing the BHN is as follows:

$$BHN = \frac{L}{\frac{\pi D}{2}\left(D - \sqrt{D^2 - d^2}\right)}$$

In this formula L is the load in kilograms, D is the diameter of the ball in millimeters, and d is the diameter of the indentation in millimeters, thus the units for BHN are kg/mm^2. The smaller the area of indentation, the harder the material and the larger the BHN value. Tables of Brinell hardness values have been developed from this formula for indentations of

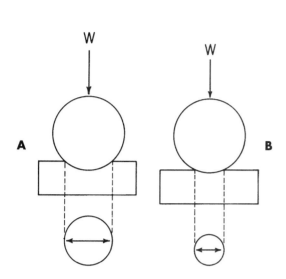

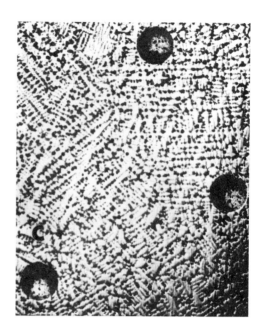

Fig. 4-33 Brinell hardness test. **A,** Indentation in soft material. **B,** Indentation in harder material. **C,** Microscopic view of indentations.

different diameters. The Brinell hardness test yields a relatively large indentation area, and as a result, this test is good for determining average hardness values and poor for determining very localized values. The Brinell hardnesses of some dental casting alloys and condensed gold are listed in Table 4-14.

Knoop hardness test

The Knoop hardness test was developed to fulfill the needs of a microindentation test method. A load is applied to a carefully prepared diamond indenting tool with a pyramid shape, and the lengths of the diagonals of the resulting indentation in the material are measured. The shape of the indenter and the resulting indentation are illustrated in Fig. 4-34, *A.* The Knoop hardness number (KHN) is the ratio of the load applied to the area of the indentation calculated from the following formula:

$$KHN = \frac{L}{l^2 C_p}$$

In this equation L is the load applied, l is the length of the long diagonal of the indentation, and C_p is a constant relating l to the projected area of the indentation. The units for KHN are also kg/mm^2.

TABLE 4-14 Brinell Hardness Number (BHN) of Some Dental Casting Alloys and Condensed Gold

Material	BHN (kg/mm^2)
Condensed gold	
Foil	69
Powdered	46
Gold alloys*	
Type I	45
Type II	95
Type III	120
Type IV	220
40% Au-Ag-Cu	252
99% noble alloy†	165

*Alloys that are hardenable by heat treatment are in the hard condition.
†For metal-ceramic restorations.

Similar to the Brinell method, higher values for KHN represent harder materials.

The Knoop method is designed so that varying loads may be applied to the indenting instrument. The resulting indentation area therefore varies according to the load applied as well as to the nature

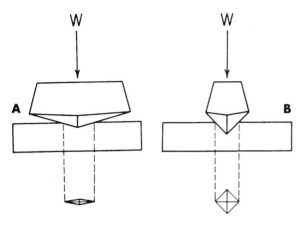

Fig. 4-34 Principle of the Knoop hardness measurement, **A**, and the diamond pyramid (Vickers) indentation test, **B**.

TABLE 4-15   Knoop Hardness Number (KHN) of Dental Materials

Material	KHN (kg/mm²)
Silicon carbide abrasive	2480
Feldspathic porcelain	460
Cobalt-chromium partial denture alloy	391
Enamel	343
Gold foil	69
Dentin	68
Cementum	40
Zinc phosphate cement	38
Denture acrylic	21

of the material tested. The advantage of this method is that materials can be tested with a great range of hardness simply by varying the test load. Because very light load applications produce extremely delicate microindentations, this method of testing can be employed to examine materials that vary in area hardness. For example, the Knoop method has been used extensively in testing the hardness of both enamel and dentin in extracted teeth and in determining the hardness of metals and alloys that have isolated hard and soft phases throughout the material. The chief disadvantages of the method are the need for a highly polished and flat test sample and the time required to complete the test operation, which is considerably greater than that required for some other, less precisely controlled methods. The KHNs of some dental materials are listed in Table 4-15.

Vickers hardness test

The 136-degree diamond pyramid, or Vickers hardness test, is also suitable for testing the surface hardness of materials. It has been used to a limited degree as a means of testing the hardness of restorative dental materials. The method is similar in principle to the Knoop and Brinell tests except that a 136-degree diamond pyramid-shaped indenter is forced into the material with a definite load application. The indenter produces a square indentation, the diagonals of which are measured as shown in Fig. 4-34, *B*. Equipment for Knoop hardness testing has been adapted to use the 136-degree indenter.

Loads are varied from 1 to 120 kg, depending on the hardness of the tested material. The Vickers test is especially useful in measuring the hardness of small areas and for very hard materials.

Rockwell hardness test

The Rockwell hardness test was developed as a rapid method for hardness determinations. A ball or metal cone indenter is normally used, and the depth of the indentation is measured with a sensitive dial micrometer. The indenter balls or cones are of several different diameters, as well as different load applications (60 to 150 kg), with each combination described as a special Rockwell scale, Rockwell A-G, denoted R_A, R_B, etc.

The superficial Rockwell method has been used to test plastics used in dentistry. This method uses a relatively light (30 kg) load and a large-diameter (12.7 mm) ball in comparison with the standard Rockwell methods. The test is made by first applying a preload (minor load) of 3 kg. A major load of 30 kg then is applied to the sample for 10 minutes before a reading is taken. Because dental plastics are viscoelastic, recovery of the indentation occurs once the major load has been removed. The percent recovery can be determined on the same specimen by the following equation:

$$\text{Percent recovery} = \frac{A - B}{A} \times 100\%$$

where *A* is the depth of the indentation caused by application of the major load for 10 minutes, and *B*

TABLE 4-16 Indentation Depth and Percent Recovery of Some Dental Plastics

Material	Indentation Depth (μm)	% Recovery
Unfilled restorative resin	113	74
Acrylic denture teeth	93	88
Pit and fissure sealants	85-158	74-86
Composite resin	56-72	70-83

TABLE 4-17 Values of Shore A Hardness for Some Dental Materials

Material	Shore A Hardness
Resilient denture liners	48-85
Polyvinylacetate-polyethylene mouth protector	67
Silicone maxillofacial elastomer	25

is the depth of the indentation after the major load has been removed for 10 minutes. Values of indentation depth and percent recovery for some dental plastics are listed in Table 4-16. The advantages of the Rockwell hardness test are that hardness is read directly and it is good for testing viscoelastic materials. The disadvantages are that a preload is needed, greater time is required, and the indentation may disappear immediately when the load is removed.

Shore A hardness

The hardness measurements described previously cannot be used to determine the hardness of rubbers because the indentation disappears after the removal of the load. An instrument called a Shore A Durometer is used in the rubber industry to determine the relative hardness of elastomers. The instrument consists of a blunt-pointed indenter 0.8 mm in diameter that tapers to a cylinder 1.6 mm. The indenter is attached by a lever to a scale that is graduated from 0 to 100 units. If the indenter completely penetrates the sample, a reading of 0 is obtained, and if no penetration occurs, a reading of 100 units results. Because rubber is viscoelastic, an accurate reading is difficult to obtain because the indenter continues to penetrate the rubber as a function of time. The usual method is to press down firmly and quickly on the indenter and record the maximum reading as the Shore A hardness. The test has been used to evaluate soft denture liners, mouth protectors, and maxillofacial elastomers, values of which are listed in Table 4-17.

Friction

Friction is the resistance to motion of one material body over another. If an attempt is made to

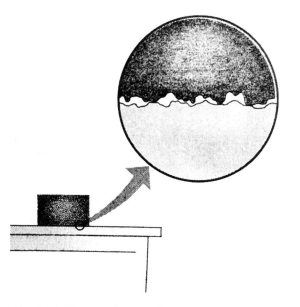

Fig. 4-35 Microscopic area of contact between two objects. The frictional force, which resists motion, is proportional to the normal force and the coefficient of friction. (Adapted from Tipler PA: *Physics*, 1976, Worth, p 156.)

move one body over the surface of another, a restraining force to resist motion is produced (Fig. 4-35). This restraining force is the (static) frictional force and results from the molecules of the two objects bonding where their surfaces are in close contact. The frictional force, F_s, is proportional to the normal force $(F_\perp)$ between the surfaces and the (static) coefficient of friction (μ_s).

$$F_s = \mu_s \times F_\perp$$

The coefficient of friction varies between 0 and 1 and is a function of the two materials in contact, their composition, surface finish, and lubrication. Similar materials have a greater coefficient of friction, and if a lubricating medium exists at the interface, the coefficient of friction is reduced.

The conditions for motion are for the applied force to be greater than F_s.

Once motion occurs, molecular bonds are made and broken, and microscopic pieces break off from the surfaces. With motion, a sliding or kinetic friction is produced, and the force of kinetic friction opposes the motion.

$$F_k = \mu_k \times F_\perp$$

Frictional behavior therefore arises from surfaces that, because of microroughness, have a small real contact area (Fig. 4-35). These small surface areas result in high contact stresses, which lead to local yielding. The resistance to shear failure of the junctions results in the frictional force. When static friction is overcome and relative motion takes place, it is accompanied by the modification of the interface through kinetic friction and wear.

An example of the importance of friction in dentistry lies in the concept of roughening the surface of a dental implant to reduce motion between the implant and adjacent tissue. It is perceived that a rough surface and resultant less motion will provide better osseointegration.

Wear

Wear is a loss of material resulting from removal and relocation of materials through the contact of two or more materials. When two solid materials are in contact, they only touch at the tips of their highest asperities (Fig. 4-35). Wear is usually undesirable, but under controlled conditions during finishing and polishing procedures, wear is highly beneficial.

Several factors make wear of biomaterials unique. Most importantly, wear can produce biologically active particles, which can excite an inflammatory response. The wear process can also produce shape changes that can affect function. For example, wear in the oral cavity is characterized by the loss of the original anatomical form of the material. Wear of tooth structure and restorative materials may result from mechanical, physiological, or pathological conditions. Normal mastication may cause attrition of tooth structure or materials, particularly in populations that consume unprocessed foods. Bruxism is an example of a pathological form of wear in which opposing surfaces slide against each other. If improperly performed, toothbrushing with dentifrices may cause an abrasive form of wear.

Wear is a function of a number of material and environmental factors, including the nature of wearing surfaces (i.e., inhomogeneity, crystal orientation, phases, and inclusions present); the microscopic contact; interaction between sliding surfaces (i.e., elevated stress, temperature, and flow at contact points, leading to localized yielding, melting, and hardening); lubrication; and different material combinations. In general, wear is a function of both opposing materials and the interface between them. The presence of a lubricating film, such as saliva, separates surfaces during relative motion and reduces frictional forces and wear.

In general, there are four types of wear: (1) adhesive wear; (2) corrosive wear; (3) surface fatigue wear; and (4) abrasive wear. Adhesive wear is characterized by the formation and disruption of microjunctions. The volume of wear debris, V, is determined by

$$V = \frac{kF_\perp x}{3p}$$

where x is the total sliding distance, k is the wear coefficient, $F_\perp$ is the perpendicular force, and p is the surface hardness (of the softer material).

Abrasive wear involves a soft surface in contact with a harder surface. In this type of wear, particles are pulled off of one surface and adhere to the other during sliding. There can be two types of abrasive wear—two- and three-body abrasion (wear). This type of wear can be minimized if surfaces are smooth and hard and if particles are kept off the surfaces. Corrosive wear is secondary to physical removal of a protective layer and is therefore related to the chemical activity of the wear surfaces. The sliding action of the surfaces removes any surface barriers and causes accelerated corrosion. In surface fatigue wear, stresses are produced by asperities or free particles, leading to the formation of surface or subsurface cracks. Particles break off under cyclic loading and sliding.

In general, metals are susceptible to adhesive, corrosive and three-body wear, whereas polymers are susceptible to abrasive and fatigue wear.

Wear has been studied by (1) service or clinical testing, (2) simulated service measurements, (3) model systems using various wear machines, (4) measurements of related mechanical properties such as hardness, and (5) examination of the amount and type of surface failure from a single or low number of sliding strokes.

Two-body abrasion tests have been used to rank the wear resistance of restorative materials. As shown in Table 4-18, the resistance of composite resins to abrasion depends on the nature of the filler particles (glass or quartz) and on silanation of the filler. Three-body abrasion tests often are used to compare the abrasion resistance of tooth structure to dentifrices and prophylaxis materials. Enamel is about 5 to 20 times more resistant to abrasion than dentin. Cementum is the least resistant to abrasion. Measurements of enamel loss during a 30-second prophylaxis have shown that fluoride is removed from the enamel surface and have allowed estimation of the removal of enamel to be 0.6 to 4 μm depending on the abrasive.

Unfortunately, a 1:1 ratio between clinically observed wear and that measured in the laboratory seldom exists. Thus most tests strive to rank materials in an order that is seen clinically. Traditional wear tests measure the volume of material lost but do not reveal mechanisms of wear, whereas a single-pass sliding technic may characterize modes of surface failure. In general, wear data do not correlate well with other mechanical property data.

In the study and evaluation of wear, note that multiple processes occur simultaneously, and materials, mechanics, and environment have combined effects on wear. Most important is the fate of the wear particles. Are these particles dissolved or distributed? If they are distributed, is their migration local or systemic, and what biological consequences can arise?

■ STRESS ANALYSIS AND DESIGN OF DENTAL STRUCTURES

The mechanical properties of dental restoration materials must be able to withstand the stresses and strains caused by the repetitive forces of mastication. The design of dental restorations is particularly important if the best advantage of a material is to be taken. The necessary designs are those that do not result in stresses or strains that exceed the strength properties of a material under clinical conditions.

Stresses in dental structures have been studied by such technics as brittle coatings, strain gages, holography, two- and three-dimensional photoelasticity, finite element analysis and other numerical methods. Stress analysis studies of inlays, crowns, bases supporting restorations, fixed bridges, complete dentures, partial dentures, endodontic posts, and implants have been reported, as well as studies of teeth, bone, and oral soft tissues. The stress analysis literature is too extensive and beyond the scope of this text to review. Only brief summaries of two-dimensional photoelasticity and finite element analysis, and the advantages and disadvantages of both, are provided.

Two-Dimensional Photoelasticity

The procedure for two-dimensional models is to prepare a transparent plastic or other isotropic model of the restoration or appliance. The material becomes anisotropic (its properties exhibit a directional dependence) when stressed, and so the behavior of light is affected by the direction it takes. As a result of the applied stress, the plastic model exhibits double refraction because of its anisotropic structure. The light from a source passes through a polarizer, which transmits light waves parallel to the polarizing

TABLE 4-18   Two-Body Abrasion of Restorative Dental Materials

Material	Two-Body Abrasion (10^{-4} mm^3/mm of Travel)
Amalgam	
Spherical	7.0
AgSn + AgCu	5.6
Composite resin	
Glass-filled	7.7
Glass-filled–no silane	13.8
Quartz-filled	3.8
Quartz-filled–no silane	5.6
Microfilled	12.0
Diacrylate resin	17.0
Pit and fissure sealant	21.5
Unfilled acrylic resin	13.3

axis, known as plane polarized light. The plane polarized light is converted to circularly polarized light by a quarter-wave plate, and this polarized beam is split into two components traveling along the directions of principal stress in the model. Depending on the state of stress in the model, the two beams travel at different rates. After the light emerges from the model, it passes through a second quarter-wave plate, which is crossed with respect to the first, and an analyzer that is most frequently perpendicular to the polarizer. The interference pattern may be recorded photographically as shown in Fig. 4-36, which is an isochromatic fringe pattern. These isochromatic fringes, or dark lines, represent locations where the difference in the principal stresses is a constant. The magnitude of the stress can be determined by identifying the order of the isochromatic fringes. Some of the fringe orders (numbers) are indicated on Fig. 4-36. The fringe order multiplied by a constant and divided by the thickness of the model gives the value of the differences in the principal stresses. Areas in the model where the fringes are close together are under higher stress gradients than areas where there are fewer fringes, and areas containing fringes of higher order are under higher stress than those having fringes of lower order.

The advantages of using photoelasticity are that it can quantify stresses throughout a three-dimensional structure and determine stress gradients. However, a birefringent material is needed and the technic is more difficult with complex geometries.

Finite Element Analysis

The finite element method is a numerical method and offers considerable advantages over photoelasticity. The method is valuable for analyzing complex geometries, and it can determine stresses and strains throughout a three-dimensional component. In this method, a finite number of discrete structural elements are interconnected at a finite number of points or nodes. These finite elements are formed when the original structure is divided into a number of appropriately shaped sections, with the sections retaining the actual properties of the real materials. The information needed to calculate the stresses and displacements in a finite element model is (1) the total number of nodal points and elements, (2) a numbering system for identifying each nodal point and element, (3) the elastic moduli and Poisson's ratio for the materials associated with each element, (4) the coordinates of each nodal point, (5) the type of boundary constraints, and (6) the evaluation of the forces applied to the external nodes. Note that finite element methods are purely numerical methods, are based on many limiting assumptions, and are potentially costly. Much more research is needed in this area before the numerical values can be accepted without question. In general, the finite element method is best suited for predicting trends and performing parametric analyses. There is an increased awareness that detailed knowledge of anisotropic material properties and constitutive relations is important in building a valid finite element model. There is also an increased emphasis on experimental validation of numerical results.

Summary

The physical properties of oral restorations must adequately withstand the stresses of mastication. Several means may be used to ensure proper strength of a restoration. With a constant force, the stress is

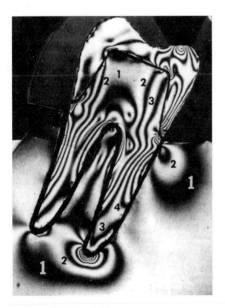

Fig. 4-36 Isochromatic fringes in a two-dimensional photoelastic model of a molar with a full crown under a concentrated force of 266 N; the numbers represent the fringe order of the isochromatic fringes. (From Hood JAA, Farah JW, Craig RG: *J Prosthet Dent* 34:415, 1975.)

inversely proportional to the contact area; therefore stresses may be reduced by increasing the area over which the force is distributed. In areas of high stress, materials having high elastic moduli and strength properties should be used if possible. If a weaker material has desirable properties, such as esthetic qualities, one may minimize the stress by increasing the bulk of the material when possible.

As an example, consider cement bases used under amalgam restorations. Occlusal forces on the amalgam restoration create tensile stresses in the amalgam adjacent to the cement base. The tensile strength of amalgam is low, and if the cement base has a low modulus, it allows deflection of the amalgam adjacent to the cement base resulting in tensile stresses that are sufficient to initiate fracture of the amalgam. The use of zinc phosphate cement as a base rather than zinc oxide–eugenol cement reduces the probability of fracture of the amalgam because the zinc phosphate cement has a higher modulus. If zinc oxide–eugenol cement is necessary to protect the pulp, a minimum amount should be used, followed by the use of a zinc phosphate cement base to provide resistance to deflection.

Restorations and appliances should be designed so that the resulting forces of mastication are distributed as uniformly as possible. Also, sharp line angles, nonuniform areas, and notched, scratched, or pitted surfaces should be avoided to minimize stress concentrations. For example, in the construction of a complete maxillary denture, the midline notch between the central incisors should remain at a minimum. This area is under repetitive stress during mastication as a result of the transverse bending of the denture. If a sharp notch is present in this area, the denture will be less resistant to fatigue or impact forces.

The maximum tensile stress in a metal partial-denture circumferential clasp is near the midpoint of the inside surface. Because brittle materials are generally weak in tension, this is a likely area of failure when a force is applied to the tip of the clasp. Other factors such as the uniformity of the taper of the clasp, porosity in the clasp, or notches and scratches on the surface of the metal may alter the stress pattern. If a thin or porous area exists between the junction and the tip of the clasp, failure may occur at this site rather than at the midpoint. Notched or scratched areas are especially subject to fracture from fatigue or impact. Because a partial denture clasp is flexed a great number of times at values well below the yield point, failure by fatigue is particularly significant.

The dentist is often concerned not so much with the fracture of an appliance as with the deflection that occurs when a force is applied. This is the case with a fixed bridge, which may be cast as a single unit or may consist of soldered units. As discussed earlier in this chapter, the deflection of a beam, or in this case a bridge, supported on each end with a concentrated load in the center depends directly on the cube of the beam length and indirectly on the cube of the beam thickness. Therefore doubling the length of the beam increases the deflection by eight times. This also indicates that decreasing the thickness of the beam by one-half increases the deflection by eight times. If too much bulk is required to develop the stiffness desired, changing to a material with a higher elastic modulus would be beneficial. This is one advantage that nickel-chromium or cobalt-chromium alloys have over gold, because the elastic modulus is greater than 200 GPa, whereas the modulus of gold alloys is less than 100 GPa.

These isolated examples of applied knowledge of biting forces and stresses in dental structures indicate why an understanding of this subject is necessary to the practicing dentist.

In summary, three interrelated factors are important in the long-term function of dental restorative materials: (1) material choice, (2) component geometry (e.g., to minimize stress concentrations), and (3) component design (e.g., to distribute stresses as uniformly as possible). It should be noted that failures can and do occur. In such instances, several questions should be asked: (1) why did it fail?; (2) how did it fail?; (3) whose fault is it?; and (4) can such failures be prevented in the future? Lastly, remember that dental material behavior is dependent on the interrelated physical, chemical, optical, mechanical, thermal, electrical, and biological properties, and improvement of one specific property often leads to a reduction in another property.

■ SPECIFICATIONS FOR RESTORATIVE MATERIALS

The properties described in this and previous chapters serve as the basis for a series of specifications that have been developed for restorative materials, instruments, and equipment. One group is the American National Standards Institute/American Dental Association Specifications (ANSI/ADA). The Council on Scientific Affairs of the ADA sponsors Accredited Standards Committee MD156, which has responsibility for the specifications. Presently 52 specifications have been adopted and another 30 are being developed. Also, task groups are actively developing standards for corrosion testing and athletic mouth protectors. A larger group called Federal Specifications and Standards is designed to regulate requirements of federal government service agencies for the purchase and use of materials. Specifications of this type have been available for the past quarter of a century, and additional specifications continue to be added in each group. A series of similar specifications is available for products in Australia, Japan, and several other countries. In 1963 a program for international specifications was established that combined the efforts of the Fédération Dentaire Internationale and the International Organization for Standardization. The practice of using physical test controls through methods of applied specifications is well established and will likely continue. Both the dental student and the practitioner must not only recognize that specifications for certain materials are available but learn to some extent the qualities that are controlled by each specification. Through the specifications the quality of each product is maintained and improved.

American Dental Association Specifications

The first of the American Dental Association Specifications was for amalgam alloy, formulated and reported in 1930. Since that time other specifications have been or are being formulated, as indicated in Table 4-19.

Copies of the specifications and worksheets, to assist in the recording of the required data, are available from the Council on Scientific Affairs of the American Dental Association in Chicago. The Council periodically publishes *Clinical Products in Dentistry: A Desktop Reference*, which lists the trade names and manufacturers of accepted dental products. This publication can also be obtained from the American Dental Association.

An examination of each specification reveals a general pattern of standardization common to each material.

1. These features include an item on scope and classification of the material, which defines the application and general nature of each material.
2. Each specification includes information on other applicable specifications.
3. The requirements of each material consider such factors as uniformity, color, or general working characteristics of the material, as well as the general limitations of test values.
4. The methods of sampling, inspection, and testing procedures include details of sample preparation and physical tests to be performed.
5. Each specification includes information on preparation for delivery, with instructions concerning packaging, instructions for use, and the marking with lot numbers and the date of manufacture.
6. Each specification includes notes that provide additional information on intended uses, and references to the literature or other special items.

The important features of each of these specifications are described appropriately in later chapters.

American Dental Association Acceptance Program

The American Denatal Association, through the Council on Scientific Affairs, maintains an acceptance program for dental materials, instruments and equipment. All ANSI/ADA Specifications are incorporated into general category guidelines. The categories are restorative materials, prosthodontic materials, instruments, equipment, and infection control products. Generally, if a specification exists, the manufacturer need only comply with the requirements of the guidelines. If a specification does not exist, the guidelines require clinical evidence of safety and efficacy in order to comply with the guidelines. When the product meets the criteria in the guideline, its name is placed on the Accepted List and the manufacturer is allowed to place the Seal of Acceptance of the American Dental Association on the product.

Index of Federal Specifications and Standards

The Index of Federal Specifications and Standards includes specifications for a number of restorative

TABLE 4-19   List of American National Standards Institute/American Dental Association Specifications on Dental Materials, Instruments, and Equipment

Number	Title	Date of Specification or Latest Revision, Addendum, or Reaffirmation
1	Alloy for dental amalgam	1993
2	Gypsum-bonded casting investment for dental gold alloy	1995
3	Dental impression compound	1994
4	Dental inlay casting wax	1994
5	Dental casting alloys	1988
6	Dental mercury	1995
7	Dental wrought gold wire alloy	1989
11	Dental agar impression material	1995
12	Denture base resins	1987
13	Denture cold-curing repair resin	1987
14	Dental base metal casting alloys	1989
15	Synthetic resin teeth	1992
16	Dental impression paste–zinc oxide eugenol material	1989
17	Denture base temporary relining resin	1990
18	Dental alginate impression material	1992
19	Elastomeric dental impression material	1993
20	Dental duplicating material	1995
22	Intraoral dental radiographic film	1972
23	Dental excavating burs	1993
24	Dental baseplate wax	1991
25	Dental gypsum products	1989
26	Dental x-ray equipment and accessory devices	1991
27	Direct filling resins	1993
28	Endodontic files and reamers	1996
29	Hand instruments	1994
30	Zinc oxide–eugenol and non-eugenol cements	1996
32	Orthodontic wires not containing precious metals	1989
33	Dental terminology	1990
34	Aspirating syringes	1987
35*	High speed air-driven handpieces	–
36*	Diamond rotary cutting instruments	–
37	Dental abrasive powders	1994
38	Metal-ceramic systems	1991
39	Pit and fissure sealants	1992
40A*	Unalloyed titanium for dental implants	–
40B*	Cast cobalt-chromium-molybdenum alloys for dental implants	–
41	Recommended standard practices for biological evaluation of dental materials	1989
42*	Phosphate-bonded investments	–
43	Electrically powered dental amalgamators	1995
44	Dental electrosurgical equipment	1986
45*	Dental porcelain teeth	–
46	Dental chairs	1996
47	Dental units	1996

*Specifications in the process of development.

TABLE 4-19, cont'd.   List of American National Standards Institute/American Dental Association Specifications on Dental Materials, Instruments, and Equipment

Number	Title	Date of Specification or Latest Revision, Addendum, or Reaffirmation
48	Dental activator, disclosing and transillumination devices	1989
49*	Analgesia equipment	–
53*	Crown and bridge plastics	–
54	Double-pointed, parenteral, single use needles in dentistry	1986
55	Dispensers of alloy and mercury for dental amalgam	1992
57	Endodontic filling materials	1993
58	Root canal files, type H (Hedström)	1988
59	Portable steam sterilizers for use in dentistry	1992
62*	Dental abrasive pastes	–
63	Rasps and barbed broaches	1989
64	Dental explorers	1994
65*	Low speed handpieces	–
69	Dental ceramic	1991
70*	Dental x-ray protective aprons and accessory devices	–
71*	Root canal filling condensors and spreaders	1995
73	Dental absorbent points	1993
74*	Dental stools	–
75*	Resilient denture liners	–
76	Non-sterile latex gloves for dentistry	1991
77*	Stiffness of tufted area of toothbrushes	–
78	Dental obturating points	1994
79*	Dental vacuum pumps	–
80	Color stability test procedure	1989
81*	Magnets and keepers used for intraoral and extraoral retainers for prosthetic restorations	–
82*	Combined reversible/irreversible hydrocolloid impression materials	–
85*	Prophy angles	–
87	Impression trays	1995
88*	Dental brazing alloys	–
89*	Dental operating lights	–
90*	Dental rubber dam	–
91*	Ethyl silicate investments	–
92*	Refractory die materials	–
93*	Soldering investments	–
94	Dental compressed air quality	1996
95*	Root canal enlargers	–
96	Dental water-based cements	1994
97*	Corrosion	–
98*	Designation system for teeth and areas of the oral cavity	–
99*	Athletic mouth protector materials	–

dental materials not described elsewhere. These specifications are used primarily by the federal services to maintain some quality control of dental products and are valuable for suppliers of these materials. In a few instances reference is made to specific federal specifications and standards in later chapters.

SELECTED PROBLEMS

Problem 1. With an average biting force of 565 N on the first or second molar, how is it possible for a patient to fracture a gold alloy bridge in service when the alloy has a tensile strength of 690 MPa?

Solution. The stress produced by the biting force is a function of the cross section of the bridge and the size of the contact area over which the force is applied. When the contact area from the opposing tooth is very small and located near a portion of the bridge having a small cross section, bending produces tensile stresses that can exceed the tensile strength of the gold alloy. For example, in the above problem, relating the biting force of 565 N to the tensile strength of 690 MPa indicates that a minimum area of 0.82 mm^2 is necessary in this bridge:

$$\text{Area} = \text{Force/Stress} = 565 \text{ N/690 MPa}$$
$$= 8.2 \times 10^{-7} \text{ m}^2 = 0.82 \text{ mm}^2$$

Problem 2. Why is the yield strength of a restorative material such an important property?

Solution. The yield strength defines the stress at the point at which the material changes from elastic to plastic behavior. In the elastic range, stresses and strains return to zero after biting forces are removed, whereas in the plastic range some permanent deformation results on removal of the force. Significant permanent deformation may result in a functional failure of a restoration even though fracture does not occur.

Problem 3. Why is the elongation value for a casting alloy not always an indication of the burnishability of the margins of the casting?

Solution. Although the elongation of an alloy gives an indication of its ductility, or ability to be drawn into a wire without fracturing, to burnish a margin of a casting, sufficient force must be applied to exceed the yield strength. Therefore alloys with high yield strengths are difficult to burnish even though they have high values for elongation.

Problem 4. Why does a mesial-occlusal-distal (MOD) amalgam fail in tension when compressive biting forces are applied from the opposing teeth?

Solution. The compressive load produces bending of the MOD amalgam, which results in compressive stress

on the occlusal surface and tensile stresses at the base of the restoration. Amalgam is a brittle solid with much lower tensile than compressive strength and therefore fails first at the base of the restoration with the crack progressing to the occlusal surface of the amalgam.

Problem 5. Because the modulus of nickel-chromium alloys is about twice that of gold alloys, why is it not correct to reduce the thickness by one-half and have the same deflection in bending?

Solution. Although the deflection in the bending equation is directly proportional to the modulus, it is inversely proportional to the cube of the thickness. Therefore only minimal reductions in thickness are possible for the nickel-chromium alloy to maintain the same deflection.

Problem 6. How is it possible to use a single rubber impression material and yet have the correct viscosity for use in the syringe and the tray?

Solution. Correct compounding of the polymer and filler produces a material that has the quality described as shear thinning. Such a material decreases in viscosity at high shear rates, such as during spatulation or syringing, and has a higher viscosity at low shear rates as when it is placed and used as a tray material.

Problem 7. After an orthodontic latex band is extended and placed, the force applied decreases with time more than expected for the distance the tooth moves. Why?

Solution. Latex rubber bands behave elastically, viscoelastically, and viscously. It is principally the viscous deformation that is not recoverable that accounts for the greater than expected decrease in force as the band shortens from the movement of the tooth. This effect is even more pronounced when plastic rather than latex bands are used.

Problem 8. If dental manufacturers showed you the compliance versus time curve for their rubber impression material and pointed out that it had a high elastic compliance, a moderate viscoelastic compliance, and a very low viscous compliance, how would you characterize the product?

Solution. The material would be highly flexible, should recover from deformation moderately rapidly, and the recovery from deformation should be nearly complete.

Problem 9. If you wished to measure the surface hardness of a material that had small isolated areas of widely varying hardnesses, which hardness test would be most appropriate and why?

Solution. Diamond pyramid hardness. Only the Knoop and diamond pyramid are appropriate for surface hardness and a wide range of hardness. The selection of the diamond pyramid over the Knoop test is based on the information that there were isolated areas of different hardness and the diamond pyramid indentation can be placed in smaller areas.

Problem 10. Why is the selection of a cement base with a high modulus so important for an amalgam restoration, whereas the selection is not as critical for a composite restoration?

Solution. The cement base under an amalgam should have a high modulus (stiffness) to provide support and prevent bending and thus minimize tensile stresses. Also, low-stress gradients occur across the amalgam-cement base interface when the modulus values are similar. The composite has greater tensile strength than does amalgam and a lower modulus, allowing the use of a cement base with a somewhat lower modulus.

■ REFERENCES

Forces on Dental Structures

Black GV: An investigation of the physical characters of the human teeth in relation to their diseases, and to practical dental operations, together with the physical characters of filling materials, *Dent Cosmos* 37:469, 1895.

Burstone CJ, Baldwin JJ, Lawless DT: The application of continuous forces in orthodontics, *Angle Orthod* 31:1, 1961.

Caputo AA, Standlee JP: *Biomechanics in clinical dentistry,* Chicago, 1987, Quintessence.

Dechow PC, Carlson DS: A method of bite force measurement in primates, *J Biomech* 16:797, 1983.

Koolstra JH, van Euden TMGJ: Application and validation of a three-dimensional mathematical model of the human masticatory system *in vivo, J Biomech* 25:175, 1992.

Plesh O, Bishop B, McCall WD, Jr: Kinematics of jaw movements during chewing at different frequencies, *J Biomech* 26:243, 1993.

Southard TE, Southard KA, Stiles RN: Factors influencing the anterior composnet of occlusal force, *J Biomech* 23:1199, 1990.

Stress Analysis and Design of Dental Structures

Chen J, Xu L: A finite element analysis of the human temporomandibular joint, *J Biomech Engr* 116:401, 1994.

Craig RG: Dental mechanics. In Kardestuncer H: *Finite element handbook,* New York, 1987, McGraw-Hill.

Craig RG, Farah JW: Stress analysis and design of single restorations and fixed bridges, *Oral Sci Rev* 10:45, 1977.

Craig RG, Farah JW: Stresses from loading distal-extension removable partial dentures, *J Prosthet Dent* 39:274, 1978.

Farah JW, Craig RG: Distribution of stresses in porcelain-fused-to-metal and porcelain jacket crowns, *J Dent Res* 54:255, 1975.

Farah JW, Craig RG, Sikarskie DL: Photoelastic and finite element stress analysis of a restored axisymmetric first molar, *J Biomech* 6:511, 1973.

Farah JW, Hood JAA, Craig RG: Effects of cement bases on the stresses in amalgam restorations, *J Dent Res* 54:10, 1975.

Farah JW, Powers JM, Dennison JB, Craig RG, Spencer J: Effects of cement bases on the stresses and deflections in composite restorations, *J Dent Res* 55:115, 1976.

Hart RT, Hennebel VV, Thonpreda N, Van Buskirk WC, Anderson RC: Modeling the biomechanics of the mandible: a three-dimensional finite element study, *J Biomech* 25:261, 1992.

Hylander WL: Mandibular function in galago crassicaudatus and macaca fascicularis: an *in vivo* approach to stress analysis of the mandible, *J Morph* 159:253, 1979.

Koran A, Craig RG: Three-dimensional photoelastic stress analysis of maxillary and mandibular complete dentures, *J Oral Rehabil* 1:361, 1974.

Korioth TWP, Hannam AG: Deformation of the human mandible during simulated tooth clenching, *J Dent Res* 73:56, 1994.

Properties from Stress-Strain Curves

Andrews CW: Effect of temperature on the modulus of elasticity, *Metals Prog* 58:85, 1950.

Berenbaum R, Brodie J: Measurement of tensile strength of brittle materials, *Br J Appl Physics* 10:281, 1959.

Bryant RW, Mahler DB: Modulus of elasticity in bending of composites and amalgams, *J Prosthet Dent* 56:243, 1986.

Campbell JB: What tensile properties of metals mean in design, *Mater Meth* 31:49, 1950.

Cooke FW, editor: Biomaterials: bulk characterization. In von Recum AF: *Handbook of biomaterials evaluation; scientific, technical, and clinical testing of implant materials,* New York, 1986, Macmillan.

Dorn JE, Tietz TE: The modulus of elasticity—a review of metallurgical factors, *Metals Prog* 58:81, 1950.

Hayden HW, Moffatt WG, Wulff J: *The structure and properties of materials,* vol 3, Mechanical behavior, New York, 1965, John Wiley & Sons.

Roberts JC, Powers JM, Craig RG: Fracture toughness and critical strain energy release rate of dental amalgam, *J Mater Sci* 13:965, 1978.

Roberts JC, Powers JM, Craig RG: Fracture toughness of composite and unfilled restorative resins, *J Dent Res* 56:748, 1977.

Rudnick G, Hunter GR, Holden FC: An analysis of the diametral-compression test, *Mater Res Standards* 3:283, 1963.

Smyd ES: Mechanics of dental structures: guide to teaching dental engineering at undergraduate level, *J Prosthet Dent* 2:668, 1952.

Swann PR: Stress-corrosion failure, *Sci Am* 214:72, 1966.

Titelman AS, McEvily AJ, Jr: *Fracture of structural materials,* New York, 1967, John Wiley & Sons.

Fracture Toughness

Cruickshanks-Boyd DW, Lock WR: Fracture toughness of dental amalgams, *Biomaterials* 4:234, 1983.

de Groot R, Van Elst HC, Peters MCRB: Fracture mechanics parameters for failure prediction of composite resins, *J Dent Res* 67:919, 1988.

Dhuru VB, Lloyd CH: The fracture toughness of repaired composite, *J Oral Rehabil* 13:413, 1986.

El Mowafy OM, Watts DC: Fracture toughness of human dentin, *J Dent Res* 65:677, 1986.

Ferracane JL, Antonio RC, Matsumoto H: Variables affecting the fracture toughness of dental composites, *J Dent Res* 66:1140, 1987.

Ferracane JL, Berge HX: Fracture toughness of experimental dental composites aged in ethanol, *J Dent Res* 74:1418, 1995.

Ferracane JL, Marker VA: Solvent degradation and reduced fracture toughness in aged composites, *J Dent Res* 71:13, 1992.

Hassan R, Vaidyanathan TK, Schulman A: Fracture toughness determination of dental amalgams through microindentation, *J Biomed Mater Res* 20:135, 1986.

Hill RG, Bates JF, Lewis TT, Rees N: Fracture toughness of acrylic denture base, *Biomat* 4:112, 1983.

Kon M, Ishikawa K, Kuwayam N: Effects of zirconia addition on fracture toughness and bending strength of dental porcelains, *Dent Mater J* 9:181, 1990.

Kusy RP: Morphology of polycrystalline alumina brackets and its relationship to fracture toughness and strength, *Angle Orthod* 58:197, 1988.

Lloyd CH: The fracture toughness of dental composites. II. The environmental and temperature dependence of the stress intensification factor (K'_{IC}), *J Oral Rehabil* 9:133, 1982.

Lloyd CH: The fracture toughness of dental composites. III. The effect of environment upon the stress intensification factor (K'_{IC}) after extended storage, *J Oral Rehabil* 11:393, 1984.

Lloyd CH: Resistance to fracture in posterior composites: Measurement of their fracture toughness and a comparison with other restorative materials, *Br Dent J* 155:411, 1983.

Lloyd CH, Adamson M: The development of fracture toughness and fracture strength in posterior restorative materials, *Dent Mater* 3:225, 1987.

Lloyd CH, Adamson M: The fracture toughness (K_{IC}) of amalgam, *J Oral Rehabil* 12:59, 1985.

Lloyd CH, Anderson JN: The strength and fracture toughness of calcium hydroxide preparations, *J Oral Rehabil* 7:155, 1980.

Lloyd CH, Dhuru VB: Effect of a commercial bonding agent upon the fracture toughness (K'_{IC}) of repaired heavily filled composite, *Dent Mater* 1:83, 1985.

Lloyd CH, Iannetta RV: The fracture toughness of dental composites. I. The development of strength and fracture toughness, *J Oral Rehabil* 9:55, 1982.

Lloyd CH, Mitchell L: The fracture toughness of tooth coloured restorative materials, *J Oral Rehabil* 11:257, 1984.

Mair LH, Vowles R: The effect of thermal cycling on the fracture toughness of seven composite restorative materials, *Dent Mater* 5:23, 1989.

Marcos Montes-G G, Draughn RA: Slow crack propagation in composite restorative materials, *J Biomed Mater Res* 21:629, 1987.

Morena R, Lockwood PE, Fairhurst CW: Fracture toughness of commercial dental porcelains, *Dent Mater* 2:58, 1986.

Mueller HJ: Fracture toughness and fractography of dental cements, lining, build-up, and filling materials, *Scanning Microsc* 4:297, 1990.

Neihart TR, Li SH, Flinton RJ: Measuring fracture toughness of high-impact poly(methyl methacrylate) with the short rod method, *J Prosthet Dent* 60:249, 1988.

Pilliar RM, Smith DC, Maric B: Fracture toughness of dental composites determined using the short-rod fracture toughness test, *J Dent Res* 65:1308, 1986.

Pilliar RM, Vowles R, Williams DF: The effect of environmental aging on the fracture toughness of dental composites, *J Dent Res* 66:722, 1987.

Roberts JC, Powers JM, Craig RG: Fracture toughness of composite and unfilled restorative resins, *J Dent Res* 56:748, 1977.

Rosenstiel SF, Porter SS: Apparent fracture toughness of all-ceramic crown systems, *J Prosthet Dent* 62:529, 1989.

Rosenstiel SF, Porter SS: Apparent fracture toughness of metal ceramic restorations with different manipulative variables, *J Prosthet Dent* 61:185, 1989.

Scott GE Jr: Fracture toughness and surface cracks–the key to understanding ceramic brackets, *Angle Orthod* 58:5, 1988.

Sih GC, Berman AT: Fracture toughness concept applied to methyl methacrylate, *J Biomed Mater Res* 14:311, 1980.

Stafford GD, Huggett R, Causton BE: Fracture toughness of denture base acrylics, *J Biomed Mater Res* 14:359, 1980.

Taira M, Nomura Y, Wakasa K, Yamaki M, Matsui A: Studies on fracture toughness of dental ceramics, *J Oral Rehabil* 17:551, 1990.

Uctasli S, Harrington E, Wilson HJ: The fracture resistance of dental materials, *J Oral Rehabil* 22:877, 1995.

Shear Strength

Black J: "Push-out" tests, *J Biomed Mater Res* 23:1243, 1989.

Johnston WM, O'Brien WJ: The shear strength of dental porcelain, *J Dent Res* 59:1409, 1980.

Smith DC, Cooper WEG: The determination of shear strength–a method using a micro-punch apparatus, *Br Dent J* 130:333, 1971.

Bending and Torsion

Asgharnia MK, Brantley WA: Comparison of bending and torsion tests for orthodontic wires, *Am J Orthodont* 89:228, 1986.

Brantley WA, Augat WS, Myers CL, Winders RV: Bending deformation studies of orthodontic wires, *J Dent Res* 57:609, 1978.

Council on Dental Materials and Devices: New American Dental Association Specification No. 28 for endodontic files and reamers, *J Am Dent Assoc* 93:813, 1976.

Council on Dental Materials and Devices: New American Dental Association Specification No. 32 for orthodontic wire not containing precious metals, *J Am Dent Assoc* 95:1169, 1977.

Craig RG, McIlwain ED, Peyton FA: Bending and torsion properties of endodontic instruments, *Oral Surg* 25:239, 1968.

Dolan DW, Craig RG: Bending and torsion of endodontic files with rhombus cross sections, *J Endodont* 8:260, 1982.

Johnston EP, Nicholls JI, Smith DE: Flexural fatigue of 10 commonly used denture base resins, *J Prosthet Dent* 46:478, 1981.

Krupp JD, Brantley WA, Gerstein H: An investigation of the torsional and bending properties of seven brands of endodontic files, *J Endodont* 10:372, 1984.

Ruyter IE, Svendsen SA: Flexural properties of denture base polymers, *J Prosthet Dent* 43:95, 1980.

Viscosity

Combe EC, Moser JB: The rheological characteristics of elastomeric impression materials, *J Dent Res* 57:221, 1978.

Herfort TW, Gerberich WW, Macosko CW, Goodkind RJ: Viscosity of elastomeric impression materials, *J Prosthet Dent* 38:396, 1977.

Koran A, Powers JM, Craig RG: Apparent viscosity of materials used for making edentulous impressions, *J Am Dent Assoc* 95:75, 1977.

Vermilyea SG, Huget EF, de Simon LB: Apparent viscosities of setting elastomers, *J Dent Res* 59:1149, 1980.

Vermilyea SG, Powers JM, Craig RG: Rotational viscometry of a zinc phosphate and a zinc polyacrylate cement, *J Dent Res* 56:762, 1977.

Vermilyea SG, Powers JM, Koran A: The rheological properties of fluid denture-base resins, *J Dent Res* 57:227, 1978.

Viscoelasticity

Bertolotti RL, Moffa JP: Creep rate of porcelain-bonding alloys as a function of temperature, *J Dent Res* 59:2062, 1980.

Cook WD: Permanent set and stress relaxation in elastomeric impression materials, *J Biomed Mater Res* 15:449, 1981.

Duran RL, Powers JM, Craig RG: Viscoelastic and dynamic properties of soft liners and tissue conditioners, *J Dent Res* 58:1801, 1979.

Ellis B, Al-Nabash S: The composition and rheology of denture adhesives, *J Dent* 8:109, 1980.

Ferracane JL, Moser JB, Greener EH: Rheology of composite restoratives, *J Dent Res* 60:1678, 1981.

Goldberg AJ: Viscoelastic properties of silicone, polysulfide, and polyether impression materials, *J Dent Res* 53:1033, 1974.

McCabe JF, Bowman AJ: The rheological properties of dental impression materials, *Br Dent J* 151:179, 1981.

Morris HF, Asgar K, Tillitson EW: Stress-relaxation testing. Part I: A new approach to the testing of removable partial denture alloys, wrought wires, and clasp behavior, *J Prosthet Dent* 46:133, 1981.

Nikolai RJ, Crouthers RC: On the relaxation of orthodontic traction elements under interrupted loads, *J Dent Res* 59:1071, 1980.

Oglesby PL: Viscoelastic behavior. In Dickson G, Cassel JM, editors: *National Bureau of Standards Special Publication* 354, July 1972.

Park JB: *Biomaterials science and engineering,* New York, 1984, Plenum Press.

Ruyter IE, Espevik S: Compressive creep of denture base polymers, *Acta Odont Scand* 38:169, 1980.

Tolley LG, Craig RG: Viscoelastic properties of elastomeric impression materials: polysulphide, silicone and polyether rubbers, *J Oral Rehabil* 5:121, 1978.

Wills DJ, Manderson RD: Biomechanical aspects of the support of partial dentures, *J Dent* 5:310, 1977.

Dynamic Properties

Godwin WC, Koran A, Craig RG: Evaluation of the dynamic and static physical properties of mouth protectors, *J Dent Res* 53(Special Issue):67, 1974.

Impact resistance of plastics and electrical insulating material, D 256-92. In ASTM Standards 1993, Vol. 8.01, Philadelphia, American Society for Testing and Materials, 1993.

Koran A, Craig RG: Dynamic mechanical properties of maxillofacial materials, *J Dent Res* 54:1216, 1975.

Soni PM, Powers JM, Craig RG: Physical and mechanical properties of acrylic and modified acrylic denture resins, *J Mich Dent Assoc* 59:418, 1977.

Properties of Composite Materials

Braem MJA, Davidson CL, Lambrechts P, Vanherle G: In vitro flexural fatigue limits of dental composites, *J Biomed Mater Res* 28:1397, 1994.

Braem M, Van Doren VE, Lambrechts P, Vanherle G: Determination of Young's modulus of dental composites: a phenomenological model, *J Mater Sci* 22:2037, 1987.

Goldberg AJ, Burstone CJ, Hadjinikolaou I, Jancar J: Screening of matrices and fibers for reinforced thermoplastics intended for dental applications, *J Biomed Mater Res* 28:167, 1994.

Holliday L, editor: *Composite materials,* New York, 1966, Elsevier.

Van der Varst PGT, Brekelmans WAM, De Vree JHP, de Groot R: Mechanical performance of a dental composite: probabilistic failure prediction, *J Dent Res* 72:1249, 1993.

Whiting R, Jacobsen PH: A non-destructive method of evaluating the elastic properties of anterior restorative materials, *J Dent Res* 59:1978, 1980.

Willems G, Lambrechts P, Braem M, Vanherle G: Composite resins in the 21st century, *Quint Int* 24:641, 1993.

Tear Strength and Tear Energy

Herfort TW, Gerberich WW, Macosko CW, Goodkind RJ: Tear strength of elastomeric impression materials, *J Prosthet Dent* 39:59, 1978.

MacPherson GW, Craig RG, Peyton FA: Mechanical properties of hydrocolloid and rubber impression materials, *J Dent Res* 46:714, 1967.

Strength of conventional vulcanized rubber and thermoplastic elastomers, D 624-91. In ASTM Standards 1994, Vol. 9.01, Philadelphia, American Society for Testing and Materials, 1994.

Webber RL, Ryge G: The determination of tear energy of extensible materials of dental interest, *J Biomed Mater Res* 2:231, 1968.

Hardness

DeBellis A: Fundamentals of Rockwell hardness testing. In Hardness Testing Reprints, WD-673, Wilson Instrument Division, Bridgeport, Conn, 1967.

Lysaght VE: How to make and interpret hardness tests on plastics. In Hardness Testing Reprints, WD-673, Wilson Instrument Division, Bridgeport, Conn, 1967.

Lysaght VE: *Indentation hardness testing,* New York, 1949, Reinhold.

Lysaght VE, DeBellis A: Microhardness testing. In Hardness Testing Reprints, WD-673, Wilson Instrument Division, Bridgeport, Conn, 1967.

Specifications

Council on Dental Materials, Instruments and Equipment: *Dentist's desk reference: materials, instruments and equipment,* 2d ed., Chicago, 1983, American Dental Association.

Council on Scientific Affairs: *Clinical products in dentistry: a desktop reference,* Chicago, 1996, American Dental Association.

United States General Services Administration: *Index of Federal Specifications and Standards,* Washington, DC, 1994, Superintendent of Documents, US Government Printing Office.

Wear

Barbakow F, Lutz F, Imfeld T: A review of methods to determine the relative abrasion of dentifrices and prophylaxis pastes, *Quintessence Internat* 18:23, 1987.

Craig RG, Powers JM: Wear of dental tissues and materials, *Int Dent J* 26:121, 1976.

Draughn RA, Harrison A: Relationship between abrasive wear and microstructure of composite resins, *J Prosthet Dent* 40:220, 1978.

Powers JM, Craig RG: Wear of dental tissues and restorative materials. In Proceedings of national symposium on wear and corrosion, June 4–6, Washington, DC, 1979, American Chemical Society.

Powers JM, Fan PL, Craig RG: Wear of dental restorative resins. In Gebelein CG, Koblitz FF, editors: *Biomedical and dental applications of polymers: Polymer science and technology,* vol 14, New York, 1981, Plenum Press.

Roberts JC, Powers JM, Craig RG: Wear of dental amalgam, *J Biomed Mater Res* 11:513, 1977.

Stookey GK: In vitro estimates of enamel and dentin abrasion associated with a prophylaxis, *J Dent Res* 57:36, 1978.

Wu W, McKinney JE: Influence of chemicals on wear of dental composites, *J Dent Res* 61:1180, 1982.

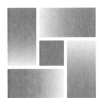

5 Nature of Metals and Alloys

GENERAL CHARACTERISTICS OF METALS

A metal is any element that ionizes positively in solution. (Metals are the majority of elements on the periodic table left of the heavy zigzagging diagonal line in Fig. 14-1.) They have certain typical and characteristic properties that distinguish them from the nonmetallic elements. The optical properties, metallic luster and high opacity, physical property of high ductility, and high thermal and electrical conductivity are used to identify metals. The extensive use of metals and their alloys in mechanical and structural applications is a result of the good mechanical properties and workability of many metals. Metals have widely varying properties, which makes it necessary to use a variety of different metals.

Another important group of elements are the semiconductors or metalloids, such as carbon, silicon, boron, and others (located between the metals and nonmetals on the periodic table). These elements do not ionize in solution to become positive charges but are good conductors of heat and electricity. These are often added to metals to improve selected properties.

Metals in the pure state are used to a greater extent in dentistry than in most other arts or industries. Extreme ductility is sometimes desirable in metals used in dentistry, and this property predominates in pure metals rather than in mixtures of metals. The chemical properties of the metals used in dentistry are important because a metal that is readily corroded or tarnished cannot be used in the mouth. This is also an area where some pure metals excel. The pure metals that are commonly used in dentistry are gold and platinum in the form of foil for use in restorations; liquid mercury for making amalgam, and electroplated silver and copper for preparing dies. Usually the ideal combination of physical and chemical properties cannot be found in any one metal. Consequently a limited number of pure metals can be used in addition to an extensive group of mixtures of metals, which are called alloys.

Metallic Bonding and Properties of Alloys

Primary bonds have been classified as ionic, covalent, and metallic; secondary bonds have been classified as London forces, van der Waals' forces, and hydrogen bonding. Of these, metallic bonding is most important with metals.

Metallic bonding is responsible for the unique properties of metals. Metal atoms have valence electrons that are rather loosely held, and these electrons are free to travel throughout the solid. This diffuse nature is responsible for the easy deformability of metals and their high thermal and electrical conductivities. They are opaque because the valence electrons absorb light, and they are reflective or lustrous because the electrons reemit the light. As the number of valence electrons increases, they become more localized and the metal develops some covalent character, which partly accounts for the higher melting points of such metals as iron and nickel.

CRYSTAL STRUCTURE OF METALS

Six different crystal systems have been recognized: cubic, tetragonal, orthorhombic, monoclinic, triclinic, and hexagonal. They can be seen in Fig. 5-1, where the XYZ coordinate system is shown. In the cubic system the distance between atoms on the X, Y, and Z axes is the same, and the angles α, β, and γ formed by the axes are 90 degrees. The tetragonal system differs from the cubic system in that the distance between the atoms on the Z axis is different from the

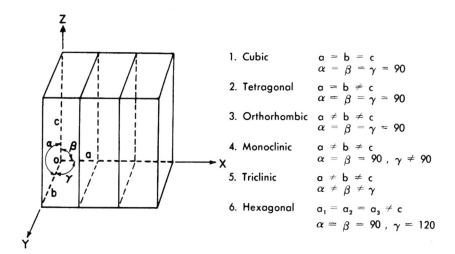

Fig. 5-1 Crystal structure systems.

distance on the X and Y axes. In the monoclinic system, the distances between atoms on the X, Y, and Z axes are all different, and the angle γ is not 90 degrees. The orthorhombic and triclinic systems are also described. The hexagonal system is not as obvious, but the shape can be thought of as a hexagonal right prism, although the real shape is a pie-shaped prism only one-sixth of the hexagonal prism. Thus this pie-shaped prism consists of an equilateral triangle as a base ($a_1 = a_2 = a_3$), and the length of the prism is c, which does not equal a_1. The angles α and β equal 90 degrees, but γ equals 120 degrees.

Atoms can be arranged in the six crystal systems in only 14 different arrays: (1) simple cubic, (2) face-centered cubic, (3) body-centered cubic, (4) simple tetragonal, (5) body-centered tetragonal, (6) rhombohedric, (7) simple orthorhombic, (8) base-centered orthorhombic, (9) face-centered orthorhombic, (10) body-centered orthorhombic, (11) simple monoclinic, (12) base-centered monoclinic, (13) triclinic, and (14) hexagonal.

Fig. 5-2 shows the three most common arrays for the metals used in dentistry: body-centered cubic, face-centered cubic, and hexagonal close packed. These simple arrays are called unit cells and are the basis of the crystal structures. In the body-centered cubic unit cell, atoms are located at each corner, and one atom is located in the center. This is the unit cell of iron and of its many alloys that are used in dentistry. With the face-centered cubic unit cell,

atoms are located at each corner, as with the body-centered cubic, but no atom is in the center, and atoms are located in the center of each of the six faces of the cube. The face-centered cubic is the structure found in most of the pure metals and alloys used in dentistry, including the gold, palladium, cobalt, and nickel alloys. A few metals used in dentistry have the more complex hexagonal close packed structure; a notable example is titanium.

If one of these unit cells is extended in all directions, a perfect single crystal results, called a space lattice. A portion of a space lattice with a simple cubic structure is shown in Fig. 5-3. It is defined as a set of geometric points superimposed on the crystalline substance in such a manner that the atoms surrounding any point in the set is the same as the group surrounding any other point in the set.

Physical Properties and Crystal Structure

If a person examines the crystal structure of a metal shown in Fig. 5-3 and imagines moving from atom to atom, he or she would find that in any one direction the distance between atoms is the same and that the arrangement of nearby atoms remains unchanged. However the distance between adjacent atoms will vary depending on the direction the observer moves. Occasionally a defect or a missing atom would occur, but in general, the structure would be regular.

A crystal observed from different directions, perhaps diagonally through the unit cell or along an

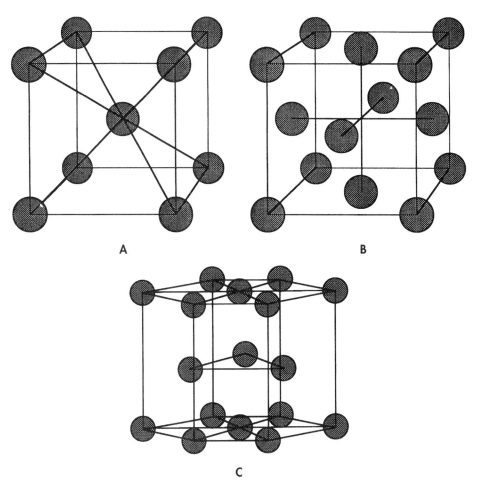

Fig. 5-2 A, Body-centered cubic unit cell. **B,** Face-centered cubic unit cell. **C,** Hexagonal close packed unit cell. The atoms in all three cases would actually be larger and touching each other. They were drawn smaller to make the structures easier to visualize.

edge, appears different because the distance between opposite corners of a cube is longer than along the edge. Crystals also have different properties in different directions, and this can be demonstrated when the strength of large single crystals of copper are tested in different directions. Also, it has been found that iron crystals are easier to magnetize in one direction and that zinc crystals conduct heat faster in one direction. Another example is that different faces on the crystal have different energies and wear properties. Many other properties are dependent on crystal directions.

These changes in properties along different crystal directions are not usually observed in pieces of metal or other solids large enough for practical use because they are polycrystalline. Polycrystalline materials are made up of large numbers of single crystals, called grains, that are bonded together at their boundaries. Each grain is oriented more or less randomly with respect to its neighbors; thus the variation in properties with crystal direction averages out. The material as a whole therefore exhibits identical properties in all directions.

Deformation of Metals

The arrangement of atoms also affects the mechanical properties. The effect of elastic strain is discussed briefly in Chapter 4, and another example

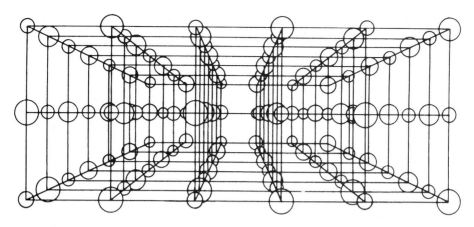

Fig. 5-3 Space lattice of an alloy.

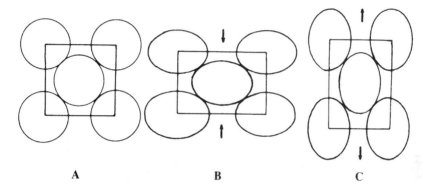

Fig. 5-4 A, Normal atoms in a lattice. **B,** System under compressive stress. **C,** System under tensile stress.

is given in Fig. 5-4. The crystal represented by *A* shows the atoms in their normal relationship; when it is loaded in compression, *B*, or tension, *C*, the atoms are deformed and strain results. Calculations based on the assumption of perfect crystals and the strength of metallic bonds indicate that metals should be hundreds of times stronger than they are in reality. However, real crystals usually contain a variety of defects. Dislocations are a type of crystal defect and are important because they provide a mechanism for metals to deform at much lower stress levels than theory would predict. Formation and propagation of a dislocation by shear stress is shown in Fig. 5-5. An extra plane of atoms appears, and the region at its base is called an edge dislocation. This dislocation moves across the crystal, as shown in *C*, deforming it in a series of single steps, and the dislocation finally moves out of the crystal

as shown in *D*. Dislocations allow metals to deform by moving one plane of atoms at a time instead of moving many planes at the same time. They also permit metals to deform at lower stress levels. An analogy is moving a large heavy rug by forming a small fold or kink in the rug and pushing the fold from one end of the rug to the other. This would require much less force than sliding the entire rug at once. Another type of dislocation is the screw dislocation, which is shown schematically in Fig. 5-6. A dislocation can move through a crystal as an edge dislocation, a screw dislocation, or as a combination of both.

All the technics for improving the strength of metals impede the motion of dislocations. Treatments, which will be discussed later, including alloying, precipitation hardening, grain refining, and cold working, can hinder dislocation movement. For

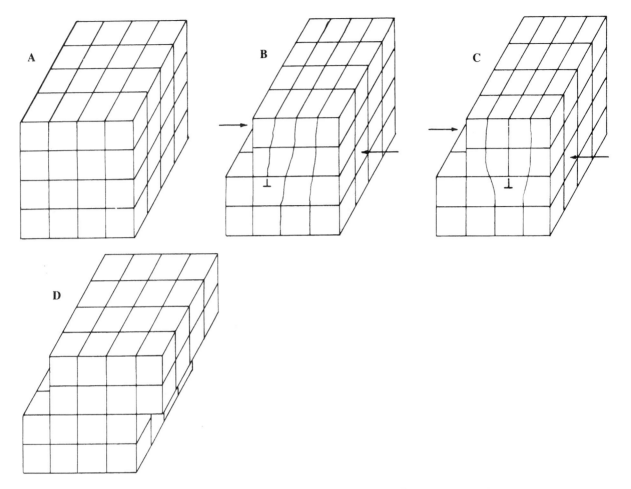

Fig. 5-5 Sketches representing a crystal and the mechanism of slip as a result of the movement of a dislocation.

example, metals are grain refined to produce finer grain sizes. When a dislocation moves through a grain-refined metal it will encounter more grain boundaries than with a material with coarser grains. Dislocations become stuck on grain boundaries, thereby preventing further dislocation motion and strengthening the metal.

Fracture of Solids

Plastic shearing in a crystal lattice is a frequent source of fracture. Fig. 5-7, *A, B,* and *C* show the successive displacement of rows of atoms by an applied force and facilitated by a dislocation shown by the extra half plane of black atoms. The broken lines indicate successively ruptured bonds. Fig. 5-7, *D, E,* and *F* show the same event with the disloca-

tion blocked by a strongly bonded group of shaded impurity atoms. The blocking causes a concentration of stresses that may cause a crack to open (the wedge in Fig. 5-7, *E*). A second shearing event in Fig. 5-7, *F*, enlarges the crack by pushing another dislocation against the obstacle, and complete fracture soon follows.

Although most metallic crystals and some nonmetallic crystals may have no cracks initially, they often contain dislocations that allow them to flow plastically. These dislocations make the crystals vulnerable to crack formation through the mechanism just illustrated. Crystals deform plastically by the sliding of one part of a crystal over the rest, rather like the sliding of the cards in a deck over one another. If the sliding occurs freely, the result is just

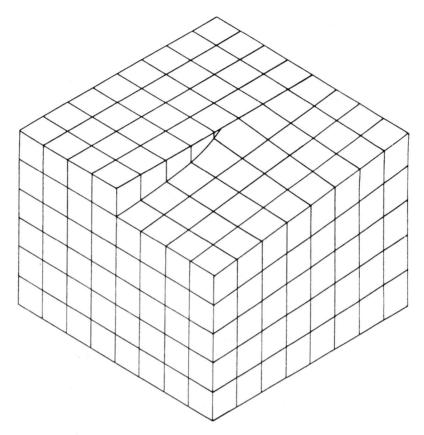

Fig. 5-6 Sketch representing a screw dislocation in a crystal.

a change in the shape of a crystal. However, if the sliding is blocked by a hard particle inside a crystal or at the grain boundary between crystals, a high concentration of stress collects at the place where the sliding is blocked. The bonds at this location are under great stress, and they stretch beyond their limit and rupture, forming a tiny crack.

Once a crack is well started, it takes very little force to propagate to a complete fracture. Because the force depends on the length of the crack, a specific case must be examined to state how much force is involved. For example, consider a plate of steel that is 15 cm wide and 6 mm thick. Suppose it has a 5-cm crack running into one side. The force required to make the crack run the remaining 10 cm would be only about 180 kg. Without the aid of the crack, a force of 230,000 kg would be required to pull the plate apart if it were made of the best commercially available steel, and a force of about 4.5 million kg if

it were made of a single crystal. A large leverage effect like this makes it possible for a relatively small force to fracture an entire sample.

■ NATURE OF ALLOYS

An alloy is any combination of two or more metals. An alloy system is a blend of two or more metals in all possible combinations. For example, the gold-copper system includes all the possible alloys of gold and copper. This is a binary system, which involves only two metals and considers all different possible combinations. Likewise, a ternary system includes three metals.

A structurally homogeneous material has the same structure throughout and is called a one-phase system. On the other hand, heterogeneous substances contain two or more distinct homogeneous regions; these distinct regions, separated by surface

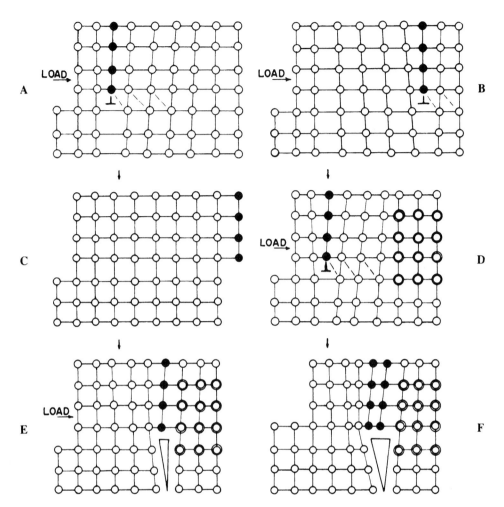

Fig. 5-7 Sketches describing plastic shearing and crack formation as a result of dislocations piling up at a location containing an impurity.

boundaries, are called phases. Each phase has a distinct composition or arrangement of atoms (crystal structure). For example, a mixture of ice and water is a two-phase system; even though the ice may be in many pieces, it is still one phase, and the water is the other phase. Although the ice and water have the same composition, one has a crystalline atomic structure, whereas the other has the random atomic structure of a liquid.

Classification of Alloy Systems

To form an alloy, two or more metals are heated to a homogeneous liquid state. However, a few combinations of metals are not miscible in the liquid state and will not form alloys. When immiscible metals are melted, two layers are formed with little or no mixing of atoms of one metal with those of the other metal, a situation similar to mixing oil and water. In the liquid state the metal with the lower density will float over the denser one. After solidification they will form two separate layers, each layer containing one of the two metals. Therefore whenever two metals are not completely miscible in the liquid state, they cannot form any type of alloy. Two of the more common examples are copper with lead and zinc with lead, as shown in Fig. 5-8.

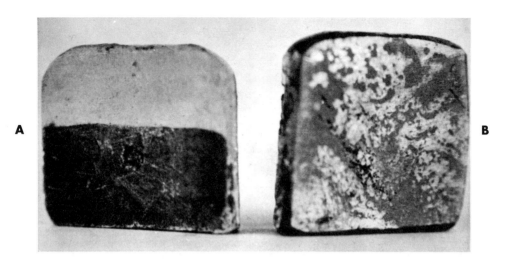

Fig. 5-8 Zinc-lead, **A,** and copper-lead, **B,** mixtures melted together and allowed to solidify, showing separation of ingredient metals.

When a combination of two metals is completely miscible in the liquid state, the two metals are capable of forming an alloy. When such a combination is cooled, one of three microstructures may form: a solid solution, a mixture of intermetallic compounds, or an eutectic mixture.

Solid solution

When two metals are completely miscible in the liquid state, and they remain completely mixed on solidification, the alloy formed is called a solid solution. The copper and gold combination crystallizes in such a manner that the atoms of copper are scattered randomly throughout the crystal structure (space lattice) of gold, resulting in a single-phase system. Such a combination is called a solid solution because it is a solid but has the properties of a solution. These single-phase solid solutions always have a range of possible compositions, never a fixed composition; for example the solid phase in the copper-gold system has a wide range of compositions between 100% Cu and 100% Au.

Intermetallic compounds

Intermetallic compounds are also formed on cooling liquid metal solutions. However, the resulting phase has a fixed chemical composition or a narrow range of compositions. As far as the space lattice is concerned, the atoms of one metal occupy a definite position in relation to every point on the space lattice. For example, if an alloy of silver and tin containing 73.2% Ag and 26.8% Sn by weight is heated above 650° C, it is a single-phase liquid system. When the alloy is cooled below 480° C, it solidifies to form a compound with the fixed composition Ag_3Sn, with silver and tin atoms occupying definite positions in the space lattice. Such an alloy is called an intermetallic compound and is present in dental amalgam alloys.

The products of the setting reaction of Ag_3Sn low-copper dental amalgam alloys with mercury are also intermetallic compounds Ag_2Hg_3 and $Sn_{7-8}Hg$. These phases have distinctly different structures and are seen on the surface of a set amalgam under magnification, as in Fig. 5-9.

Eutectic mixture

Eutectic mixtures occur when the metals are miscible in the liquid state but separate into two phases in the solid state. The two phases usually precipitate as alternating very fine layers of one phase over the other; such a combination is called an eutectic mixture. An example of such a combination is 72% Ag and 28% Cu, which is used as one of the components in some dental amalgams. With this alloy the eutectic is composed of fine, alternating layers of high-silver and high-copper phases.

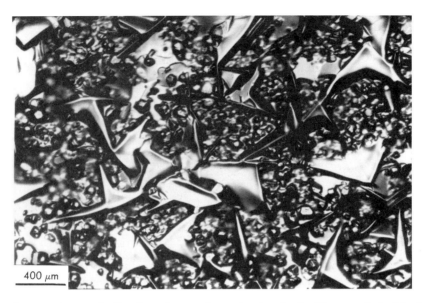

400 μm

Fig. 5-9 Scanning electron micrograph of surface of set amalgam showing the Ag_2Hg_3 crystals (polyhedra) and $Sn_{7.8}Hg$ weblike plate-shaped phase γ_2. (From O'Brien WJ, Johnston WM, Heinkel DE: *J Am Dent Assoc* 94:893, 1977. Copyright by the American Dental Association. Reprinted by permission.)

PHASE DIAGRAMS

Phase diagrams are maps of phases as a function of composition and temperature (and sometimes pressure). Each elemental metal and each alloy combination has its own characteristic phase diagram, which may be relatively simple in some instances and exceedingly complex in others. Only the less complex examples of phase diagrams are presented.

An example of a phase diagram is the salt-water phase diagram shown in Fig. 5-10. While it does not show metallic phases, the phases shown are familiar to everyone. Salt, brine, and ice, in addition to mixtures of these phases, are present in this diagram. It is comparable to a map with composition replacing longitude and temperature replacing latitude. If we want to find what phases are present we only have to look at a specified composition and temperature on the phase diagram. A well-known position on this phase diagram is 0% NaCl (100% H_2O) at 0° C (position *a*) where liquid water transforms to ice on cooling. The diagram also shows that when NaCl is added to this ice at –5° C, shown by moving horizontally to the right on the diagram, a mixture of ice and brine is formed (*b*). If more NaCl is added to give a composition of 15% NaCl our mixture will

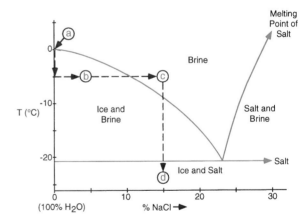

Fig. 5-10 A portion of the NaCl–H_2O phase diagram showing the freezing point of water *a*, ice and brine mixture *b*, brine *c*, and solid ice and solid salt mixture *d*.

transform to a single phase–brine (*c*). If we were to cool our brine below 21° C–by moving straight downward on the phase diagram–our material would form a mixture of solid ice and salt phases (*d*). Similar phase diagrams show the phases of metal alloys.

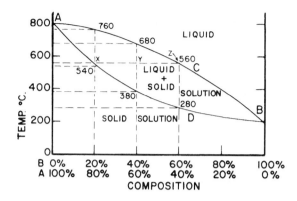

Fig. 5-11 Phase diagram for the alloy system *AB*.

TABLE 5-1 Composition of Liquid and Solid Phases at Various Temperatures for the Alloy System *AB*

Temperature (° C)	80% *A* and 20% *B*	
	Liquid	Solid
>760	80% *A*	None
760	80% *A*	97% *A*
680	60% *A*	90% *A*
560	40% *A*	80% *A*
<540	None	80% *A*

Types of Phase Diagrams

Solid solutions

The phase diagram for metals *A* and *B* that form solid solutions is shown in Fig. 5-11. All compositions above the line *ACB* are liquid (liquidus line), and those below line *ADB* are solid (solidus line); solid and liquid exist in the area between the liquidus and solidus lines. If an alloy of 80% *A* and 20% *B* is melted and then cooled, it remains liquid until 760° C, at which point the solid, having the composition of 97% *A* and 3% *B*, begins to precipitate. The composition of the solid and liquid for this alloy during cooling is listed in Table 5-1. Further cooling to 680° C results in the solid with the composition 90% *A* and 10% *B* and the liquid with the composition 60% *A* and 40% *B*. These values are obtained by drawing a horizontal line through the temperature and noting the composition where this line crosses the solidus and liquidus lines. When the temperature reaches 560° C, the solid is 80% *A* and

the liquid contains 40% *A*; below 540° C there is no liquid and the solid is 80% *A*. The relative amounts of the two phases in the liquid-solid region can be determined at a given temperature by the inverse lever rule; the fraction of the material that is liquid at 560° C for 60% *A* and 40% *B* composition is *XY/XZ* and the fraction that is solid is *YZ/XZ*.

The liquidus and solidus lines are shown in Fig. 5-12 for the silver-gold system. The interpretation of this phase diagram is similar to the one just described for alloy *AB*. One of the most important alloy systems in dentistry is the gold-copper system, in which a series of solid solutions are formed. This system is described in greater detail in Chapter 14.

Eutectic alloy

A phase diagram of an eutectic mixture of the alloy system *AB* is shown in Fig. 5-13. This diagram is similar to the NaCl-H_2O diagram discussed earlier. When the composition of 90% *A* and 10% *B* is heated to position *x*, the system is liquid. On cooling to x', crystals of *A* form. As cooling is continued, more *A* crystallizes until the eutectic temperature, *f*, is reached, and the entire system solidifies and consists of crystals of *A* in a matrix of eutectic. A similar situation exists when a composition of 20% *A* and 80% *B* is cooled from *y*. At *y'* crystals of *B* form in the melt, and when solidification is complete, the solid consists of crystals of *B* in a matrix of eutectic. If an eutectic composition of 37% *A* and 63% *B* is cooled from the liquid state, it solidifies at *e*, and the solid is completely eutectic. Notice the extremely narrow (vertical line) phase field at 100% *A*, below *F.P.*, and a similar one on the right side of the diagram at 100%. In other eutectic phase diagrams the phase fields along each side may be solid solutions and are represented by wider fields.

As seen in the eutectic phase diagram in Fig. 5-14, when a 70% Pb and 30% Sn alloy is cooled from the liquid state, pure lead precipitates at 265° C; continued cooling to 215° C causes more lead to precipitate and the liquid composition is 50% Pb. Cooling to just the eutectic temperature results in a liquid containing 38% Pb, and further cooling results in no liquid and a solid having 70% Pb. When cooled below the eutectic temperature, no lead or tin crystallizes, but a homogeneous mixture of lead and tin crystallizes. The liquidus line for the

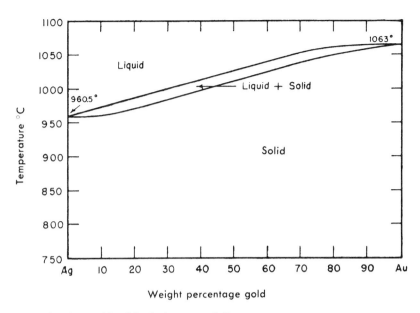

Fig. 5-12 Phase diagram of a silver-gold solid-solution type of alloy.

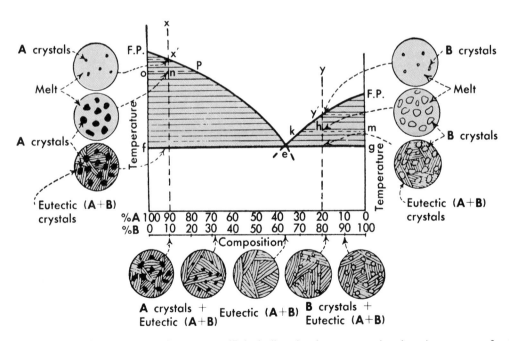

Fig. 5-13 Phase diagram for the eutectic alloy system *AB*, including sketches representing the microstructure for the various compositions at different temperatures.

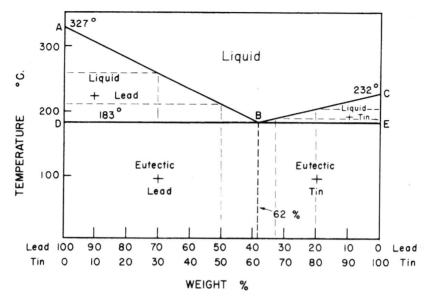

Fig. 5-14 Typical eutectic phase diagram of tin and lead.

lead-tin system is *ABC* and the solidus line is *ADBEC*. No effort has been made to show the limited solubility of tin in lead or lead in tin that may occur on prolonged heating of solid alloys. The lead-tin eutectic alloys are important because they are used as soft solders.

The silver-copper phase diagram is shown in Fig. 5-15. It should be noticed that a small amount of solid solution exists in the narrow phase fields on each side of the diagram. The liquidus line is *ABC* and the solidus line is *ADBEC*. The silver and copper form an eutectic at 779.4° C with a composition of 71.9% Ag and 28.1% Cu. At 779.4° C a maximum of 8.8% Cu and 8% Ag can remain in solid solution. The compositions of the liquid and solid at various temperatures for 95% Ag–5% Cu and an 80% Ag–20% Cu alloy are listed in Table 5-2. The 95% Ag and 5% Cu alloy is solid below 871° C, and it is in the solid solution form between 871° C and 654° C. If it is allowed to cool slowly from 654° C to room temperature, the alloy will be a mixture of eutectic and solid solution. If quenched from any temperature from 871° to 654° C, the alloy will be a solid solution because time has not been allowed for equilibrium to occur.

An alloy of 80% Ag and 20% Cu at 779.4° C will contain some solid and some liquid; the liquid will have the eutectic composition, and the solid will be a

solid solution of 8.8% Cu in 91.2% Ag. An alloy of 80% Ag and 20% Cu at any temperature below 779.4° C is a solid, consisting of an eutectic mixture and a solid solution regardless of the method of cooling.

A photomicrograph of a silver-copper eutectic mixture shows that silver and copper have separated as mixtures rather than as homogeneous solutions of silver and copper. Evidence of a mixture is shown by the light and dark areas in Fig. 5-16; this appearance is typical of eutectic alloys.

Intermetallic compounds

Phase diagrams can be developed from a series of cooling curves for two metals that form compounds in the same manner that they are developed for eutectic and solid-solution alloys. These diagrams generally are more complex than those for eutectic and solid-solution alloys. Such a diagram for the silver-tin system, showing the compound Ag_3Sn, is represented in Fig. 9-2.

Ternary Phase Diagrams

The phase diagram for ternary alloys can be prepared from cooling curves in a manner similar to that used for binary alloys. The three pure metals may be represented as the vertices of an equilateral triangle, with the temperature indicated by the

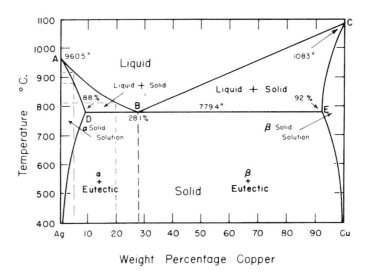

Fig. 5-15 Silver-copper phase diagram of eutectic alloy.

TABLE 5-2   Composition of Liquid and Solid Phases at Various Temperatures for Two Silver-Copper Alloys

Temperature (° C)	95% Ag and 5% Cu		Temperature (° C)	80% Ag and 20% Cu	
	Liquid	Solid		Liquid	Solid
>920	95% Ag	None	>819	80% Ag	None
920	95% Ag	97% Ag	819	80% Ag	92% Ag
881	89% Ag	95% Ag	779.4	72% Ag	91.2% Ag
<881	None	95% Ag	<779.4	None	80% Ag

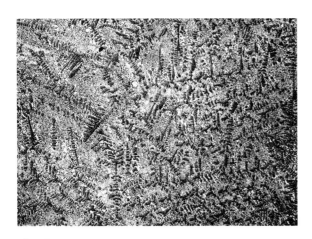

Fig. 5-16 Microscopic view of silver (71.9%) and copper (28.1%) eutectic mixture. (About ×50.)

length of a vertical line perpendicular to the plane of the triangle. The complete diagram must be constructed as a three-dimensional model as shown in Fig. 5-17. Ternary diagrams have not been developed to the extent of binary diagrams because of the difficulty in their preparation.

Construction of Phase Diagrams

Phase diagrams are frequently constructed from cooling curves, which show the temperatures of phase changes. These phase changes are then used to position the lines on phase diagrams. In Fig. 5-18, *A,* as a pure metal is cooled from the liquid phase (position *a*) the temperature falls off smoothly until the freezing point (more commonly referred to as the melting point) is reached (*b*). At the freezing

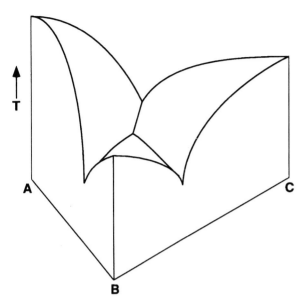

Fig. 5-17 Ternary phase diagram showing the liquid-solid surface formed between components *A, B,* and *C.* The vertical axis represents increasing temperature.

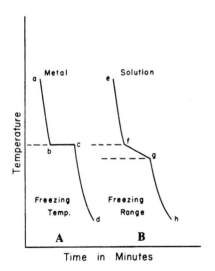

Fig. 5-18 Time-temperature cooling curve of a pure metal, *A,* and a solution type of alloy, *B.*

point the temperature stops falling and remains constant until all metal has solidified (*b-c*). Only then does the temperature continue to drop. By monitoring the temperature of a melt and the delay in cooling, the melting point and its position on a phase diagram are determined. In a similar manner the

changes in the cooling curve for a metal solution can be determined (Fig. 5-18, *B*). Here the delay in cooling is not at a fixed temperature but occurs over a freezing range. Solutions associated with eutectic alloys show cooling curves and freezing points like that of the pure metal at the eutectic composition.

■ PROPERTIES OF ALLOYS

Solid-Solution Alloys

In general, the properties of the solid solutions resemble those of the metals forming the alloy, with certain exceptions. Solid-solution alloys often have higher strength and hardness and lower ductility than either pure metal. This is the basis of solid-solution strengthening. From a theoretical perspective the alloying atoms are absorbed into dislocations, thereby preventing dislocation movement and improving strength. Solid solutions also possess melting ranges rather than melting points and always melt below the melting point of the highest fusing metal and sometimes below the melting points of both metals. These alloys are commonly used in dentistry because they have higher corrosion resistance than multiphased alloys. Also, in a few cases solid solutions have higher corrosion resistance than the pure metals. A notable example is the addition of chromium to iron in solid solution to make the corrosion-resistant alloy "stainless steel." However, in the case of gold, addition of other elements reduces the corrosion resistance.

Eutectic Alloys

Eutectic mixtures are usually harder and stronger than the metals used to form the alloy and are often quite brittle. They possess a melting point at the eutectic composition, not a melting range, and any other combination of the alloy system has a higher fusion temperature than the melting point of the eutectic mixture. Eutectic mixtures, along with other two-phase microstructures, often have poor corrosion resistance. Galvanic action between the two phases at a microscopic level can accelerate corrosion as described in Chapter 3.

Intermetallic Compounds

The intermetallic compounds formed in some alloy systems are usually very hard and brittle.

Their properties rarely resemble those of metals making up the alloy. For example, Ag_2Hg_3 is an intermetallic compound formed in dental amalgam that has properties completely different from those of pure silver or mercury.

■ MICROSTRUCTURE OF METALS AND ALLOYS

The study of the internal structure of metals and alloys is known as the science of metallography. There are two internal structures present in all metals, the microstructure and the crystal structure or nanostructure. The microstructure is composed of grains and phases, which may vary in size from ultramicroscopic particles to grains that can be seen without a microscope. The microstructure is commonly viewed by light or electron microscopy. The crystal structure is the arrangement of atoms in the material. It can be determined by x-ray diffraction methods or viewed by high-resolution electron microscopy and other advanced microscopic technics. The physical properties of alloys are strongly dependent on the microstructure, the crystal structure, and the type of bonding between atoms.

Solidification of Metals

Virtually all metals solidify in crystalline form when they are allowed to cool from the molten state. The crystals of metals are called grains because they seldom exhibit the familiar form of crystals grown from solutions or gases. When crystals of metals solidify, they grow until they contact each other, thereby preventing the formation of the complete crystal. Some metal grains may be seen with the unaided eye after they are polished and etched with suitable chemical reagents, but magnification is usually necessary to make them visible. The grain structure is altered by changing alloy composition, heat treating, and deforming the metal.

A pure metal, when cooled from a temperature at which it was liquid, eventually reaches a temperature at which crystal nuclei form throughout the liquid. The number of these nuclei depends on a variety of factors, such as the purity of the metal, rate of crystallization, rate of cooling, agitation during cooling, and shape of the mold. Assuming all other factors to be constant, the number of grains in the final

solid is proportional to the rate of cooling. As heat is lost, more solid metal forms, which deposits on the original nuclei in a regular manner to build larger grains. This action continues until all the liquid material has solidified, which results in an aggregate of grains, the number depending on the number of original crystal nuclei that formed. The shape of the grains will seldom be regular because they often are in a freely solidifying substance containing excess liquid. During the solidification of metals the crystallization is usually so rapid that large, individual grains with definite geometric form are seldom obtained. The location of the final liquid when it solidifies will determine the boundary of the crystals or grains, so that their shape will depend on the manner in which the grains have developed toward each other. The grains of solidified pure gold and 22k alloy are shown in Fig. 5-19.

The outline of the grains depends entirely on chance because each grain is built to retain the same orientation as that of the original nucleus. If adjoining grains have the same orientation, they will merge into one grain; if they have a different orientation, a boundary between adjoining grains will be produced because of the different axial directions.

Dendrites form during solidification when the metal builds rapidly in the direction of one of the major axes to produce an elongated grain. Branches from the original grain form before the remaining metal has time to solidify, and a skeleton grain is produced. If the first metal to solidify has a composition different from the remaining liquid, these skeletons will not have the same composition as the surrounding metal. An artist's conception of the skeletal structure of a dendrite is shown in Fig. 5-20. This shows how the crystal develops in three directions from the central nucleus where crystallization first begins. Eventually all the liquid metal between the branches solidifies with the whole dendrite forming a single grain. Insoluble impurities such as oxides, if present in the metal, usually remain in the liquid until they become entrapped between the branches in the final portion and solidify. Microscopic examination of a metal often shows these imperfections in structure and may indicate the type of impurity present and its relative amount. Pure metals also solidify with a dendritic structure, but this structure

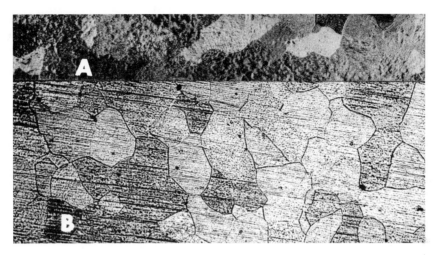

Fig. 5-19 Typical grain structure of pure gold, **A,** and 22k alloy, **B,** when viewed at low magnification.

presence is not revealed by etching and microscopic examination unless the metal has been contaminated.

The dendritic (treelike) pattern of crystallization is common in dental alloys and often appears on the surface of solidified sprue buttons of dental castings. Such a sprue button is shown, only slightly magnified, in Fig. 5-21. Etching reagents have a differential action on the components of the alloys so that microscopically the dendrite outline of the internal structure may be observed as shown in Fig. 5-22.

Solidification of Alloys

Sections of annealed solid-solution alloys, when properly prepared, etched, and examined, show structures similar to those for pure metals, as was illustrated in Fig. 5-19. Each grain usually has a different shade as a result of the amount of light reflected from the surface to the eye; this is caused by variation in grain orientation. The number of crystal nuclei formed during initial solidification determines the number of individual grains and the final grain size. By reference to the phase diagram of a solid solution, one can follow the process of crystallization.

An alloy forming an eutectic produces a different type of structure during solidification, as illustrated in Fig. 5-16. The structure of this alloy would not be homogeneous as that of a simple solid solution. The initially solidified crystals appear scattered throughout an eutectic matrix. At higher magnification the

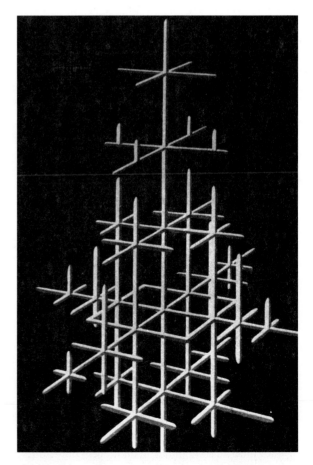

Fig. 5-20 Sketch of dendritic structure of a crystal.

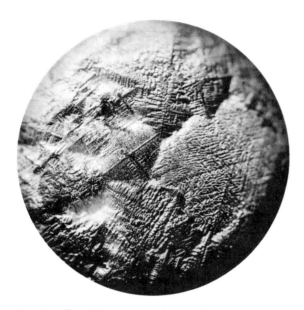

Fig. 5-21 Dendritic structure developed in a sprue button of a gold alloy casting as seen without polishing or etching. (×5.)

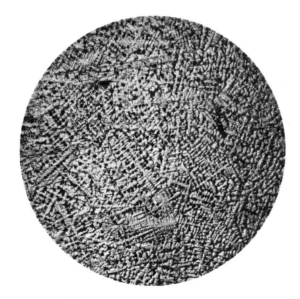

Fig. 5-22 Microscopic view of internal dendritic structure as revealed by suitable polishing and etching action. (About ×50.)

structure of the eutectic is also found to be heterogeneous because it is a mixture of two components.

Intermetallic compounds in alloys generally appear as homogeneous grains. They occasionally solidify with a more definite grain outline than pure metals or solid solutions and may appear as almost perfect geometric forms, especially during slow solidification of the alloy.

Cast Microstructures

The size and shape of the grains may reveal the history of the metal. For example, large grains suggest pure metals or simple alloys and a slow rate of solidification. Deforming an alloy at room temperature (cold working) develops a distinctive type of structure. Heating and holding this cold-worked alloy at a high temperature (annealing) produces characteristic grains of recrystallized alloy. The size of the grains after annealing suggests the temperature and time of heating if a certain amount of cold working is assumed.

The size of the grains in a cast alloy not only depends on the casting environment and general composition but also is affected by traces of impurities. These may be present unintentionally in dental gold or chromium-cobalt-nickel alloys, but occasionally they are added to control the grain size or crystal transformation rate. The addition of small amounts (0.005% to 0.1%) of platinum group metals, especially iridium and ruthenium, produces grain refinement in gold alloys. These high-melting elements form many nuclei on which grains form during cooling and solidification.

Impurities in metals often change the microscopic structure. If the impurities are soluble in the metal in the solid state, little change in grain structure may be noted. Impurities that are soluble in the liquid and insoluble in the solid metal are usually deposited at the grain boundary or in the eutectic mixture. Such impurities as oxides or slag material may become trapped in the casting and usually can be detected as foreign particles.

Other defects in cast metals and alloys may include small internal pits caused by gas inclusion. Often these are invisible without the aid of a microscope, and many times in bulky restorations they may not be harmful to the finished restoration. However they may contribute to fracture in delicate clasps that are subjected to bending or alternating stresses. Numerous microscopic pits at the surface of a casting may contribute to corrosion and tarnish. The pitted restoration may also be discolored by collecting organic material from the mouth.

Imperfections in castings such as shrinkage voids may result from an improper casting technic. Dental alloys shrink when changing from a liquid to a solid state, and voids are likely to be produced unless the molten metal is allowed to flow into the mold throughout the entire process of solidification. The supply of metal may be cut off by premature solidification, or isolated portions of the casting may be enclosed by solidified metal before the interior is completely crystalline. Voids produced in this manner can usually be distinguished from other types by microscopic examination.

Uniformly shaped grains, described as being equiaxed, are illustrated in Fig. 5-19. Equiaxed grains tend to form more readily in a hot mold with the metal and mold cooled slowly. In this way the grains have an opportunity to grow from a few centers distributed throughout the mass of the casting. A slight increase in the rate of cooling tends to develop a greater number of nuclei, which results in smaller grain size.

When a mass of metal is poured, or cast, into a cold mold, the metal at the mold wall is the first to drop below the freezing temperature, and nuclei form in this area, with crystallization proceeding toward the center of the mass. Such grain growth is described as columnar, with the grain boundaries projecting from the mold wall to the center of the casting. Fig. 5-23 shows a column structure that developed when a cobalt-chromium alloy was poured into a cold hexagonal mold; it also shows how the grains growing simultaneously from the six mold faces produce interference boundaries in the solidified metal. Such boundaries act as planes of weakness and potential sources of failure if the casting is subjected to bending or cold working. Sharp corners in the casting design and impurities in the metal that concentrate in the boundary planes are both sources of weakness in the finished casting and should be avoided.

Cold-Worked Microstructures

Metals and alloys are cast for two quite different purposes. In one instance the casting serves as the final structure. In the second, it serves as an object that is further manipulated to form wires, sheets, bars, or similar fabricated structures. A typical cast structure in dentistry is an inlay or bridge restora-

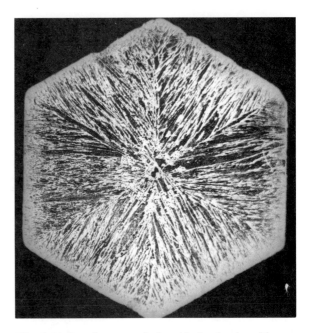

Fig. 5-23 Interference grain boundaries developed by an alloy poured into a hexagonally shaped mold. (×5.)

tion, which is not given further mechanical treatment except for polishing or marginal adaptation by hand operations. This limited treatment does not significantly modify the microstructure of the casting. Such a casting is designed to form to precision measurements, and the properties of the structure are those displayed by the cast metal or alloy.

When the metal is to be used for wires, bands, bars, or other types of wrought structures, it is first cast into ingots that are then subjected to rolling, swaging, or wire-drawing operations, which produce severe mechanical deformation of the metal. Such operations are described as hot or cold working of the metal, depending on the temperature at which the operation is performed. Many dental structures such as orthodontic wires and bands are formed by cold-working operations. The finished product is often described as a wrought structure to denote that it has been formed by severe working or shaping operations. The properties of wrought structures are quite different from those of cast structures in both internal appearance and mechanical characteristics.

The microscopic appearance of a cast metal is a crystalline and sometimes dendritic structure, as shown in Fig. 5-24. When this metal is subjected to

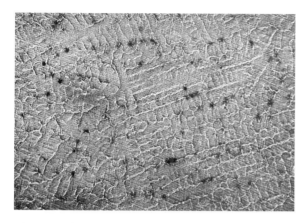

Fig. 5-24 Characteristic microscopic structure of a cast dental gold alloy.

Fig. 5-25 Typical internal structure of a dental gold alloy in wire form, showing fibrous structure.

cold-working operations, such as drawing into a wire, the grains are broken down, entangled in each other, and elongated to develop a fibrous structure or appearance that is characteristic of wrought forms, as shown in Fig. 5-25. This change in internal appearance is accompanied by a change in mechanical properties. In general, mechanical properties of the wrought structure are superior to those of a casting prepared from the same metal or alloy. It should be emphasized that in cast dental structures such as inlays, the mechanical properties of strength and hardness are not modified appreciably by simple polishing or marginal adaptation operations.

Recrystallization and Grain Growth

Metals or alloys that have been cold worked in the process of forming wires or bands change their internal structure and properties when heated or annealed. The characteristic fibrous structure of the wrought mass is gradually lost, and a grain or crystalline structure reappears. The process is known as recrystallization or grain growth. The degree of recrystallization is related not only to the alloy composition and mechanical treatment or strain hardening received during fabrication but also to the temperature and the duration of the heating operation. High temperatures and long heating periods produce the greatest amount of recrystallization. It is not uncommon to find that during a soldering or annealing operation of a practical appliance the temperature applied to the wire or band material was sufficient to cause recrystallization of the wrought structure. Recrystallization of a segment of wire adjacent to a soldered joint is shown in Fig. 5-26. Because the strength is usually reduced in recrystallized wrought structures (ductility often increases), it is necessary to guard against excessive heating during the assembly of a wrought metal appliance. Although the tendency for recrystallization is more prevalent in some wires than others, it can be kept to a minimum when the time and temperature of heating are kept as low as possible.

Even though there is probably some tendency for cast metal structures to recrystallize when heated after casting, the grain growth does not become evident when the structure is heated within the range of practical operations. Under excessive conditions of heating there is some evidence of recrystallization in cast alloys, but the significance is not so pronounced as in the case of wrought forms. Within practical limits of operation this characteristic of recrystallization and grain growth is limited therefore to wrought structures.

The cause for grain growth in the wrought structure is related to the tendency for metals to maintain a crystalline internal orientation of the component atoms. During the formation of the wrought structure, the original grains produced during the crystallization of the original casting were deformed and broken into small units. The deformation of the metal mass occurred by slippage of one portion past another along definite crystallization planes.

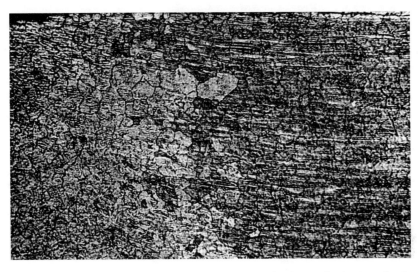

Fig. 5-26 Dental gold wire showing evidence of recrystallization as a result of excessive heat application, with loss of fibrous structure.

The deformation and slippage occurred in various directions to distort the grain boundaries. The greater the degree of cold working, the greater the degree of grain boundary deformation. This deformed structure is unstable in nature, with greater internal energy than one that is in the cast condition. Accordingly, it possesses modified physical properties and the tendency to recrystallize when heated.

Stress relieving, annealing, recrystallization, and grain growth can be illustrated by a series of sketches as in Fig. 5-27. A wrought wire that has been bent beyond the proportional limit and that contains tensile and compressive stresses at the upper and lower boundaries is shown in Fig. 5-27, *A*; the wire has the typical fibrous structure and a deformed crystal lattice. Moderate temperatures cause the release of these stresses, as shown in Fig. 5-27, *B*, without other changes. Higher heating at annealing temperatures (Fig. 5-27, *C*) causes the disrupted crystal structure to contain sufficient energy to return to its normal crystal structure, but the fibrous wrought structure is still evident; under this condition the corrosion resistance is increased. Further increases in temperature or time or both, as seen in Fig. 5-27, *D*, permit recrystallization with grains appearing and the fibrous structure disappearing. Finally in Fig. 5-27, *E*, grain growth occurs.

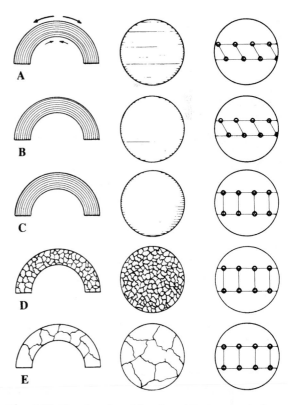

Fig. 5-27 Sketches describing the microstructure and crystal structure of a wrought wire that was bent, **A,** stress-relieved, **B,** and annealed, **C.** Further heating caused recrystallization, **D,** and grain growth, **E.**

■ TECHNIQUES TO STRENGTHEN METALS AND ALLOYS

To strengthen a metal we must make it more difficult for the metal to deform. Because metals deform by dislocation, the metal must be modified to impede the motion of dislocations. Alloying elements are added to impede dislocation motion by several mechanisms. The most important alloy-strengthening mechanisms are solid-solution strengthening, precipitation hardening, and grain refining. In addition, all metals and alloys can be strengthened by cold working. All of these mechanisms can be combined to produce alloys with optimal properties.

Most dental alloys are solid solution strengthened. Solid solutions contain atoms of different sizes. Even slightly dissimilar metal atoms can stabilize dislocations and make it more difficult for the dislocations to move. In the center of a dislocation are regions where the atoms are packed tightly and where replacement of some of the atoms by smaller atoms would result in a less-strained crystal structure. There are also regions where larger atoms would fit into the structure and fill excess space. In both cases the dislocation is stabilized and becomes less mobile. When many dislocations are stabilized the metal becomes stronger.

The precipitation of a phase such as an intermetallic compound from solid solution is widely used for strengthening alloys. This phase or precipitate acts as an obstacle to the movement of dislocations. To carry out precipitation hardening, alloys are heat treated at temperatures where the phase diagrams indicate that precipitation will be produced. The most effective precipitation strengthening occurs at an early stage before a precipitate is visible in the microstructure. In this initial stage, a coherent precipitate is formed that is still part of the alloy lattice (Fig. 5-28). The strain produced by the coherent precipitate within the lattice effectively prevents dislocation movement and therefore hardens and strengthens the alloy. Further growth of the precipitate during heat treatment results in the formation of a precipitate as a separate phase with a decrease in strength. The precipitation of the compound $FePt_3$ by heat treatment of gold-platinum-iron alloys provided the strength necessary for the first bridges constructed from porcelain fused to metal. A high-magnification electron micrograph of the precipitate is shown in Fig. 5-29. The effect of the iron

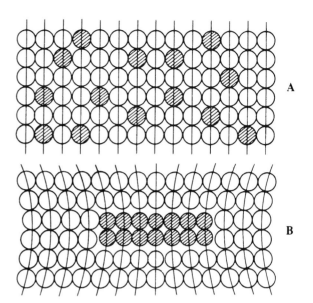

Fig. 5-28 Formation of a coherent precipitate. **A,** Supersaturated solution of B atoms (dark circles) in a matrix of A atoms (light circles). **B,** Coherent precipitate particle formed by clustering of B atoms but still part of the lattice. (From Reed-Hill RE: *Physical metallurgy principles,* ed 2, © 1973, Litton Educational Publishing. Reprinted by permission of PWS-KENT.)

content and heat-treatment time on hardness is shown in Fig. 5-30.

To have effective precipitation hardening the fine precipitate must be dispersed throughout the alloy and not along grain boundaries. Precipitation that occurs at grain boundaries often has a detrimental effect on mechanical properties, commonly making the alloy brittle. To avoid this kind of precipitate, heat treatment must be carefully controlled.

Modifying metals and alloys to produce finer grains always leads to improved mechanical properties. It is one of the best ways to improve the mechanical properties of metals and alloys because the strength and hardness are improved without sacrificing ductility. Reduced grain size can be achieved by adding grain-refining alloying elements to cast alloys or by cold working.

Grain refining by adding trace amounts of elements has been used successfully with gold alloys. Small quantities (0.005%) of iridium are added to the alloys during their formulation. On subsequent castings of these alloys, iridium functions as a nucleating agent and produces about 125 times the grains

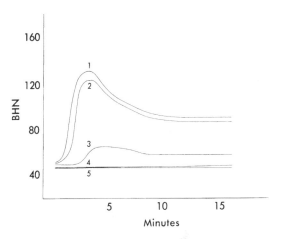

Fig. 5-30 Brinell hardness numbers (BHN) of gold-platinum alloys with the addition of small amounts of iron as a result of heating for various times at 700° C. Percentage iron content was: *1,* 0.16; *2,* 0.08; *3,* 0.04; *4,* 0.02; and *5,* 0.01. (From Fuys RA, Fairhurst CW, O'Brien WJ: *J Biomed Mater Res* 7:471, 1973.)

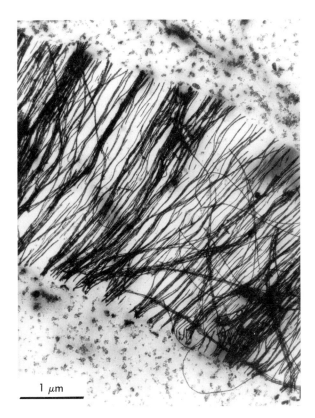

Fig. 5-29 Electron micrograph of FePt$_3$ formed in a gold platinum alloy containing 0.08 wt% iron. (From Sims JR, Jr, Blumenthal RN, O'Brien WJ: *J Biomed Mater Res* 7:497, 1973.)

per unit volume. As a result, the average grain size is reduced from a diameter of 350 to 70 μm.

In general, cold working improves mechanical properties of metals and alloys if the operation is not too severe. If cold worked too much, the metal may form fine cracks and the strength may be severely decreased. The operations of rolling into sheets, drawing into wires, and swaging into special shapes represent the principal processes of deformation that make alloys more useful in structural applications. Many alloys are capable of considerable deformation before rupture when the deformation is performed in a suitable manner. The resulting worked, or wrought, structures have the size and shape of the modified grain structure, which results in the normal increase in strength and hardness.

A cast gold alloy having an ultimate tensile strength of approximately 517 MPa and a hardness of 160 BHN in the softened condition is increased in strength to approximately 690 MPa with a hardness of 175 BHN when converted to a wire. Other mechanical properties are modified in a similar manner. Further comparisons between cast and wrought alloys are made in Chapter 15.

If a metal or alloy is recrystallized after cold working the resulting grain size is usually much finer than the grain size before the metal was cold worked. This sequence, cold working followed by recrystallization, is often used to create finer grain sizes for improved mechanical properties. If heating is continued, grain growth occurs as shown in Fig. 5-27, *E.* As recrystallization and grain growth occur, the strength is greatly reduced, and the elongation and ductility are increased.

SELECTED PROBLEMS

Problem 1. What methods can be used to improve the mechanical properties of a dental casting alloy?

Solution. Perhaps the best approach is to add grain-refining elements to the alloy. Fine grain size generally improves all mechanical properties, including the ductility. Another method that can be used is solid-solution strengthening. Strength and hardness can be dramatically improved by small additions of alloying metals, which go into solution. However, with solid-solution strengthening the ductility may be reduced. Other technics, such as alloying to form second phases to produce eutectic structures or precipitation hardening, are less desirable for use in dentistry because of increased susceptibility to corrosion. Finally, cold working a casting is generally impractical because the shape would be affected.

Problem 2. In the lead-tin alloy system, which compositions will show melting points and which will show melting ranges (refer to Fig. 5-14)?

Solution. The pure metals always have melting points. With eutectic alloys the eutectic composition will also have a melting point. So we have melting points at 100% Pb, 100% Sn, and 38% Pb-62% Sn. All other compositions will show melting ranges.

Problem 3. An alloy composed of 30% Ag and 70% Cu is melted and cast. The casting is cooled and a specimen is prepared for metallography. Using the Ag-Cu phase diagram, describe the microstructure (refer to Fig. 5-15).

Solution. Alloys are usually heated to about 100° C above the liquidus before casting (about 1050° C for this alloy). After casting and as the alloy cools, the first solid crystals will form just below the liquidus at about 950° C. These high copper crystals β continue to grow as the alloy is cooled. At the temperature just above the eutectic (779.4° C) solid crystals and liquid alloy are present. As the temperature drops below the eutectic temperature the crystals are retained but all of the liquid becomes a fine-grained eutectic mixture of α and β. So a microscope would show a microstructure of high copper crystals β surrounded by a fine eutectic.

Problem 4. A stainless steel wire of an orthodontic appliance was found to be weak and to deform easily after an annealing heat treatment over a flame. What caused the change in properties?

Solution. Annealing a wrought appliance causes several changes in the crystal structure and microstructure. Initially, residual stresses are relieved, but further heating will cause major changes in the microstructure and properties. If the alloy is overheated, recrystallization (and perhaps grain growth) will occur and this will reduce the wire's strength. The annealing treatment must be carefully controlled to avoid overheating the metal.

■ REFERENCES

Asgar K, Peyton FA: Pits on inner surface of cast gold crowns, *J Prosthet Dent* 9:448, 1959.

ASM metals handbook, ed 7, Cleveland, 1948, American Society for Metals. (See also ed 8, vol 1, 1961, and ed 9, vol 1, 1978.)

Bush SH, Taylor DF, Peyton FA: A comparison of the mechanical properties, chemical composition, and microstructures of dental gold wires, *J Prosthet Dent* 1:177, 1951.

Coleman RL: Physical properties of dental materials, research paper no 32, *J Res Nat Bur Stand* 1:867, 1928.

Crawford WH: Selection and use of investments, sprues, casting equipment and gold alloys in making small castings, *J Am Dent Assoc* 27:1459, 1940.

Doan GE, Mahla EM: *The principles of physical metallurgy,* ed 2, New York, 1941, McGraw-Hill.

Flinn RA, Trojan PK: *Engineering materials and their applications,* ed 2, Boston, 1981, Houghton Mifflin.

Lane JR: A survey of dental alloys, *J Am Dent Assoc* 39:414, 1949.

Nielsen JP, Tuccillo JJ: Grain size in cast gold alloys, *J Dent Res* 45:964, 1966.

Peyton FA: Restorative materials. In Gabel AB, editor: *The American textbook of operative dentistry,* ed 9, Philadelphia, 1954, Lea & Febiger.

Phillips RW: Studies on the density of castings as related to their position in the ring, *J Am Dent Assoc* 35:329, 1947.

Reed-Hill RE: *Physical metallurgy principles,* ed 2, New York, 1973, D Van Nostrand.

Ryge G, Kozak SF, Fairhurst CW: Porosities in dental gold castings, *J Am Dent Assoc* 54:746, 1957.

Shell JS: Metallography of precious metals, *J Am Dent Assoc* 12:794, 1925.

Shell JS: Microscopic comparison of two gold alloys, *J Am Dent Assoc* 12:801, 1925.

Souder W, Paffenbarger GC: *Physical properties of dental materials,* National Bureau of Standards Circular No C433, Washington DC, 1942, US Government Printing Office.

Strickland WB, Sturdevant CM: Porosity in the full cast crown, *J Am Dent Assoc* 58:69, 1959.

Taylor DF, Peyton FA: A comparison of the tensile and bending properties of dental gold wires, *J Dent Res* 30:290, 1951.

Udah K-I, Yasuda K, Ohta M: Age-hardening characteristics in an 18 carat gold commercial dental alloy containing palladium, *J Less-common Metals,* 118:249, 1986.

Vines RF: *The platinum metals and their alloys,* New York, 1941, The International Nickel Co.

Wise EM, Crowell WS, Eash JT: The role of platinum metals in dental alloys, *Trans Am Inst of Mech Engineers, Inst Met Div* 99:363, 1932.

Wise EM, Eash JT: The role of platinum metals in dental alloys, *Trans Am Inst of Mech Engineers, Inst Met Div* 104:276, 1933.

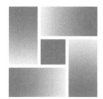

6 Polymers and Polymerization

Before the introduction of acrylic polymers to dentistry in 1937, the principal polymer used for denture bases was vulcanized rubber. Polymers introduced, since then have included vinyl acrylics, polystyrene, epoxies, polycarbonates, polyvinylacetate-polyethylene, *cis-* and *trans-* polyisoprene, polysulfides, silicones, polyethers, and polyacrylic acids. In addition, oligomers from bisphenol A and glycidyl methacrylate (such as dimethacrylates) and urethane dimethacrylates have been applied.

In terms of quantity, the primary use of polymers has been in the construction of prosthetic appliances such as denture bases. However, they have been used for highly important applications such as artificial teeth, tooth restoratives, cements, orthodontic space maintainers and elastics, crown and bridge facings, obturators for cleft palates, inlay patterns, implants, impressions, dies, temporary crowns, endodontic fillings, and athletic mouth protectors.

■ BASIC NATURE OF POLYMERS

Chemical Composition

The term *polymer* denotes a molecule that is made up of many (poly) parts (mers). The *mer* ending represents the simplest repeating chemical structural unit from which the polymer is composed. Thus poly(methyl methacrylate) is a polymer having chemical structural units derived from methyl methacrylate, as indicated by the simplified reaction and structural formula I below.

The molecules from which the polymer is constructed are called monomers (one part). Polymer molecules may be prepared from a mixture of different types of monomers. They are called copolymers if they contain two or more different chemical units and terpolymers if they contain three different units, as indicated by the structural formulas II and III on the next page.

As a convenience in expressing the structural formulas of polymers, the mer units are enclosed in

I

Methyl methacrylate   Poly(methyl methacrylate)

127

II

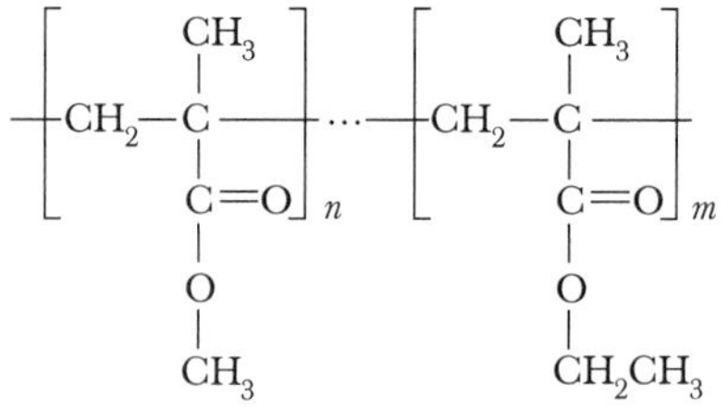

Methyl methacrylate–ethyl methacrylate copolymer

III

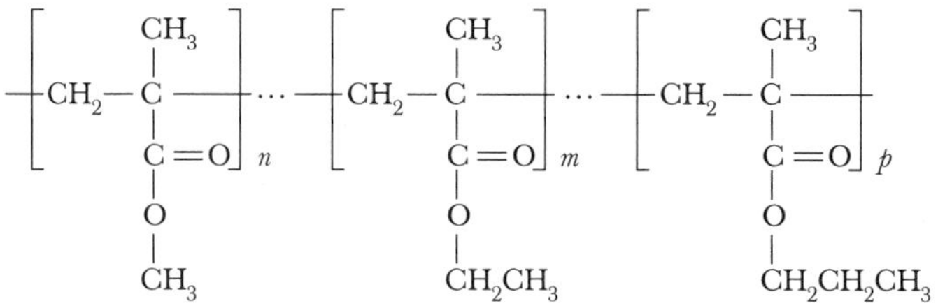

Methyl-, ethyl-, propyl methacrylate copolymer or terpolymer

brackets, and subscripts such as *n, m,* and *p* represent the average number of the various mer units that make up the polymer molecules. Notice that in normal polymers the mer units are spaced in a random orientation along the polymer chain. It is possible, however, to produce copolymers with mer units arranged so that a large number of one mer type is connected to a larger number of another mer type. This special type of polymer is called a block polymer. It also is possible to produce polymers having mer units with a special spatial arrangement with respect to the adjacent units, and these are called stereospecific polymers.

Molecular Weight

The molecular weight of the polymer molecule equals the molecular weight of the various mers multiplied by the number of the mers and may range from thousands to millions of molecular weight units, depending on the preparation conditions. The higher the molecular weight of the polymer made from a single monomer, the higher the degree of polymerization. The term *polymerization* is often used in a qualitative sense, but the degree of polymerization is defined as the total number of mers in a polymer molecule.

In general, the molecular weight of a polymer is reported as the average molecular weight because the number of repeating units may vary greatly from one molecule to another. As would be expected, the fraction of low, medium, and high molecular weight molecules in a material or, in other words, the molecular weight distribution, has as pronounced an effect on the physical properties as the average molecular weight does. Therefore two poly(methyl methacrylate) samples can have the same chemical composition but greatly different physical properties because one of the samples has a high percentage of low molecular weight molecules, whereas the other has a high percentage of high molecular weight molecules. Variation in the molecular weight distribution may be obtained by altering the polymerization procedure. These materials therefore, do not possess any precise physical constants, such as melting point, as ordinary small molecules do. For example, the higher the molecular weight, the higher the softening and melting points and the stiffer the plastic.

Spatial Structure

In addition to chemical composition and molecular weight, the physical or spatial structure of the poly-

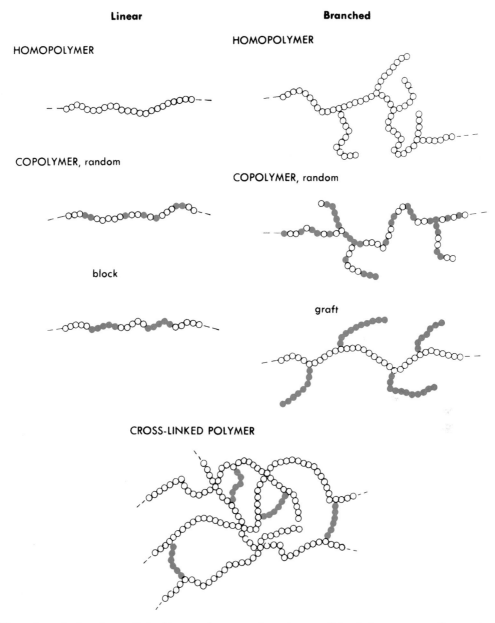

Fig. 6-1 Linear, branched, and cross-linked homopolymers and copolymers; light circles, one type of mer unit; dark circles, another type of mer unit; dotted lines, only a segment of the polymer.

mer molecules is also important in determining the properties of the polymer. There are three basic types of structures: linear, branched, and cross-linked. They are illustrated in Fig. 6-1 as segments of linear, branched, and cross-linked polymers. The linear homopolymer has mer units of the same type, and the random copolymer of the linear type has the two mer units randomly distributed along the chain. The linear block copolymer has segments, or blocks, along the chain where the mer units are the same. The branched homopolymer again consists of the same mer units, whereas the graft-branched copolymer consists of one type of mer unit on the main chain and another mer for the branches. The cross-linked polymer shown is made up of a homopolymer cross-linked with a single cross-linking agent.

The linear and branched molecules are separate and discrete, whereas the cross-linked molecules are a network structure that may result in the polymer becoming one giant molecule. The spatial structure of polymers has an effect on their flow properties, but generalizations are difficult to make because either the interaction between linear polymer molecules or the length of the branches on the branched molecules may be more important in a particular example. In general, however, the cross-linked polymers flow at higher temperatures than linear or branched polymers. Another distinguishing feature of some cross-linked polymers is that they do not absorb liquids as readily as either the linear or branched materials.

An additional method of classifying polymers other than by their spatial structure is according to whether they are thermoplastic or thermosetting. The term *thermoplastic* refers to polymers that soften when heated and solidify when cooled. (The process is repeatable.) Typical examples of polymers of this type are poly(methyl methacrylate), polyvinyl acrylics, and polystyrene. The term *thermosetting* refers to plastics that solidify during fabrication but cannot be softened by reheating. These polymers generally become nonfusible because of a cross-linking reaction and the formation of a spacial structure. Typical dental examples are cross-linked poly(methyl methacrylate), silicones, *cis*-polyisoprene, and bisphenol A-diacrylates.

As a class polymers have unique properties, and by varying the chemical composition, the molecular weight, the molecular weight distribution, or the spatial arrangement of the mer units, the physical and mechanical properties of the polymers may be altered.

■ PREPARATION OF POLYMERS

Polymers are prepared by a process called polymerization, which consists of the monomer units becoming chemically linked to form high molecular weight molecules. The polymerization process may take place by several different mechanisms, but most polymerization reactions fall into two basic types: addition polymerization and condensation polymerization. Important addition polymerization reactions are free radical, ring opening, and ionic reactions.

Addition Polymerization

Free-radical polymerization

Free-radical polymerization reactions usually occur with unsaturated molecules containing double bonds as indicated by the following equation, where R represents any organic group, chlorine, or hydrogen.

$$n \ CH_2{=}CH{-}\underset{R}{|} \xrightarrow{\text{Initiator}} \left[CH_2{-}\underset{R}{\overset{H}{\underset{|}{\overset{|}{C}}}} \right]_n$$

In this type of reaction no by-product is obtained. The reaction takes place in three stages called the initiation, propagation, and termination stages. The reaction may be accelerated by heat, light, and traces of peroxides, as well as trialkyl borane and other chemicals. In any case, the reaction is initiated by a free radical, which may be produced by any of the methods mentioned, as shown in the equation on p. 131, top.

Sufficient free radicals for polymerization may be produced at room temperatures by the reaction of a chemical accelerator such as a tertiary amine or a sulfinic acid with the organic peroxide. N,N-dihydroxyethyl-para-toluidine

$$CH_3{-}\langle\!\bigcirc\!\rangle{-}N\!\!\begin{array}{c} CH_2CH_2OH \\ \\ CH_2CH_2OH \end{array}$$

has commonly been used as an accelerator in dental products.

The initiation stage is followed by the rapid addition of other monomer molecules to the free radical and the shifting of the free electron to the end of the growing chain (see reactions on p. 131), which describes the propagation stage.

This propagation reaction continues until the growing free radical is terminated. The termination stage may take place in several ways as indicated, where M represents the mer unit and n and m represent the number of mer units.

Initiation stage

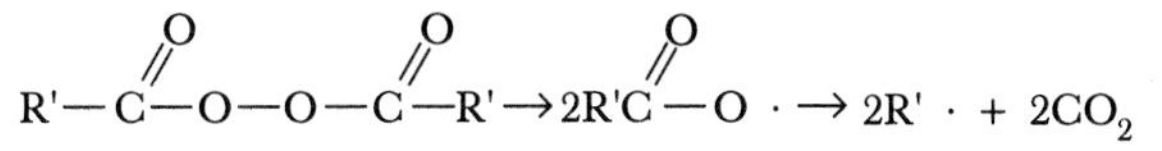

$$R'-\overset{\overset{O}{\|}}{C}-O-O-\overset{\overset{O}{\|}}{C}-R' \rightarrow 2R'\overset{\overset{O}{\|}}{C}-O\ \cdot\ \rightarrow 2R'\ \cdot\ +\ 2CO_2$$

Organic peroxide   Free radical

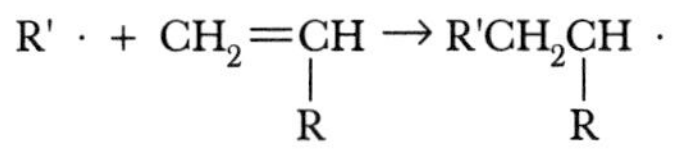

$$R'\ \cdot\ +\ CH_2{=}\underset{\underset{R}{|}}{CH} \rightarrow R'CH_2\underset{\underset{R}{|}}{CH}\ \cdot$$

Propagation stage

$$R'CH_2\underset{\underset{R}{|}}{CH}\ \cdot\ +\ CH_2{=}\underset{\underset{R}{|}}{CH} \rightarrow R'CH_2\underset{\underset{R}{|}}{CH}{-}CH_2{-}\underset{\underset{R}{|}}{CH}\ \cdot\ \rightarrow\ etc.$$

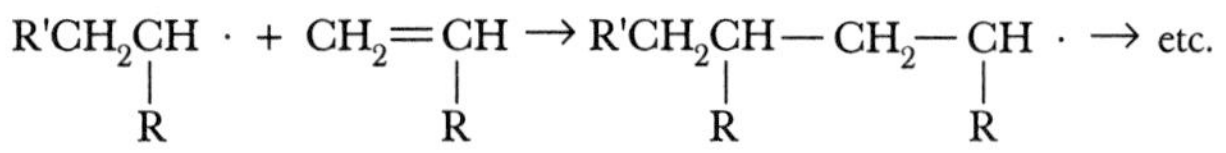

Termination stage

$$R'M_n\ \cdot\ +\ \cdot\ M_mR \rightarrow R'M_nM_mR$$

Annihilation reaction

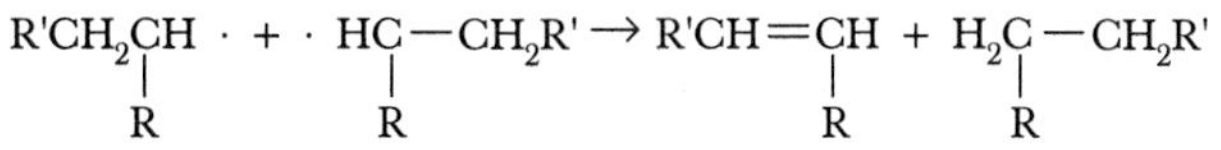

$$R'CH_2\underset{\underset{R}{|}}{CH}\ \cdot\ +\ \cdot\ \underset{\underset{R}{|}}{HC}{-}CH_2R' \rightarrow R'CH{=}\underset{\underset{R}{|}}{CH}\ +\ H_2\underset{\underset{R}{|}}{C}{-}CH_2R'$$

Disproportionation reaction

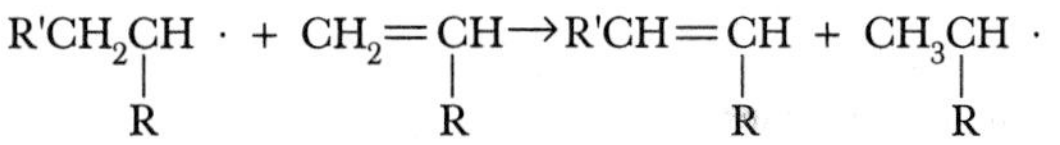

$$R'CH_2\underset{\underset{R}{|}}{CH}\ \cdot\ +\ CH_2{=}\underset{\underset{R}{|}}{CH} \rightarrow R'CH{=}\underset{\underset{R}{|}}{CH}\ +\ CH_3\underset{\underset{R}{|}}{CH}\ \cdot$$

Transfer reaction

A study of these termination reactions reveals how branched and cross-linked polymer molecules may be obtained.

Free-radical polymerization reactions can be inhibited by the presence of any material that will react with a free radical, thus decreasing the rate of initiation or increasing the rate of termination. Decreasing the rate of initiation results in a retarding of the polymerization reaction, and increasing the rate of termination decreases the degree of polymerization or the molecular weight of the final polymer. Such materials as hydroquinone, eugenol, or large amounts of oxygen will inhibit or retard the polymerization. Small amounts of hydroquinone are used to protect the methyl methacrylate monomer from premature polymerization, which prolongs the shelf life of the monomer.

Another important free-radical polymerization reaction is responsible for the setting of resin restorative composites. The manufacturer prepares a compound from one molecule of bisphenol A and two molecules of glycidyl methacrylate called 2,2-*bis*[4(2-hydroxy-3 methacryloyloxy-propyloxy)-phenyl] propane (see Chapter 10). The acronym Bis-GMA has been used to identify this compound. Because it is not, strictly speaking, a monomer, it is called an oligomer. A simplified structural formula is shown below:

Lower molecular weight difunctional monomers such as triethyleneglycol dimethacrylate are added to reduce the viscosity, and polymerization is accom-

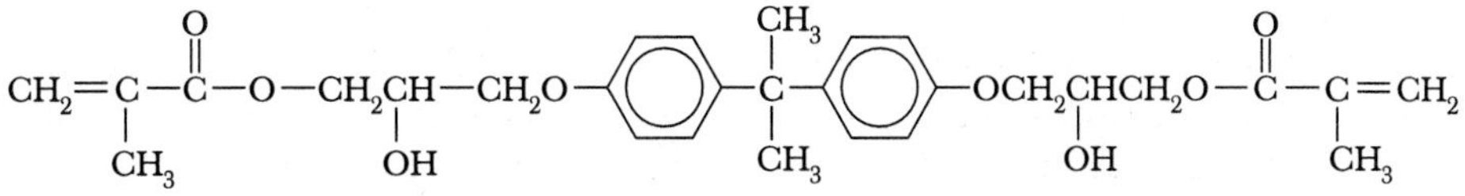

$$CH_2{=}\underset{\underset{CH_3}{|}}{C}-\overset{\overset{O}{\|}}{C}-O-CH_2\underset{\underset{OH}{|}}{CH}-CH_2O-\bigcirc-\underset{\underset{CH_3}{|}}{\overset{\overset{CH_3}{|}}{C}}-\bigcirc-OCH_2\underset{\underset{OH}{|}}{CH}CH_2O-\overset{\overset{O}{\|}}{C}-\underset{\underset{CH_3}{|}}{C}{=}CH_2$$

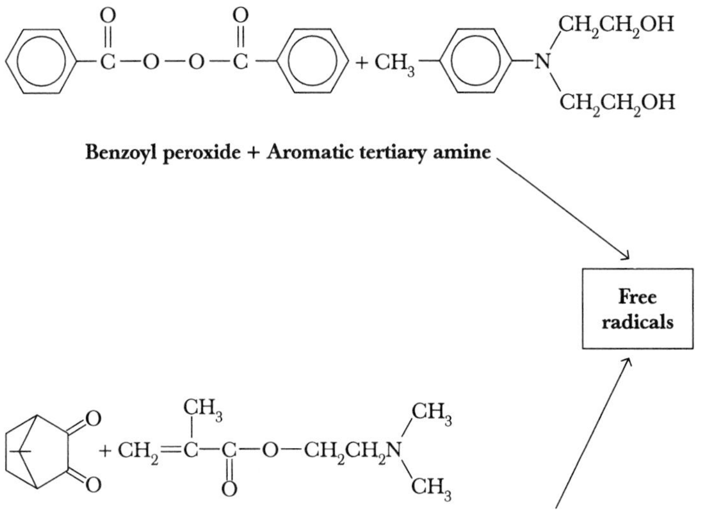

Benzoyl peroxide + Aromatic tertiary amine

Free radicals

A diketone such as camphoroquinone + Aliphatic amine + Visible light (460 nm)

plished using free radicals. Because the Bis-GMA has reactive double bonds at each end of the molecule just as the added lower molecular weight monomers do, a highly cross-linked polymer is obtained.

Free radicals needed to initiate the reaction are produced in composites by one of the two methods shown above.

Some composites contain oligomers that are urethane dimethacrylates such as that shown below.

Polymerization is accomplished by free-radical initiation with a peroxide-amine system or a diketone-amine system and exposure to blue visible light.

The free-radical polymerization of monomers or oligomers with unsaturated double bonds does not result in all the double bonds reacting. The term *degree of conversion* describes the percentage of double bonds that react, and, depending on the conditions, the value may vary from 35% (at the air inhibited layer) to 80%.

Photo-initiation polymerization has become highly popular in dentistry and it has been shown that the degree of conversion ranges from about 65 to 80% while chemical initiation results in values from 60 to 75%. Systems used to cement restorations frequently use both photo- and chemical-initiation (dual curing) because it often is difficult to expose the material to

sufficient light to reach the maximum degree of conversion and thus maximum strength. With these dual curing materials maximum degrees of conversion of 80% have been reported.

Ring-opening polymerization

Two important ring-opening polymerizations in dentistry are the epoxy and ethylene imine reactions. The former is used to produce dies from rubber impressions, and the latter is used in the setting reaction of polyether rubber impression materials.

The reactants for the epoxy system are a difunctional epoxide oligomer and a difunctional amine as shown in the following simplified equation:

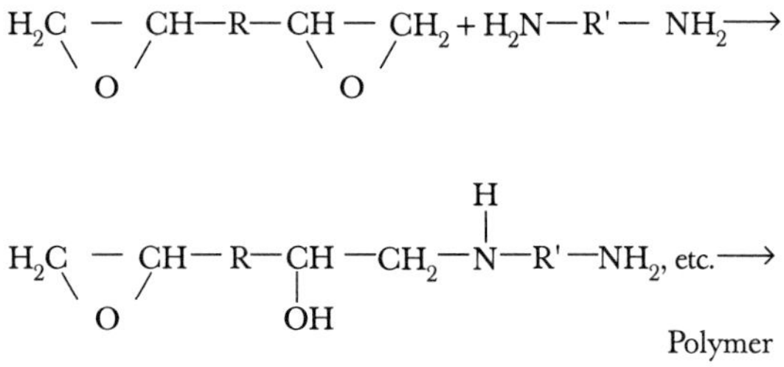

$$H_2C \underset{O}{-} CH - R - CH \underset{O}{-} CH_2 + H_2N - R' - NH_2 \longrightarrow$$

$$H_2C \underset{O}{-} CH - R - \underset{OH}{CH} - CH_2 - \overset{H}{N} - R' - NH_2, \text{ etc.} \longrightarrow$$

Polymer

The amine opens the ring and cross-linking results in a rigid polymer. Water interferes with the

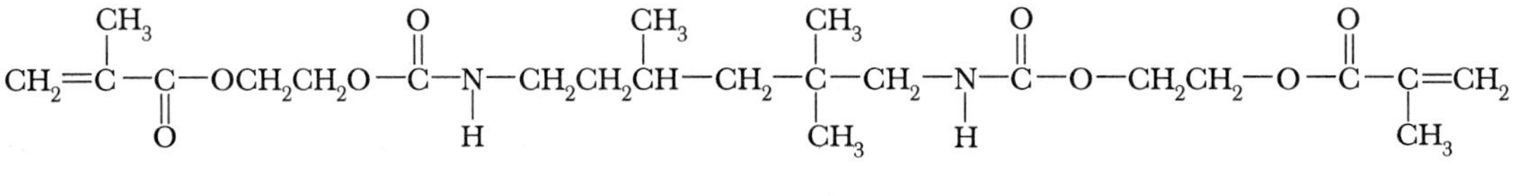

$$CH_3-\underset{\underset{\displaystyle CH_2-CH_2}{\overset{|}{N}}}{\overset{\displaystyle \overset{H}{|}}{C}}-R-\left[CH(CH_2)_n-O\right]_m-R-\underset{\underset{\displaystyle CH_2-CH_2}{\overset{|}{N}}}{\overset{\displaystyle \overset{H}{|}}{C}}-CH_3 + \text{(aryl sulfonate)} \longrightarrow$$

Polyether   **Catalyst**

$$CH_3-\underset{\underset{\displaystyle CH_2-CH_2}{\overset{|}{N}}}{\overset{\displaystyle \overset{H}{|}}{C}}-R-\left[CH(CH_2)_n-O\right]_m-R-\underset{\underset{\displaystyle \overset{|}{CH_2}}{\underset{\displaystyle CH_2}{}}}{\overset{\displaystyle \overset{H}{|}}{\underset{\displaystyle R''-N}{C}}}-CH_3, \text{ etc. } \longrightarrow \textbf{Polymer}$$

setting reaction because it will react with the epoxide. Therefore agar and alginate impressions are incompatible with this die material.

The polyether oligomer has a three-membered ring containing nitrogen as shown above. The ring is opened by the alkyl benzenesulfonate catalyst, and polymerization results in a cross-linked rubber.

Ionic polymerization

One final example of an addition reaction is with a vinyl-terminated silicone and a silane (–H)-containing siloxane as shown below. In this instance the H_2PtCl_6 attacks the hydrogen in the silane-containing dimethyl siloxane, and this complex reacts with the vinyl-terminated dimethyl siloxane to form a cross-linked silicone rubber. Compounds used in the vul-

canization of latex surgical gloves interfere in the polymerization of addition silicones, and thus contact should be avoided.

Condensation Polymerization

Condensation reactions result in polymerization plus the production of low molecular weight by-products. Polysulfide rubbers are formed by a condensation reaction, the most general reaction being between low molecular weight polysulfide polymers having mercaptan (–SH) groups and lead dioxide as shown below by the simplified reactions.

Water and lead sulfide are by-products of the reaction. Mercaptan groups are also along the chain and thus cross-linking occurs. The rate of the reaction is proportional to –SH, PbO_2, and H_2O.

$$CH_2{=}CH-\underset{\underset{\displaystyle CH_3}{|}}{\overset{\overset{\displaystyle CH_3}{|}}{Si}}-O-\left[\underset{\underset{\displaystyle CH_3}{|}}{\overset{\overset{\displaystyle CH_3}{|}}{Si}}-O\right]_x-\underset{\underset{\displaystyle CH_3}{|}}{\overset{\overset{\displaystyle CH_3}{|}}{Si}}-CH{=}CH_2 + \left[\underset{\underset{\displaystyle CH_3}{|}}{\overset{\overset{\displaystyle H}{|}}{Si}}-O\right]_y\cdots\left[\underset{\underset{\displaystyle CH_3}{|}}{\overset{\overset{\displaystyle CH_3}{|}}{Si}}-O\right]_z + H_2PtCl_6 \longrightarrow$$

Vinyl-terminated siloxane   **Silane-containing siloxane**

$$\cdots\underset{\underset{\displaystyle CH_3}{|}}{\overset{\overset{\displaystyle CH_3}{|}}{Si}}-CH_2CH_2-\underset{\underset{\displaystyle O}{|}}{\overset{\overset{\displaystyle CH_3}{|}}{Si}}-\cdots, \text{ etc.} \longrightarrow \begin{array}{l}\textbf{Silicone}\\\textbf{rubber}\end{array}$$

$$HS-R-SH + PbO_2 \longrightarrow HS-R-SS-R-SH + PbO + H_2O, \text{ etc.}$$
$$HS-R-SH + PbO \longrightarrow HS-R-S-Pb-S-R-SH + H_2O$$
$$HS-R-S-Pb-S-R-SH + S \longrightarrow HS-R-SS-R-SH + PbS, \text{ etc.} \longrightarrow \text{Rubber}$$

Condensation polymerization of the mercaptan groups can also be accomplished by use of a $Cu(OH)_2$ or an organic hydroperoxide $R'-OOH$ as shown by the following simplified reactions:

$$HS-R-SH + Cu(OH)_2 \longrightarrow$$
$$HS-R-S-Cu-S-R-SH + H_2O$$

$$HS-R-S-Cu-S-R-SH \longrightarrow$$
$$CuS + HS-R-SS-R-SH, \text{ etc.}$$

and

$$HS-R-SH + R'-OOH \longrightarrow$$
$$HS-R-SS-R + R'-OH + H_2O, \text{ etc.}$$

The polymerization with peroxides results in greater shrinkage on setting than when metal oxides are used, and thus PbO_2 and $Cu(OH)_2$ are preferred.

Silicones may be polymerized by a condensation reaction if they contain terminal hydroxy groups as shown by the reaction below.

Metal esters used have been stannous octoate and dibutyl tin dilaurate. The ortho-ethyl silicate is used as a cross-linking agent and is more stable if not combined with the metal ester. Ethyl alcohol is the by-product, and its evaporation from the set rubber accounts for a significant portion of the shrinkage of condensation silicones after setting. Organosilicon compounds with only two ethoxy groups can be substituted for the ortho-ethyl silicate, thus reducing the by-product and shrinkage on setting.

Polymer acids are used successfully in dentistry to react with hydrated metal ions such as Zn^{+2}, Ca^{+2}, or Al^{+3}. A copolymer of acrylic acid and itaconic acid in water is reacted with zinc oxide in an acid-base reaction to form a cement called zinc polyacrylate as outlined:

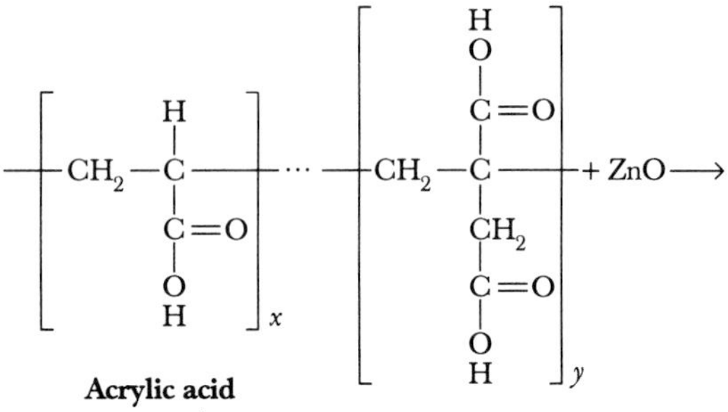

Acrylic acid mer unit

Itaconic acid mer unit

or simplified:

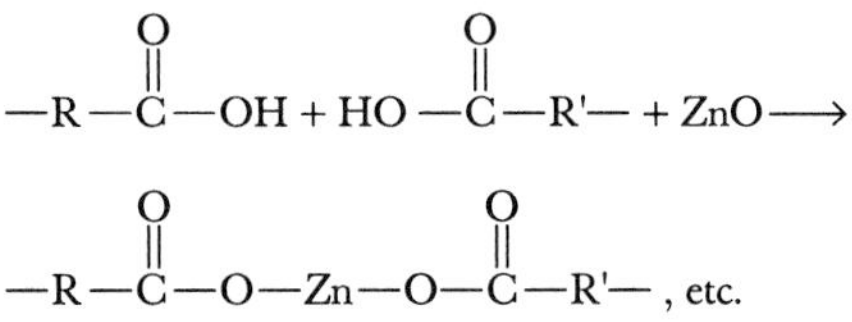

The copolymer acid can also be freeze-dried and included with the ZnO powder, and then only water is mixed with the powder.

A similar reaction with a copolymer of acrylic and itaconic acid is used with an aluminosilicate glass. Tartaric acid is also present in the formulation:

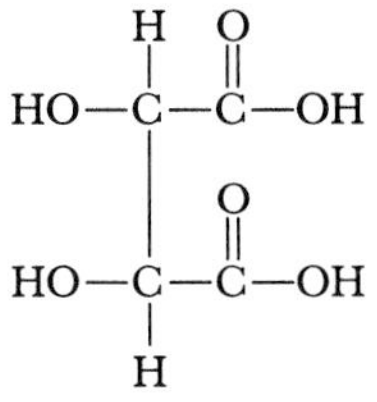

Tartaric acid

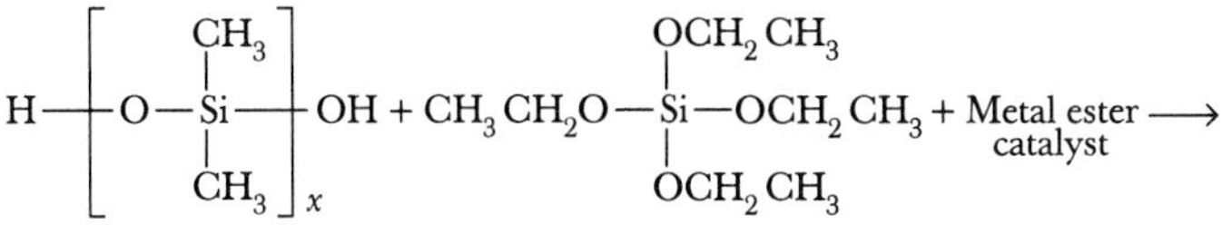

Hydroxyl-terminated siloxane   ***ortho*-Ethyl silicate**

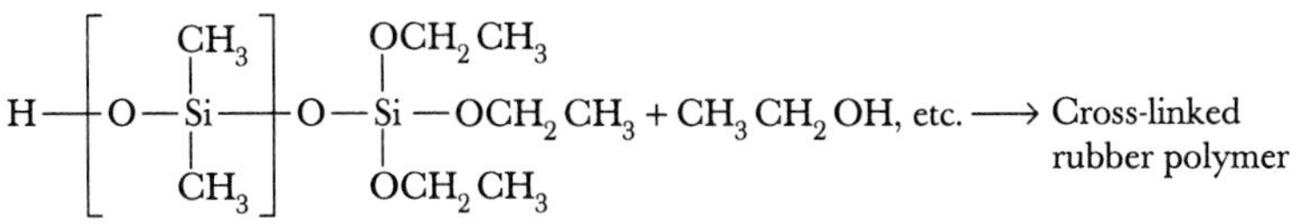

The copolymer acid reacts first with Ca^{+2} and then $Al+3$ dissolved out of the glass by an ionic reaction to form metal esters. The material is called an ionomer and is used as both a restorative and a cement.

Materials are available that use a combination of the ionomer reaction and free-radical polymerization. The polyacrylic acid molecules containing pendant methacrylate groups are dissolved in water along with 2-hydroxyethylmethacrylate and tartaric acid. The powder contains a glass and microencapsulated potassium persulfate and ascorbic acid catalyst. On mixing the powder and liquid an acid-base ionomer reaction accompanied by a free-radical methacrylate reaction occurs.

Other Polymers

A variety of polymers are used in fully polymerized form without any polymerization reaction carried out by the dentist or laboratory technician. Polyisoprene is available in two forms, *cis* and *trans,* and both are natural rubbers. These structures are shown as follows:

cis-Polyisoprene

trans-Polyisoprene

Notice that for the *cis* type the $-CH_3$ and $-H$ are on the same *(cis)* side, whereas for the *trans* type they are on opposite *(trans)* sides. *cis*-Polyisoprene is cross-linked by the process of vulcanization with sulfur or other chemicals such as peroxides. In the vulcanized form it is very flexible and is used as surgical gloves, rubber dams for the restorative procedures, and elastics for orthodontic applications. *trans*-Polyisoprene is rigid and is compounded mainly with zinc oxide but also with some waxes and zinc silicate and is used for endodontic points as part of the filling material for root canals. For this application it is called gutta-percha.

A copolymer of ethylene and vinyl acetate has the structural formula that follows.

Copolymers containing 18% to 33% vinyl acetate are sold in fully polymerized sheets and are heated to about 90° C and vacuum or hand formed over gypsum dental models to produce athletic mouth protectors. The manufacturer uses a free-radical polymerization method to produce the polymer, which is then molded into sheets. No polymerization occurs in the dental processing of the mouth protector, and they are processed as thermoplastics.

SELECTED PROBLEMS

Problem 1. Two samples of poly(methyl methacrylate) were listed by the manufacturer to be 100% pure, which was true, yet one had a significantly lower softening temperature than the other. Why?

Solution. The two samples could have had different average molecular weights, different molecular weight distributions, or different spatial structures (linear, branched, or cross-linked).

Problem 2. The hardness and stiffness of two samples of ethylene-vinyl acetate copolymer used to fabricate athletic mouth protectors were found to be substantially different at body temperature. What is the most likely cause of the difference?

Solution. It is probable that the ratio of ethylene to vinyl acetate in the samples was different, with the softer and less stiff sample containing less vinyl acetate. It is also possible that the average molecular weights or their distributions were different.

Problem 3. Two denture base poly(methyl methacrylate) products were heated. One sample softened and flowed, whereas the second decomposed rather than melted. What is the most likely reason for this observation?

Solution. The former poly(methyl methacrylate) sample was most likely a linear polymer, whereas the latter was a cross-linked poly(methyl methacrylate).

Problem 4. An experimenter determined the degree of polymerization of a poly(methyl methacrylate) material and used this information to calculate the degree of conversion. Would this procedure give a correct result?

Solution. No. The degree of polymerization measures the number of mer units in the polymer molecule, whereas the degree of conversion measures the number of unreacted carbon double bonds.

Problem 5. The dimensional change during polymerization of condensation silicone rubber impression material is significantly greater than that during polymerization of addition silicone rubber impression materials. Why?

Solution. During the polymerization of condensation silicones and the rearrangement of chemical bonds, ethyl alcohol is released as a by-product, but during the polymerization of addition silicones, the hydrogen of one silicone polymer adds to the carbon double bond of the second silicone polymer with no by-product being formed.

Problem 6. Polyisoprene is available in two forms, one highly elastic and the other brittle. Why?

Solution. The *cis*-form has a spatial structure, with the methyl and hydrogen on the same side of the carbon double bond, that allows less intramolecular attraction than the *trans*-form, with the methyl carbon and the hydrogen on opposite sides of the carbon double bond.

■ REFERENCES

Allen JG, Dart EC, Jones E, Nemcek, J: Photochemistry. In Jones DG: *ICI Corporate Laboratory,* Chemistry and Industry, no 3, Feb 7, 1976.

Asmussen E: NMR–analysis of monomers in restorative resins, *Acta Odontol Scand* 33:129, 1975.

Braden M: Characterization of the setting process in dental polysulfide rubbers, *J Dent Res* 45:1065, 1966.

Braden M, Causton B, Clarke RL: A polyether impression rubber, *J Dent Res* 51:889, 1972.

Braden M, Elliott JC: Characterization of the setting process of silicone dental rubbers, *J Dent Res* 45:1016, 1966.

Brauer GM, Antonucci JM: Dental applications. In *Encyclopedia of polymer science and engineering,* vol 4, ed 2, New York, 1986, Wiley.

Cook WD: Photopolymerization kinetics of dimethacrylates using camphoroquinone/amine initiator system, *Polymer* 33:600, 1992.

Cook WD: Rheological studies of the polymerization of elastomeric impression materials. I. Network structure of the set state, *J Biomed Mater Res* 16:315, 1982.

Cook WD: Rheological studies of the polymerization of elastomeric impression materials. II. Viscosity measurements, *J Biomed Mater Res* 16:331, 1982.

Cook WD: Rheological studies of the polymerization of elastomeric impression materials. III. Dynamic stress relaxation modulus, *J Biomed Mater Res* 16:345, 1982.

Craig RG: Chemistry, composition, and properties of composite resins, *Dent Clin North Am* 25:219, 1981.

Craig RG: Photopolymerization of dental composite systems. In Leinfelder KF, Taylor DF, editors: *Posterior composites,* Proceedings of the International Symposium on Posterior Composite Resins, Chapel Hill, NC, 1982, DF Taylor, 1984.

Darr AN, Jacobsen PH: Conversion of dual cure luting cements, *J Oral Rehabil* 22:43, 1995.

Harashima I, Nomata T, Hirasawa T: Degree of conversion of dual cured composite luting agents, *Dent Mater* 10:8, 1991.

Higashi S, Yasuda S, Horie K, Yamada H, Takeda K, Miyajima T, Ishikawa S: Studies on rubber base impression materials. Discussions on the setting mechanism of polysulfide rubber as the dental impression material, chiefly viewed from variations of viscosity and molecular weight, *J Nihon Univ Sch Dent* 13:33, 1971.

Joos RW, McCue EC, Nachtsheim HG: Polymerization kinetics of two paste resin composites, *Int Assoc Dent Res Program and Abstracts,* 1971.

Kitian RJ: The application of photochemistry to dental materials. In Gebelein CG, Koblitz FF, editors: *Polymer science and technology,* vol 14, *Biochemical and dental applications of polymers,* New York, 1981, Plenum.

McCabe JR, Wilson HJ: Addition curing silicone rubber impression materials, *Br Dent J* 145:17, 1978.

Pappas SP, Chattopadhyay AK, Carlblom LH: Benzoin ether photoinitiated polymerization of acrylates. In Labana SS, editor: *Ultraviolet light induced reactions of polymer,* ACS Symposium Ser 25, Washington, DC, 1976, American Chemical Society.

Phillips D: Polymer photochemistry. In Bryce-Smith D, editor: *Photochemistry,* vol 1, London, 1970, The Chemical Society, Burlington House.

Ruyter IE: Monomer systems and polymerization. In Vanherle G, Smith DC: International symposium on posterior composite resin dental restorative materials, *Peter Szulc Publ* 6:109, Netherlands, 1985.

Williams JR, Craig RG: Physical properties of addition silicones as a function of composition, *J Oral Rehabil* 15:639, 1988.

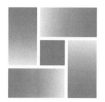

7 Biocompatibility of Dental Materials

Biocompatibility is defined as the compatibility of manufactured materials and devices with body tissues and fluids. The field of dental materials shares the problem of biocompatibility with other fields of biotechnology. Today, in the development of an intraoral material one must consider not only the strength, esthetics, or functional aspects of the material, but its biocompatibility as well. Thus, biocompatibility is important to manufacturers and materials scientists. The field of biocompatibility is broad, and encompasses the development of new testing methodologies, the survey of materials *in vitro* for potential biocompatibility in different biological contexts, and the evaluation of materials in a clinical setting.

Interactions of materials with tissues may alter normal metabolism and physiological processes. These interactions may be physical or chemical, with cells going through stages of degeneration, death, and necrosis (Table 7-1). There are three stages of injury to cells and tissues by any agent. In chronological order, these are (1) the biochemical lesion, (2) the functional lesion, and (3) the morphological lesion (Table 7-1). An example of injury is an infarct of tissue resulting from ischemia (i.e., acute loss of circulation and oxygen). A reduced O_2 supply to individual cells results in a suppression of oxidative phosphorylation and adenosine triphosphate (ATP) production within seconds to minutes (biochemical lesion), followed by decreased function of the sodium pump of the cell membrane. Failure of the pump results in cellular swelling from retention of sodium and water and in reduced function (e.g., reduced protein synthesis or mobility [functional lesion]). Finally, losses in the integrity of the cell and nuclear membranes and release of lysosomal enzymes occur (morphological lesion of necro-

sis). These chemical and physical injuries lead further to a sequence of connective tissue changes classified as inflammatory reactions, immunological reactions, and repair (Table 7-2). All the events shown in Table 7-1 are initial events (within about 24 hours of injury) in Table 7-2.

A variety of *in vitro* cytotoxicity assays (also called screening tests) are shown at the bottom of Table 7-1. The *in vitro* assays parallel specific events during the degenerative (reversible) and necrotic (irreversible) stages of cell and tissue injury. However, these tests do not measure whether materials degrade over long periods as a result of the physical and chemical environment. Other short-term *in vitro* screening tests that may help to determine inflammatory and immune system-stimulating potentials of materials are shown at the bottom of Table 7-2. These include tests for chemotaxis of white blood cells or connective tissue cells, the development of an inflammatory response, or the stimulation of the immune system. Finally, tests for regulation of differentiation as well as mutagenesis determine the frequency of DNA alterations that occur in the presence of various chemicals.

Tables 7-1 and 7-2 emphasize *in vitro* screening tests, or tests done outside of an animal system. However, biocompatibility is also assessed with secondary or usage tests *in vivo* (in animals). Although *in vivo* tests give a more complete picture of the biological response to a material than *in vitro* tests, it is usually very difficult to understand the biological response to a material using *in vivo* tests. The difficulty arises because the biological response may involve many simultaneous reactions. Screening tests are able, by design, to dissect a single response (e.g., suppressed proliferation or migration, enhanced chemotaxis or immune reaction, and increased DNA

TABLE 7-1 Stages of Cell Response after Injury

Type of injury	Degenerative Changes — BIOCHEMICAL	Degenerative Changes — FUNCTIONAL	Degenerative Changes — MORPHOLOGICAL	Cell Death	Necrotic Changes — MORPHOLOGICAL
Ischemia	*A few seconds* O_2 deprivation, ⇓ Oxidative phosphorylation	*< 60 seconds* ⇓ Mitochondrial function, ⇓ ATP* production, ⇓ Na^+ pump → ⇑ Glycolysis, ⇑ Na^+/K^+ ratio within cell, ⇑ Ca^{++}/Mg^{++} ratio within cell, Earliest signs of chromatin clumping	*Several hours* ⇓ Glycogen stores, ⇑ Lactate, ⇓ pH, Cellular swelling, Chromatin clumping, Mitochondrial contraction, Mitochondrial degranulation, ER dilation, ⇓ Protein synthesis → Mitochondrial swelling, Lysosomal swelling, Degranulation of RER, ⇑ Membrane permeability, Pyknotic nuclei		*12-24 hours* ⇑ Lysosome permeability, Release of hydrolases, Release of intracellular enzymes, Permeability to external molecules / Karyolysis, "Myelin" forms derived from cell membranes, Cellular debris, Digestion of cell components
CCl₄	Conversion to CCl_3 radical by P450 oxidase system of mitochondria, Oxidation of membranes	Oxidation/damage to cell membrane lipids, ⇓ Mitochondrial function, ⇓ ATP production / ⇑ Glycolysis, ⇑ Na^+/K^+ ratio within cell, ⇑ Ca^{++}/Mg^{++} ratio within cell, Release of lipid peroxidation products	Cellular swelling, ER dilation, ⇓ Protein synthesis / Mitochondrial swelling, Degranulation of RER, ⇑ Denatured protein, ⇑ Lipid deposits, Pyknotic nuclei		Karyolysis
Screening tests	Mitochondrial enzyme function	Other cellular enzyme functions / ——— Assays for DNA and protein synthesis ——→	Light and electron microscopy ——→		^{51}Cr release assay, Trypan blue uptake, Neutral red uptake (agar overlay), Lysosome enzyme assays / Microscopy ——→

Adapted from Trump BF, Mergner WJ: Cell injury. In Zweifach BW, Grant L, McCluskey RT, editors: *The inflammatory process*, vol 1, ed 2, New York, 1974, Academic press, pp 115-127; Robbins SL, Cotran RS, Kumar V: *Pathologic basis of disease*, ed 3 Philadelphia, 1984, WB Saunders, pp 1-39.

*ATP–adenosine triphosphate; ER–endoplasmic reticulum; RER–rough endoplasmic reticulum.

TABLE 7-2 Host Tissue Morphological Changes after Injury

	Initial Events (0-12 hr)	Tissue Response (12 hr-1 wk)		Final Events (1 wk-6 wk)
	Cell Degeneration, Death, and Necrosis	**Inflammation**	**Immune**	**Regeneration and Repair**
Host responses	Cell swelling Loss of enzyme function Loss of semipermeability of membranes Pyknosis and loss of nuclei	Fluid exudate from capillaries (ions and serum molecules) Cellular exudates and infiltrates Neutrophils Fibroblasts Angioblasts	Lymphocytes Plasma cells Macrophages	Parenchymal regeneration OR → Scar (e.g., fibrous capsule)
Relevant biocompatibility tests	Screening tests Attachment, growth, and macromolecular synthesis Membrane permeability Enzyme assays Secondary tests Usage tests	Screening tests Neutrophilic chemotaxis Lymphocyte chemotaxis Fibroblast chemotaxis Lymphocyte transformation Secondary tests Usage tests		Screening tests None Secondary tests Usage tests

139

fragmentation) from the multitude of responses occurring in the whole animal.

This chapter surveys the tests used for evaluating biocompatibility of dental materials, the specifications that govern such testing, and the strengths and weaknesses of the testing methods. In addition, the biocompatibility of various materials used in dentistry are discussed. Because understanding biocompatibility requires understanding the biological system into which materials are placed, this chapter will first summarize the developmental, anatomical, and pathological aspects of the oral tissues.

BIOLOGY AND INFLAMMATORY RESPONSE OF ORAL TISSUE TO INJURY

The Tooth

Enamel

Mature human enamel is highly mineralized (96% by weight), with only 1% of its weight being organic molecules and 3% being water. The organic matrix of enamel consists of at least two types of glycoproteins, the amelogenins and the enamelins. During development, the organic matrix supports the growth of highly organized hydroxyapatite crystals, which eventually replace most of this matrix and squeeze the remaining matrix to the periphery to form the organic sheaths of the enamel prisms. After synthesis by ameloblasts, the calcified organic matrix of enamel does not appear to be maintained in any way by cellular synthetic mechanisms, contrary to other calcified tissues such as dentin, bone, and cementum. Because of its high mineral (hydroxyapatite) content, enamel is much more brittle than dentin and is solubilized to a greater extent by acid solutions.

Dentin and pulp

Odontoblasts and the dentin matrix are formed from interactions between the dental lamina (and later the dental organ) and the dental papilla. The terminally differentiated odontoblast, which forms first, controls the secretion of the dentin matrix and its subsequent mineralization in both primary and secondary dentin. The dentin matrix contains many proteins, which include collagenous proteins (mainly Type I collagen with smaller amounts of Type V and Type I trimer collagens), noncollagenous dentin-specific proteins (phosphophoryns, dentin sialoprotein, and dentin matrix protein-1) and several nonspecific proteins associated with mineralized tissues (e.g., osteocalcin and osteopontin). Dentin matrix (both calcified and uncalcified dentinoid) forms the greatest bulk of the tooth. Calcified dentin is about 20% organic, 70% inorganic, and 10% aqueous by weight. Collagen constitutes approximately 85% of the organic portion of dentin, and hydroxyapatite is the main inorganic compound. This matrix surrounds dentinal tubules that are filled with the odontoblastic processes that secreted the dentin matrix during formation of the dentin. These tubules traverse the region between the dentoenamel junction (DEJ) and the pulp. The numbers of tubules per cross-sectional area range from about 20,000/mm^2 near the DEJ to 50,000/mm^2 near the pulp. Also, the tubule diameter varies from about 0.5 µm at the DEJ to about 2.5 µm near the pulp (Fig. 7-1). Some odontoblastic processes extend through the dentin tubules to the DEJ. The percentage of processes that reach the DEJ is a matter of some conjecture.

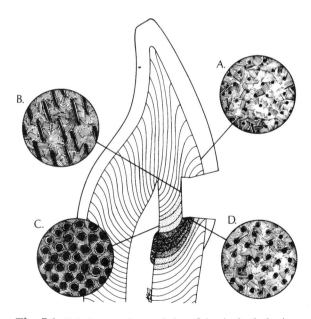

Fig. 7-1 Relative number and size of dentinal tubules in various portions of a tooth. (Courtesy Avery JK: Ann Arbor, 1987, University of Michigan School of Dentistry.)

A serumlike fluid surrounds the odontoblastic processes and fills the dentinal tubules when these processes are absent. This fluid has continuity with the extracellular fluid of the pulp tissue. The pulpal circulation maintains an intercellular hydraulic pressure of about 24 mm Hg (32.5 cm H_2O), which causes fluid flow in the tubules to be directed from the pulp outward toward the DEJ when enamel is removed. External hydrostatic and osmotic pressures can also cause fluid movement toward or away from the pulp. The positive or negative displacement of this fluid through exposed dentinal tubules is capable of affecting either odontoblasts or pulpal nerve endings. These effects are the basis of the hydrodynamic theory of hyperalgesia (pulpal hypersensitivity).

During cavity preparation by the dentist, a "smear layer" is formed by the action of the bur or hand instruments on the calcified dentin matrix (Fig. 7-2). This mat of organic and inorganic particles occludes the dentinal tubules to some extent. The smear layer is quite effective in reducing hydrostatic pressures, but less effective in reducing diffusion, especially if the layer is interrupted or defective. The smear layer can be removed by acid etching, which also demineralizes the openings of the tubules (Fig. 7-3). The dentinal tubules establish continuity with the pulpal fluid to facilitate the diffusion of molecules, both natural or from materials, into and out of the pulp.

Deep cavity preparation can destroy the majority of the dentin and kill the primary odontoblasts. A number of investigators think that the extracellular matrix (ECM) of dentin and pulp is largely responsible for differentiation of secondary odontoblasts that form reparative dentin. The source of secondary odontoblasts is not known, but much of the proliferative activity of granulation tissue following pulpal insult is found in perivascular areas proximal to the core of the pulp. In monkeys the minimal amount of time between pulp injury and replacement odontoblast differentiation is about 5 days. Nerves and blood vessels, which arborize from the core of the pulp as they approach the odontoblastic layer, may influence the extent of the inflammatory response and the amount of new dentin matrix that is formed during dentin repair.

In the absence of a smear layer, chemical and bacterial products diffuse toward the pulp against the pressure gradient (diffusional permeability). Bacteria can be visualized occasionally within tubules below a carious lesion or at the base of a prepared cavity with or without a restoration (Fig. 7-4). When toxic bacterial or chemical products traverse the dentin, odontoblasts and the pulpal connective tissue usually respond first by focal necrosis (0 to 12 hours), which may be followed by an acute, but more widespread, pulpitis (12 hours to several days). This response may resolve naturally if the injurious agent is removed or the tubules are blocked. If the pulpitis does not resolve, it may spread to more completely involve the pulp in liquefaction necrosis (especially if the pulpitis results from bacterial products) or in

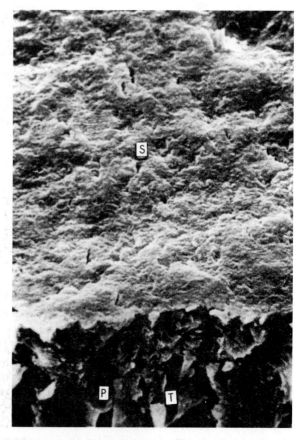

Fig. 7-2 The ground dentinal surface, *S*, has been cleansed only with water spray. The smear layer consisting of powdered dentin obscures the tubule orifices, *T*. A debris plug, *P*, appears in one tubule. (From Brännström M: *Dentin and pulp in restorative dentistry*, Stockholm, 1981, Dental Therapeutics AB.)

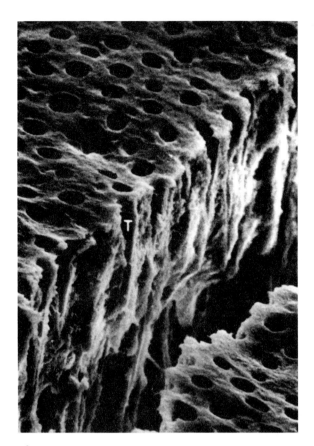

Fig. 7-3 Dentinal surface etched with 37% phosphoric acid for 5 seconds. The dentinal tubules, *T,* are open and enlarged. (From Brännström M: *Dentin and pulp in restorative dentistry,* Stockholm, 1981, Dental Therapeutics AB.)

chronic inflammation. Finally, both acute complete pulpitis and acute exacerbation of chronic pulpitis may lead to sequelae such as dental periapical lesions and osteomyelitis, which may be reviewed in oral pathology textbooks.

Dentin permeability

Much has been learned about dentin permeability in the last two decades. In practical terms, two types of dentin permeability occur. The first is fluid convection, which is movement of fluid through the dentinal tubules. Fluid convection toward the pulp will occur under positive hydraulic pressure when a crown or inlay is being seated. If the dentinal tubules are open, this produces a sharp, localized pain in the pulp from stimulation of A-fibers. Fluid convection

away from the pulp will occur with negative osmotic pressures when concentrated solutions, such as sucrose or saturated calcium chloride, are exposed to open dentinal tubules. Clinically this situation occurs with cervical abrasion or carious lesions. Convection of fluids across dentin varies with the fourth power of the radius of the dentinal tubule (r^4) and thus is very sensitive to the diameter of the tubules. In general, coronal dentin exhibits greater convective permeability than root dentin. Axial wall dentin is more permeable than dentin in the floor of cavities, and dentin near pulp horns (where tubule diameter is greatest) is more permeable than dentin at a distance from the pulp horns. The presence of a smear layer or of cavity liners, sealers, crystals such as calcium oxalate, and even debris and bacteria in the dentinal tubules can dramatically reduce fluid convection.

The second type of dentin permeability is diffusion. Patent dentinal tubules, no matter how small the diameter, establish a diffusion gradient through which ions and molecules can move, even against positive hydraulic pressure. Diffusion is proportional to the length of the dentinal tubules and thus, roughly, to the thickness of the dentin between cavity preparation and the pulp. Smear layers created in cavity preparation are better than cavity liners and sealers at limiting diffusional permeability. However, if the smear layer is incomplete, interrupted or removed, or if there is a disruption in a cavity liner, sealer, or base, then diffusion of molecules toward the pulp will occur.

Diffusion of many molecules through dentin has been studied. In general, diffusion through a given thickness of dentin is proportional to the molecular size of the molecule. Consequently, molecules the size (molecular weight [mw]) of urea (mw 60), phenol (mw 94), and glucose (mw 180) diffuse more easily than molecules the size of dextran (mw 20,000) and albumin (bovine serum albumin, mw 68,000). Through diffusion, small or globular molecules such as albumin, gamma globulin, and the Bis-GMA oligomer are diluted 2000 to 10,000 times on the pulpal side of the dentin by 0.3 to 0.4 mm of dentin. Large, fibrous molecules such as fibrinogen are diluted 25,000 to 125,000 times by the same dentin thickness. Most molecules are probably adsorbed to some extent by dentin. Some molecules and atoms or ions, such as tetracycline, zinc, H_2O_2, and fluorescein, are adsorbed to a greater extent than the

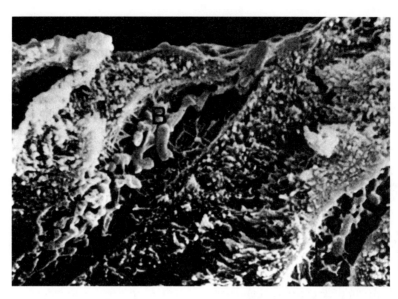

Fig. 7-4 Scanning electron micrograph of bacteria, *B,* in dentinal tubules. (From Brännström M: *Dentin and pulp in restorative dentistry,* Stockholm, 1981, Dental Therapeutics AB, and London, 1982, Wolfe Medical.)

biological molecules and resin monomers just mentioned. Finally, the capillary beds and vascular dynamics in most healthy pulps are probably capable of removing relatively large amounts of cytotoxic chemicals and bacterial products once they diffuse through the dentin. However, if the pulp is already damaged (inflamed because of caries or trauma), edema and sluggish circulation probably compromise the removal of these materials. Much still needs to be learned about the dynamics and significance of diffusion and adsorption of both host and foreign molecules through dentin.

Bone

Bone is an extracellular matrix (ECM) with accompanying cells and tissue. The ECM of bone is a mineralized tissue composed of about 23% organic substances and about 77% hydroxyapatite. Like dentin, most (86%) of this organic matrix is Type I collagen, which gives elastic and viscoelastic qualities to bone. The hydroxyapatite crystals are smaller and less well formed than those in dentin. Because of the vascularity of bone, the mineral phase serves as a major reservoir of both calcium and phosphate ions for the body's metabolic processes. In the oral cavity, maxillary and mandibular alveolar bone support the teeth through a connective tissue called the periodontal ligament. Branches of the trigeminal nerve and the external carotid artery, which supply the teeth, pass through the alveolar bone and supply the bone. The maxilla, premaxilla, and mandible (except for the condylar head) all are formed by membranous bone formation, whereas most long bones of the body are the product of endochondral bone formation.

Membranous bone formation

In membranous bone formation, the ECM of bone (osteoid) is synthesized by osteoblasts that constitute the innermost layer of the periosteum and endosteum. The osteoblasts also initiate mineralization of this ECM. As bone is formed, osteoblasts are trapped within the ECM and become osteocytes that reside in lacunae, communicate with cells in other lacunae through canaliculi, and maintain the vitality of bone. These cells die if surgical manipulation destroys the vascular supply or heats the bone above 45° C for more than a few minutes. Another bone cell type, the osteoclast, decalcifies the ECM and resorbs the organic portion of bone. It also responds to both physiological stimuli and injury. The coupling of osteoblastic and osteoclastic activity directs remodeling and occurs almost continuously throughout life.

If bone injuries are small and periosteal or endosteal damage is not severe, the usual mechanism for bone repair is membranous bone formation. Granulation tissue is formed from the surrounding vascularized connective tissue to fill the bony defect. New osteoblasts, derived from precursor cells in residual periosteum or endosteum, secrete collagen-rich osteoid, which is subsequently mineralized and remodeled. At a clean fracture site, there are two remodeling surfaces: the periosteum, into which ligaments and tendons insert on the outside of bone, and the endosteum, which lines the cavities of spongy or medullary (cancellous) bone. If the injury, such as a fracture, is complicated by bacterial infection, then acute inflammatory cells (neutrophils) and their hydrolytic products complicate bone healing in the subsequent acute osteomyelitis. Osteomyelitis may be reduced by the body's defenses, curettage and debridement, or antibiotics. The osteomyelitis may be resolved through a healing stage exhibiting chronic mononuclear inflammatory cells. On the other hand, residual nonpyogenic microorganisms or toxins may cause a residual low-grade chronic inflammation with persistent mononuclear cell infiltration, which is described as chronic osteomyelitis. Ironically, bone and scar tissue may be stimulated to grow more densely in these sites (sclerotic bone).

In defects caused by tooth extraction or bone fracture, the site initially fills with blood. The fibrin cascade results in a blood clot that fills this site and attaches to the walls of the alveolar bony socket. Subsequently, mesenchymal cells and endothelial cells grow into the blood clot from the surrounding connective tissue of the alveolar bone and create a young, vascular granulation tissue. With succeeding weeks and months, new osteoblasts differentiate from the granulation tissue and elaborate an ECM that gradually mineralizes. Through osteoblastic and osteoclastic influence, the new bone subsequently remodels itself to the general shape and architecture of the surrounding bone. Alveolar bony mass and height are gradually lost, however, because of the lack of tensile forces from teeth and functional periodontal ligament.

Endochondral bone formation

Large bony defects are usually replaced by endochondral bone formation. Connective tissue cells in the region fill the defect and differentiate temporarily into chondroblasts that secrete a cartilaginous scaffolding that lends integrity to the bone. With time, this cartilage is covered and replaced with osteoid that calcifies as the cartilage and bone remodel. This process is under the direction of bone morphogenic proteins. Although remodeling and minor adjustments from physiological stress usually occur by membranous mechanisms, one may occasionally observe centers of cartilage formation in fracture sites, healing wounds, and extraction sites in the maxilla and mandible.

An issue that faces dentists, and particularly implantologists, is the development of materials for implants that are physically and biologically compatible with alveolar bone. Ideally, bone does not respond to the material as a foreign substance by forming a fibrous tissue capsule around it, but rather should integrate the material, substance, or device into the remodeled bone structure. Under optimum circumstances, bone differentiation should occur directly adjacent to the material (osseointegration).

Periodontium

The periodontium is a combination of tissues, including the periodontal ligament (PDL), cementum, and alveolar bone. The cementum and alveolar bone are mineralized extracellular matrices with the associated cells that are responsible for generating and maintaining them.

Collagenous fibers of the PDL extend from cementum to fibrous connective tissue above the alveolar crest, to alveolar cortical bone, or to cementum of the adjacent teeth. The ends of these collagenous fibers are anchored in a calcified ECM synthesized either by cementoblasts (cementoid) or osteoblasts (osteoid). The orientation of the fibers translates compressive forces of mastication to tensile forces on the cementum and alveolar bone. The tensile stress stimulates low-grade cementogenesis and osteogenesis and maintains fairly constant alveolar bone heights, cementum thicknesses, and PDL widths. The exact mechanisms involved in these processes remain largely unknown and are of great interest in the fields of periodontology and implantology, as well as in orthopedic surgery. In contrast, direct pressure (compression) on alveolar bone and cementum (e.g., in orthodontic movement) results in PDL, alveolar bone necrosis, and an active biological resorption that removes portions of alveolar bone, as well as cementum and dentin, from the tooth root. The necrosis is caused by ischemia of PDL and alveolar bone.

The PDL and its attachments to alveolar bone and teeth are maintained by cellular synthetic processes. At least in some animal species, there appears to be some compartmentalization of differentiated cells within the PDL, with fibroblasts in the tooth half of the PDL moving mesially with the constantly erupting incisor. Thus, specific populations of differentiated, predifferentiated, or precursor cells probably give rise to and maintain the matrices of cementum, alveolar bone, and PDL. When cells that maintain the PDL are destroyed during injury and have no source of progenitor cells, ankylosis may result between tooth and bone (e.g., after tooth transplantation or placement of dental implant).

Regeneration of PDL, epithelial attachment, and alveolar bone around periodontally diseased teeth is an important issue in dentistry. In an attempt at regeneration, gingival epithelium replaces crevicular epithelium, which was originally responsible for the epithelial attachment of the tooth. Following scaling and currettage of periodontal pockets, this gingival epithelium proliferates faster than the PDL fibers can reattach in newly formed cementum. Although fibrous reattachment to alveolar bone appears to occur quite readily, the original orientation of fiber to the tooth surface seems quite difficult to achieve. This results in epithelial-lined subcrestal pockets in the PDL space between alveolar bone and tooth surface. When this process advances, it exfoliates the tooth. Investigators have made efforts to limit epithelial down-growth of the gingiva, to enhance PDL reattachment to tooth and bone surfaces by chemical and surgical means, and to use implant materials that maximize both epithelial and connective tissue cell attachment and limit the apical migration of epithelial cells.

Gingiva and Mucosa

The linings of the oral cavity are composed of gingiva and oral mucosa. The gingiva is a connective tissue with an epithelial surface that covers the alveolar ridge, surrounds the crevices of the teeth, and fills interproximal spaces between teeth. Gingiva is divided into attached and free gingiva. The attached gingiva forms a junction with the alveolar oral mucosa toward the vestibule of the mouth and also with the free gingival margin toward the crowns of the teeth. The free gingiva fuses with the attachment epithelium, which surrounds the tooth at its cervix in the young, healthy tooth. Some of the crevicular epithelium and all the attachment epithelium, at least in the young individual, are derived embryologically from reduced enamel epithelium. The oral mucosa is composed of a loose fibroelastic connective tissue with a well vascularized and innervated lamina propria and submucosa and is covered mainly by a parakeratinized stratified squamous epithelium.

The oral mucous membrane can be injured chemically or physically. If the injury is short-termed (acute) and leads to loss of tissue but does not involve infection by pathogenic microorganisms, the connective tissue defect is filled in with granulation tissue within 3 to 4 days and epithelium regenerates over the surface within a week. The tissue is remodeled to nearly normal by the end of 2 to 3 weeks. As with other body tissues, the ability to heal depends on the metabolic status of the patient and the removal of external irritating factors. Occasionally, immune hypersensitivity to materials or pharmaceutical agents may delay the healing response. The presence of microorganisms or immune hypersensitivity reactions results in an infiltration of acute or chronic inflammatory cells and delay of healing.

The gingival response to injury may be complicated by its association with the tooth. Calculus deposition on the tooth, malocclusion, and faulty restorations may enhance the destructive effects of microorganisms. The crevicular epithelium then becomes vulnerable to endotoxin and various exogenous and endogenous chemicals. The resulting breakdown of tissue leads to an acute inflammatory response by the gingival connective tissue called acute gingivitis. This condition is often reversible if the injurious agent is removed and the reaction is limited to the connective tissue above the alveolar bony crest. If the insult continues, the inflammatory infiltrate becomes mixed and then predominantly mononuclear. Inflamed epithelial-lined granulation tissue gradually spreads apically to and below the alveolar bony crest. At this point the condition is described as chronic periodontal disease, a non-self-limiting disease process that is probably reinforced by immune mechanisms. Chronic periodontal disease can only be altered clinically by removing all irritating factors such as plaque and calculus, removing epithelial-lined granuation tissue from the walls of the periodontal pocket, and administering professional and home dental hygiene measures on a regular basis. If teeth are lost because of pulpal and periapical pathological lesions or advanced (severe) periodontal disease, then the edentulous gingiva responds to injury much like the rest of the oral mucosa.

The reaction of gingival tissues to oral implants is an important area of research. Permucosal implants present special problems including epithelial ingrowth, encystification, and exfoliation of the implant. Additionally, there is the problem of maintaining a close epithelial attachment between the implant and soft tissue that excludes bacteria. Thus, the implant material should ideally encourage firm attachment of epithelial cells on its surface, but only limited growth and migration of these cells. At present, a major problem is encouraging connective tissue fibroblasts to attach firmly to the surface of the implant or tooth and to migrate and proliferate at rates faster than the epithelium.

Oral mucosa and gingiva are susceptible to immune hypersensitivity reactions when subjected to synthetic or natural materials that are antigenic. Local binding of antigens to membranes of white blood cells (i.e., lymphocytes, macrophages, basophils, mast cells) or Langerhans' cells of skin and oral mucosal epithelium play a role in activating these various reactions. Although a few of the mucosal reactions are documented as Type I reactions (wherein vasoactive substances are released from mast cells because of antigen-IgE reactions), most reactions to dental materials are classified as Type IV (T-cell-mediated) reactions. This type of reaction is sometimes called contact mucositis. Skin testing can be used to help document both Type I and Type IV reactions to environmental antigens, metallic elements used in alloys, and by-products from polymers. *In vitro* tests for cell-mediated hyperimmunity are occasionally performed and include transformation of the patient's lymphocytes and production of a migration inhibition factor by these cells in response to the antigenic stimulus. The most common metal sensitivities are those to nickel, cobalt, and chromium, but sensitivities to other metallic elements are possible. The reaction is to a metal-protein complex, usually formed when the metal contacts the epithelium, giving rise to a Type IV reaction much like that of poison ivy. Persons with metal sensitivity usually do not react to an alloy containing the metallic elements unless the alloy corrodes. However, minute amounts of corrosion products can cause hypersensitivity, and the corrosion may not be visible.

Summary

All the degenerative, necrotic, inflammatory, and immune reactions that occur in other tissues of the body from body-material contact can also occur when such materials are placed in contact with oral tissues such as alveolar bone, periodontium, gingiva, or mucosal connective tissue. However, some variations in the structures of the oral tissues, such as the tubular structure of dentin, alter the local responses to insults from materials or bacteria.

■ TYPES OF BIOCOMPATIBILITY TESTS

The first efforts of the American Dental Association (ADA) to establish guidelines for dental materials came in 1926 when scientists at the National Bureau of Standards, now the National Institute of Science and Technology (NIST), developed specifications for dental amalgam. Unfortunately, recommendations on materials and conditions for biological compatibility have not kept pace with the technological development of dental materials. Reasons for this are (1) the fast advance of cellular and molecular biology, (2) the variety of tests available for assessing biocompatibility of materials, and (3) the lack of standardization of these tests. Standardization is a difficult and lengthy process, made more difficult by disagreement on the appropriateness and significance of particular tests. One of the early attempts to develop a uniform test for all materials was the study by Dixon and Rickert in 1933, in which toxicity of most of the dental materials in use at that time was investigated by implanting the materials into pockets in subdermal tissue. Small standard-sized pieces of gold, amalgam, guttapercha, silicates, and copper amalgam were sterilized and placed in uniformly sized pockets within skeletal muscle tissue. Biopsy specimens were evaluated microscopically after 6 months. Other early attempts to standardize techniques were carried out by Mitchell (1959) on connective tissue and by Massler (1958) on tooth pulp. Not until the passage of the Medical Device Bill by Congress in 1976 was biological testing for all medical devices (including dental materials) given a high priority.

In 1972 the Council on Dental Materials, Instruments, and Equipment of the American National Standards Institute/American Dental Association (ANSI/ADA) approved Document No. 41 for Recommended Standard Practices for Biological Evaluation of Dental Materials. The committee that developed this document recognized the need for standardized methods of testing and for sequential testing of materials to reduce the number of compounds that would need to be tested clinically. In 1982, an addendum was made to this document, including an update of the Ames' Test for mutagenic activity. Recently, several multinational working groups, including scientists from ANSI and the International Standards Organization (ISO), were formed to develop international standards for biomedical materials and devices. The final document (ISO 10993), which will service the European Community, has been only partially published. A complete version is due in 1996. ISO 10993 will contain "initial" and "supplementary" tests to assess the biological reaction to materials. In particular, ISO 10993 will greatly expand the choices of mutangenicity tests. (The current working version of this standard is available from the Association for the Advancement of Medical Instrumentation [AAMI], 3330 Washington Blvd., Suite 400, Arlington, VA 22201-4598.) ADA/ANSI Document No. 41 is also being revised to conform to the ISO 10993 standard, and should be completed sometime in 1996. Unlike the ISO standard, which covers all biomedical devices, the ADA/ANSI document is limited to dental devices, and the new version will probably contain special emphasis on dental applications, which are absent from ISO 10993. However, there will be many similarities between the two standards in both philosophy and application. Currently the 1982 version of the ADA/ANSI document governs biocompatibility testing in the United States. The 1982 version is available from the Council on Dental Materials, Instruments and Equipment, American Dental Association, 211 E. Chicago Avenue, Chicago, IL 60611.

Three categories of tests are described in the 1982 ADA/ANSI document: "initial," "secondary," and "usage" tests. The "initial" tests include *in vitro* assays for cytotoxicity, red blood cell membrane lysis (hemolysis), mutagenesis and carcinogenesis at the cellular level, and *in vivo* acute physiological distress and death at the level of the whole organism. Based on the results of these initial tests, promising materials are tested by one or more "secondary" tests in small animals (*in vivo*) for inflammatory or immunogenic potential (e.g., dermal irritation, subcutaneous and bony implantation, and hypersensitivity tests). Finally, materials that pass secondary tests and still hold potential are subjected to one or more *in vivo* "usage" tests (placement of the materials in their intended contexts, first in larger animals, often primates, and finally, with Food and Drug Administration approval, in humans). This strategy of screening materials through a series of tiered tests is widely recognized by manufacturers and researchers as important for reducing the workload and the costs of product development in the field of dental materials and in other areas of biotechnology.

Initial Tests

Cytotoxicity assays

In general, cytotoxicity tests measure the effect of a material on (1) cell number or growth, (2) integrity of cell membranes, (3) biosynthesis or enzyme activity, or (4) the genetic material of the cell. Cytotoxicity tests have the advantages of (1) testing for a specific function of cell metabolism in isolation from other events, (2) screening large numbers of samples quickly and inexpensively, (3) quantifying results, (4) giving greater sensitivity to toxic materials than usage tests, and (5) having potential for standardization of test methods. Disadvantages of the *in vitro* cytotoxicity tests include (1) limitation of testing to only one cell type at a time, (2) dissimilarity of test cells to host cells, and (3) lack of inflammatory and other tissue protective mechanisms in tissue culture.

If a material is highly cytotoxic, there are several ways to improve it: (1) reduce the level of toxic substances leached, (2) consider a use for the material in which the leachable product will not affect the individual, or (3) use a different formula for the material. In all cytotoxicity tests, the test system itself must be nontoxic, sterile, and reproducible so as not to interfere with the analysis of the materials. It should be emphasized that cytotoxicity tests alone cannot predict the overall biocompatibility of a material.

Cell number and growth tests assess the cytotoxicity of a material by measuring cell number or growth after exposure to a material. Cells are plated in a well of a cell culture dish where they attach. The material is then placed in the test system. If the material is not cytotoxic, the cells will remain attached to the well and will proliferate with time. If the material is cytotoxic, the cells may stop growing, exhibit cytopathic features (Figs. 7-5 and 7-6), or may detach from the well. If the material is a solid, then the density (number of cells per unit area) of cells may be assessed at different distances from the material, and a "zone" of inhibited cell growth may be described (Fig. 7-7, *A*). The cell density can be assessed either qualitatively, semiquantitatively, or quantitatively. Often, the viability of the cells around the material are determined using other biosynthetic or membrane integrity tests. Substances such as Teflon can be used as negative (noncytotoxic) controls, whereas materials such as plasticized polyvinyl chloride can be used as positive (cytotoxic) controls. Control materials should be well defined and commercially available to facilitate comparisons among testing laboratories.

Another group of tests is used to measure cell status by a change in *membrane permeability* (Fig. 7-7, *B*). Membrane permeability is the ease with which a dye can pass through a cell membrane. There are two basic types of dyes used. Vital dyes are actively transported into viable cells, where they are retained unless cytotoxic effects increase the permeability of the membrane. It is important to establish that the dye itself does not exhibit cytotoxicity during the time frame of the test. Nonvital dyes are not actively transported, and are only taken up if membrane permeability has been compromised by cytotoxicity. Many types of vital dyes have been used, including neutral red and $Na_2{}^{51}CrO_4$, which are both particularly advantageous because they are neither synthesized nor metabolized by the cell. The ^{51}Cr assay is the only cytotoxicity assay presently described in ANSI/ADA Document 41. It involves incubating ^{51}Cr-loaded suspensions of cells with the material for either 4 or 24 hours and comparing the release of ^{51}Cr (a gamma radiation emitter) from test samples with that from positive (phenol) and negative (untreated) controls. The ^{51}Cr-release technique appears to be a fairly consistent quantitative assay with good guidelines for interpreting cytotoxicity where intimate contact occurs between tissue and test material. Disadvantages of this test include the necessity of managing radioactive isotopes. Examples of nonvital dyes include trypan blue and propidium iodide.

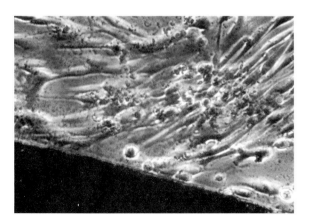

Fig. 7-5 Human periodontal ligament fibroblasts growing adjacent to resin-containing calcium hydroxide pulp-capping agent (dark image at bottom of picture). This is a noncytotoxic reaction.

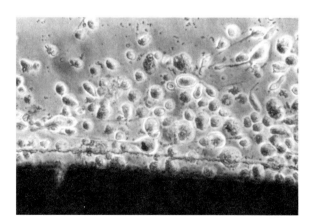

Fig. 7-6 Human periodontal ligament fibroblasts adjacent to a second resin-containing calcium hydroxide pulp cavity agent (dark image at bottom of picture). This is a severe cytotoxic reaction.

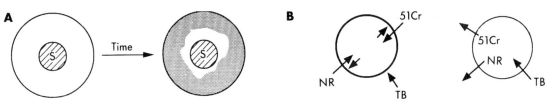

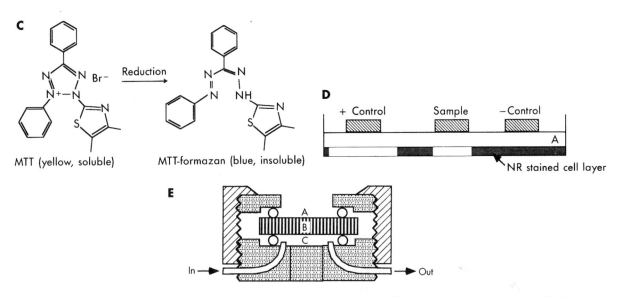

Fig. 7-7 Methods of *in vitro* testing of dental materials. **A,** A material sample (*S*) is placed in the center of a cell culture well, and cells and medium are added. After 1 to 3 days, the cells have multiplied in areas where the material has not inhibited their growth. The area devoid of growth is often referred to as a ring of inhibition. Several methods are available to assess the amount of cellular growth around the samples. **B,** The selective permeability of cell membranes is the basis for several cytotoxicity tests. Compounds such as $Na^{51}CrO_4$ (^{51}Cr), and neutral red (*NR*) are actively sequestered by healthy cells. These compounds will leach out of the cell if the cell is injured and cannot maintain its membrane integrity. Other compounds such as trypan blue (*TB*) are excluded by a healthy cell, but can diffuse through the membrane of an injured cell. **C,** MTT is a yellow-soluble molecule that can be used to assess cellular enzymatic activity. If the cell is able to reduce the MTT, the resulting formazan is blue and insoluble and deposits in the cell. The amount of formazan formed is proportional to the enzymatic activity. The activity of a number of cellular enzymes can be assessed in this manner. **D,** The agar overlay method has been used to evaluate the cytotoxicity of dental materials. The cell layer, which has been previously stained with neutral red (*NR*), is covered with a thin layer of agar (*A*). Samples are placed on top of the agar for a time. If the material is cytotoxic, it will injure the cells, and the neutral red will be released, leaving a zone of inhibition. **E,** A dentin disk has been used as a barrier in cytotoxicity tests that attempt to predict the toxicity of materials placed on dentin *in vivo*. The material is placed on one side (*A*) of the dentin disk (*B*) in the device used to hold the dentin disk. Collection fluid (cell culture medium or saline) is on the other side of the disk (*C*). Cells can also be grown in the collection side. Components from the material may diffuse through the dentin and the effect of the medium on cell metabolism can then be measured. Cell metabolism can be measured by any of the methods described in **A** through **D**. To assess the rate of diffusion, the collection fluid can be circulated into and out of the collection chamber (*C*).

A third type of cytotoxicity test uses *biosynthetic or enzymatic activity* of cells to assess cytotoxic response. The measurement of DNA synthesis or protein synthesis is a common example of this type of test. Analysis of synthesis of DNA or protein by cells is usually performed by adding radioisotope-labeled precursors to the medium followed by quantification of radioisotope (e.g., ^{3}H-thymidine or ^{3}H-leucine) incorporated into DNA or protein. A commonly used enzymatic test for cytotoxicity is the MTT test. This test measures the activity of cellular dehydrogenases, which convert the MTT, via several cellular reducing agents, to a blue, insoluble formazan compound (Fig. 7-7, *C*). If the dehydrogenases are not active because of cytotoxic effects, the formazan will not form. The production of formazan can be quantified by dissolving it and measuring the optical density of the resulting solution. Alternatively, the formazan can be localized around the test sample by light or electron microscopy. Many other enzymatic activities of cells can be followed qualitatively or quantitatively.

Most of the cytotoxicity tests presented thus far are performed with the material in direct contact with the cell culture. Researchers have long recognized that *in vivo* direct contact often does not exist between cells and the materials. Separation of cells and materials may occur from keratinized epithelium, dentin, or extracellular matrix. Thus, several *in vitro* barrier tests have been developed to mimic the *in vivo* conditions. One such test is the agar overlay method (Fig. 7-7, *D*) in which a monolayer of cultured cells is established before adding 1% agar or agarose (low-melting temperature) plus a vital stain, such as neutral red, to fresh culture media. The agar forms a barrier between the cells and the material, which is placed on top of the agar. Nutrients, gas, and soluble toxic substances can diffuse through the agar. Solid test samples or liquid samples adsorbed onto filter paper can be tested with this assay for up to 24 hours. This assay correlates positively with the direct-contact assays described above and the intramuscular implantation test in rabbits. However, the agar may not adequately represent barriers that occur *in vivo*. Furthermore, because of variability of the agar's diffusion properties, it is difficult to correlate the intensity of color or width of the zone around a material with the concentration of leachable toxic products.

A second barrier assay is the Millipore filter assay. This technique establishes a monolayer of cells on filters made of cellulose esters. Then the culture medium is replaced with a medium containing about 1% agar, and this mixture is allowed to gel over the cells. Finally, the filter-monolayer-gel is detached and turned over so that the filter is on top for placement of solid or soluble test samples for 2 or more hours. After exposure to the test samples, the filter is removed and an assay is used to determine the effect of the sample on some cell metabolic activity. The succinyl dehydrogenase assay described previously can be used with this test. Like the agar overlay test and the cell contact tests, toxicity in the Millipore filter test is assessed by the width of the cytotoxic zone around each test sample. This test also has the drawback of arbitrarily influencing the diffusion of leachable products from the test material. Both the agar diffusion and Millipore filter tests can provide, at best, a cytotoxic ranking among materials.

Dentin barrier tests have shown improved correlation with the cytotoxicity of dental materials in usage tests in teeth and are gradually being developed for screening purposes (Fig. 7-7, *E*). A number of studies have shown that dentin forms a barrier through which toxic materials must diffuse to reach pulpal tissue. Thus pulpal reaction to zinc oxide–eugenol is relatively mild as compared with the more severe reactions to the same material in direct contact with cells in *in vitro* assays and tissue in implantation tests. The thickness of the dentin correlates directly with the protection offered to the pulp. Thus, assays have been developed that incorporate dentin disks between the test sample and the cell assay system. The dentin disks offer the added advantage of directional diffusion between the restorative material and the culture medium.

Standardization of cytotoxicity tests is a primary concern of those trying to evaluate materials. Two types of cells can be used for cytotoxicity assays. Primary cells are cells taken directly from an animal into culture. These cells will grow only a limited time in culture but retain many of the characteristics of cells *in vivo*. Continuous cells are primary cells that have been transformed to allow them to grow more or less indefinitely in culture. Because of their transformation, these cells may not retain all *in vivo* characteristics. Primary cell cultures would seemingly be more relevant than continuous cell lines for measuring cytotoxicity of materials. However, there appears to be little difference in the metabolic responses of continuous and primary cell lines to cytotoxic compounds. Furthermore, the genetic and metabolic stability of continuous cell lines contributes significantly toward standardizing assay methods. The standardization of controls and reference materials is another area of concern for researchers.

Cytotoxicity tests are appropriate to measure initial reactions by cells to materials. As such, the cytotoxic reactions of cells should mimic closely the early cytotoxic reactions (degeneration and necrosis) to these materials *in vivo*. The shortcomings of cytotoxicity assays are that they cannot measure long-term reactions or the effects of inflammation, immune responses, mutagenesis, or carcinogenesis.

Mutagenesis assays

Mutagenesis assays assess the effect of materials on a cell's genetic material. There are a wide range of mechanisms by which materials can affect the genetic material of the cell. *Genotoxic mutagens* directly alter the DNA of the cell through various types of mutations. Each chemical may be associated with a specific type of DNA mutation. Genotoxic chemicals may either be mutagens in their native states, or may require activation or biotransformation to be mutagens, in which case they are called promutagens. *Epigenetic mutagens* do not alter the DNA themselves, but support tumor growth by altering the cell's biochemistry, altering the immune system, acting as hormones, or other mechanisms. Carcinogenesis is the ability to cause cancer *in vivo*. Mutagens may or may not be carcinogens, and carcinogens may or may not be mutagens. Thus the quantification and relevance of tests that attempt to measure mutagenesis and carcinogenesis are extremely complex. A number of government-sponsored programs evaluate the ability of *in vitro* mutagenesis assays to predict carcinogenicity.

Many tests that measure the mutagenic and carcinogenic properties of materials have been developed by toxicologists. These tests are employed with a strategy called the decision-point approach. Using this strategy, tests are applied in a specific order, and testing is stopped when any one indicates mutagenic potential of the material or chemical. The validity of any of these tests may be effected by issues of species,

tissue, gender, and other factors. Tests are generally divided into *in vitro* genotoxic short-term tests (STTs), limited-term *in vivo* tests, and long-term or lifetime tests. *In vitro* tests may include tests that measure bacterial or mammalian mutagenesis, those that measure cytogenesis or visible chromosomal damage, those that measure transformation of cell growth properties such as loss of contact inhibition, and those that measure damage to sperm. Limited-term *in vivo* tests measure altered liver function or increased tumor induction when animals are exposed to the chemicals for a fraction of their lifetimes. Long-term *in vivo* tests are performed by keeping the chemical in contact with the animal over the majority of its lifetime.

The ANSI/ADA Document 41, 1982 Addendum, had only two assays for mutagenesis, the *Ames' test* and the *Styles' cell transformation test*. The ISO Standard 10993 will include a series of *in vitro* genotoxicity tests, *in vivo* genotoxicity tests, and carcinogenicity tests, and will suggest that one or more of these tests be run on a particular material. The number and types of tests that will be required will depend on the location of the material, its duration of contact with the organism, and whether it is implanted in the animal or not. It is suggested that at least three assays be included, and at least two of these should use mammalian cells. The *in vitro* tests should include three levels of genotoxic effects: DNA effects, gene mutations and chromosomal aberrations. Further carcinogenicity testing is suggested for resorbable materials and devices, materials and devices where *in vitro* mammalian tests have shown genetic damage.

The Ames' test is the most widely used short-term mutagenesis test and the only short-term test that is considered to be thoroughly validated. It uses mutant stocks of *Salmonella typhimurium* that require exogenous histidine. Native stocks of bacteria do not require exogenous histidine. Exclusion of histidine from the culture medium allows a chemical to be tested for its ability to convert the mutant strain to a native strain. Chemicals that significantly increase the frequency of reversion back to the native state have a reportedly high probability of being carcinogenic in mammals because the chemicals significantly alter the genetic material. Performance of this test requires experience in the field and special strains of *Salmonella* to produce meaningful results.

A second test for mutagenesis described in ANSI/ADA Document 41 is the Styles' cell Transformation test. This test on mammalian cells was developed to offer an alternative to bacterial tests (Ames test), which may not be relevant to mammalian systems. This assay quantifies the ability of potential carcinogens to transform standardized cell lines so that they will grow in soft agar. Untransformed fibroblasts normally will not grow within an agar gel, whereas genetically transformed cells will grow below the gel surface. This characteristic of transformed fibroblasts is the only characteristic that correlates with the ability of cells to produce tumors *in vivo*. At least four different continuous cell lines (Chang, BHK, HeLa, WI-38) have been used. In 1978, Styles claimed 94% "accuracy in determining carcinogenic or noncarcinogenic activity" when testing 120 compounds in two cell lines. However, there has been some difficulty in reproducing these results.

In a recent report, four short-term tests (STTs) for gene toxicity were compared (Table 7-3). The Ames test was the most specific (86% of noncarcinogens yielding a negative result). The Ames test also had the highest positive predictability (83% of positives were actually carcinogens) and displayed nega-tive predictability equal to that of other STTs (i.e., 51% of all Ames test negatives were noncarcinogenic). However, the results were in agreement (concordance) with rodent carcinogenicity tests for only 62% of the chemicals. Also, the Ames test was sensitive to only 45% of the carcinogens; that is, it missed over half of the known carcinogens. The other three STTs were assays for chromosomal aberration, sister chromatid exchange in CHO cells, and the mouse lymphoma L5178Y cell mutagenesis assay. The sister chromatid exchange method, the mouse lymphoma mutagenesis assay, and the Ames test had 73%, 70%, and 45% sensitivity, respectively. However, because the Ames test is widely used, extensively described in the literature, and technically easier to conduct in a testing laboratory than the other tests, it is most often conducted in a screening program. These studies suggest that not all carcinogens are genotoxic (mutagenic) and not all mutagens are carcinogenic. Thus, although STTs for mutagenesis are helpful for predicting some carcinogens, STTs cannot predict all of them.

Other assays

Assays to measure immune function or other tissue reactions have also been used. Assays of immune

TABLE 7-3   Comparison of *In Vitro* Mutagenesis Tests

Test Parameter	Parameter Description	Test Results (average %)			
		Ames*	SCE*	MOLY	ABS
Specificity	Known noncarcinogenic material gives negative test result	86	45	45	69
Sensitivity	Known carcinogenic material gives positive test result	45	73	70	55
Positive predictability	Positive test accurately predicts a carcinogen	83	67	66	73
Negative predictability	Negative test accurately predicts a noncarcinogen	51	52	50	50
Concordance	Percent of qualitative agreements between STT and rodent carcinogenicity tests	62	62	60	60

Adapted from Tennant RW, Margolin BH, Shelby MD, et al: Prediction of chemical carcinogenicity in rodents from *in vitro* genetic toxicity assays, *Science* 236:933, 1987.
*SCE = Sister chromatid exchange test; *MOLY* = mouse lymphoma assay; *ABS* = chromosome aberration test; *STT* = short-term test.

cell function are not described in ANSI/ADA Document 41 and are not used to a great extent at the present time. However, several kinds of *in vitro* assays are available to determine if materials alter immune function. The *in vivo* significance of these assays is yet to be ascertained. These assays measure cytokine production by lymphocytes and macrophages, lymphocyte proliferation, chemotaxis, or T-cell rosetting to sheep red blood cells. Other tests measure the ability of a material to alter the cell cycle or activate complement. The activation of complement is of particular concern to researchers working on artificial or "engineered" blood vessels and other tissues in direct contact with blood. Materials that activate complement may generate inflammation or thrombi, and also may propagate a chronic inflammatory response. Whereas concerns about complement activation by dental materials are fewer, it is possible that activation of complement by resins or metals or their corrosion products may prolong inflammation in the gingiva or pulp.

Other initial assays are included in Document 41. Various materials or chemicals that can damage red blood cell membranes cause hemolysis. Hemolysis is especially important when the material contacts blood or enters blood vessels in the connective tissue. This phenomenon is also an indicator of the destructive effects on the cell membrane. The oral and intraperitoneal LD_{50} test determines acute lethal effects of agents administered either orally or intraperitoneally to rats. These acute *in vivo* toxicity tests are carried out by dissolving or suspending the material in water, aqueous methylcellulose, propylene glycol, or food-grade vegetable oil. The mixture is then administered into the stomach or peritoneum of albino rats at different concentrations. Toxic effects are recorded daily for 2 weeks. The LD_{50}, or dose required to kill 50% of the animals, is calculated. If the LD_{50} is less than 1 g/kg body weight, the material is considered to exhibit acute systemic toxicity.

Secondary or Intermediate Tests

After materials have been assessed by initial tests, a series of longer-term tests are conducted to identify inflammatory reactions or immune reactions to the material. These are performed mainly in mice, rats, rabbits, hamsters, or guinea pigs.

The *mucous membrane irritation test* determines if a material causes inflammation to mucous membranes or abraded skin. This test is conducted by placing the test materials and positive and negative controls into contact with hamster cheek pouch tissue or rabbit oral tissue. After several weeks of contact, both the controls and the test sites are examined, and the gross tissue reactions in the living animals are recorded and photographed in color. The animals are then sacrificed, and biopsy specimens are prepared for histological evaluation of inflammatory changes.

In the *skin sensitization test in guinea pigs* (guinea pig maximization test), the materials are injected intradermally to test for development of skin hypersensitivity reactions. Freund's adjuvant can be used to augment the reaction. This injection is followed by secondary treatment with adhesive patches containing the test substance. If hypersensitivity developed from the initial injection, then the patch will elicit an inflammatory response. The skin patch test can result in a spectrum from no reaction to intense redness and swelling. The degree of reaction in the patch test and the percentage of animals that show a reaction are the bases for estimating the allergenicity of the material.

Implantation tests are used to evaluate materials that will contact subcutaneous tissue or bone. The location of the implant site is determined by the use of the material, and may include connective tissue, bone, or muscle. Although amalgams and alloys are tested because the margins of the restorative materials contact the gingiva, most subcutaneous tests are used for materials that will directly contact soft tissue during implantation, endodontic, or periodontal treatment. Short-term implantation is studied by aseptically placing the compounds in small, open-ended, polyethylene tubes into the tissue. The test samples and controls are placed at separate sites, and allowed to remain for 1 to 11 weeks. Alternatively, an empty tube is embedded first, and the inflammatory reaction from surgery is allowed to subside. The implant site is then reopened, and the test material is placed into this healed site or is packed into the tube that was placed previously. At the appropriate time, the areas are excised and prepared for microscopic examination and interpretation. The tissue response can be evaluated by normal histological, histochemical, or immunohistochemical methods. Implantation tests of longer duration, for identification of either chronic inflammation or tumor formation, are performed in a manner similar to that of short-term tests except the materials remain in place for 1 to 2 years before examination.

Although the present ADA specifications suggest placing the materials in polyethylene tubes, recent findings indicate that some plastics may themselves be the source of tissue reaction. Consequently, many investigators today implant a uniformly sized pellet of material into the tissue. For example, the test material may be cut or formed into a thin cylinder and placed into a beveled point of a large hypodermic needle, which is introduced into muscle tissue. Improvements on direct application of materials into dermal, subcutaneous, muscle, or bone tissue have also been reported.

Usage Tests in Animals

Usage tests are performed to identify all the effects of dental materials on the tissues in which they will be used. Usage tests differ from secondary tests because the material must be placed into the same function in the animal as it will be in the human. In contrast, secondary tests do not require that the material function. The dental pulp, the periodontium, and gingival or mucosal tissues are generally the tissues that are of concern in dentistry.

Dental pulp irritation tests

According to the ANSI/ADA Document 41, materials to be tested on the dental pulp are placed in class 5 cavity preparations in intact, noncarious teeth of monkeys or other suitable animals. Care is taken to prepare uniformly sized cavities. After anesthesia and a thorough prophylaxis of teeth, cavities are prepared under sterile conditions with an efficient water-spray coolant to ensure minimal trauma to the pulp. The compounds are placed in an equal number of anterior and posterior teeth of the maxilla and mandible to ensure uniform distribution in all types of teeth. The materials are left in place from 1 to 8 weeks. Zinc oxide–eugenol and silicate cement have been used as negative and positive control materials, respectively.

At the conclusion of the study, the teeth are removed and sectioned for microscopic examination. The tissue sections are evaluated by the investigators without knowledge of the identity of the materials, and necrotic and inflammatory reactions are classified according to the intensity of the response. Measurements of thicknesses of remaining dentin and reparative dentin are recorded for all histological specimens by a photomicrometer. Evaluation of the response of the pulp is based on its appearance after treatment. The severity of the lesions are based on disruption of the structure of the tissue and the number of inflammatory cells (usually both acute and chronic) present. Pulpal response is classified as either slight (mild hyperemia, few inflammatory cells, slight hemorrhage in odontoblastic zone), moderate (definite increase in number of inflammatory cells, hyperemia, and slight disruption of odontoblastic zone), or severe (decided inflammatory infiltrate, hyperemia, total disruption of odontoblastic layer in the zone of cavity preparation, reduction or absence of predentin, and perhaps even localized abscesses). Just as with dental caries, the mononuclear cells are usually most prominent in the inflammatory response. If neutrophils are present, the presence of bacteria or bacterial products must be suspected. Some investigators now use ZOE cements to "surface-seal" the restorations to eliminate the effects of microleakage on the pulp.

Until recently, most dental pulp irritation tests have involved intact and noncarious teeth, without inflamed pulps. There has been increased concern that inflamed dental pulp tissue may respond differently than normal pulps to liners, cements, and restorative agents. Efforts have been made to develop techniques that identify bacterial insults to the pulp. Studying teeth with induced pulpitis for usage tests allows evaluation of types and amount of reparative dentin formed and will probably continue to be developed.

Dental implants into bone

At present, the best estimations of the success and failure of implants are gained from three tests: (1) penetration of a periodontal probe along the side of the implant, (2) mobility of the implant, and (3) radiographs indicating either osseous integration or radiolucencies around the implant. Currently, an implant is considered successful if it exhibits no mobility, no radiographic evidence of peri-implant radiolucency, minimal vertical bone loss, and absence of persistent peri-implant soft tissue complications. Previously, investigators argued that formation of a fibrous connective tissue capsule around a sub-periosteal implant or root cylinder was the natural reaction of the body to a material. They argued that this was actually an attachment similar to the periodontal ligament and should be considered a sign of an acceptable material. However, in most cases it resembled the wall of a cyst, which is the body's attempt to isolate the implanted material as the material slowly degrades and leaches its components into tissue. Currently, for implants in bone, implants should be completely encased in bone, the most differentiated state of that tissue. Fibrous capsule formation is a sign of irritation and chronic inflammation.

Mucosa and gingival usage tests

Because various dental materials contact gingival and mucosal tissues, the tissue response to these materials must be measured. Materials are placed in cavity preparations with subgingival extensions. The materials' effects on gingival tissues are observed at 7 days and again after 30 days. Responses are categorized as slight, moderate, or severe. A slight response is characterized by a few mononuclear inflammatory cells (mainly lymphocytes) in the epithelium and adjacent connective tissue. A moderate response is indicated by numerous mononuclear cells in the connective tissue and a few neutrophils in the epithelium. A severe reaction evokes a significant mononuclear and neutrophilic infiltrate, as well as thinned or absent epithelium.

A difficulty with this type of study is the frequent presence of some degree of preexisting inflammation in gingival tissue. Bacterial plaque is the most important factor in causing this inflammation. Secondary factors are the surface roughness restorative material, open or overhanging margins, and overcontouring or undercontouring of the restoration. One way to reduce the interference of inflammation caused by plaque is to perform dental prophylaxis before cavity preparation and placement of the material. However, the prophylaxis and preparation of the cavity preparation will themselves cause some inflammation of the soft tissues. Thus if margins are placed subgingivally, time for healing (typically 8 to 14 days) must be allowed before assessment of the effects of the restorative agents.

Correlation among Screening and Usage Tests

In the field of biocompatibility, some scientists question the usefulness of screening tests in light of the apparent lack of correlation with secondary and usage tests. However, the lack of correlation is really not surprising in light of the differences among these tests. As explained previously (Tables 7-1 and 7-2), *in vitro* cytotoxicity tests can at best estimate the initial degenerative and necrotic events (first 12 to 24 hours) but not the inflammatory or chronic reactions of tissue. Conversely, secondary and usage tests measure host cell degeneration and necrosis, as well as inflammatory and immune reactions. Furthermore, barriers between the material and tissues may exist in usage tests that may not exist in screening tests. Thus it is important to remember that each type of test has been designed to measure different aspects of the biological reponse to materials, and correlations may not always be expected.

The best example of a barrier that occurs in usage but not screening tests is the dentin barrier. When restorative materials are placed in teeth, dentin will generally be interposed between the material and the pulp. The dentin barrier, although possibly only a fraction of a millimeter thick, is effective in modulating the effects of dental materials. The effect of the dentin barrier is illustrated by the following classic study (Table 7-4). Four *in vitro* methods were used to evaluate the following materials: a zinc oxide–eugenol (ZOE) cement, a composite material, and a silicate cement. These methods included (1) four different cell culture tests, (2) an

TABLE 7-4   Comparison of Reactions of Three Materials by Screening and Usage Tests

Material	Cell Culture	Implantation in Connective Tissue	Pulp Response
Silicate	+	+	++
Composite	++	++	+
ZOE	+++	+	0

From Mjör IA, Hensten-Pettersen A, Skogedal O: *Int Dent J* 27:127, 1977.
+++ = Severe; ++ = Moderate; + = Slight; 0 = No reaction; *ZOE,* zinc oxide–eugenol.

implantation test, and (3) a usage test in class 5 cavity preparations in monkey teeth. The results of the four cell culture tests were relatively consistent, with silicate having only a slight effect on cultured cells, composite, a moderate effect, and ZOE, a severe effect. These three materials were also embedded subcutaneously in connective tissue in polyethylene tubes (secondary test), and observations were made at 7, 30, and 90 days. Reactions at 7 days could not be determined because of inflammation caused by the operative procedure. At 30 days, ZOE appeared to cause a more severe reaction than silicate cement. The inflammatory reactions at 90 days caused by ZOE and silicate were slight, and the reaction to composite materials was moderate. When the three materials were evaluated in class 5 cavity preparations under prescribed conditions of cavity size and depth (usage test), the results were quite different from those obtained by the screening methods. The silicate was found to have the most severe inflammatory reaction, the composite had a moderate to slight reaction, and the ZOE had little or no effect.

The apparent contradictions in this study may be explained by considering the components that were released from the materials and the environments into which they were released. The silicate cement released hydrogen ions that were probably buffered in the cell culture and implantation tests but may not have been buffered by the dentin in the usage tests. Microleakage of bacteria or bacterial products also may have added to the inflammatory reaction in the usage test. Thus this material appeared most toxic in the usage test. The composites released low molecular weight resins, and the ZOE released eugenol and zinc ions. In the cell culture tests, these compounds had direct access to cells and probably caused the moderate to severe cytotoxicity. In the implantation tests, the released components may have caused some cytotoxicity, but the severity may have been reduced because of the capacity of the surrounding tissue to disperse the toxins. In usage tests, these materials probably were less toxic because the diffusion gradient of the dentin barrier reduced concentrations of the released molecules to low levels. The slight reaction observed with the composites may also have been caused in part by microleakage around these restorations. The ZOE did not show this reaction, however, because the eugenol probably killed bacteria in the cavity, and the surface-seal of the ZOE prevented microleakage of bacteria into the cavities.

Another example of this lack of correlation of usage tests with implantation tests is the inflammatory response of the gingiva at the gingival and interproximal margins of restorations that accumulate bacterial plaque and calculus. Plaque and calculus cannot accumulate on implanted materials and therefore the implantation test cannot hope to duplicate the usage test. However, connective tissue implantation tests are of great value in demonstrating cytotoxic effects of materials and evaluating materials that will be used in contact with alveolar bone and apical periodontal connective tissues. In these cases, the implant site and the usage sites are sufficiently similar to compare the test results of the two sites.

Summary

Tests to evaluate the biological response to dental materials can be divided into initial, secondary, and usage tests. Each test level gives additional information about the biocompatibility of the material. In this way, the initial tests, which are quicker and less expensive to perform, can screen potential materials before more complex secondary and usage tests are used. The initial tests can also delineate the components of materials that might be causing adverse reactions in the *in vivo* tests. Although there are problems with the correlation among initial, secondary, and usage tests, and although one type of test cannot be substituted for another at present, each type of test gives important information about the effect of materials on cell and tissue function. Continuing efforts to develop further correlation between screening and usage tests are in progress.

■ BIOCOMPATIBILITY OF VARIOUS DENTAL MATERIALS

Reactions of Pulp

Microleakage

There is evidence that restorative materials may not bond to enamel or dentin with sufficient strength to resist the forces of contraction on polymerization, wear, or thermal cycling. When debonding occurs, bacteria, food debris, or saliva may be drawn into the gap between the restoration and the tooth by capillary action. This effect has been termed *microleakage*. The importance of microleakage in pulpal irritation has been extensively studied. Early studies reported that various dental restorative materials irritated pulpal tissue in animal tests. However, other studies hypothesized that it was often the products of microleakage, not the restorative materials, that caused the pulpal irritation. Subsequently, numerous studies showed that bacteria were present under restorations and in dentinal tubules, which might be responsible for pulpal irritation. Other studies showed that bacteria or bacterial products such as lipopolysaccharides could cause pulpal irritation within hours of being applied to dentin. Finally, a classic animal study shed light on the roles of restorative materials and microleakage on pulpal irritation. Amalgam, composite, zinc phosphate cement, and silicate cement were used as restorative materials in class 5 cavity preparations in monkey teeth. The materials were placed directly on pulpal tissues. Half of the restorations were surface-sealed with zinc oxide–eugenol (ZOE) cement. Although some pulpal irritation was evident in all restorations at 7 days, after 21 days the sealed restorations showed less pulpal irritation than those not sealed, presumably because microleakage had been eliminated. Only zinc phosphate cement elicited a long-term inflammatory response. Furthermore, the sealed teeth exhibited a much higher rate of dentin bridging under the material. Only amalgam seemed to prevent bridging. From this study it appeared that microleakage plays a significant role in pulpal irritation, but that the materials can also alter normal pulpal and dentinal repair.

The full biological effects of restorative materials on the pulp are still not clear. Restorative materials may directly affect pulpal tissues, or may play an auxiliary role by causing sublethal changes in pulpal cells, which make them more susceptible to bacterial or neutrophillic damage. It is clear, however, that the design of tests that measure pulpal irritation must include provisions for eliminating bacteria, bacterial products, or other microleakage. Furthermore, the role of dentin in mitigating the effects of microleakage remains to be fully revealed.

Dentin bonding

In restorative dentistry, it may be desireable to bond restorative materials to enamel or dentin. Traditionally, bond strengths to enamel have been higher than those to dentin. Bonding to dentin has proven more difficult because of its composition (being both organic and inorganic), wetness, and lower mineral content. Because the dentinal tubules and their resident odontoblasts are extensions of the pulp, bonding to dentin also involves biocompatibility issues. Thus the majority of the following paragraphs will focus on dentin bonding.

When the dentin surface is cut as in a cavity preparation, the surface that remains is covered by a 1-2 μm layer of organic and inorganic debris. This layer has been named the smear layer (see Fig. 7-2). In addition to covering the surface of the dentin, the smear layer debris is also deposited into the tubules to form dentinal plugs. The smear layer and dentinal plugs appear impermeable when viewed by electron microscopy and reduce the flow of fluid (convective transport) significantly. However, more recent evidence has shown that diffusion of molecules as large as albumin (66 kDa) will occur through the smear layer. The presence of the smear layer is important to the strength of bonds of restorative materials and to the biocompatibility of those bonded materials. Numerous studies have shown that removal of the smear layer improves the strength of the bond between dentin and restorative materials with contemporary dentin bonding agents, although earlier research with older bonding agents showed the opposite. A variety of agents have been used to remove the smear layer including acids, chelating agents such as EDTA, sodium hypochlorite, and proteolytic enzymes. Removal of the smear layer increases the wetness of the dentin and demands that the bonding agent be able to wet dentin and displace dentinal fluid. The mechanism by which bonding occurs remains unclear, but currently, it appears that the most successful bonding agents are able to penetrate into the layer of collagen that remains after acid etching, creating a "hybrid layer" of resin and collagen in intimate contact with dentin and dentinal tubules. The strength of the collagen itself has also been shown to be important to bond strengths.

From the standpoint of biocompatibility, the removal of the smear layer may pose a threat to the pulpal tissues for three reasons. First, its removal juxtaposes resin materials and dentin without a barrier, and therefore increases the risk that these materials can diffuse and cause pulpal irritation. Second, the removal of the smear layer makes any microleakage more significant because a significant barrier to the diffusion of bacteria or bacterial products toward the pulp is removed. Third, the acids used to remove the smear layer are a potential source of irritation themselves. Nevertheless, removal of the smear layer is now routine because of the superior bond strengths that can be achieved.

The biocompatibility of acids used to remove the smear layer have been extensively studied. Numerous acids have been used to remove the smear layer, including phosphoric, hydrochloric, citric, and lactic acids. The effect of the acids on pulpal tissues depends on a number of factors including the thickness of dentin between the restoration and the pulp, the strength of the acid, and the degree of etching. Most studies have shown that dentin is a very efficient buffer of protons, and most of the acid may never reach the pulp if sufficient dentin remains. A dentin thickness of 0.5 mm has proven adequate in this regard. Citric or lactic acids are less well buffered, probably because these weaker acids do not dissociate as efficiently. Usage tests that have studied the effects of acids have shown that phosphoric, pyruvic, and citric acids all produce moderate pulpal inflammatory responses, which resolve after 8 weeks. Recent research has shown that in most cases the penetration of acids into the dentin is probably less than 100 μm. However, the possibility of adverse effects of these acids cannot be ruled out because odontoblastic processes in the tubules may be affected even though the acids do not reach the pulp itself.

Dentin bonding agents

A variety of dentin bonding agents have been developed including: (1) *carboxylic acids* and derivatives in combination with resin-based wetting agents (e.g., NPG-GMA with PMDM); (2) phosphonates in combination with resin-based wetting agents (e.g., chlorophosphonate esters of Bis-GMA and of hydroxyethyl methacrylate (HEMA)); (3) *isocyanate* groups in acrylates and polyurethanes; and (4) *aldehydes* and ketones in combination with resin-based wetting agents (e.g., glutaraldehyde with HEMA). Bonding agents must provide a sufficient bond strength to prevent debonding of the resin restorative material from the tooth as polymerization contraction of the resin, thermocycling of the restoration, and wear of the restoration occur. Early dentin bonding systems were applied directly to smear layers, and bond strengths were much lower than strengths obtained on enamel etched by acid. To improve bond strength, smear layers were removed and bonding systems were applied directly to etched dentin. Initially, this did not improve bond strengths, largely because of cavity wetness from convection of fluids from positive pulp fluid pressures. More recently, either removal of the smear layer or the penetration of the smear layer by hydrophilic resins, such as HEMA or 4-methacryloxyethyl-trimellitic acid anhydride (4-META), have been included in the procedures of many bonding systems, and this has resulted in some bond strengths approaching the tensile or shear bond strengths needed to resist debonding.

There have been relatively few studies on biocompatibility of dentin bonding systems. The Bowen system, which consists of treatment of dentin with ferric oxalate, then with NPG-GMA or NTG-GMA (reaction products of N-phenyl glycine or N-tolyl glycine with glycidyl methacrylate) and finally PMDM (reaction product of pyromellitic acid dianhydride and 2-hydroxyethyl methacrylate), has been reported most extensively. All these reagents, except PMDM, were cytotoxic for cells in culture if tested alone. However, when placed on dentin and rinsed with tap water between applications of subsequent reagents as prescribed, cytotoxicity was eliminated. This suggests residual unbound reagents were the cause of the cytotoxicity. Individual components did not cause red blood cell hemolysis or toxicity to mice when given orally, and they did not reduce mouse fibroblast cloning efficiency or cause mutagenesis as determined by the Ames test. Finally, usage tests in class 5 cavity preparations in monkey teeth indicated that under clinical conditions, this system was as biocompatible as ZOE covered by cavity varnish and finished with an amalgam restoration. At 4 to 25 days, there were only slight inflammatory infiltrates, but these were minimal at 59 days. The removal of the smear layer before applying the ferric oxalate is now recommended.

There have been a few studies of the biological effects of other resin-based dentin bonding agents. HEMA, a hydrophilic resin contained in several bonding systems, is at least 100 times less cytotoxic in tissue culture than Bis-GMA. These effects are reduced even more by the presence of a dentin barrier. Clinical studies have shown few or no viable bacterial cells in cavity preparations treated with this system, and no or only slight inflammatory reactions in the pulp. However, if the dentin in the floor of the cavity preparation is thin ($<$ 0.1 mm), there is some evidence that HEMA may be cytotoxic *in vivo*. There are also studies that have established the cytotoxicity *in vitro* of most of the common resins in dentin bonding agents such as Bis-GMA, triethylene glycol dimethacrylate (TEGDMA), urethane dimethacrylate (UDMA), and others. Other studies have shown that combinations of HEMA and other resins that are found in dentin bonding agents may act synergistically to cause cytotoxic effects *in vitro*. However, there have been essentially no clinical studies on the diffusion of hydrophilic and hydrophobic resin components through dentin. The risk of using these agents, and therefore their *in vivo* biocompatibility, cannot be completely defined until this information is obtained.

Resin-based materials

For tooth restoration, resin-based materials have been used as cements and restorative materials. Because they are a combination of organic and inorganic phases, these materials are called resin composites. The organic phase of these materials consists of Bis-GMA or UDMA resins diluted with TEGDMA. Organic initiators and accelerators are also present in smaller concentrations. The inorganic phase consists of particulate glasses coated with agents to promote bonding with the organic phase (silane coupling agents). Cements and restorative materials have similar basic compositions but differ in the amount and size of the inorganic filler. These materials set either chemically through a peroxide-amine system, or by visible light.

In vitro, freshly set, chemically cured, and light-cured resins cause moderate cytotoxic reactions in cultured cells. The cytotoxicity is significantly reduced 24 to 48 hours after setting and by the presence of a dentin barrier. Evidence indicates that the light-cured resins are less cytotoxic than chemically cured systems. This may result from the use of different initiators and accelerators in the light-cured systems. *In vivo* usage tests have been used to identify toxic components of Bis-GMA resins. Eight ingredients of Bis-GMA resins were placed individually into surface-sealed class 5 cavity preparations in monkey teeth for 21 days. Only three materials (2-hydroxy-4-benzophenone, benzoyl peroxide and methyl ester of benzoin) caused pulpal reactions. In addition, moderate inflammation usually occurred only in specimens with a remaining dentin thickness of 1 mm or less. The only exception was 2-hydroxy-4-methoxy benzophenone (a UV absorber), which irritated pulpal tissue through almost 3 mm of dentin. Benzoyl peroxide and the methyl ester of benzoin caused hemorrhage (necrosis of blood vessels) of the pulp in which remaining dentin was approximately 1 mm. These investigators suggested that the individual unreacted ingredients of these resins are not responsible for the tissue reactions that sometimes occur with resin composite restorations with over 1 mm remaining dentin thickness. In earlier usage tests, the pulpal inflammatory response to both chemically cured and light-cured resin composites was low to moderate after 3 days when they were placed in cavities with approximately 0.5 mm of remaining dentin. This reaction diminished as the postoperative periods increased to 5 to 8 weeks and was accompanied by an increase in reparative dentin (Fig. 7-8). With a protective liner or a bonding agent, the reaction of the pulp to resin composite materials is minimal.

Amalgams and cast alloys

Amalgams have been used extensively for dental restorations. The biocompatibility of amalgams is thought to be determined largely by corrosion products that are released while in service. Early dental amalgams were mixed by combining particles of Ag_3Sn with an excess of mercury. This resulted in a material containing γ_2, a phase that contains tin and mercury. The presence of the γ_2 phase was important because it was the most corrodible of the phases in the set mass, and it was continuous throughout the mass. Today's dental amalgams generally have higher amounts of copper. The copper is either added as a separate silver-copper particle (giving an admixed amalgam) or incorporated as Cu_3Sn within

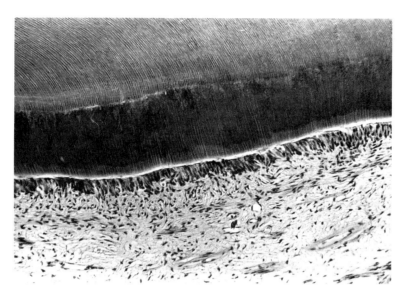

Fig. 7-8 A slight response is usually seen under unlined composites at 5 and 8 weeks. Few, if any, inflammatory cells are present, and regular-appearing reparative dentin is seen underlying the cavity. (Courtesy Avery JK: Ann Arbor, 1987, University of Michigan School of Dentistry.)

the Ag_3Sn particles (giving a unicompositional amalgam). Set high-copper amalgams have no γ_2 phase. Instead the Cu_6Sn_5 phase is formed, which is less corrodible and not continuous. This results in an amalgam that corrodes less in the oral environment. Tin oxide, a product of amalgam surface oxidation, protects the surface of amalgams from corrosion at pH 7.0. Thus, on surfaces exposed to oxygen and at a neutral pH, the corrosion process is said to be passivated. In crevices, stress cracks, open margins, and under dental plaque, the pH of the electrolytic fluids can become very acidic, which depassivates the amalgam surface and leads to corrosion. Corrosion becomes a continuous process, releasing products including oxides, hydroxides, and oxychlorides of tin, as well as ions of zinc and copper, which can be detected in dentin beneath amalgams. Abrasion can also remove the passive surface and encourage corrosion. Mercury can also be detected beneath amalgams for a few days after placement.

In cell culture screening tests, free or unreacted mercury from amalgam is toxic, but low-copper amalgam that has set for 24 hours does not inhibit cell growth. With the addition of copper, amalgams become toxic to cells in culture. Implantation tests show that low-copper amalgams are well tolerated,

but high-copper amalgams cause severe reactions when in direct contact with tissue. In usage tests the response of the pulp to amalgam in shallow cavities or in deeper but lined cavities is minimal. In deep cavities (0.5 mm or less of remaining dentin) pain results from using amalgams in unlined cavity preparations. An inflammatory response is seen after both 3 days and 5 weeks. In cavities with 0.5 to 1.0 mm of dentin remaining in the floor, the cavity preparation should be lined for two other reasons. First, thermal conductivity with amalgam is significant and can be a problem clinically. Second, margins of newly placed amalgam restorations show significant microleakage. Marginal leakage of both corrosion and microbial products are probably enhanced by the natural thermal cycling that occurs daily in the oral cavity. The short-term pulpal response is significantly reduced when the cavity is lined, and amalgam rarely causes irreversible damage to the pulp. Long-term sealing of the margins occurs through the buildup of corrosion products.

A number of high-copper amalgams are currently in clinical use. Usage tests reported that at 3 days the pulpal responses elicited by these materials appear similar to those elicited by low-copper amalgams in deep, unlined cavities. At 5 weeks they elicited only slight pulpal response. At 8 weeks the inflammatory response was reduced. Bacterial tests on the high-copper amalgam pellets have revealed little inhibitory effect on serotypes of *S. mutans,* thus suggesting that the elements were not released in amounts necessary to kill these microorganisms. Although the high-copper amalgams seem biologically acceptable in usage tests, liners are suggested for all deep cavities.

Amalgams based on gallium rather than mercury have been developed to provide direct restorative materials that are free of mercury. In cell culture, these alloys appear to be no more cytotoxic than traditional high-copper amalgams. These restorations release significant amounts of gallium *in vitro*, but the importance of this release is not known. In implantation tests, gallium alloys caused a significant foreign body reaction. Clinically, these materials show much higher corrosion rates than amalgams, leading to roughness and discoloration. There are few reports of pulpal responses to these materials.

Cast alloys have been used for single restorations, bridges, porcelain-fused-to-metal crowns, and partial dentures. The gold content in these alloys ranges from 0% to 85% (percentage by weight). These alloys contain several other noble and nonnoble metals that may have an adverse effect on cells if they are released from the alloys. However, released metals are most likely to contact gingival and mucosal tissues, and the pulp is more likely to be affected by the cement retaining the restoration.

Glass ionomers

Glass ionomers are another type of material that have been used both as a cement (luting agent) and as a restorative material. The material is a product of the reaction of a polymer acid and a fluoride-containing calcium aluminosilicate glass. The acid either is used as an aqueous solution or dehydrated and coated onto the glass particles. In the latter case, the liquid used is often a dilute solution of tartaric acid. Copolymers of acrylic, maleic, and itaconic acids have been used in some systems. Unreacted glass particles give strength and abrasion resistance to these materials, and the polymeric acids bond to these particles, as well as to enamel, dentin, and some alloys. Release of fluorides from the set material reduces the effect of acidic attacks on enamel or dentin. Light-cured ionomer systems have been introduced and these systems use Bis-GMA or other oligomers as pendant chains on the polyacrylate main chain. In screening tests, freshly prepared ionomer is mildly cytotoxic, but this effect is reduced with increased times after setting. Some researchers have reported that some systems are more cytotoxic than others, but the reasons for this observation are not clear. The overall pulpal biocompatibility of these materials has been attributed to the weak nature of the polyacrylic acid, which is unable to diffuse through dentin because of its high molecular weight. In usage tests the pulp reaction to glass ionomer cements is mild. Histological studies in usage tests show that any inflammatory infiltrate from ionomer is minimal or absent after 1 month. There have been several reports of pulpal hyperalgesia for short periods (days) of time after placing glass ionomers in cervical cavities. This effect is probably the result of increased dentin permeability after acid etching.

Liners, varnishes, and nonresin cements

Calcium hydroxide cavity liners come in many forms, ranging from saline suspensions with a very alkaline pH (above 12) to modified forms containing zinc oxide, titanium oxide, and resins. Resin-containing preparations can be polymerized chemically, but light-activated systems have also been introduced. The high pH of calcium hydroxide in suspension leads to extreme cytotoxicity in screening tests. Calcium hydroxide cements containing resins cause mild-to-moderate cytotoxic effects in tissue culture in both the freshly set and long-term set conditions. The inhibition of cell metabolism is reversible in tissue culture by high levels of serum proteins, suggesting that protein binding or buffering in inflamed pulpal tissue may play an important role in detoxifying these materials *in vivo*. The initial response of exposed pulpal tissue to the highly alkaline aqueous pulp-capping agents is necrosis to a depth of 1 mm or more. The alkaline pH also helps to coagulate any hemorrhagic exudate of the superficial pulp. Shortly after necrosis occurs, neutrophils infiltrate into the subnecrotic zone. Eventually, after 5 to 8 weeks, only a slight inflammatory response remains. Within weeks to months, the necrotic zone undergoes dystrophic calcification, which appears to be a stimulus for dentin bridge formation. When resins are incorporated into the formulae, these calcium hydroxide compounds become less irritating and are able to stimulate reparative dentin bridge formation more quickly than the $Ca(OH)_2$ suspensions, and with no zone of necrosis. Therefore, reparative dentin is laid down adjacent to the liner (Fig. 7-9), an indication that the replacement odontoblasts form the dentin bridge in contact with the liner. However, some of these materials evidently break down with time and create a gap between the

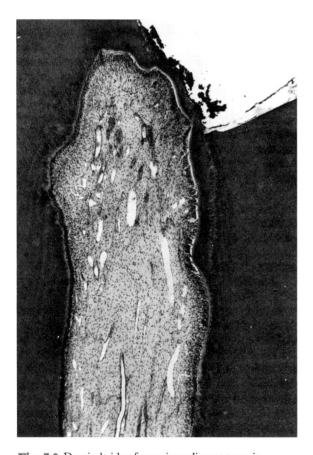

Fig. 7-9 Dentin bridge formation adjacent to resin-containing calcium hydroxide pulp-capping agent. Pulp exposure of young adult monkey was made 5 weeks before extraction and histologic evaluation of pulp reaction. There is a minimal inflammatory response to this procedure. Dilated blood vessels were caused by perfusion. (Courtesy Heys DR: Ann Arbor, 1987, University of Michigan School of Dentistry.)

restoration and the cavity wall. Resin-containing calcium hydroxide pulp-capping agents are the most effective liners now available for treating pulp exposures. After pulp exposure, the uninfected pulp undergoes a relatively uncomplicated wound-healing process. There are studies in progress to determine the feasibility of using bone morphogenic protein-coated demineralized bone or dentin matrix as potential pulp-capping agents.

Numerous investigators have analyzed the effects of applying thin liners such as copal *varnishes* and polystyrenes under restorations. These materials are not generally used under resin-based materials because resin components dissolve the thin film of varnish. Because liners are used in such thin layers, they do not provide thermal insulation, but they initially isolate the dentinal tubule contents from the cavity preparation. They may also reduce penetration of bacteria or chemical substances for a time. However, because of the thinness of the film and formation of pinpoint holes, the integrity of these materials is not as reliable as that of other cavity liners.

Zinc phosphate has been the most widely used dental cement for castings, orthodontic bands and to base cavity preparations. Because the thermal conductivity of this cement is approximately equal to that of enamel and considerably less than that of metals, it has also been used to build up the remaining tooth structure. The fluid component of this cement consists of about 40% aqueous solution of orthophosphoric acid and small amounts of ionized aluminum and zinc. The powder contains zinc oxide with a small amount of magnesium oxide. The set reaction product is hydrated amorphous zinc phosphate containing unreacted zinc oxide particles. *In vitro* screening tests indicate that these cements elicit strong-to-moderate cytotoxic reactions that decrease with increased time after setting. Leaching of zinc ions and a low pH may explain these effects. The dilution of leached cement products by dentin filtration has been shown to protect the pulp from most of these cytotoxic effects. Focal necrosis, observed in implantation tests with zinc phosphate cements injected into rat pulp, confirm the cytotoxic effects of this cement where it contacts tissue. In usage tests in deep cavity preparations, moderate-to-severe localized pulpal damage is produced within the first 3 days, probably because of the initial low pH on setting (4.2 at

3 minutes). The pH of the set cement approaches neutrality after 48 hours. By 5 to 8 weeks, only mild chronic inflammation is present, and reparative dentin has usually formed. Because of the initially painful and damaging effects on the pulp of this cement when placed in deep cavity preparations, a protective layer of ZOE, varnish, or calcium hydroxide is recommended under the cement. Other formulae have included calcium hydroxide in the powder, lowering the concentrations of phosphoric acid in the liquid, or included materials such as copper and fluoride ions that may function as antimicrobial agents. However, copper ions have proven extremely toxic to cells in culture and in implantation tests.

Zinc polyacrylate cements (polycarboxylate cements) were developed to combine the strength of zinc phosphate cements with the adhesiveness and biocompatibility of zinc oxide–eugenol (ZOE). Aqueous polyacrylic acid is mixed with zinc oxide to form a zinc polyacrylate. As with glass ionomers, adhesion presumably occurs through the reaction of acid groups with calcium in the tooth structure. In short-term tissue culture tests, cytotoxicity of freshly set and completely set cements has correlated both with the release of zinc and fluorides into the culture medium and with a reduced pH. Some researchers suggest that this cytotoxicity is an artifact of tissue culture because the phosphate buffers in the culture medium encourage zinc ions to leach from the cement. Supporting this theory, cell growth inhibition can be reversed if EDTA (which chelates zinc) is added to the culture medium. Furthermore, inhibition of cells decreases as the cement sets. In addition, concentrations of polyacrylic acid above 1% appear to be cytotoxic in tissue culture tests. On the other hand, subcutaneous and bone implant tests over a 1-year period have not indicated long-term cytotoxicity of these cements. Thus, other mechanisms such as buffering and protein-binding of these materials may neutralize these effects *in vivo* over time. Polyacrylic cements cause a pulpal response similar to that caused by ZOE, with a slight-to-moderate response after 3 days and only mild, chronic inflammation after 5 weeks. Reparative dentin formation is minimal with these cements, and thus they are recommended only in cavities with intact dentin in the floors of the cavity preparations.

Zinc oxide–eugenol cements (ZOE) have been used in dentistry for many years. *In vitro* eugenol from ZOE fixes cells, depresses cell respiration, and reduces nerve transmission with direct contact. Surprisingly, it is relatively innocuous in usage tests in class 5 cavity preparations. This is not contradictory for a number of reasons. The effects of eugenol are dose dependent, and diffusion through dentin dilutes eugenol by several orders of magnitude. Thus, although the concentration of eugenol in the cavity preparations just below the ZOE has been reported to be 10^{-2} M (bactericidal), the concentration on the pulpal side of the dentin may be 10^{-4} M or less. This lower concentration reportedly suppresses nerve transmission and inhibits synthesis of prostaglandins and leukotrienes (antiinflammatory). In addition and as described before, ZOE may form a temporary seal against bacterial invasion. In cavity preparations in primate teeth (usage tests), ZOE caused only a slight-to-moderate inflammatory reaction within the first week, and this was reduced to a mild, chronic inflammatory reaction, with some reparative dentin formation when cavities were deep, within 5 to 8 weeks. For this reason, it has been used as a negative control substance for comparison with restorative procedures in usage tests.

Bleaching agents

Bleaching agents have been used on nonvital and vital teeth for many years, but their use on vital teeth has increased dramatically. These agents usually contain some form of peroxide (generally carbamide peroxide) in a gel that can be applied to the teeth either by the dentist or at home by the patient. The agents may be in contact with teeth for several minutes to several hours depending on the formulation of the material. *In vitro* studies have shown that peroxides can rapidly (within minutes) traverse the dentin in sufficient concentrations to be cytotoxic. The cytotoxicity depends to a large extent on the concentration of the peroxide in the bleaching agent. *In vivo*, there are few studies that have demonstrated adverse pulpal effects from bleaching, but most reports agree that a legitimate concern exists about the long-term use of these products on vital teeth.

Reaction of Other Oral Soft Tissues to Restorative Materials

Restorative materials may cause reactions in the oral soft tissues such as gingiva. At present, it is not clear how much of the *in vivo* cytotoxicity observed is caused by the restorative materials and how much is caused by products of bacterial plaque that accumulate on teeth and restorations. In general, conditions that promote retention of plaque, such as rough surfaces or open margins, increase inflammatory reactions in gingiva around these materials. However, released products of restorative materials also contribute either directly or indirectly to this inflammation, particularly in areas where the washing effects of saliva are less, such as in interproximal areas, in deep gingival pockets, or under removable appliances. Several studies have documented increased inflammation or recession of gingiva adjacent to restorations where plaque indexes are low. In these studies, released products from materials could cause inflammation in the absence of plaque or could inhibit formation of plaque and cause inflammation in gingiva.

Cements exhibit some cytotoxicity in the freshly set state, but this decreases substantially with time. The buffering and protein-binding effects of saliva appear to mitigate against the cytotoxic effects. Resin cements and glass ionomer cements that have been eluted for several days have exhibited essentially nontoxic reactions when tested in fibroblastic cell culture. On the other hand, the eugenol that is released from ZOE cements fixes cells in culture so that they exhibit no mitochondrial enzyme activity. Thus, gingival tissues that are exposed to significant amounts of eugenol would be expected to exhibit a localized area of coagulation necrosis.

Amalgam restorations carried into the gingival crevice may cause inflammation of the gingiva because of either products of corrosion or bacterial plaque. Seven days after placement of an amalgam, a few inflammatory cells appear in the gingival connective tissue, and hydropic degeneration of some epithelial cells may be seen. Some proliferation of epithelial cells into the connective tissue may also occur by 30 days, and chronic mononuclear cell infiltration of connective tissue is evident. Increased vascularity persists, with more epithelial cells invaginating into the connective tissue. Some of these changes may be a chronic response of gingiva to plaque on the margins of the amalgams. Nevertheless, corrosion products from amalgam cannot be ruled out at this time because implanted amalgams produce similar responses in connective tissues in animals. In addition, although copper enhances the physical properties of amalgam and is bactericidal, it is also toxic to host cells and causes severe tissue reactions in implantation tests. Animal implantation studies have also shown severe reactions to gallium-based alloys, which have been used as amalgam replacements.

There is a report in the literature in which amalgam and resin composite restorations were placed in cavity preparations in monkey central incisors that had been extracted for less than one hour. The cavities, with depths of about 2 mm, were placed halfway between the cementoenamel junction and the root tip. The teeth were immediately reimplanted after restoration, and the animals were sacrificed at intervals up to 6 months. Repair of the PDL took place in a normal fashion except for the presence of an intense inflammatory infiltrate in the PDL adjacent to the amalgams through 2 weeks, but to the resin composites through 3 to 6 months. This result suggests that both resin composites and amalgam release cytotoxic materials that are the cause of tissue responses, at least at sites of implantation. For materials placed where they are rinsed in saliva, these cytotoxic agents are probably washed away before they harm the gingiva. However, rough surfaces on these types of restorations have been associated with increased inflammation *in vivo*. Usage tests in which restorations were extended into the gingival crevice have shown that finished materials gave a much milder inflammatory response than unfinished materials. The detrimental effect of surface roughness has been attributed to the increased plaque retention on these surfaces. However, rough surfaces on alloy restorations also caused increased cytotoxic effects in *in vitro* experiments where plaque was absent. This and other *in vitro* studies again would suggest that the cytotoxic response to alloys may be associated with release of elements from the alloys. The increased surface area of a rough surface may enhance release of these elements.

Denture base materials, especially methacrylates, have been associated with immune hypersensitivity reactions of gingiva and mucosa probably more than any other dental material. The greatest potential for hypersensitization is for dental and laboratory personnel who are exposed repeatedly to a variety of unreacted components. Hypersensitivity has been documented to the acrylic and diacrylic monomers, certain curing agents, antioxidants, amines, and formaldehyde. For the patient, however, most of these materials have reacted in the polymerization reaction, and the incidence of hypersensitization is quite low. Screening tests for sensitization potential include testing of unreacted ingredients, the polymeric substance after reaction, and oil, saline, or aqueous extracts of the polymer in both *in vitro* tests described previously and in skin tests in animals. In addition to hypersensitivity, visibly light-cured denture base resins and denture base resin sealants have been shown to be cytotoxic to epithelial cells in culture.

Soft tissue responses to *soft denture liners and adhesives* is of concern because of the intimate contact between these materials and the gingiva. Plasticizers, which are incorporated into some materials to make them soft and flexible, have been shown to be released *in vivo* and *in vitro*. Cell culture tests have shown that some of these materials are extremely cytotoxic. In animal tests, several of these materials have caused significant epithelial changes, presumably from the released plasticizers. In usage the effects of the released plasticizers are probably often masked by the inflammation already present in the tissues onto which these materials are placed. Denture adhesives have been evaluated *in vitro* and show severe cytotoxic reactions. Several had substantial formaldehyde content. The adhesives also allowed significant microbial growth.

Reaction of Bone and Soft Tissues to Implant Materials

There are 50 to 60 million extractions yearly, and there are some 20 million edentulous people in the United States. The recent development of new biomaterials has promoted interest in tooth replacement. To date, at least six different categories of implants are used by the profession: (1) subperiosteal implants, (2) transosteal implants, (3) ramus bars, (4) endosteal blades and anchors, (5) root replicas and cylinders, and (6) alveolar ridge augmentation. Implant failure may result from the following: physical properties of design, the material from which the implant is fabricated, and local and systemic biological problems with the health of the patient. Because this chapter is not a comprehensive review, it focuses on the biological compatibility of the materials. There are four basic materials used in implant fabrication: ceramics, carbon, metals, and polymers (and combinations of the above).

Reactions to ceramic implant materials

Ceramics have the general formula of quartz, feldspar, and kaolin. Ceramics are a combination of metal oxides, including SiO_2, Al_2O_3 (alumina), MgO (magnesia), $MgAl_2O_3$ (spinel), and many others (see Chapter 17 on ceramics). These materials are used mainly for fabricating endosteal bars, coating metallic endosteal blades, or making root cylinders. The carbons, single quartz crystals and a formula called Bioglass, consisting of Na_2O, CaO, and SiO_2, also fit into this category. In addition, hydroxyapatite $(Ca_{10}[PO_4]_6[OH]_2)$ and tricalcium phosphate $(\beta\text{-}Ca_3[PO_4]_2)$, which continue to be tested for bone augmentation, are ceramic materials.

Most ceramic materials have very low toxic effects on tissues, either because they are in an oxidized state or are corrosion resistant. As a group, they have low toxicity and are nonimmunogenic and noncarcinogenic. Their disadvantages are that they are brittle and lack impact and shear strength. Thus, these materials have been used as coatings on metals or other materials. These coatings have been used in either porous or dense forms. If the root surface porosities are over 150 μm in diameter, the implants often become firmly bound to bone (ankylosis, osseointegration), especially if they are taken out of occlusion for a time. If the porosities are smaller, the tissue usually forms only fibrous ingrowth. Dense ceramics are also used as root replicas or bone screws. Made of either single crystal (sapphire) or polycrystalline aluminum oxide, they become osseointegrated and provide excellent stability if left unloaded for a time. In one study, 60% of the restorations still performed adequately after 6 years in place.

Hydroxyapatite, a relatively nonresorbable form of calcium phosphate, has been used with some success as a coating material for titanium implants and as a ridge augmentation material. Studies indicate that the hydroxyapatite increases the rate of bony ingrowth toward the implant. However, the long-term corrosion of these coatings and the stability of the bond of the coating to the substrate are still controversial. Beta-tricalcium phosphate, another form of calcium phosphate, has been used in situations where resorption of the material is desirable, such as repair of bony defects. Carbon has been used as a coating and in bulk forms for implants. Although the biological response to carbon coatings can be favorable, they have been supplanted by titanium, aluminum oxide bulk materials, and hydroxyapatite coatings. Finally, Bioglass forms a surface gel that reacts favorably with connective tissue, allowing bone formation adjacent to it.

Reactions to pure metals and alloys

Pure metals and alloys are the oldest type of oral implant materials. All metal implants share the quality of strength. Initially, metallic materials were selected on the basis of ease of fabrication. However, with time, biocompatibility with bone and soft tissue, as well as longevity of the implant, have become more important. A variety of implant materials have been used, including stainless steel, chromium-cobalt-molybdenum, and titanium and its alloys. These materials have been used in a variety of forms, including root forms, subperiosteal, and transosteal implants.

Stainless steel was used a great deal in the past because it was inexpensive, easily available, and strong. In addition, it could be cast or wrought, which meant it could be fabricated into many forms such as endosteal blades and ramus bars. However, stainless steel is very susceptible to corrosion in a saline environment such as tissue fluid. With corrosion, stainless steel undergoes metal fatigue, a major reason for failure of the implant. Furthermore, it is believed that the corrosion products that are released from stainless steel cause adverse inflammatory reactions. In endosseous implants (those in bone), this inflammation discourages osseointegration and promotes fibrous capsule formation.

Cobalt-chromium-molybdenum alloys are castable and were the mainstay of the metallic implants for many years in dentistry and orthopedics. In dentistry, they have been used as subperiosteal saddles, endosteal blades, and transosteal implants for about 40 years. The surface of this alloy has also been coated (sintered) with a porous ceramic or porous carbon. However, connective tissue forms a fibrous capsule around these implants within weeks to months after placement. This fibrous reaction, although less

intense than for stainless steel, is thought to be due to elements that are released from the implants. Studies have shown that these elements accumulate locally and in systemic organs, such as the lung, liver, and kidney, over a period of years. However, controversy remains about the significant of the presence of these elements in tissues.

Titanium is a pure metal, at least when first cast. Within a short time (less than a second) the surface forms a thin film of titanium oxide, which is corrosion resistant and allows bone to grow to within 100 Å of the implant. The major disadvantage of this metal is that it is difficult to cast. It has been wrought into endosteal blades and root forms, but this process introduces metallic impurities into the surface that may adversely effect bony response unless extreme care is taken during manufacturing. Titanium implants have been used with success as root forms that are left unloaded under the mucosa for several months before they are used to support a prosthesis. With frequent recall and good oral hygiene, the implants have been maintained in healthy tissue for up to two decades. Titanium-aluminum-vanadium alloys (Ti6Al4V) have been used successfully in this regard as well, but questions remain about the liability of the aluminum and vanadium that are released. Although titanium and titanium alloy implants have corrosion rates that are markedly less than other metallic implants, they do release titanium into the body. However, currently there is no evidence that these released elements are a problem locally or systemically. The issue remains controversial.

In the soft tissue, epithelium will form a bond with the titanium that is morphologically similar to that with the tooth, but this interface has not been fully characterized. Connective tissue apparently does not bond to the titanium, but does form a tight seal, which seems to limit ingress of bacteria and bacterial products. Techniques are being developed to limit downgrowth of the epithelium and loss of bone height around the implant, which ultimately causes implant failure.

Reactions to other materials

Polymers are not currently used for endosseous implant materials, but are used in dentistry for maxillofacial prosthetics. In orthopedics polymer cements have been used for many years for fixation. The most common of these is polymethyl methacrylate (PMMA) cement. These cements are quite similar chemically to denture base resin materials. The biological response to PMMA cements is generally not favorable because the monomer is quite toxic to the bone tissue and heat generated during the setting can kill tissue. Nevertheless, these cements have been used with remarkable success. Glass ionomer bone cements are being developed for fixation in orthopedics, but are not currently used in implantology in dentistry.

Polymers of glutamic acid (PGA) and lactic acid (PLA) are used as implants in nondental applications as biodegradable materials that can deliver drugs at a precise rate or hold space for normal tissue development. These materials have been used for resorbably sutures. The resorption rate can be controlled by the composition of the polymers, and copolymers are often used. Although these materials are currently not used in dentistry as restorative materials, it is conceivable that they could find application for the delivery of drugs or repair of tissues.

Summary

The biocompatibility of a dental material depends on the composition of the material and the location and interactions of the material with the oral cavity. Metal, ceramic, and polymer materials all elicit different biological responses because of their differences in composition. Furthermore, diverse biological responses to these materials depend on whether they release their components and if those components are toxic, immunogenic, or mutagenic at the released concentrations. The location of a material in the oral cavity also partially determines its biocompatibility. Materials that appear biocompatible when in contact with the oral mucosal surface may cause adverse reactions if they are implanted beneath it. Materials that are toxic when in direct contact with the pulp may be essentially innocuous if placed on dentin or enamel. Finally, interactions between the material and the body influence the biocompatibility of the material. The material's response to changes in pH, the application of force, or the degradative effects of biological fluids can alter its biocompatibility. Features of a material's surface that promote or discourage the attachment of bacteria, host cells, or biological molecules determine whether the material will promote plaque retention, integrate with bone, or adhere to dentin.

SELECTED PROBLEMS

Problem 1. You have a group of six materials, all of which can be classified as posterior composites, but each of which has a slightly different formula. To determine which of these freshly set materials is *least* toxic in the least expensive, least time-consuming manner, what would you do?

Solution. You may choose an *in vitro* cell growth test. The materials would be formed into disks of equal dimensions, and there should be at least six disks per material. The disks should be stabilized on the bottoms of cell culture wells. Cells are then placed into the wells with the materials and are incubated in an appropriate incubation medium and environment for 24 hours or more. Then the disks and wells are observed and photographed under phase-contrast microscopy, taking special note of zone width of cytopathic effects around each disk for semiquantitative results.

Other options are the agar overlay test and the Millipore filter test.

Problem 2. If you have the same situation as in Problem 1, but you want to quantify your results, what are your options?

Solution. You may choose the same test model as in the solution for Problem 1, but you would measure the cellular response quantitatively rather then by visual observation. There are several options: you could (1) measure the area of cytopathic effect around each sample, (2) measure the membrane permeability of the cells that remain around the disks using neutral red or ^{51}Cr (see Fig. 7-7), or (3) measure some aspect of cellular biosynthesis or metabolism (MTT test, DNA synthesis). Otherwise, you might choose other models such as extracting the sample for 1 to 3 days in given volumes of solvent and then treating a cell with serial dilutions of the elutants.

Problem 3. With the same situation as in Problem 1, you want to know the effect of the setting reaction or time on the toxicity of the material. What would you do?

Solution. Usually the material is made into disks and allowed to set for varying periods (from 1 to several days). Then, for each period, the set disks are placed into tissue culture wells or are extracted with a solvent that is placed into tissue culture wells. Then your options are the same as those in the solutions for 1 or 2.

Problem 4. If you have a series of composites and you want to rank them according to the toxicity they may have specifically for pulpal cells, what would you do?

Solution. You should choose a test model in which dentin is interspaced between material and cell test system.

Problem 5. One of your six composite materials is associated fairly consistently with pulpitis when used by you and your fellow clinicians. The cytotoxicity test that you chose indicates that this material is not much more toxic than the other materials. How can you better understand what is causing the pulpitis?

Solution. The pulpitis may be caused by microleakage of bacteria or by the material's ability to cause an inflammatory (vs. toxicity) response. If the facilities are available, you may do *in vitro* chemotaxis tests, using human peripheral leukocytes (PMNs) with the test sample to determine which materials might be responsible for the inflammation. If the material does not show an inflammatory response in these tests, then usage tests in animals could be used to verify the pulpitis *in vivo* in a more controlled environment. Then, if usage tests in animals substantiate the pulpitis, you should be highly suspicious of microleakage of environmental materials or bacteria products. To confirm this suspicion, additional usage tests could be used where the margins of the restoration are surface-sealed to prevent microleakage.

Problem 6. You have a new polymeric substance that you believe might function well as a root cylinder implant. What kinds of tests should you conduct to answer questions of safety according to the FDA standards, and how long will this take?

Solution. Initial tests should include cytotoxicity tests, a hemolysis test, some test for mutagenesis or gene toxicity, and probably an oral LD_{50} test. (All tests except mutagenesis can be performed and analyzed in about 2 to 3 weeks if run concurrently. The mutagenesis tests may require between 1 and 3 months for performance analysis.)

Secondary tests might include implantation into bone and soft tissue of small animals, tests for mucous membrane irritation, and hypersensitivity tests. If done concurrently, this will take about 1 month before histological preparation of tissue is begun. Time required for histology and reading of slides may vary, depending on the size of the project.

Usage tests (percutaneous implants) in jaws of larger animals may require that the implants remain in place for 1 to 2 years, followed by histological processing and evaluation.

Problem 7. You are a dentist who has been practicing for 20 years, and you like to do a lot of your own laboratory work. You have noticed that when you handle methacrylate denture base and monomer, you develop a rash on your hands. What is the problem, and what can you do about it?

Solution. You are probably hypersensitive to the monomer and should wear rubber gloves around monomer and freshly polymerized methacrylate. Try to avoid contact, because monomer can penetrate latex rubber.

Problem 8. You have a patient who has an endosteal blade that had been implanted by her previous prosthodontist before she moved to town. The implant has been in place 1 year and appears to be somewhat mobile. What are your options for analyzing the problem?

Solution. Radiographs of the implant and tissue in the region should be done to look for areas of radiolucencies, both at the cervix and at the mesial and distal tips of the blade. A periodontal probe may be used gently to determine if there is tissue attachment around the implant. However, if the implant is mobile at all, failure is probably imminent.

■ REFERENCES

Screening Tests

AAMI Standards and Recommended Practices: *Biological Evaluation of Medical Devices,* vol 4, Arlington, VA, Association for the Advancement of Medical Instrumentation, 1994.

American Dental Association: Addendum to American National Standards/American Dental Association Document No. 41 for recommended standard practices for biological evaluation for dental materials, Chicago, 1982, American Dental Association.

American Dental Association: American National Standards Institute/American Dental Association Document No. 41 for recommended standard practices for biological evaluation of dental materials, *J Am Dent Assoc* 99:697, 1979.

Barile FA: *In vitro cytotoxicity: mechanisms and methods.* Boca Raton, 1994, CRC Press.

Bumgardner JD, Lucas LC, Tilden AB: Toxicity of copper-based dental alloys in cell culture, *J Biomed Mater Res* 23:1103, 1989.

Caughman WF, Caughman GB, Dominy WT, Schuster GS: Glass ionomer and composite resin cements: effects on oral cells, *J Prosthet Dent* 63:513, 1990.

Craig RG, Hanks CT: Cytotoxicity of experimental casting alloys evaluated by cell culture, *J Dent Res* 69:1539, 1990.

Ecobichon, DJ: *The basis of toxicity testing.* Boca Raton, 1992, CRC Press.

Guess WL, Rosenbluth SA, Schmidt B, Autian J: Agar diffusion method for toxicity screening of plastics on cultured cell monolayers, *J Pharm Sci* 54:1545, 1965.

Hanks CT, Anderson M, Craig RG: Cytotoxic effect of dental cements on two cell culture systems, *J Oral Pathol* 10:101, 1981.

Hanks CT, Bergenholtz G, Kim J-S: Protein synthesis *in vitro* in the presence of $Ca(OH)_2$-containing pulp-capping medicaments, *J Oral Pathol* 12:356, 1983.

Hanks CT, Strawn SE, Wataha JC, Craig RG: Cytotoxic effects of resin components on cultured mammalian fibroblasts, *J Dent Res* 70:1450, 1991.

Hanks CT, Syed SA, Craig RG, Hartrick JM: Modeling bacterial damage to pulpal cells *in vitro*, *J Endodontol* 17:21, 1991.

Hume WR: A new technique for screening chemical toxicity to the pulp from dental restorative materials and procedures, *J Dent Res* 64:1322, 1985.

Hume WR, Mount GJ: *In vitro* studies on the potential for pulpal cytotoxicity of glass ionomer cements, *J Dent Res* 67:915, 1988.

Kaga M, Seale NS, Hanawa T, Okabe T: Cytotoxicity of amalgams, alloys and their elements and phases, *Dent Mater* 7:68, 1991.

Kawahara H, Yamagami A, Nakamura M: Biological testing of dental materials by means of tissue culture, *Int Dent J* 18:443, 1968.

Meryon SD: The influence of dentine on the *in vitro* cytotoxicity testing of dental restorative materials, *J Biomed Mater Res* 18:771, 1984.

Meryon SD, Riches DW: A comparison of the *in vitro* cytotoxicity of four restorative materials assessed by changes in enzyme levels in two cell types, *J Biomed Mater Res* 16:519, 1982.

Mjör IA: Usage tests for restorative materials, *J Endodont* 4:308, 1978.

Mjör IA, Hensten-Pettersen A, Skogedal O: Biologic evaluation of filling materials: a comparison of results using cell culture techniques, implantation tests and pulp studies, *Int Dent J* 27:124, 1977.

Müller J, Hörz W, Bruckner G, Kraft E: An experimental study on the biocompatibility of lining cements based on glass ionomer as compared with calcium hydroxide, *Dent Mater* 6:35, 1990.

Neimi L, Hensten-Pettersen A: *In vitro* cytotoxicity of Ag-Pd-Cu based casting alloys, *J Biomed Mater Res* 19:549, 1985.

Okita N, Hensten-Pettersen A: *In vitro* cytotoxicity of tissue conditioners, *J Prosthet Dent* 66:656, 1991.

Rathbun MA, Craig RG, Hanks CT, Filisko FE: Cytotoxicity of a Bis-GMA dental composite before and after leaching in organic solvents, *J Biomed Mater Res* 25:443, 1991.

Schmalz G: A reproducibility study on the agar diffusion test, *J Dent Res* 61:577, 1982.

Spängberg L: Kinetic and quantitative evaluation of material cytotoxicity *in vitro*, *Oral Surg* 35:389, 1973.

Styles JA: Tissue culture methods of evaluating biocompatibility of polymers. In Williams DF, editor: *Systemic aspects of biocompatibility,* vol 2, Boca Raton, 1981, CRC Press.

Tennant RW, Margolin BH, Shelby MD, Zeigler E, Haseman JK, Spalding J, Caspary W, Resnick M, Stasiewicz S, Anderson B, Minor R: Prediction of chemical carcinogenicity in rodents from *in vitro* genetic toxicity assays, *Science* 236:933, 1987.

Tronstad L, Wennberg A, Hasselgren G: Screening tests for dental materials, *J Endodont* 4:304, 1978.

Trump BF, Mergner WJ: Cell injury. In Zweifach BW, Grant L, McCluskey RT, editors: *The inflammatory process,* vol 1, ed 2, New York, 1974, Academic Press.

Tyas M: A method for the testing of dental materials, *J Dent Res* 10:1285, 1977.

Wataha JC, Hanks CT, Craig RG: Precision of and new methods for testing *in vitro* alloy cytotoxicity, *Dent Mater* 8:65–71, 1992.

Wennberg A: *In vitro* assessment of the biocompatibility of dental materials: the Millipore filter method, *Int Endod J* 21:67, 1988.

Wennberg A, Mjör IA, Hensten-Pettersen A: Biological evaluation of dental restorative materials: a comparison of different test methods, *J Biomed Mater Res* 17:23, 1983.

Williams GM and Weisburger, JH: Chemical carcinogens. In Amdur, MO et al., editors: *Casarett and Doull's toxicology: the basic science of poisons,* ed. 4, New York, Pergamon Press, 1991.

Pulp

Brännström M: *Dentin and pulp in restorative dentistry,* London, 1982, Wolfe Medical.

Brännström M: Reaction of the pulp to amalgam fillings, *Odontol Rev* 14:244, 1964.

Cox CF, Keall CL, Keall HJ, Ostro EO: Biocompatibility of surface-sealed dental materials against exposed pulps, *J Prosthet Dent* 57:1, 1987.

El-Kafrawy AH, Dickey DM, Mitchell DF, Phillips RW: Pulp reaction to a polycarboxylate cement in monkeys, *J Dent Res* 53:15, 1974.

Espevik S, Mjör IA: Corrosion and toxicology of dental amalgams. In Smith DC, Williams DF, editors: *Biocompatibility of dental materials,* vol 3, Boca Raton, 1982, CRC Press.

Felton D, Bergenholtz G, Cox CF: Inhibition of bacterial growth under composite restorations following GLUMA pretreatment, *J Dent Res* 68:491, 1989.

Going RE: Cavity liners and dentin treatment, *J Am Dent Assoc* 69:415, 1964.

Heys DR, Cox CF, Heys RJ, Loesche WJ, Avery JK: Histopathologic and bacterial evaluation of conventional and new copper amalgam, *J Oral Pathol* 8:65, 1979.

Heys DR, Heys RJ, Cox CF, Avery JK: Experimental observations on the biocompatibility of composite resins. In Smith DC, Williams DF, editors: *Biocompatibility of dental materials,* vol 3, Boca Raton, 1982, CRC Press.

Heys DR, Heys RJ, Cox CF, Avery JK: Histopathologic evaluation of the effects of four calcium hydroxide liners on monkey pulps, *J Oral Pathol* 5:129, 1976.

Heys DR, Heys RJ, Cox CF, Avery JK: Histological evaluation of two calcium hydroxide compounds on inflamed pulps, *J Dent Res* 56:A63, 1977.

Heys DR, Heys RJ, Cox CF, Avery JK: Pulpal response to acid etching agents, *Mich Dent Assoc J* 58:221, 1976.

Jendresen MD, Trowbridge HO: Biologic and physical properties of a zinc polycarboxylate cement, *J Prosthet Dent* 28:264, 1972.

Lervik T: The effect of zinc phosphate and carboxylate cements on the healing of experimentally induced pulpitis, *Oral Surg* 45:123, 1978.

McComb D: Tissue reaction to silicate, silico-phosphate and glass ionomer cements and restorative materials. In Smith DC, Williams DF, editors: *Biocompatability of dental materials,* vol 3, Boca Raton, 1982, CRC Press.

Mjör IA, Tronstad L: Experimentally induced pulpitis, *Oral Surg* 34:102, 1972.

Müller J, Bruckner G, Kraft E, Hörz W: Reaction of cultured pulp cells to eight different cements based on glass ionomers, *Dent Mater* 6:172, 1990.

Pashley DH: Smear layer: physiological considerations, *Oper Dent* suppl 3:13, 1984.

Pashley DH: The effects of acid etching on the pulpodentin complex, *Oper Dent* 17:229, 1992.

Pathobiology of the dentin/pulp complex, International Conference, The University of North Carolina at Charlotte, 1991, *Proc Finn Dent Soc* 88(suppl 1), 1992.

Proceedings of an International Workshop on the biology of dentin and pulp, The University of North Carolina at Charlotte, 1984, *J Dent Res* 64(spec issue):481, 1985.

Proceedings of the First World Conference on dental and pulpal pain: mechanisms and management, *J Endodont* 12:435, 1986.

Smith DC: Tissue reaction to cements. In Smith DC, Williams DF, editors: *Biocompatibility of dental materials,* vol 2, Boca Raton, 1982, CRC Press.

Swerdlow H, Stanley HR: Response of the human dental pulp to amalgam restorations, *Oral Surg* 15:499, 1962.

Torstenson B, Nordenvall J-J, Brännström M: Pulpal reaction and microorganisms under Clearfil composite resin in deep cavities with acid etched dentin, *Swed Dent J* 6:167, 1982.

Trowbridge HO: Pathogenesis of pulpitis resulting from dental caries, *J of Endodont* 7:52, 1981.

Gingival Tissue

App GR: Effect of silicate, amalgam and cast gold on the gingiva, *J Prosthet Dent* 11:522, 1961.

Carranza FA, Jr, Romanelli JH: The effects of fillings and prosthetic appliances on the marginal gingiva, *Int Dent J* 23:64, 1973.

Ducheyne P: Bioceramics: material characteristics versus *in vivo* behavior, *J Biomed Mater Res:App Biomat* 21(A2):219, 1987.

Harsanyi BB, Foong WC, Howell RE, Jones DW: Hamster cheek-pouch testing of dental soft polymers, *J Dent Res* 70:991, 1991.

Hensten-Pettersen A, Nilner K, Möller B: Guinea pig maximization test with a polyether impression material, *Scand J Dent Res* 98:356, 1990.

Karlsen K: Gingival reactions to dental restorations, *Acta Odontol Scand* 28:895, 1970.

Klotzer WT: Oral mucosal usage tests, *J Endodont* 4:312, 1978.

Klotzer WT: Reactions of the gingiva to dental materials, *Rev Belge Med Dent* 31:253, 1976.

Lorato DC: Influence of a composite resin restoration on the gingiva, *J Prosthet Dent* 28:402, 1972.

Merritt K: Immunological testing of biomaterials. In Williams DF, editor: *Techniques in biocompatibility testing,* vol 2, Boca Raton, 1986, CRC Press.

Smith DC: Tissue reaction to cements. In Smith DC, Williams DF, editors: *Biocompatibility of dental materials,* vol 2, Boca Raton, 1982, CRC Press.

Smith DC: Tissue reaction to noble and base alloys. In Smith DC, Williams DF, editors: *Biocompatibility of dental materials,* vol 4, Boca Raton, 1982, CRC Press.

Sotres LS, Van Haysen G, Gilmore HW: A histologic study of gingival tissue response to amalgam, silicate and resin restorations, *J Periodontol* 40:543, 1969.

Trivedi SC, Talim ST: The response of human gingiva to restorative materials, *J Prosthet Dent* 29:73, 1973.

Waerhaug J: Effect of rough surfaces upon gingival tissue, *J Dent Res* 35:323, 1956.

Watson IB: The effect of complete dentures on oral mucosa, *J Dent* 6:171, 1978.

Williams DF: Toxicology of ceramics. In Williams DF, editor: *Fundamental aspects of biocompatibility,* vol 2, Boca Raton, 1981, CRC Press.

Bonding and Etching

Beech D: Adhesion in the oral environment: biophysical and biochemical considerations, *Int Dent J* 28:388, 1978.

Hörsted-Bindslev P: Monkey pulp reactions to cavities treated with GLUMA dentin bond and restored with a microfilled composite, *Scand J Dent Res* 95:347, 1987.

Causton BE, Samara-Wickrama DYD, Johnson NW: Effect of calcifying fluids on bonding of cements and composites to dentin *in vitro*, *Br Dent J* 140:339, 1976.

Council on Dental Materials, Instruments, and Equipment: Dentin bonding systems: an update, *J Amer Dent Assoc* 114:91, 1987.

Meryon SD, Brook AM: *In vitro* cytotoxicity of three dentine bonding agents, *J Dent* 17:279, 1989.

Munksgaard EC, Asmussen E: Methacrylate-bonding to dentin. In Thylstrup A, Leach SA, and Qvist V, editors: *Dentine and dentine reactions in the oral cavity: proceedings of a workshop,* Oxford, 1987, IRL Press Limited.

Nakabayashi N, Kojima K, Masuhara E: The promotion of adhesion by the infiltration of monomers into tooth substrates, *J Biomed Mater Res* 16: 265-273, 1982.

Pashley DH: Dentin bonding agents, *Curr Opin Dent* 2:46-51, 1992.

Pashley DH: Smear layer: Overview of structure and function, *Proc Finn Dent Soc* 88(Suppl. 1): 215-224, 1992.

Retief DH: Standardizing laboratory adhesion tests, *Amer J Dent* 4: 231-236, 1991.

Rueggeberg F: Substrate for adhesion testing to toothstructure—review of the literature, *Dent Mater* 7: 2-10, 1991.

Stanley HR: Guest editorial: an urgent plea for a standardized bonding (adhesion) test, *J Dent Res* 72: 1362-1363, 1993.

Stanley HR, Bowen RL, Cobb EN: Pulp response to a dentin and enamel adhesive bonding procedure, *Oper Dent* 13:107, 1988.

Implants

Adell R, Lekholm U, Rockler B, Bränemark PI: A 15-year study of osseointegrated implants in the treatment of the edentulous jaw, *Int J Oral Surg* 10:387, 1981.

Brunette DM, Kenner GS, Gould TRL: Grooved titanium surfaces orient growth and migration of cells from human gingival implants, *J Dent Res* 62:1045, 1983.

Bryan B: Bioactive glasses, aluminum oxide, and titanium: biochemistry of the interface. In Ducheyne P, Lemons JE, editors: *Bioceramics: material characteristics versus in vivo behavior,* New York, 1988, New York Academy of Sciences.

Clark AE, Hench LL, Paschall HA: The influence of surface chemistry on implant interface histology: a theoretical basis for implant materials selection, *J Biomed Mater Res* 10:161, 1976.

Köndell PA, Söder P-O, Landt H, Frithiof L, Anneroth G, Engström P-E, Olsson M-L: Gingival fluid and tissues around successful titanium and ceramic implants, *Acta Odont Scand* 49:169, 1991.

McKinney RV, Steflick DE, Koth DL, Suigh BB: The scientific basis for dental implant therapy, *J Dent Educ* 52:696, 1988.

Melcher AH: Summary of biological considerations, *J Dent Educ* 52:812, 1988.

National Institutes of Health: Consensus development statement on dental implants, June 13-15, 1988, *J Dent Educ* 52:824, 1988.

Pazzaglia UE, Zatti G, Cherubino P, Frick W: Bone reaction to the implant of intermedullary pins of three different metals in rat femur, *J Mater Sci: Mater Med* 2:77, 1991.

Pedley RB, Meachim G, Williams DF: Tumor induction by implant materials. In Williams DF, editor: *Fundamental aspects of biocompatibility,* Boca Raton, 1981, CRC Press.

Schnitman PA, Natiella JR, Young FA: Dental implants. In Reese JA, Valega TM, editors: *Restorative dental materials, an overview,* vol 1, Chicago, 1985, Quintessence.

Schroeder A, van der Zypen E, Stich H, Sutter F: The reactions of bone, connective tissue and epithelium to endosteal implants with titanium-sprayed surfaces, *J Maxillofac Surg* 9:15, 1981.

Steflik DE, McKinney RV, Koth DL: A statistical analysis of the clinical response to the single-crystal sapphire endosseous dental implant in dog jaws, *J Dent Res* 62:1212, 1983.

Zarb GA, Schmitt A: Osseointegration and the edentulous predicament: the 10-year old Toronto study, *Br Dent J* 170:439, 1991.

General Reading

Avery JK, editor: *Oral development and histology,* Philadelphia, 1988, BC Decker.

Hodgson E, Levi PE, editors: *A textbook of modern toxicology,* New York, 1987, Elsevier Science.

Robbins SL, Cotran RS, Kumar V: *Pathologic basis of disease,* ed 3, Philadelphia, 1984, WB Saunders.

TenCate AR, editor: *Oral histology: development, structure and function,* ed 4, St Louis, 1994, Mosby.

8 Cement

A variety of cements have been used in dentistry through the years. In general, cements are employed for two primary purposes: to serve as a restorative filling material either alone or with other materials, and to retain restorations or appliances in a fixed position within the mouth. Certain other cements, however, are used for specialized purposes in the restorative, endodontic, orthodontic, periodontic, and surgical fields of dentistry.

When the properties of the dental cements are compared with those of other restorative materials, such as amalgam, gold, or porcelain, the cements exhibit less favorable strength, solubility, and resistance to the conditions within the oral cavity. As a result, the general use of cements for restorations exposed to the oral environment is quite limited.

The zinc phosphate, glass ionomer, and zinc oxide–eugenol (ZOE) types can be applied as a base in deep cavities to insulate the pulp from possible chemical and thermal trauma. A metallic, ceramic, or resin filling material then may be placed over such a cement base in sufficient bulk and in proper adaptation to the cavity walls to form the final restoration. The sedative nature of the ZOE mixtures has made them valuable for a variety of applications. The ability of the glass and hybrid ionomer cements to release fluoride and to bond chemically to tooth structure has resulted in their uses as bases and for cementation of orthodontic bands. The resin cements are used for retention of orthodontic brackets, veneers, all-ceramic crowns and inlays, and resin-bonded bridges because of their strength and bonding to acid-etched enamel.

The following is a classification of dental cements, based on their chief chemical ingredients and application:

Zinc Phosphate

Retention of restorations
Retention of orthodontic bands
High-strength base
Temporary restoration

Zinc Oxide–Eugenol

Low- and high-strength bases
Temporary restorations
Temporary and permanent retention of restorations

Zinc Oxide–Non-Eugenol

Temporary retention of restorations
Root canal sealer
Gingival tissue pack
Surgical dressing

Zinc Polyacrylate

Retention of restorations
Retention of orthodontic bands
High-strength base

Glass and Hybrid Ionomers

Class 5 restorations (see Chapter 10)
Retention of restorations
Retention of orthodontic bands
High-strength base
Interim restoration

Resin, Composite, and Adhesive Resin Cements

Retention of conventional crowns and bridges
Retention of ceramic and composite inlays and onlays
Retention of temporary restorations
Retention of orthodontic brackets
Retention of posts
Retention of resin-bonded bridges
High-strength base

Calcium Hydroxide

Low-strength base

Ten types of materials are currently available. Although members of the profession are not in unanimous agreement regarding the purposes for each cement or the necessity for all the types, the cements are available to the dental profession and have been employed principally in the ways listed.

■ ZINC PHOSPHATE CEMENT

Through the years the refinement in formulation and compounding of the zinc phosphate cements and the increase in standards brought about by the adoption of former ADA Specification No. 8 in 1935 have resulted in a valuable, widely employed material in dentistry. The zinc phosphate cement is supplied as a powder and as a liquid, both of which are carefully compounded to react with one another during the mixing to develop a mass of cement possessing desirable physical characteristics.

Composition

Powder

The principal ingredient of the zinc phosphate cement powder is zinc oxide. Magnesium oxide, silicon dioxide, bismuth trioxide, and other minor ingredients are used in some products to alter the working characteristics and final properties of the mixed cement. A typical formulation of a zinc phosphate cement powder and liquid is shown in Table 8-1. The magnesium oxide, in quantities usually of about 10%, is added to the zinc oxide to reduce the temperature of the calcination process. The silicon dioxide is an inactive filler in the powder and during manufacture aids in the calcination process. Although the bismuth trioxide is believed to impart a smoothness to the freshly mixed cement mass, in large amounts it may also lengthen the setting time. Tannin-fluoride may be added to provide a source of fluoride ions in some products. Other modifiers in lesser amounts appear not to be essential in making a satisfactory cement powder.

The ingredients of the powder are heated together at temperatures ranging from 1000° to 1300° C for approximately 4 to 8 hours or longer, depending on the temperature. This calcination results in a fused or sintered mass. The mass is then ground and pulverized to a fine powder, which is sieved to recover selected particle sizes. The degree

TABLE 8-1 Typical Composition of Zinc Phosphate Cement Powder and Liquid

Composition	Weight (%)
Powder	
ZnO	90.2
MgO	8.2
SiO_2	1.4
Bi_2O_3	0.1
Misc. BaO, Ba_2SO_4, CaO	0.1
Liquid	
H_3PO_4 (free acid)	38.2
H_3PO_4 (combined with Al and Zn)	16.2
Al	2.5
Zn	7.1
H_2O	36.0

Adapted from Paffenbarger GC, Sweeney WT, Issacs A: *J Am Dent Assoc* 20:1960, 1933.

of calcination, the fineness of particle size, and the composition determine the reactivity the powder will have with the liquid.

Liquid

Zinc phosphate cement liquids are produced by adding aluminum and sometimes zinc, or their compounds, to an orthophosphoric acid solution. Although the original acid solution contains about 85% phosphoric acid and is a syrupy fluid, the resulting cement liquid usually contains about one-third water, as shown in Table 8-1. The partial neutralization of the phosphoric acid by the aluminum and zinc tempers the reactivity of the liquid and is described as buffering. This reduced rate of reaction aids in establishing a smooth, nongranular, workable cement mass during the mixing procedure. The setting time for the mixed cement may be modified by the proper dilution of the phosphoric acid with water. The presence of additional water shortens the setting time, whereas an insufficient amount of water prolongs the setting time. The zinc phosphate cement liquid therefore is adjusted by both partial neutralizing or buffering and dilution so that it reacts with its powder to produce a cement mass with proper setting time and mechanical qualities.

Chemistry of the Setting Reaction

When an excess of zinc phosphate cement powder is brought into contact with the liquid to begin the cement mix, wetting occurs and a chemical reaction is initiated. The surface of the alkaline powder is dissolved by the acid liquid, resulting in an exothermic reaction.

The set zinc phosphate cement is essentially a hydrated amorphous network of zinc phosphate that surrounds incompletely dissolved particles of zinc oxide. This amorphous phase is extremely porous. There is no evidence that the magnesium oxide present in the powder reacts with the phosphoric acid. Although no crystalline phosphate is involved in the setting process of the cement, there can be subsequent growth of crystalline hopeite, $Zn_3(PO_4)_2 \cdot 4H_2O$, in the presence of excess moisture during setting.

Manipulation

The manner in which the reaction between the zinc phosphate cement powder and liquid is permitted to occur determines to a large extent the working characteristics and properties of the cement mass. The proper amount of powder should be slowly incorporated into the liquid on a cool slab (approximately 21° C) to attain the desired consistency of cement. Certain requirements must be met to carry out this type of manipulation.

Mixing slab

Most chemical reactions are accelerated by the presence of heat because of an increase in molecular activity of the reactants. Because the combination of the modified zinc oxide and phosphoric acid results in the liberation of heat in the immediate environment of the reaction, this heat must be dissipated readily or the reaction will proceed too fast toward completion. Should this rapid reaction occur, ample working time is not available for proper manipulation of the cement before hardening or setting occurs.

A properly cooled glass slab thick enough that it is not readily influenced by the environment will dissipate the heat of the reaction. The mixing slab temperature should be low enough to be effective in cooling the cement mass but must not be below the dew point unless the frozen slab technic is used; this method is described subsequently. A temperature of 18° to 24° C is indicated when room humidity permits. The moisture condensation on a slab cooled below the dew point contaminates the mix, diluting the liquid and shortening the setting time. The ability of the mixing slab to be cooled and yet be free of moisture greatly influences proper control of the reaction rate of the zinc phosphate cement.

Powder/liquid ratio

The amount of powder that can be incorporated into a given quantity of liquid greatly determines the properties of the mixed mass of cement. Because an increase in the ratio of powder to liquid generally provides more desirable properties, as much powder as possible should be used to obtain a particular consistency.

Care of the liquid

The zinc phosphate cement liquid consists of the partially neutralized diluted phosphoric acid. When this liquid is exposed to a humid atmosphere, it will absorb water, whereas exposure to dry air tends to result in a loss of water.

While using some dispensing bottles of liquid, the cap is off for a sufficient period of time to significantly affect the water content of the liquid if exposure has been made to an unfavorable atmospheric humidity. Leaving the cap off the bottle unnecessarily may result in a rapid change of water content in the liquid. Therefore keeping the bottle tightly closed when not used is good practice. The polyethylene squeeze bottles do not require removal of a dropper and therefore eliminate the tendency for gain or loss of water from the liquid.

The setting time of the mixed cement is quite noticeably affected by water addition or subtraction from the cement liquid. The addition of water causes a more rapid reaction with the powder, resulting in a shorter setting time. A loss of water from the liquid results in a lengthened setting time.

Mixing procedure

By the initial incorporation of small portions of powder into the liquid, minimal heat is liberated and easily dissipated. The heat of the reaction is most effectively dissipated when the cement is mixed over a large area of the cooled slab. A relatively long, narrow-bladed stainless steel spatula may be used conveniently to spread the cement across this large area, thereby controlling the temperature of the mass and its setting time.

During the neutralization of the liquid by the powder, the temperature of the mixing site is inversely proportional to the time consumed in accomplishing the mix. Thus if a large volume of powder is carried to the liquid all at once rather than spatulated over a large area of the slab for a sufficient time, the temperature at the site of the reaction becomes higher. This temperature rise speeds the reaction and hinders control over the consistency. In this case the consistency of the mass is achieved by the rapid approach of the initial setting rather than by the establishment of a higher powder/liquid ratio under more ideal mixing conditions.

During the middle of the mixing period, larger amounts of powder may be incorporated to further saturate the liquid with the newly forming complex zinc phosphates. The quantity of unreacted acid is less at this time because of the prior neutralization gained from adding small increments of initial powder. The amount of heat liberated will likewise be less, and it can be dissipated adequately by the cooled slab.

Finally, smaller increments of powder again are incorporated, so that the desired ultimate consistency of the cement is not exceeded. Thus the mixing procedure begins and ends with small increments, first to achieve slow neutralization of the liquid with the attendant control of the reaction and last to gain a critical consistency.

Depending on the product, 60 to 90 seconds of mixing appears to be adequate to accomplish a proper zinc phosphate cementing mass. Because the setting time is measured from the beginning of the mix, continued spatulation of the cement merely extends this time. When the mixing time is unduly long, the cementing mass may be ultimately weakened by the breaking down of the matrix because it tends to form and bind the undissolved powder particles together.

Frozen slab method

The mixes used in the normal mixing procedure have adequate working and setting times for the cementation of inlays and crowns. However, in the cementation of orthodontic bands the short working time of normal mixes allows the cementation of only a few bands with one mix, and the setting times are too long for clinical convenience. The frozen slab method has been developed to overcome these difficulties. In this method a glass slab is cooled in a refrigerator at 6° C or a freezer at –10° C. No attempt is made to prevent moisture from condensing on the slab when it is brought to room conditions. Cement is mixed on the cold slab by adding the powder until the correct consistency is reached. The amount of powder incorporated with the frozen slab method is 50% to 75% more than with the normal procedures. The compressive and tensile strengths of cements prepared by the frozen slab method are not significantly different from those prepared from normal mixes, however, because incorporation of condensed moisture into the mix in the frozen slab method counteracts the higher powder/liquid ratio. No difference exists in the solubility of frozen slab and normal mixes.

The advantages of the frozen slab method are a substantial increase in the working time of the mix on the slab and a shorter setting time of the mix after placement into the mouth. Increases in working times of 4 and 11 minutes are not unusual for slab temperatures of 6° C and –10° C compared with the working time for a slab temperature of 23° C. Setting times of mixes prepared by the frozen slab method are shortened from 20% to 40% compared with those of normal mixes. This method has been advocated for cementation of bridges with multiple pins.

Characteristic Properties

ANSI/ADA Specification No. 96 for dental water-based cements

Zinc phosphate cements exhibit certain properties during their setting reaction and in their hardened state that determine the success with which they may be used. The more important of the properties are included in ANSI/ADA Specification No. 96 (ISO 9917) approved in 1994. A summary of these requirements is given in Table 8-2.

Selected properties of a typical zinc phosphate cement together with those of other luting materials are listed in Tables 8-3 and 8-4.

Consistency and film thickness

The desired consistency of the zinc phosphate cement mix depends on the particular purpose of

TABLE 8-2 Specification Requirements for Dental Water-Based Cements

Cement	Film Thickness, Maximum (μm)	Net Setting Time (min)	Compressive Strength (MPa)	Acid Erosion, Maximum (mm/hour)	Opacity, $C_{0.70}$	Acid-Soluble Arsenic Content (mg/kg)	Acid-Soluble Lead Content (mg/kg)
Glass ionomer (luting)	25	2.5-8.0	70	0.05	—	2	100
Zinc phosphate (luting)	25	2.5-8.0	70	0.1	—	2	100
Zinc polycarboxylate (luting)	25	2.5-8.0	70	2.0	—	2	100
Glass ionomer (base/liner)	—	2.5-6.0	70	0.05	—	2	100
Zinc phosphate (base/liner)	—	2.5-6.0	70	0.1	—	2	100
Zinc polycarboxylate (base/liner)	—	2.5-6.0	70	2.0	—	2	100
Glass ionomer (restorative)	—	2.5-6.0	130	0.05	0.35-0.90	2	100

Modified from ANSI/ADA Specification No. 96 for dental water-based cements.

TABLE 8-3   Mechanical Properties of Luting Cements

	Compressive Strength (MPa)	Tensile Strength (MPa)	Elastic Modulus (GPa)	Bond Strength to Dentin (MPa)
CEMENTS FOR FINAL CEMENTATION				
Adhesive resin	52-224	37-41	1.2-10.7	11-24 with bonding agent
Composite resin	180-265	34-37	4.4-6.5	18-30 with bonding agent
Glass ionomer	93-226	4.2-5.3	3.5-6.4	3-5
Hybrid ionomer	85-126	13-24	2.5-7.8	10-12 without bonding agent, 14-20 with bonding agent
Zinc oxide–eugenol (Type II)				
EBA-alumina	64	6.9	5.4	0
Polymer-modified	37	3.8	2.7	0
Zinc phosphate	96-133	3.1-4.5	9.3-13.4	0
Zinc polyacrylate	57-99	3.6-6.3	4.0-4.7	2.1
CEMENTS FOR TEMPORARY CEMENTATION				
Non-eugenol–zinc oxide	2.7-4.8	0.39-0.94	–	0
Composite resin	25-70	–	–	0
Zinc oxide–eugenol unmodified (Type I)	2.0-14	0.32-2.1	0.22	0

TABLE 8-4   Physical Properties of Luting Cements

Cements	Solubility in H_2O (% in 24 hr)	Setting Time at 37° C (100% Humidity) (min)	Film Thickness (μm)
Composite resin	0.13	4-5	13-20
Glass ionomer	0.4-1.5	6-8	22-24
Hybrid ionomer	0.07-0.40	5.5-6.0	10-22
Zinc oxide–eugenol			
Polymer-modified	0.08	9	25
EBA-alumina	0.02-0.04	7-9	25-35
Zinc polyacrylate	<0.05	7-9	25-48
Zinc phosphate	0.2 maximum	5-9	25 maximum

the material and the working convenience needed as expressed by the setting time. Two arbitrary consistencies, termed *inlay seating,* or luting, and *cement base,* or filling, are in general use. A third consistency of zinc phosphate cement, which lies midway between the inlay seating and the cement base, is used for the retention of orthodontic bands and has been termed a *band-seating consistency.*

The inlay-seating consistency of zinc phosphate cement is used to retain restorations. Although the unhardened zinc phosphate cement is somewhat tenacious, the retaining action in its hardened state is one of mechanical interlocking between the surface irregularities of the tooth and the restoration. This interlocking is illustrated in the photomicrograph of the interface of a gold casting and the opposing dentin and enamel wall shown in Fig. 8-1. The gold casting and the dentin are separated slightly and mechanically locked by cement.

The film thickness of the zinc phosphate cement greatly determines the adaptation of the casting to the tooth. The strength of the retention bond may

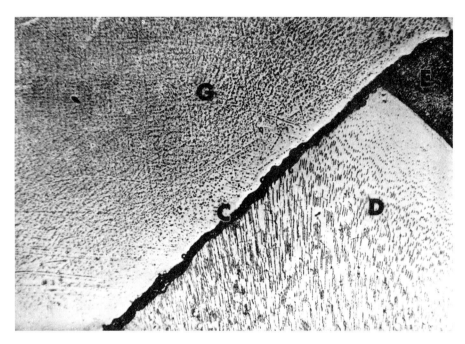

Fig. 8-1 Cement film between gold inlay and tooth. *G,* Gold inlay; *C,* cement; *D,* dentin; *E,* enamel.

also be influenced by the film thickness. ANSI/ADA Specification No. 96 has requirements for cements designed for the seating of precision appliances. The maximum film thickness is 25 μm. The heavier the consistency, the greater the film thickness, as shown in Fig. 8-2, and the less complete the seating of the restoration. The ultimate film thickness that a well-mixed, nongranular cement attains depends on, first, the particle size of the powder and, second, the concentration of the powder in the liquid, or the consistency of the cement. The film thickness also varies with the amount of force and the manner in which this force is applied to a casting during the cementation. The type of restoration being cemented influences the ease of escapement of the cement from around the margins of the restoration. A full crown casting apparently presents the greatest problem in obtaining maximum displacement of the cement.

Obviously the consistency of the zinc phosphate cement to be used in the cementation of a casting is critical. An increased amount of powder incorporated into the liquid will increase the consistency of the cement mass. The diameter of a disk formed when a total weight of 1.2 N is placed on a 0.5 ml volume of freshly mixed cement, as shown in Fig. 8-3, illustrates

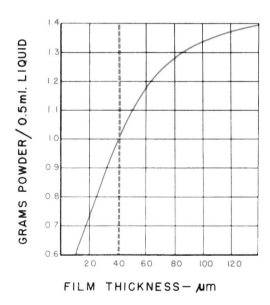

Fig. 8-2 Relation of powder/liquid ratio to film thickness.

the change in consistency caused by variations in the powder/liquid ratio. The heavier-than-normal inlay-seating consistencies of cement are more difficult to express from under a casting, and incomplete seating of the inlay or crown may result from their

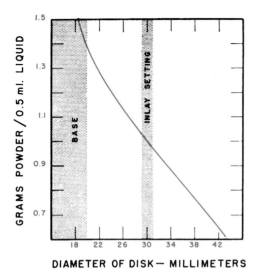

Fig. 8-3 Influence of powder/liquid ratio on consistency.

use. Although the approximate powder/liquid ratio, the manner of mixing, and the mixing time are guides to obtaining proper consistency, the operator must frequently test each mass as the end of the mixing time is approached. The final consistency will be fluid, yet the cement will string up from the slab on the spatula about 2 to 3 cm as the spatula is lifted away from the mass.

A heavy, puttylike consistency of zinc phosphate cement is used both as a thermal and chemical insulating barrier over thin dentin and as a high-strength base. This same consistency may also serve as a fairly durable temporary filling material. As such, the cement is exposed to dissolution in saliva, abrasion of mastication, and other oral conditions for an extended period of time. The cement base or filling consistency is achieved when using a powder/liquid ratio higher than that used for the inlay-seating or band-seating consistency, as shown in Fig. 8-3. Although the manner of mixing the cement base consistency is similar to the procedures already described, the greater quantity of powder to be incorporated may require slightly longer than the usual 90 seconds.

Viscosity

The consistency of cements can be quantified by measurement of the viscosity. The initial viscosity of mixes of zinc phosphate cements of inlay consis-

tency is shown in Fig. 8-4 for mixes made at 18°, 20°, and 25° C. A small but significant increase in viscosity is seen at the higher temperatures. The viscosities of the mixes 2 minutes after reaching the completion of mixing are also shown. In all instances pronounced increases in viscosity occurred during this time interval, with greater increases at the higher temperatures. Values for mixes of zinc polyacrylate cements are also listed. The rapid increase in viscosity demonstrates that restorations should be cemented promptly after completion of the mixing to take advantage of the lower viscosity of the cement. Delays in cementation can result in considerably larger film thicknesses and insufficient seating of the restoration.

Setting time

Of equal importance to the consistency of the cement is its setting time. A sufficient period of time must be available after the mixing to seat and finally adapt the margins of a casting, to seat and adjust a series of orthodontic bands, or to properly contour a base or temporary restoration. Adequate working time is expressed by proper net setting time, which, as determined by ANSI/ADA Specification No. 96 and based on an inlay-setting consistency, is between 2.5 and 8 minutes at a body temperature of 37° C. The first 60 to 90 seconds are consumed by the mixing of the powder and liquid, so the net setting time is the time elapsed between the end of mixing and the time of setting as measured by resistance to a standard indentor. The setting time at mouth temperature of one brand of zinc phosphate cement, as the powder/liquid ratio is increased, is shown in Fig. 8-5.

The setting time for the band-seating or cement base consistency is only slightly shorter because of the greater quantity of powder used to establish the heavier consistency.

Several factors influence the rate of set of the zinc phosphate cement. Those factors under the control of the manufacturer and the operator are listed in Tables 8-5 and 8-6. Although the manufacturer initially adjusts the setting time, improper handling of the powder and liquid can greatly modify the setting time. Anything that tends to speed the rate of reaction will shorten the setting time.

Effect of powder/liquid ratio. When a greater surface area of powder is allowed to react

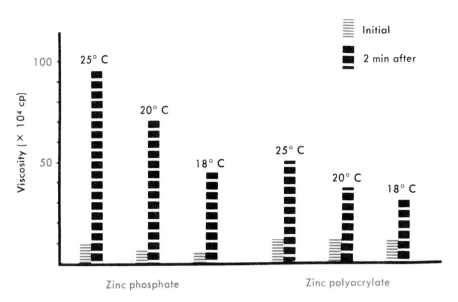

Fig. 8-4 Viscosity of zinc phosphate and zinc polyacrylate cements as a function of temperature and time. (Modified from Vermilyea SG, Powers JM, Craig RG: *J Dent Res* 56:762, 1977.)

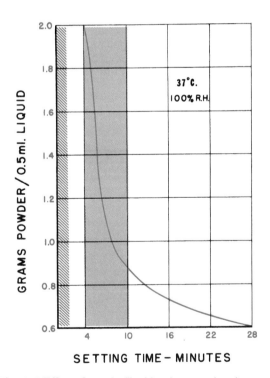

Fig. 8-5 Effect of powder/liquid ratio on setting time.

TABLE 8-5   Factors Governing the Rate of Set of Zinc Phosphate Cement

Controlled by Manufacturer	Controlled by Operator
Powder composition	Powder/liquid ratio
Degree of powder calcination	Rate of powder incorporation
Particle size of powder	Mixing temperature
Buffering of liquid	Manner of spatulation
Water content of liquid	Water contamination or loss from liquid

with the liquid, the reaction will terminate more readily when all other factors are constant. This effect can be obtained by using a smaller particle size, a more rapid rate of incorporation of the powder, and a higher powder/liquid ratio. The last two of these factors are under the control of the operator.

Temperature of the mixing slab. Because an increase in temperature accelerates a chemical reaction, the rise in temperature of the mass of cement during manipulation tends to cause the cement to set more rapidly. Failure to mix on a cooled slab, incorporation of relatively large initial amounts of powder, and failure to distribute the partially mixed cement over a wide area of the slab to dissipate the evolved heat will all shorten the setting time.

TABLE 8-6   Effects of Manipulative Variables on Selected Properties of Zinc Phosphate Cement

Manipulative Variables	Property				
	Compressive Strength	Film Thickness	Solubility	Initial Acidity	Setting Time
Decreased powder/liquid ratio	Decrease	Decrease	Increase	Increase	Lengthen
Increased rate of powder incorporation	Decrease	Increase	Increase	Increase	Shorten
Increased mixing temperature	Decrease	Increase	Increase	Increase	Shorten
Water contamination	Decrease	Increase	Increase	Increase	Shorten

From Craig RG, O'Brien WJ, Powers JM: *Dental materials: properties and manipulation,* ed 6, St Louis, 1996. Mosby.
*Water contamination should not be confused with water incorporated in the frozen slab method.

Water content of the mix. As pointed out in the previous discussion on liquid dilution, the addition of water to the liquid shortens the setting time and a concentration of the liquid prolongs the setting time. Although phosphoric acid is very soluble, it is a weak acid. If the acid is diluted, increased dissociation results. The greater dissociation provides a better chance for the acid to react with other materials.

Strength

The strength of the zinc phosphate cement is influenced by the initial powder and liquid composition, the powder/liquid ratio and manner of mixing, and the handling of the cement during its placement.

ANSI/ADA Specification No. 96 stipulates that a standard inlay-seating consistency must exhibit a minimum 24-hour compressive strength of 70 MPa. Thus any certified cement, when properly manipulated, will possess sufficient strength for the intended purpose. The crushing strength of the zinc phosphate cement develops rapidly, with the inlay-seating consistency reaching at least two-thirds of its final strength within 1 hour.

A proper mixing technic ensures a greater powder/liquid ratio for the consistency of cement desired, and this increases the compressive strength of the cement mass. A cement base consistency, when properly achieved, offers a greater resistance to crushing than the inlay-seating consistency does. A powder/liquid ratio is reached, however, when further amounts of powder do not increase the strength but may in fact decrease it because of the presence of excess unattacked powder. For this reason a mass of mixed cement should evenly incorporate the powder throughout the mix.

Solubility and disintegration

The premature contact of the incompletely set cement with water results in the dissolution and leaching of that surface. For this reason the use of the term *hydraulic* to describe any of the zinc phosphate cements is improper because they do not harden or set with desirable physical properties when submerged in water.

Prolonged contact, even of the well-hardened cement, with moisture demonstrates that some erosion and extraction of soluble material does occur from the cement. ANSI/ADA Specification No. 96 allows a maximum rate of erosion of 0.1 mm/hour when the cement is subjected to lactic acid erosion by an impinging jet technique. Even the filling cement mixes with heavier consistencies achieved by using higher powder/liquid ratios show considerable loss of material in the mouth over a period of time. Although this loss unquestionably results from a combination of other factors with the solubility and disintegration of the cement, it indicates that zinc phosphate cement can be regarded only as a temporary filling material. Wear, abrasion, and attack of food decomposition products accelerate the disintegration of the zinc phosphate cements within the oral cavity. Greater resistance to solution and disintegration is obtained by increasing the powder/liquid ratio. A thicker mix of cement therefore exhibits less solubility and disintegration than a thinner mix does.

The difference between the resistance to abrasive and chemical attack intraorally and the passive resistance to solution and disintegration in distilled water causes a different clinical observation between zinc phosphate and other cements. This lack of correlation has been demonstrated in a clinical study in which the order of solubility of cements tested in the mouth was, from least to most soluble, glass ionomer, zinc phosphate, ZOE reinforced with ethoxybenzoic acid, and polyacrylate cements. Laboratory tests in distilled water indicate that the glass ionomer cements would be the most soluble, and that the polyacrylate, ZOE, and zinc phosphate cements would be the least soluble.

ANSI/ADA Specification No. 96 specifies the maximum acid-soluble arsenic and lead contents as 2 and 100 mg/kg, respectively.

Dimensional stability

Zinc phosphate cement exhibits shrinkage on hardening. The normal dimensional change that occurs when a properly mixed cement is brought into contact with water after it has set is that of slight initial expansion, apparently from water absorption. This expansion is then followed by a slight shrinkage of 0.04% to 0.06% in 7 days as measured by a dental interferometer.

Acidity

During the formation of zinc phosphate cement, the union of the zinc oxide powder with the phosphoric acid liquid is accompanied by a change in pH as shown in Fig. 8-6. In the early manipulative stage this increase in pH is relatively rapid, with a standard mix reaching a pH of 4.2 within 3 minutes after mixing is started. At the end of 1 hour this value increases to about 6 and is nearly neutral at 48 hours.

Investigation and observation have shown that the initial acidity of the zinc phosphate cement at the time of placement into a tooth may excite a pulpal response, especially where only a thin layer of dentin exists between the cement and the pulp. In a normal, healthy tooth this response may be entirely reversible,

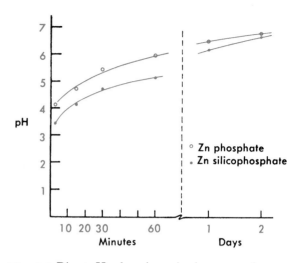

Fig. 8-6 Direct pH values determined on external surface of cements stored in humidor. Note: Zinc silicophosphate cements are no longer used commonly. (Adapted from Norman RD, Swartz ML, Phillips RW: *J Dent Res* 45:136, 1966.)

whereas in a tooth whose pulp has already been put under stress from other trauma the response may be irreversible, with pulp death ensuing. When zinc phosphate cement is to be used, precaution should be exercised in the deep cavity to protect the nearby pulp tissue from further trauma by the initial acidity of the cement. Such precautions include the use of resinous film-forming cavity varnishes, calcium hydroxide and zinc oxide suspensions, ZOE or calcium hydroxide bases, and, more recently, dentin bonding agents.

Gross decalcifications occasionally observed after the removal of orthodontic bands that have been retained in place with zinc phosphate cement are most probably attributable to the loss of the luting material between the band and the tooth, which resulted in a favorable environment for bacterial action. Although some slight decalcification might likely occur from the initial acidity of a standard cementing consistency, and especially with very thin consistencies developed from low powder/liquid ratios, proper manipulation of the cementing media appears to cause no changes of clinical significance.

Thermal and electrical conductivity

One of the primary uses of zinc phosphate cement is as an insulating base beneath metallic restorations. Recent studies have shown that as a base material this cement is an effective thermal insulator, although it is not more effective than dentin itself. Although the presence of moisture does not have a significant effect on the thermal conductivity of the cement, the moisture present under clinical conditions greatly reduces the potentially good electrical insulating properties of the material.

From the standpoint of good clinical practice, a zinc phosphate cement base is desirable to protect against thermal trauma to the pulp where a significant amount of dentin has been lost because of caries or trauma.

Applications

Zinc phosphate cement is used most commonly for luting permanent restorations and as a base. Other applications include cementation of orthodontic bands and the use of the cement as a temporary restoration.

Cementation of orthodontic bands

Zinc phosphate cement has been used for the cementation of orthodontic bands to the teeth for many years. The orthodontic consistency lies somewhere between the luting and base consistencies. Apparently the most important requirement is working time. Longer working times have been achieved by use of the frozen slab method.

■ ZINC OXIDE–EUGENOL AND NON-EUGENOL CEMENTS

When certain types of zinc oxide are mixed with eugenol, the mix sets to a hard cement that in suitable formulations is compatible with both the hard and soft tissues of the mouth. Cements of this type have been used extensively in dentistry since the 1890s. Simple mixtures of these two materials did not have great strength when compared with the zinc phosphate cements, and their use in dentistry was limited for many years to situations in which strength was not important. Quite early in their use it was found that they had a sedative effect on exposed dentin and that they made an excellent temporary restoration. For many years the cements were used as temporary restorations, as soft tissue packs in oral surgery and periodontics, and as root canal sealers.

TABLE 8-7   Formula for a Typical Zinc Oxide–Eugenol Temporary Filling Cement

Ingredients	Weight (%)
Powder	
Zinc oxide	69.0
White rosin	29.3
Zinc stearate	1.0
Zinc acetate	0.7
Liquid	
Eugenol	85.0
Olive oil	15.0

Adapted from Wallace DA, Hansen HL: *J Am Dent Assoc* 26:1536, 1933.

Recently, non-eugenol–zinc oxide cements for temporary cementation have become available. These cements are suitable for patients sensitive to eugenol.

Composition

A typical formula for a ZOE cement compounded as a temporary filling cement is shown in Table 8-7. The powder is mainly zinc oxide with the addition of white rosin to reduce the brittleness of the set cement, zinc stearate as a plasticizer, and zinc acetate to improve the strength of the cement. The liquid is eugenol with olive oil as a plasticizer. Two compositional changes have been used to increase the strength of the cement for luting purposes. In one, methyl methacrylate polymer is added to the powder, and in the other, alumina (Al_2O_3) is added to the powder and ethoxybenzoic acid (EBA) is added to the liquid.

A typical polymer-reinforced cement has 80% zinc oxide and 20% poly(methyl methacrylate) in the powder and eugenol in the liquid. These cements are sufficiently strong for final cementation of fixed prostheses and are used also as cement bases and temporary restorations. A typical EBA-alumina–reinforced ZOE cement contains 70% zinc oxide and 30% alumina by weight in the powder. In some cases rosin and copolymers may be added to reduce the brittleness and film thickness and to improve the mixing qualities. The liquid of the EBA-alumina–reinforced cements contains 62.5% ortho-EBA by weight and 37.5% eugenol by weight.

The compressive strength of a typical EBA cement is shown in Table 8-3.

The non-eugenol–zinc oxide cements typically contain an aromatic oil and zinc oxide. Other ingredients may include olive oil, petroleum jelly, oleic acid, and beeswax.

Chemistry of Setting

The chemistry of setting of the ZOE cements is similar to that of the ZOE impression materials. The reaction is not measurably exothermic, and the presence of moisture is essential for setting to occur.

Manipulation

Dispensing

The unmodified ZOE and non-eugenol–zinc oxide cements are typically two-paste systems. Equal lengths of each paste are dispensed and mixed to a uniform color.

For some cements used for temporary cementation or for temporary restorations, powder is often incorporated into a dispensed amount of liquid until a suitable consistency is achieved for the operation at hand. The dentist makes this determination from experience. A considerable amount of powder can be incorporated into the liquid by heavy spatulation with a stiff spatula. In general, the more powder incorporated, the stronger the cement and the more viscous the mixed cement.

Those cements intended for final cementation of restorations carry manufacturers' directions and measuring devices that are important to use. Because of the deceptive flow qualities of these cements, adding powder until the operator feels the mix is of suitable consistency for cementing a restoration will lead to a cement deficient in powder and a lowered strength in the set cement. To those accustomed to the handling qualities of zinc phosphate cement as a luting medium, a correctly proportioned and mixed ZOE luting cement appears far too viscous.

Mixing procedures

Because the setting reaction is not significantly exothermic, a cooled mixing slab is not required. Usually a paper mixing pad with disposable sheets, which is available in a variety of types and sizes, is used. Frequently the manufacturer supplies a mixing pad with the cement. The use of a paper pad facili-

tates the cleanup procedures after cementation. However, there is no reason why a glass slab cannot be used. A glass slab is recommended for mixing the EBA-alumina–modified cements. There is no need to incorporate the powder in small increments, and usually the bulk of the powder is incorporated in the initial step, the mix is thoroughly spatulated, and then a series of smaller amounts is added until the mix is complete. A stiff-bladed steel spatula is the most effective type. The EBA-alumina–modified cement is dispensed according to the instructions, kneaded for 30 seconds, and then stropped for 60 seconds to develop a creamy consistency. Oil of orange can be used to clean eugenol cements from instruments.

Characteristic Properties

The variety of compositions of the ZOE cements and the many uses to which they are applied make it difficult to write a specification for these cements. Revised ANSI/ADA Specification No. 30 (ISO 3107) for dental zinc oxide–eugenol cements and zinc oxide–non-eugenol cements gives standards for temporary cements, permanent cements, filling materials and bases, and cavity liners. It sets requirements for the general characteristics of the powders, liquids, and pastes used in these cements and some specific requirements for the important physical properties of setting time, compressive strength, solubility, film thickness, and acid-soluble arsenic content where these are applicable. The limiting values established for these properties for each type of cement are shown in Table 8-8.

Film thickness

Film thickness is an important factor in the complete seating of restorations at the time of cementation. Some of the early ZOE cements had a greater film thickness than desirable, but the products on the market today are able to meet the requirement that the film thickness be not more than 25 µm as determined by the specification test. This requirement is not applied to cements used for purposes other than cementation.

Setting time

The importance of the setting time for cements has been discussed in the sections related to zinc

TABLE 8-8 Specification Requirements for Zinc Oxide–Eugenol and Zinc Oxide–Non-Eugenol Cements

Cement	Setting Time at 37° C (min)	Compressive Strength (24 hr) (MPa)	Maximum Solubility and Disintegration (24 hr) (%)	Maximum Film Thickness (μm)	Maximum Acid-Soluble Arsenic Content (mg/kg)
Type I. Temporary Cement					
Class 1. Powder-liquid	4-10	35 maximum	2.5	25	2
Class 2a. Paste-paste (eugenol)	4-10	35 maximum	2.5	25	2
Class 2b. Paste-paste (non-eugenol)	4-10	35 maximum	2.5	25	2
Class 3. Paste-paste (nonsetting)	–	–	–	25	2
Type II. Permanent cement					
Class 1. Powder-liquid	4-10	35 minimum	1.5	25	2
Type III. Filling materials and bases					
Class 1. Powder-liquid	2-10	25 minimum	1.5	–	2
Class 2. Paste-paste	2-10	25 minimum	1.5	–	2
Type IV. Cavity liners					
Class 1. Powder-liquid	4-10	5 minimum	1.5	–	2
Class 2. Paste-paste	4-10	5 minimum	1.5	–	2

Modified from Revised ANSI/ADA Specification No. 30 for dental zinc oxide–eugenol cements and zinc oxide–non-eugenol cements, 1990.

phosphate cements. Similar criteria apply to the ZOE cements. For all except two of the cements, a range of setting times from 4 to 10 minutes is required. For cements intended for filling materials and bases, the preference of some operators for a faster setting cement is recognized in the specification by extending the lower end of the range to 2 minutes.

Compressive strength

A maximum value of 35 MPa is required for cements intended for temporary cementing, and a minimum of 25 MPa is required for permanent cementing and for filling materials and bases. Lining materials are required to have a minimum compressive strength of 5 MPa. Clinical studies have shown that for temporary cementing of restorations a variety of cements with compressive strengths varying from 1.38 to 20.7 MPa is desirable. The strength of a cement for temporary cementing is selected in relation to the retentive characteristics of the restoration and the expected problems of removing the restoration when the time arrives. The value of 35 MPa would be a little high as a maximum value. For permanent cementation the strongest cement possible is preferable.

Most ZOE cements for permanent cementation have compressive strength values considerably higher than the 25 MPa required by the specification. The strength of the non-eugenol–zinc oxide cements is similar to that of the unmodified ZOE cements intended for temporary cementation. A comparison of the compressive strengths of several types of cements on the market is given in Table 8-3.

Solubility

The solubility of the cements is generally regarded as less critical for cements that are to be used as interim restorations or for temporary cementation than is the case for cements used for final cementation. This is reflected in the maximum specification values for solubility and disintegration in 24 hours. A maximum value of 2.5% is acceptable for interim cementing materials, but a value of 1.5% is required for the other cements. The test used is the amount of solubility and disintegration, measured by weight loss, that occurs in a disk of the cement immersed in distilled water for 24

hours. There is no close correlation between this test and the clinical behavior of these cements, and the test serves only to compare cements of known clinical acceptability with other products. It is a useful monitoring method for evaluating new products and for ensuring quality control of manufacturing processes.

Applications

A range of ZOE and modified ZOE cements are available that are suitable for many uses in restorative dentistry, and the practitioner should become familiar with each type and its application.

Base

The materials having a compressive strength of 5.5 to 39 MPa are used as a cement base, and the strength reaches a maximum in about 12 to 15 minutes. They are normally used under zinc phosphate cement, which acquires about three times the strength in the same time. The ZOE cements have the advantage that the thermal insulating properties of the cements are excellent and are approximately the same as those for human dentin. Bases are discussed later in this chapter.

Temporary cementation

The unmodified ZOE cements are used also as luting materials for temporary crowns and for temporary cementation of gold restorations in crown and bridge prosthodontics. Laboratory studies have shown that the retention of metal restorations with the unmodified cements is proportional to the compressive strength of the cements. The unmodified ZOE cements are available in a range of compressive strengths varying from 1.38 MPa to 20.7 MPa. A clinical study of the various unmodified cements for luting of temporary crowns indicated that a cement with a compressive strength of 15.2 to 24.1 MPa was the most appropriate cement on the basis of (1) retention, (2) taste, (3) ease of removal, and (4) ease of cleaning. Another clinical study indicated that an unmodified ZOE cement with a compressive strength of 6.9 MPa was the most frequently used material for the temporary cementation of complete crown and bridge restorations, though a range of cements with compressive strengths of from 1.38 to 20.7 MPa was found to be desirable.

The non-eugenol–zinc oxide cements do not adhere as well to preformed metal crowns as the eugenol-containing cements, and they are slower setting. The non-eugenol cements, however, do not soften temporary acrylic crowns.

Temporary restorations

The EBA-alumina–modified cements have been tried as temporary restorations based on their physical properties. Clinical studies showed that these cements were handled easily and had improved carvability, which prevented chipping during trimming, and that symptomatic teeth without pulp exposure showed no symptoms. The EBA-alumina–modified cements, despite their low solubility in water, disintegrated and wore excessively in the mouth. A thick mix, 2.6 g/0.4 ml of polymer-modified ZOE, was more serviceable than the EBA-alumina–modified type, and although some chipping was observed at the margins, all temporary restorations of ZOE were serviceable for 2 to 10 months of observation.

Permanent cementation

The use of EBA-alumina–modified ZOE cements has been clinically successful for the permanent cementation of crowns and bridges. The film thickness of these cements is therefore important, and as indicated in Table 8-4, a film thickness of 25 to 35 μm is readily obtained. Other properties are shown in Tables 8-3 and 8-4.

Endodontic sealers

Endondontic ZOE preparations have been used as a root canal sealer alone and with gutta-percha and silver points. There are two major groups of products based on ZOE cements—conventional and therapeutic sealers.

Composition and setting. The conventional sealers generally are based on the formulas of Grossman or Rickert as summarized in Table 8-9. The setting reaction occurs between zinc oxide and eugenol. Resins improve the mixing characteristics and retard setting. Radiopacity is improved by the addition of barium or bismuth salts, or silver powder. The conventional sealers are used with silver points or gutta-percha points.

The therapeutic sealers usually are used without a core material and are formulated with ingredients, such as iodoform, paraformaldehyde, or trioxymethylene, that may have therapeutic value. The use of these sealers is controversial.

ANSI/ADA Specification No. 57 (ISO 6876)

This specification covers sealer cements used with cores (Type I) and filling materials used without cores or sealer cements (Type II). The physical properties specified include working time, flow, film thickness, setting time, dimensional stability, solubility and disintegration, and radiopacity. A summary of these requirements is given in Table 8-10.

TABLE 8-9   Composition of Typical Zinc Oxide–Eugenol Endodontic Sealers

Rickert's Formula		Grossman's Formula		Therapeutic Formula
POWDER	%	**POWDER**	%	**POWDER**
Zinc oxide	41*	Zinc oxide	42	Zinc oxide
Silver	30	Staybelite resin	27	Bismuth subnitrate
White rosin	17	Bismuth subcarbonate	15	Iodoform
Thymol iodide	12	Barium sulfate	15	Rosin
		Sodium borate anhydrate	1	
LIQUID		**LIQUID**		**LIQUID**
Oil of cloves	78	Eugenol	100	Eugenol
Canada balsam	22			Creosote
				Thymol

*Percent by weight.

TABLE 8-10 Specification Requirements for Types II and III Endodontic Filling Materials

Working Time	Minimum Flow (mm)	Maximum Film Thickness (μm)	Setting Time	Maximum Linear Dimensional Change at 30 Days (%)	Maximum Solubility and Disintegration (%)	Minimum Radiopacity (mm of Aluminum)
±10% of manufacturer's claimed value	25	50	±10% of manufacturer's claimed value	1.0	3.0	3.0

Adapted from ANSI/ADA Specification No. 57 for endodontic sealing materials, 1993.

Viscosity. The ability of a sealer to penetrate into irregularities and accessory canals has been termed *flow,* though *viscosity* is a more correct term. Viscosity has been shown by several different tests to decrease during the mixing procedure (an example of shear thinning). Values of viscosity range from 8 to 680×103 cp (centipoise).

Setting time. The setting time of cements is measured by a penetration test and ranges from 15 minutes to 12 hours at mouth temperature. The sealers set much more rapidly at mouth temperature than at room temperature.

Film thickness. The film thickness, as measured by ANSI/ADA Specification No. 57, is influenced by viscosity, setting time, and the size of filler particles in the cement. Lower values of film thickness are considered desirable for condensation of gutta-percha. Values range from 80 to 500 μm depending on the testing load.

Compressive strength. The strength of a sealer is an indication of its ability to support tooth structure weakened by the cleaning of the canal and its durability. Values range from 8 to 50 MPa.

Solubility. The solubility of a root canal sealer is undesirable because dissolution can cause the sealer to release components that may be biologically incompatible. Solubility has been measured in water, and typically values range from 0.10% to 3.5%.

Radiopacity. Radiopacity is desirable, and a minimum value of the equivalent of 3 mm of aluminum has been established. Values of radiolucency range from 0.10 to 0.98 among various sealers. Values for a silver point and a gutta-percha point have been measured to be 0.34 and 0.78, respectively. These are relative values with lower numbers for more radiopaque materials.

Dimensional change. Most root canal sealers shrink as a result of setting. This shrinkage affects the integrity of the bond between the sealer and the tooth or core material. Values of volume loss after 90 days in a capillary tube range from –0.7% to –5.0%.

Biological properties. These properties have been studied by *in vivo* and *in vitro* tests such as behavior of HeLa cells, human skin fibroblasts, and bovine pulp tissue; endodontic fillings in dogs, monkeys, and rats; and implants in tibias and in subcutaneous connective tissues of animals. The conventional ZOE sealers generally elicit mild to moderate reactions, whereas several of the therapeutic sealers elicit severe reactions.

Tissue management

Another variation of the ZOE cements has been necessitated by the special requirements imposed in the management of the gingival tissues. This group of cements is used in two ways: (1) to mechanically displace soft tissue or (2) to dress soft tissues after surgery. When these cements are used as a mechanical tissue pack, a thin consistency is incorporated into cotton fibers that are placed into the gingival sulcus. As a surgical dressing, this preparation affords greater comfort to the patient during eating, obtunds the surgerized tissue, promotes epithelial growth, and helps prevent the overgrowth of granulation tissue.

The setting times of these ZOE surgical cements must be quite long to facilitate the mixing of rather large quantities and to permit the proper placement and contouring of the dressing. Usually no accelerator is added to these materials. On placement of the packs in the mouth, the moisture and increased temperature tend to hasten the setting reaction. When mixed to a proper consistency, the cement must be soft enough to permit placement and contouring with gentle pressure and yet be firm enough to maintain the desired form.

The formulations generally have greater quantities of mineral, peanut, or almond oil to increase the plasticity over that of the filling cements. Cotton fibers are often added to increase the strength and durability. In addition to the normal ingredients (zinc oxide, rosin, and eugenol), tannic acid is often added as a hemostatic agent and to decelerate the setting reaction. Aromatic oils and coloring agents may be incorporated to improve the taste and color of the dressing. Chlorhexadine has also been added as an antibacterial agent.

■ ZINC POLYACRYLATE CEMENT

Composition and Setting Reaction

The zinc polyacrylate cements (also referred to as zinc polycarboxylate) are supplied as a powder and a liquid or as a powder that is mixed with water.

The liquid is a water solution of polyacrylic acid, the formula being

$$-CH_2-CH-CH_2-CH-$$
$$\qquad\quad\;\; | \qquad\qquad |$$
$$\qquad\quad\; C{=}O \qquad\; C{=}O$$
$$\qquad\quad\;\; | \qquad\qquad |$$
$$\qquad\quad\;\; O \qquad\qquad O$$
$$\qquad\quad\;\; | \qquad\qquad |$$
$$\qquad\quad\;\; H \qquad\qquad H$$

Most commercial liquids are supplied as a 32% to 42% solution of polyacrylic acid, having a molecular weight of 25,000 to 50,000. The manufacturer controls the viscosity of the cement liquid by varying the molecular weight of the polymer or by adjusting the pH by adding sodium hydroxide. Itaconic and tartaric acids may be present to stabilize the liquid, which can gel on extended storage.

The cement powder is essentially zinc oxide and magnesium oxide that have been sintered and ground to reduce the reactivity of the zinc oxide. Some cement powders contain alumina, and experimental powders containing stainless steel fibers to improve strength have been studied. The cement powder that is mixed with water contains 15% to 18% polyacrylic acid coated on the oxide particles.

The set cement is a zinc polyacrylate ionic gel matrix that unites unreacted zinc oxide particles. The gel is bound to the polyanion chains by electrostatic interactions rather than by stronger specific ion binding. The matrix appears to be amorphous. The setting reaction can be retarded by a cool environment or accelerated by a warm environment.

Manipulation

The cements supplied with the polyacrylic acid in the liquid are usually mixed at a powder/liquid ratio of 1:1 to 2:1. One cement mixed with water has a powder/liquid ratio of 5:1 for cementation consistency. The consistency of the mixes is creamy compared with that of zinc phosphate cements. The mixed cement is thixotropic; that is, the viscosity decreases as the shear rate increases, or, in other terms, the flow increases as the spatulation increases or as force is placed on the material. The correct consistency is found in a mix that is viscous but that will flow back under its own weight when drawn up with a spatula.

Dispensing of the liquid should be done immediately before mixing to prevent evaporation of water and subsequent thickening. A nonabsorptive surface, such as a glass slab or treated paper, will keep all the liquid available for the reaction and facilitate spatulation. Polyacrylate cements should be mixed within 30 to 60 seconds, with half to all of the powder incorporated at once to provide the maximum length of working time (typically 2.5 to 6 minutes). The working time can be extended to 10 to 15 minutes by mixing on a glass slab chilled to 4° C. The strength of the mixed cement is not compromised by this technic. Some manufacturers supply the cement as a precapsulated powder-liquid system for mixing in a mechanical mixer.

The polyacrylate cements have been used to cement inlays and crowns and to make bases. The best results have been obtained when the material is applied to clean cavity walls that are well isolated in a dry field. The mixed cement should be used only as long as it still appears glossy on the surface. Once the surface becomes dull, the cement develops stringiness and the film thickness becomes too great to seat a casting completely.

Properties

ANSI/ADA Specification No. 96

This specification establishes maximum values of setting time, film thickness, acid erosion, arsenic and lead content, and a minimum value of compressive strength for zinc polyacrylate cement. A summary of these requirements is given in Table 8-2.

Viscosity

The effect of temperature on the initial viscosity of zinc polyacrylate cement and the viscosity 2 minutes after mixing is shown in Fig. 8-4. The initial viscosity was essentially unaffected by the temperature increase from 18° to 25° C, although the viscosity is higher than the initial viscosity for comparable mixes of zinc phosphate cement. The viscosity of zinc polyacrylate cement 2 minutes after mixing increased modestly at all three temperatures; however, the increases in viscosity were substantially less than those for comparable zinc phosphate cement mixes. Thus the initial viscosity of zinc polyacrylate cements is higher than zinc phosphate cements, and a delay of 2 minutes in cementation reverses the situation.

Setting time

The setting time test measures the time at which the cement is sufficiently hard to resist indentation by a standard indenter. The net setting time should occur within 2.5 to 8 minutes so that final finishing procedures associated with the restoration can occur. As shown in Table 8-4, setting of the zinc polyacrylate cements usually occurs within 7 to 9 minutes from the start of mixing.

Film thickness

The film thickness test excludes materials that might have excessively large powder particles or a short working time because complete seating of a casting with zinc polyacrylate cement might not occur. The film thickness of the polyacrylate cements is slightly higher than that of zinc phosphate cements but is well within clinical limits, as shown in Table 8-4.

Strength

The compressive strength test excludes materials that have a compressive strength of less than 70 MPa. Clinical studies have shown that cements of this strength or greater will retain satisfactorily castings with a good fit.

The 24-hour compressive strength of the polyacrylate cements for luting is lower than that of the zinc phosphate cements (98 to 133 MPa compared with 57 to 99 MPa); however, the tensile strength of the polyacrylate cements is about 40% higher than that of zinc phosphate cements. The higher tensile strength may be influenced by the test method. In the diametral compression test, the zinc polyacrylate cement specimens deform somewhat before breaking. The deformation results in a higher load before fracture is recorded than would occur if fracture occurred brittlely. The modulus of elasticity of the zinc polyacrylate cements is about one-third that of the zinc phosphate cements mixed to a luting consistency.

Bond strength

An interesting feature of polyacrylate cement is its bonding to enamel and dentin, which is attributed to the ability of the carboxylate groups in the polymer molecule to chelate to calcium. The bond strength to enamel has been reported to be from 3.4 to 13 MPa, and the bond strength to dentin has been found to be 2.1 MPa. Optimum bonding, however, requires cleaned tooth surfaces. The bonding of the polyacrylate cements to gold casting alloy

is likewise highly dependent on surface preparation. Sandblasting or electrolytic etching of the gold alloy surface is necessary to achieve optimum bonding. Clinical studies have not demonstrated improved retention of crowns and bridges as a result of cementation with polyacrylate cements, however.

Because of the adhesion of polyacrylate cements to enamel, the cements were used at one time for direct bonding of orthodontic brackets to teeth. Presently, direct bonding is accomplished with acrylic or composite resin cements.

Solubility and disintegration

The solubility and disintegration test excludes materials that are excessively soluble in distilled water. Solubility in distilled water does not always correlate with solubility *in vivo*. Solubility in water at 1 day varies from 0.12% to 0.25% for typical zinc polyacrylate cements. One cement tested increased in solubility from 0.25% at 1 day to 0.60% at 1 month in water. Other cements were not affected by longer-term storage. ANSI/ADA Specification No. 96 specifies the maximum rate of acid erosion of zinc polyacrylate cements as 2.0 mm/hour.

Dimensional stability

The zinc polyacrylate cements show a linear contraction when setting at 37° C. The amount of contraction varies from 1% for a wet specimen at 1 day to 6% for a dry specimen at 14 days. These contractions are more pronounced than those observed for zinc phosphate cements and start earlier.

Acidity

Zinc polyacrylate cements are slightly more acidic than zinc phosphate cements when first mixed, but the acid is only weakly dissociated, and penetration of the high molecular weight polymer molecules toward pulpal tissue is minimal. Histological reactions to polyacrylate cements appear to be similar to those of ZOE cements, although the production of reparative dentin under the polyacrylate cements is more evident.

Applications

Zinc polyacrylate cements are used primarily for luting permanent restorations and as bases. These cements have also been used in orthodontics for cementation of bands and at one time for direct bonding of brackets and in endodontics as a root canal filling material.

GLASS IONOMER CEMENT

Composition and Setting Reaction

The glass ionomer cements are supplied as a powder and a liquid or as a powder that is mixed with water. Several products are encapsulated. The liquid typically is a 47.5% solution of 2:1 polyacrylic acid/itaconic acid copolymer (average molecular weight 10,000) in water. The itaconic acid reduces the viscosity of the liquid and inhibits gelation caused by intermolecular hydrogen bonding; D(+) tartaric acid (5%, the optically active isomer) in the liquid serves as an accelerator by facilitating the extraction of ions from the glass powder.

The powder of a glass ionomer cement is a calcium fluoroaluminosilicate glass with a formula of

$$SiO_2 - Al_2O_3 - CaF_2 - Na_3AlF_6 - AlPO_4$$

The nominal composition of the glass is listed in Table 8-11. The maximum grain size of the powder appears to be between 13 and 19 μm. The powder is described as an ion-leachable glass that is susceptible to acid attack when the Si/Al atomic ratio is less than 2:1. Barium glass or zinc oxide may be added to some powders to provide radiopacity.

In some products the polyacrylic acid is formulated in the powder. The liquids of these products may be water or a dilute solution of tartaric acid in water. The setting reaction is an acid-base reaction between the acidic polyelectrolyte and the aluminosilicate glass as diagrammed below.

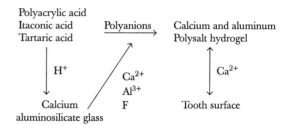

The polyacid attacks the glass to release cations and fluoride ions. These ions, probably as metal fluoride complexes, react with the polyanions to form a salt gel matrix. The Al^{3+} ions appear to be site bound, resulting in a matrix resistant to flow unlike the zinc polyacrylate matrix. During the initial setting reaction in the first 3 hours, calcium ions react with the polycarboxylate chains. Subsequently, the trivalent aluminum ions react for at least 48 hours. Between 20% and 30% of the glass is decomposed by the proton attack. The fluoride and phosphate ions form insoluble salts and complexes. The sodium ions form a silica gel. The structure of the fully set cement is a composite of glass particles surrounded by silica gel in a matrix of polyanions crosslinked by ionic bridges. Within the matrix are small particles of silica gel containing fluorite crystallites.

The glass ionomer cements chemically bond to enamel and dentin during the setting process. The mechanism of bonding appears to involve an ionic interaction with calcium and/or phosphate ions from the surface of the enamel or dentin. Bonding is more effective with a cleaned surface provided that the cleansing process does not remove an excessive amount of calcium ions. Treatment of dentin with a dilute solution of ferric chloride preceded by an acidic cleaner improves the bonding. The cleansing agent removes the smeared layer of dentin while the Fe^{3+} ions are deposited and increase the ionic interaction between the cement and dentin.

Manipulation

The cements mixed with the more viscous carboxylic acid liquids have a powder/liquid ratio of 1.3:1 to 1.35:1, whereas those mixed with water or a liquid with a consistency like that of water have a

TABLE 8-11 Nominal Composition of Calcium Fluoroaluminosilicate Glass Used in Powder of Glass Ionomer Cement

Chemical	Percent by Weight
SiO_2	29.0
Al_2O_3	16.6
CaF_2	34.3
Na_3AlF_6	5.0
AlF_3	5.3
$AlPO_4$	9.8

Adapted from Prosser HJ, Richards CP, Wilson AD: *J Biomed Mater Res* 16:431, 1982.

powder/liquid ratio of 3.3:1 to 3.4:1. The powder and liquid are dispensed onto a paper or glass slab, and the powder is divided into two equal portions. The first portion is incorporated into the liquid with a stiff spatula before the second portion is added. The mixing time is 30 to 60 seconds. Encapsulated products typically are mixed for 10 seconds in a mechanical mixer and dispensed directly onto the tooth and restoration. The cement must be used immediately because the working time after mixing is about 2 minutes at room temperature (23° C). An extension of the working time to 9 minutes can be achieved by mixing on a cold slab (3° C), but a reduction in compressive strength and in the modulus of elasticity is observed; thus the technic is not recommended. The cement should not be used once a "skin" forms on the surface or when the viscosity increases noticeably.

The glass ionomer cements are very sensitive to contact with water during setting. The field must be isolated completely. Once the cement has achieved its initial set (about 7 minutes), the cement margins should be coated with the coating agent supplied with the cement.

Properties

Requirements of ANSI/ADA Specification No. 96 approved in 1994 are given in Table 8-2.

Film thickness

The film thickness of the glass ionomer cements is similar to or less than that of zinc phosphate cement (see Table 8-4) and is suitable for cementation.

Setting time

The glass ionomer cements set within 6 to 8 minutes from the start of mixing. The setting can be slowed when the cement is mixed on a cold slab, but this technic has an adverse effect on the strength.

Strength

The 24-hour compressive strength of the glass ionomer cements ranges from 90 to 230 MPa and is greater than that of zinc phosphate cement. Values of tensile strength are similar to those of zinc phosphate cement. Unlike the zinc polyacrylate cements, the glass ionomer cements demonstrate brittle failure in the diametral compression test. The elastic modulus

of the glass ionomer cements is less than that of zinc phosphate cement, but more than that of zinc polyacrylate cement. The rigidity of the glass ionomer cement is improved by the glass particles and the ionic nature of the bonding between polymer chains.

The compressive strength of the glass ionomer cements increases between 24 hours and 1 year, unlike that of zinc polyacrylate cement. A glass ionomer cement formulated as a filling material showed an increase from 160 to 280 MPa over this period. The strength of the glass ionomer cements improves more rapidly when the cement is isolated from moisture during its early life.

Bond strength

The glass ionomer cements bond to dentin with values of tensile bond strength reported between 1 and 3 MPa. The bond strength of the glass ionomer cements to dentin is somewhat lower than that of zinc polyacrylate cements, perhaps because of the sensitivity of the glass ionomer cements to moisture during setting. The bond strength has been improved by treatment of the dentin with an acidic cleaning agent followed by an application of a dilute aqueous solution of $FeCl_3$. The glass ionomer cements bond well to enamel, stainless steel, tin oxide-plated platinum, and gold alloy.

Solubility and disintegration

Values of solubility and disintegration of the glass ionomer cements as measured in water by an ADA test are substantially higher than those measured for other cements (see Table 8-4). However, when these cements are tested in acid (0.001 N lactic acid), the values are quite low compared with values for zinc phosphate and zinc polyacrylate cements. The rankings determined by solubility and disintegration tests in acid correlate well with clinical evaluations.

ANSI/ADA Specification No. 96 specifies the maximum acid erosion rate as 0.05 mm/hour. This specification also sets limits on the acid-soluble arsenic content and lead content (Table 8-2).

Biological properties

Biological evaluations of the glass ionomer cements have been done by tissue culture and animal tests. The culture cells showed a weaker reaction to glass ionomer cement than to ZOE or zinc polyacrylate cements. Pulp tissue reactions of monkeys tested *in vivo* showed no difference between glass ionomer and ZOE cements. These reactions have been described as mild.

Glass ionomer luting cements may cause prolonged hypersensitivity, varying from mild to severe. Microleakage has been suggested as an explanation, but a recent study showed no increase in bacterial counts 56 days after cementation of crowns with a glass ionomer cement. These cements may be bacteriostatic or bactericidal, however, because of fluoride release. Good isolation appears to be essential when glass ionomer cements are used. The use of the proper powder/liquid ratio and the application of a calcium hydroxide base in areas closest to the pulp are recommended.

Applications

The glass ionomer cements are used primarily for permanent cement, as a base, and as a class 5 filling material (see Chapter 10). The cement has been evaluated as a pit and fissure sealant and as an endodontic sealer. The sensitivity of the cement to moisture and desiccation may minimize its use in these latter applications. Glass ionomer cements are being used clinically for cementation of orthodontic bands because of their ability to minimize decalcification of enamel during orthodontic treatment.

■ HYBRID IONOMER CEMENT

Both self- and light-cured hybrid ionomers (also called resin-modified glass ionomers) have been introduced recently for cementation. The hybrid ionomer restorative materials are described in Chapter 10.

Composition

One self-cured cement powder contains a radiopaque, fluoroaluminosilicate glass and a microencapsulated potassium persulfate and ascorbic acid catalyst system. The liquid is an aqueous solution of polycarboxylic acid modified with pendant methacrylate groups. It also contains 2-hydroxyethylmethacrylate (HEMA) and tartaric acid. Another self-cured cement contains a mixture of fluoroaluminosilicate and borosilicate glasses in the powder. Its liquid is a complex monomer con-

taining carboxylic acid groups that can undergo an acid-base reaction with glass and vinyl groups that can polymerize when chemically activated. A light-cured cement contains fluoroaluminosilicate glass in the powder and a copolymer of acrylic and maleic acids, HEMA, water, camphoroquinone, and an activator in the liquid.

Chemistry of Setting

Curing results from an acid-base glass ionomer reaction and self-cured or light-cured polymerization of the pendant methacrylate groups.

Manipulation

The powder is fluffed before dispensing. The liquid is dispensed by keeping the vial vertical to the mixing pad. For one product, the powder/liquid ratio is 1.6 g of powder to 1.0 g of liquid, and the powder is incorporated into the liquid within 30 seconds to give a mousselike consistency. The working time is 2.5 minutes. The cement is applied to a clean, dry tooth that is not desiccated. Some products recommend the use of a conditioner or bonding agent for enhanced bonding to dentin. No coating agent is needed. HEMA is a known contact allergen; therefore, use of protective gloves and a no-touch technique are recommended.

Characteristic Properties

The compressive and tensile strengths of a hybrid ionomer cement are similar to those of glass ionomer cements (see Table 8-3). The fracture toughness is higher than that of other water-based cements but lower than resin cements. The bond strength to moist dentin ranges from 10 to 14 MPa without a bonding agent, up to 20 MPa with a bonding agent and is much higher than that of most water-based cements. The hybrid ionomer cements have very low solubility when tested by lactic acid erosion. Fluoride release is similar to the glass ionomer cements. The early pH is about 3.5 and gradually rises. Field testing indicates minimal postoperative sensitivity.

Applications

The self-cured cements are indicated for permanent cementation of porcelain-fused-to-metal crowns; bridges; metal inlays, onlays, and crowns;

post cementation; and luting of orthodontic appliances. Additional uses include adhesive liner for amalgam, base, interim restoration, and cementation of porcelain restorations. Several products currently are not recommended for composite or all-porcelain inlays or crowns because of their shade. One light-cured hybrid ionomer cement is recommended for direct-bonding of orthodontic brackets.

■ RESIN, COMPOSITE, AND ADHESIVE RESIN CEMENTS

Cements based on acrylic or composite resins have been used for cementation of crowns, conventional bridges, and resin-bonded bridges; for bonding of esthetic ceramic and composite restorations to teeth; and for direct bonding of orthodontic brackets to acid-etched enamel. Recently, composite cements have been developed for cementation of temporary restorations.

Cementation of Crowns, Conventional Bridges, Resin-Bonded Bridges, and Temporary Restorations

Synthetic resin cements based on methyl methacrylate have been available since 1952 for cementation of inlays, crowns, and appliances. In the early 1970s a composite resin was introduced as a crown and bridge cement. Since 1986 resin cements have gained in popularity because of their use in the cementation of resin-bonded bridges and now esthetic restorations.

Composition and setting

The early resin cements were primarily poly(methyl methacrylate) powder with various inorganic fillers and methyl methacrylate liquid. Setting was caused by a peroxide initiator–amine accelerator system.

The self-cured composite cements are typically powder/liquid or two-paste systems. One major component is a diacrylate oligomer diluted with lower molecular weight dimethacrylate monomers. The other major component is silanated silica or glass. The initiator-accelerator system is peroxide-amine.

The adhesive resin cements are self-cured, powder-liquid systems formulated with methacryloxyethyl-phenyl phosphate or 4-methacryloxyethyl-trimellitic anhydride (4-META). The phosphonate cement, recently reformulated as a two-paste system, contains Bis-GMA resin and silanated quartz filler. The phosphonate is very sensitive to oxygen, so a gel is provided to coat the margins of a restoration until setting has occurred. The phosphate end of the phosphonate reacts with calcium of the tooth or with a metal oxide. The 4-META cement is formulated with methyl methacrylate monomer and acrylic resin filler and is catalyzed by tri-butyl-borane. The double-bonded ends of both phosphonate and 4-META cements react with other double bonds when available.

Properties

Some properties of composite and adhesive resin cements are listed in Tables 8-3 and 8-4. A comparison of bond strengths of the adhesive and conventional resin-bonded bridge cements is given in Table 8-12. The adhesive resin cements have superior bonding to sandblasted Ni-Cr-Be and Type IV gold alloys. The composite resin cements used for cementation of temporary restorations (25–70 MPa) have

TABLE 8-12   Bond Strengths of Adhesive and Conventional Resin-Bonded Bridge Cements to Various Substrates

Substrate	Bond Strength in Tension, MPa	
	Adhesive Resin Cement	Conventional Resin Cement
Dentin (unetched)	4.1	0.0
Enamel (etched)	15.0	10.0
Ni-Cr-Be alloy		
Sandblasted	24.0	14.1
Electrolytically etched	27.4	25.2
Type IV gold alloy		
Sandblasted	22.0	9.4
Tin-plated	25.5	12.8

From Powers JM, Watanabe F, Lorey RE: *In vitro* evaluation of prosthodontic adhesives. In Gettleman L, Vrijhoef MMA, Uchiyama Y: *Adhesive prosthodontics—adhesive cements and techniques,* Nijmegen, 1986, Academy of Dental Materials; and Watanabe F, Powers JM, Lorey RE: *In vitro* bonding of prosthodontic adhesives to dental alloys, *J Dent Res* 67:479, 1988.

a substantially lower compressive strength than the composite resin cements for permanent cementation (180–265 MPa).

Applications

The adhesive resin cements and composite resin cements in conjunction with dentin bonding agents (many of which are now called all-surface bonding agents) are being used as cements for posts and cores. Bond strengths of 14 MPa have been reported for silica-treated posts cemented with 4-META resin cement in extracted teeth. The use of resin-bonded bridges declined dramatically in the late 1980s.

Bonding of Esthetic Restorations

The bonding (cementation) of all-ceramic crowns, porcelain veneers, and tooth-colored inlays and onlays became popular in the late 1980s. Dual-cured composite resin cements are ideal for bonding cast or computer-aided design/computer-aided machining (CAD/CAM)–prepared ceramic restorations or composite inlays prepared by an indirect technic. Light-cured composite resin cements are useful for bonding thin porcelain veneers where achieving adequate depth of cure is not a problem.

Composition

The composite resin cements are microfilled or small-particle hybrid composites formulated primarily from Bis-GMA or urethane dimethacrylate resins and fumed silica or glass fillers (20% to 75% by weight) or both. The dual-cured cements come in a base-catalyst form and must be mixed before use. They are radiopaque for use in the posterior portion of the mouth. The light-cured composites are photoinitiated in the presence of a camphoroquinone-amine system. They are usually not radiopaque but provide a wide selection of shades, tints, and opaquers.

Manipulation

A dentin bonding agent is used to enhance bonding of the resin cement to tooth structure, whereas various surface preparations (sandblasting) and treatments (silanation or chemical softening) are used to prepare the ceramic or composite restorations for bonding. The ability of composite resin cements to bond well to post-cured composite inlays is currently under study.

Properties

Compressive strengths of the dual- and light-cured composite cements of from 180 to 265 MPa have been reported (see Table 8-3). Viscosity has been measured subjectively to range from low to high. Film thicknesses on vented crowns range from 13 to 20 μm.

Resin-Metal Bonding

Bonding composite to the metal framework of a bridge and denture acrylic to a partial denture framework can be improved by the use of silica coatings. Presently there are three processes for applying silica to either noble or base metal alloys. The most established method applies pyrogenic silica using a propane flame. Other methods use heat in an oven or ceramic blasting to coat the restoration or appliance. Bond strengths of composites to silica-coated Au-Pd or Ni-Cr-Be alloys range from 16 to 22 MPa. Silica coating of noble alloys may eliminate the need for tin plating of these alloys to improve adhesion of composites. The bond strength of denture acrylics to Ni-Cr-Be alloys range from 7 to 23 MPa when the alloy is treated with a silica coating or primed with an adhesive resin cement.

Bonding of Orthodontic Brackets

Resin cements were evaluated for direct bonding of orthodontic brackets (without bands) in the late 1960s. Advances in acid etching of enamel substantially increased the popularity of the technic in the mid-1970s. There are two major groups of resin cements—the unfilled acrylics and the composite cements. These cements are used with metal, plastic, or ceramic orthodontic brackets.

Composition and setting

The unfilled acrylic cements are monomer-polymer formulations based on methyl methacrylate and comonomers. The accelerator-initiator system typically is an amine and a peroxide, although tri–butyl borane has been used as an accelerator. Setting occurs as a result of a free radical polymerization characterized by liberation of heat and shrinkage of the polymer.

The filled composite cements are formulated from various diacrylate oligomers diluted with lower molecular weight dimethacrylate monomers and fillers of silica, glass, or colloidal silica. The highly filled cements typically contain silanated inorganic particles (more than 60% by weight) about 13 μm in diameter. The slightly filled cements contain 28% colloidal silica. The initiator-accelerator systems of these composite cements depend on the mode of initiating the polymerization. Amine-cured systems include the conventional two-paste products and the one-step products. Light-cured systems are polymerized by visible light.

Manipulation

The success of the direct bonding, resin orthodontic cements is highly dependent on proper isolation and acid etching of the enamel. The acid-etching technic involves etching the tooth for 15 to 60 seconds with a solution of phosphoric acid, and this procedure is followed by rinsing and drying. If the enamel is contaminated, reetching of the tooth is necessary. Acid etching is discussed in greater detail in Chapter 10.

Manipulation of the acrylic cements involves a brush technic in which a drop of liquid on a brush is dipped into the cement powder and then applied to the tooth and bracket base. An incremental addition technic is used to minimize shrinkage of the cement during polymerization. The acrylic cements can be used with metal, plastic, or ceramic brackets without the need for a primer.

The two-paste composite cements require mixing for 20 to 30 seconds before they are applied to the enamel and bracket base. A primer such as methyl methacrylate monomer in a solvent usually must be applied to a plastic bracket base. Sometimes a sealant formulated from an unfilled diacrylate is applied initially to the acid-etched enamel. The two-paste cements set several minutes after mixing.

The one-step cements require no mixing. A priming liquid is applied to the etched enamel, and the paste is applied to the bracket base. A plastic bracket may require a bracket primer. Polymerization is initiated when the bracket is placed on the primed tooth. The effect of film thickness on the polymerization of these cements has been investigated. Generally, there is a decrease in tensile bond strength as the thickness of no-mix cements increases. Failures are characterized by incomplete polymerization of the resin. Bond strength of one-step cements decreases if the primer is exposed to a

simulated oral environment for a minute or more, so bases should be placed promptly after the primer is applied to the teeth.

The light-cured cements are single-paste systems that require no mixing. The resin is applied to the tooth and bracket base, and polymerization is activated by the light source. A sealant may be used for bonding to the teeth, and a primer may be required for bonding to a plastic bracket. A concern with light-cured direct-bonding composites is the depth of penetration of the light and thus the completeness of the polymerization.

Properties

Two important properties of the resin direct-bonding cements are esthetics and bond strength to tooth structure and the bracket base.

Changes in color of the acrylic and composite cements can result from staining or from the formation of colored reaction products. After accelerated aging or exposure to a tea stain, the cements were darker and more chromatic. Exposure to the tea stain caused a greater change in color than the aging test. Generally, the composites changed color less than the acrylics.

The bond strength of the resin cements to tooth structure appears to be adequate clinically if proper isolation and manipulative technics are followed. Bonding to tooth structure results from the resin matrix penetrating into the etched areas of enamel.

Bonding to orthodontic bracket bases depends on the type of bracket base (metal, plastic, or ceramic) and the type of cement (hybrid ionomer, unfilled acrylic, highly filled composite, or slightly filled composite), as shown in Table 8-13. The highest-strength combinations are as follows: highly filled composite cement/metal base, unfilled acrylic resin/ceramic base, and unfilled acrylic resin/plastic base. Failures typically occur at the cement-base interface, or less frequently, within the cement or base. Bonding to the plastic bases appears to be chemical, whereas bonding to the metal and ceramic bases is mechanical. Failures at the cement-metal base interface are initiated at areas of stress concentration in the metal base, such as weld spots or damaged mesh (Fig. 8-7). Plastic brackets tend to fail at the wings rather than debonding in laboratory testing. Failure at the interface of the cement-ceramic

TABLE 8-13   Effect of Types of Cement and Bracket Base on Bond Strength of Direct-Bonding Cements

Type of Cement	Bond Strength, MPa Type of Bracket		
	Base Metal	Ceramic	Plastic
Hybrid ionomer	2.9-4.2	5.8-7.4	1.4-4.5
Unfilled acrylic	7.8	11.0	10.8
Slightly filled composite	8.8	4.6	8.3*
Highly filled composite	13.0	5.1	8.1

Adapted from Buzzitta VAJ, Hallgren SE, Powers JM: *Am J Orthod* 81:87, 1982; de Pulido LG, Powers JM: *Am J Orthod* 83:124, 1983; and Blalock KA, Powers JM: *Am J Orthod Dentofac Orthop* 107:596, 1995.
*With bracket primer.

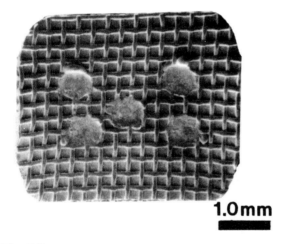

1.0mm

Fig. 8-7 Scanning electron photomicrograph of direct-bonding metal mesh base damaged by spot welds. (From Dickinson PT, Powers JM: Evaluation of fourteen direct-bonding orthodontic bases, *Am J Orthod* 78:630, 1980.)

bracket is influenced by the amount of penetration of resin into the retention ring of the base.

Improved metal bases, including photographically etched and grooved types, have been tested with surface treatments such as silanation, etching, and activation. Etching of the grooved base was most effective in improving the bond strength. Studies of the new alumina and glass-ceramic brackets indicate that high bond strengths can be attained. Most clinical failures are attributed to breakage of the wings of the ceramic brackets.

Reconditioning of metal bases by thermal treatment, by chemical treatment, and by grinding with a green stone has been evaluated. Reconditioning caused a 20% to 56% decrease in bond strength of several adhesives to a mesh metal base.

■ CAVITY VARNISHES

A cavity varnish is used to provide a barrier against the passage of irritants from cements or other restorative materials and to reduce the penetration of oral fluids at the restoration-tooth interface into the underlying dentin. Varnishes aid in the reduction of postoperative sensitivity when applied to dentinal surfaces under newly placed restorations. Cavity varnishes are rapidly being replaced by dentin bonding agents.

Composition

A cavity varnish is a solution of one or more resins from natural gums, synthetic resins, or rosin. Copal and nitrated cellulose are typical examples of a natural gum and synthetic resin ingredient. The solvents that may be used to dissolve these materials are chloroform, alcohol, acetone, benzene, toluene, ethyl acetate, and amyl acetate. Medicinal agents such as chlorobutanol, thymol, and eugenol also have been added. The volatile solvents evaporate quickly when the varnish is applied to the prepared tooth surface, thus leaving a thin resin film. The addition of fluoride to cavity varnish has not been established as effective.

Manipulation

Varnish solutions are usually applied by means of a small cotton pledget at the end of a wire or root canal reamer. Thin layers of the varnish should be applied with a partially saturated pledget. A gentle stream of air may be used for drying, but care must be taken to avoid forming ridges. A new layer is added only to a previously dried one. Two thin layers have been found to be more protective than one heavy layer. To prevent contamination of the cavity varnish, a new cotton pledget should be used for each application. Varnish solutions should be tightly capped immediately after use to minimize loss of solvent. Most varnishes are supplied with a separate bottle of pure solvent. This solvent may be used to keep the varnish from becoming too thick. The bottle should be kept half full by dilution with the solvent. Eventually the solvent will be exhausted and a new supply should be purchased. The solvent is also useful for removing varnish from external tooth surfaces.

Properties

Cavity varnishes reduce but do not prevent the passage of constituents of the phosphoric acid cements into underlying dentin. Variations in results and the mere reduction rather than the prevention of the passage of acid appear to be a result of pinpoint holes in the varnish film formed during the volatilization of the organic solvent. Greater continuity of the dried varnish film is possible by the use of successive layers of thin varnish; this technic is more effective than using just one layer of thicker varnish.

Thin films of resinous cavity varnishes have been shown to significantly reduce the leakage around the margins and walls of metallic restorations. Although the effect of the cavity varnishes is not completely known, it can be hypothesized that this reduction of fluid penetration around cavity margins would minimize postoperative sensitivity. These varnishes are applied to prepared cavity walls, including the margins. The integrity of the resin film is destroyed when restorative materials, such as the unfilled or filled resins, are placed in contact with them. The monomer contained in these resin materials dissolves the film.

Varnishes neither possess mechanical strength nor provide thermal insulation because of the thin film thickness. Values of film thickness have been measured at between 2 and 40 μm for different commercial varnishes. Contact angles of varnishes on dentin range from 53 to 106 degrees. Improved integrity of a varnish film might be achieved by improvement in the spreading of the varnish on the tooth surface.

Applications

Cavity varnishes are indicated for use (1) on dentinal surfaces to minimize the penetration of acid from zinc phosphate cements and (2) on enamel and dentinal walls to reduce the penetration of oral fluids around metallic restorations. These cavity varnishes appear also to retard the penetration of discolored corrosion products from dental amalgam into dentin. Varnishes are not used under resin or composite restorations because the monomers of these materials may disrupt the varnish film. The varnish also may prevent proper wetting of the tooth surface by the resin. A cavity varnish is applied to the dentinal walls of those tubules in direct contact with the pulp when a base of zinc phosphate cement is used. When therapeutic action is expected from a low-strength base or liner or when the cement base material itself is bland in its action on the pulp, a cavity varnish is not used on the underlying dentin. The varnish may be applied over the cement base in these situations.

■ CAVITY LINERS

A cavity liner is used like a cavity varnish to provide a barrier against the passage of irritants from cements or other restorative materials and to reduce the sensitivity of freshly cut dentin. Unlike a varnish, a liner may provide some therapeutic benefits to the tooth. Liners, however, do not set as the calcium hydroxide pulp-capping agents do.

Composition

Cavity liners are suspensions of calcium hydroxide in an organic liquid such as methyl ethyl ketone or ethyl alcohol or in an aqueous solution of methyl cellulose. The methyl cellulose functions as a thickening agent. Liners also may contain acrylic polymer beads or barium sulfate. Fluoride compounds such as calcium monofluorophosphate have been added to some liners. On evaporation of the volatile solvent, the liner forms a thin film on the prepared tooth surface.

Manipulation

Cavity liners are fluid in consistency and are easily flowed or painted over dentinal surfaces. The solvents evaporate to leave a thin film residue that protects the underlying pulp. Certain products are claimed to have better integrity and pulpal protection when used with monomer-containing restorative materials.

Properties

Like varnishes, cavity liners neither possess mechanical strength nor provide any significant thermal insulation. The calcium hydroxide liners are soluble and should not be applied at the margins of restorations.

Fluoride compounds have been added to some cavity liners to reduce the possibility of secondary caries around permanent restorations or to reduce sensitivity. Effectiveness of the fluoride for either purpose would depend on its availability to enamel and dentin through its solubility. Although *in vitro* studies with one material have shown reduced solubility of tooth tissue, clinical studies have not yet demonstrated its efficacy. However, such an investigation has shown an absence of bacteria at the resin composite–tooth tissue interface when a cavity liner containing calcium monofluorophosphate is used.

■ LOW-STRENGTH BASES

Low-strength (low-rigidity) bases are two-paste, calcium hydroxide or ZOE, cements that set to a hard mass when mixed. These cements are commonly referred to as liners, intermediary bases, or pulp-capping agents (calcium hydroxide products only). Glass ionomer, hybrid ionomer, and resin bases are discussed in the section on high-strength bases.

Composition and Chemistry of Setting

Calcium hydroxide bases

The base paste of a typical product contains calcium tungstate, tribasic calcium phosphate, and zinc oxide in glycol salicylate. The catalyst paste contains calcium hydroxide, zinc oxide, and zinc stearate in ethylene toluene sulfonamide. The ingredients responsible for setting are calcium hydroxide and a salicylate that react to form an amorphous calcium disalicylate. Fillers such as calcium tungstate or barium sulfate provide radiopacity.

A light-cured calcium hydroxide base consists of calcium hydroxide and barium sulfate dispersed in a urethane dimethacrylate resin.

Zinc oxide–eugenol bases

These bases are nonmodified (Type IV) ZOE cements as described in Revised ANSI/ADA Specification No. 30 (ISO 3107). They are typically two-paste systems in which the zinc oxide and eugenol are formulated with inert oils and fillers. The cement sets to a hard mass when mixed. The setting reaction is accelerated by moisture and an increase in temperature.

Manipulation

Both calcium hydroxide bases and ZOE low-strength bases are supplied as two-paste systems. Equal lengths of the different-colored pastes are dispensed on a paper pad and then mixed to a uniform color.

Properties

The calcium hydroxide cements are used for lining deep cavities or for direct pulp capping. The antibacterial action of calcium hydroxide makes these cements useful in indirect pulp-capping procedures involving carious dentin. The ZOE cements are used in deep cavities to retard penetration of acids and reduce possible discomfort to the pulp. Both calcium hydroxide and ZOE low-strength bases are often used with a high-strength base in restoring a tooth. Recently root canal sealers containing calcium hydroxide have been developed.

Calcium hydroxide bases

The important properties of these bases are mechanical and thermal properties, solubility, and pH. Calcium hydroxide (self-cured) bases have low values of tensile strength, compressive strength, or elastic modulus compared with the high-strength bases (Table 8-14). Although setting times vary between 2.5 and 5.5 minutes, compressive strengths of these cements continue to increase over a 24-hour period. For a group of five commercial products, compressive strengths ranged from 6.5 to 14.3 MPa at 10 minutes to from 9.8 to 26.8 MPa at 24 hours. The low elastic modulus of the calcium hydroxide bases restricts their usage to areas not critical to the support of restorations. Mechanical support should be provided by sound dentin or by a high-strength base. The calcium hydroxide bases are, however,

TABLE 8-14   Mechanical Properties of Low- and High-Strength Cement Bases

	Compressive Strength (MPa)	Tensile Strength (MPa)	Elastic Modulus (GPa)
LOW-STRENGTH (LOW-RIGIDITY) BASES			
Calcium hydroxide (light-cured)	96	38	–
Calcium hydroxide (self-cured)	12-26	1	0.4
Glass ionomer (light-cured)	90-110	11-14	3.0-4.0
Glass ionomer (self-cured)	40-175	–	1.8-2.8
Resin	160	–	2.2
Zinc oxide–eugenol (Type III)	5.5	0.41	0.3
HIGH-STRENGTH (HIGH-RIGIDITY) BASES			
Composite resin (dual-cured)	130	25	5.6
Glass ionomer (self-cured)	70-210	3.9-8.3	3.7-9.0
Hybrid ionomer (self-cured)	96-126	17-24	3.0-7.8
Polymer-reinforced zinc oxide–eugenol (Type IV)	38	3.4	2.1
Zinc phosphate	130-160	8	22
Zinc polyacrylate	80	16	5.0

considered strong enough to support the forces of condensation of amalgam.

The calcium hydroxide bases may provide some thermal insulation to the pulp if used in sufficiently thick layers. A thickness greater than 0.5 mm is not suggested. Practically, thermal protection should be provided by the overlying high-strength base.

The solubility of calcium hydroxide bases has been measured in several solvents for various periods of immersion. For a group of five commercial products, values ranged from 0.4% to 7.8% in distilled water at 37° C for 24 hours, from 0.1% to 6.2% in 35% phosphoric acid for 60 seconds, and from 0.3% to 1% in ether for 10 seconds. One product that was resistant to dissolution in water and in acid disintegrated when exposed to ether. Some solubility of the calcium hydroxide is necessary to achieve its therapeutic properties, although an optimum value is not known. Clearly the use of acid-etching procedures and varnish in the presence of calcium hydroxide bases must be done with care. Over a long term, some calcium hydroxide products seem to "disappear" from the cavity. The cause of this dissolution is unclear, but some products have been reformulated in an attempt to minimize the problem.

The pH of commercial products has been measured at between 9.2 and 11.7. Free calcium hydroxide in excess of that necessary to form the calcium disalicylate stimulates secondary dentin in proximity to the pulp and shows antibacterial activity.

One light-cured calcium hydroxide base is reported to have a surface pH of 11.9, low dissolution in acid (< 0.5%), low 24-hour solubility in water (< 1.0%), and high compressive strength (80 MPa). Whereas two-paste calcium hydroxide bases show antibacterial activity, a light-cured type did not.

Zinc oxide–eugenol bases

Revised ANSI/ADA Specification No. 30 requirements for zinc oxide–eugenol liners are listed in Table 8-8. The mechanical properties of these cements are compared with those of calcium hydroxide bases and high-strength bases (Table 8-14). The ZOE products tend to be weaker and less rigid than the calcium hydroxide pastes that set. Because the base is used in thin layers, it provides little thermal insulation. The eugenol has a sedative (obtundent) effect on the pulp. The base should not be used when a composite is to be placed because the eugenol can inhibit its polymerization.

■ HIGH-STRENGTH BASES

High-strength bases are used to provide thermal protection for the pulp and mechanical support for a restoration. Bases are usually prepared from a base or secondary consistency (higher powder/liquid ratio) of zinc phosphate or zinc polyacrylate cement. A polymer-reinforced ZOE base is also available.

Recently, self-cured and light-cured glass ionomer and hybrid ionomer cements have become available as low- and high-strength bases. The low-strength bases (liners) typically flow more readily than the high-strength bases and are less rigid as shown in Table 8-14. The new, light-cured glass ionomers are water-based cements but have a unique chemistry of setting that involves both an acid-base reaction between carboxylate ions and the glass particles and a light-accelerated polymerization of dimethacrylate oligomers. Most of the light-cured liners are premixed pastes or powder-liquid systems mixed by hand, but one recent light-cured liner is encapsulated. The composition and setting reaction of the hybrid ionomers used as bases are identical to the luting cements discussed earlier in this chapter.

Resins also are available as low- and high-strength bases. The low-strength resin base is a light-cured, urethane dimethacrylate resin with barium glass and barium sulfate fillers and dispersed sodium fluoride. The high-strength composite base is a dual-cured, paste-paste composite consisting of a Bis-GMA resin, hydrophilic diluent, fluoride-releasing glass filler, barium glass for radiopacity, and a proprietery bonding agent. Bond strengths of 14 MPa to human enamel and dentin *in vitro* have been reported. This composite also bonds to composite, porcelain, and metal.

Properties

The tensile strength, compressive strength, and elastic modulus of five types of high-strength bases are compared in Table 8-14. The secondary consistencies of these cements result in higher values of strength and elastic modulus than values obtained from mixes of a primary (luting) consistency (see Table 8-3). Zinc phosphate cements are the most rigid of the five types, whereas the polymer-modified, ZOE cements (Type III) have the lowest properties. ANSI/ADA Specification No. 96 specifies the net

setting time, minimum compressive strength, and maximum values of acid erosion, acid-soluble arsenic, and lead content for zinc phosphate, zinc polyacrylate, and glass ionomer bases as listed in Table 8-2.

The ability of a cement base to support a restoration during function has been studied by stress-analysis technics as described in Chapter 4. The thickness and elastic modulus of the base affect the deflection of the base and restoration. Mismatches in the moduli of the base and restorative material can cause tensile stresses at the cement-restoration interface that can lead to failure of either material. Studies have recommended that a zinc phosphate base be used to support an amalgam restoration, whereas zinc phosphate, glass ionomer, or zinc polyacrylate may be used to support a class 1 composite restoration.

The glass ionomer lining cements and bases are unique in their ability to bond to dentin. Bond strengths measured in tension vary from 2.0 to 4.9 MPa. These cements also can be etched to provide additional retention to a composite restoration. The so-called sandwich technic for posterior composites is discussed in Chapter 10. Glass ionomer lining cements and bases release fluoride ion and are radiopaque.

The thermal conductivity and diffusivity of dental cements (see Tables 3-4 and 3-6) are similar to those of enamel and dentin. Thus cement bases provide thermal protection to the pulp if used in a sufficiently thick layer (> 0.5 mm).

SELECTED PROBLEMS

Problem 1. A temporary acrylic crown was difficult to remove and upon removal was found to be soft. What caused these problems, and how can they be resolved?

Solution. The use of a reinforced ZOE cement makes the removal of a temporary acrylic crown difficult, and the eugenol softens the acrylic. Therefore a low-strength, non-eugenol–zinc oxide or temporary resin cement is recommended for use with acrylic crowns.

Problem 2. A low–gold content bridge with normal retention is to be temporarily cemented. Which cement is recommended for this application?

Solution. A low-strength ZOE cement is suggested to allow for easy removal and cleanup of the bridge for final cementation.

Problem 3. A low–gold content MOD inlay with normal retention is to be cemented permanently. Which cements are recommended for this application? Which are not?

Solution a. Glass ionomer, hybrid ionomer, zinc phosphate, and zinc polyacrylate cements are sufficiently strong and insoluble in oral fluids for this application.

Solution b. EBA ZOE cements are weaker and more soluble in oral fluids than are other cements and generally not recommended for final cementation.

Problem 4. A gold casting seated properly before cementation but failed to seat when cemented with zinc phosphate cement. What factors might have caused this difficulty, and how can it be corrected?

Solution a. An excessive film thickness of zinc phosphate cement may result from (1) too high a mixing temperature, (2) too high a powder/liquid ratio, (3) water contamination during mixing, (4) a glass slab temperature below the dew point, (5) too long a time between completion of mixing and cementation, and (6) cement being placed on the tooth before being placed on the casting.

Solution b. An orthodontic (medium particle size) zinc phosphate cement may have been used by mistake. A luting (fine particle size) cement should be used for accurate seating of precision appliances.

Problem 5. A clinician experienced difficulties in reproducing the consistency of mixes of a zinc polyacrylate cement. The mixes were too thick. What were the probable causes of this problem, and how can they be corrected?

Solution a. The liquid of a zinc polyacrylate cement (excluding the anhydrous type) is very viscous and difficult to dispense accurately. The dropper bottle should be held perpendicular to the mixing pad when the liquid is dispensed. Try to dispense drops of uniform size.

Solution b. The loss of water by evaporation will increase the powder/liquid ratio. The liquid should be dispensed just before mixing, and a water-resistant mixing pad should be used.

Solution c. A mixing temperature higher than 23° C or overmixing will result in a mix that is too thick. Use a cool slab for mixing, and carefully follow the recommended mixing time for more consistent mixes.

Problem 6. During the insertion of a zinc phosphate cement base into an extensive cavity preparation, the mix became dry and friable and did not adhere well to the cavity walls. What factors might be related to such a change in consistency, and how can the consistency be improved?

Solution a. The heat of reaction accelerates the setting reaction of zinc phosphate cement, thereby causing the working time to decrease. Mixing the cement with incremental additions of powder and over a large area of a cool slab will reduce the temperature rise and allow a longer working time.

Solution b. Too much powder incorporated into a mix as it approaches secondary consistency decreases the working time and causes the cement base to be weak and friable because of insufficient matrix to bind the powder together. The base should be slightly tacky after it is rolled in powder at the completion of mixing.

Problem 7. A properly mixed zinc phosphate cement base became contaminated with saliva during placement. Should there be any deleterious effect expected from the contamination?

Solution. Yes, a soft, friable surface results from the dilution of acid and leaching of the matrix of a setting cement base by saliva.

Problem 8. A calcium hydroxide base appeared to disintegrate when acid came into contact with it during an acid-etching procedure. Are there bases that can be used in conjunction with acid-etching procedures for a composite?

Solution a. Yes, acid-resistant calcium hydroxide bases containing disalicylates are available.

Solution b. Glass ionomer bases can be etched to enhance the bond between the base and the composite.

Solution c. Use a hybrid ionomer cement. Its bond to composite is not affected by etching.

Problem 9. When an amalgam is placed over a ZOE base, the cement sometimes crumbles and becomes incorporated into the amalgam mass. Should a thicker layer of ZOE cement or a different cement base be placed to provide better support?

Solution a. The ZOE base is a material with a low rigidity. Increasing its thickness will result in less rather than more support. Maintain the thickness of a low-strength base at less than 0.5 mm.

Solution b. A more rigid cement base such as zinc phosphate cement should be placed over the ZOE base to provide additional support for condensation and for the amalgam from occlusal forces.

Problem 10. A paste-primer (one-step) direct-bonding orthodontic cement failed shortly after the appliance was activated. Resin remained on both the tooth and the metal bracket. What factors might explain these observations, and how can the problem be corrected?

Solution a. The bond strength of a one-step, direct-bonding cement can be very low if too thick a layer of the paste is placed on the bracket. The primer cannot diffuse through the thick layer of paste, causing insufficient polymerization of the cement. Keep the thickness of the cement paste to less than 0.25 mm.

Solution b. The enamel primer of a one-step cement remaining in the warm, humid environment of the mouth too long before the bracket is placed will cause a decrease in the cohesive strength of the cement. Apply the brackets to the teeth within 1 minute after applying the primer.

■ REFERENCES

General

Barakat MM, Powers JM: *In vitro* bond strength of cements to treated teeth, *Aust Dent J* 31:415, 1986.

Council on Dental Materials, Instruments and Equipment, Council on Dental Therapeutics: Clinical products in dentistry. A desktop reference. American Dental Association, Chicago, IL 1993.

Craig RG, Peyton FA: Thermal conductivity of tooth structure, dental cements, and amalgam, *J Dent Res* 40:411, 1961.

Craig RG, Peyton FA, Johnson DW: Compressive properties of enamel, dental cements, and gold, *J Dent Res* 40:936, 1961.

Dennison JB, Powers JM: A review of dental cements used for permanent retention of restorations. I. Composition and manipulation, *Mich Dent Assoc J* 56:116, 1974.

McCabe JF, Wilson HJ: The use of differential scanning calorimetry for the evaluation of dental materials. I. Cements, cavity lining materials and anterior restorative materials, *J Oral Rehabil* 7:103, 1980.

Mesu FP: Degradation of luting cements measured in vitro, *J Dent Res* 61:655, 1982.

Mitchem JC, Gronas DG: Clinical evaluation of cement solubility, *J Prosthet Dent* 40:453, 1978.

Myers ML, Staffanou RS, Hembree JH, Jr, Wiseman WB: Marginal leakage of contemporary cementing agents, *J Prosthet Dent* 50:513, 1983.

Norman RD, Swartz ML, Phillips RW: Direct pH determinations of setting cements. I. A test method and the effects of storage time and media, *J Dent Res* 45:136, 1966.

Norman RD, Swartz ML, Phillips RW: Studies on film thickness, solubility, and marginal leakage of dental cements, *J Dent Res* 42:950, 1963.

Norman RD, Swartz ML, Phillips RW: Direct pH determinations of setting cements. II. The effects of prolonged storage time, powder/liquid ratio, temperature, and dentin, *J Dent Res* 45:1214, 1966.

Oilo G, Espevik S: Stress/strain behavior of some dental luting cements, *Acta Odontol Scand* 36:45, 1978.

Osborne JW, Swartz ML, Goodacre CJ, Phillips RW, Gale EN: A method for assessing the clinical solubility and disintegration of luting cements, *J Prosthet Dent* 40:413, 1978.

Paddon JM, Wilson AD: Stress relaxation studies on dental materials. I. Dental cements, *J Dent* 4:183, 1976.

Phillips LJ, Schnell RJ, Phillips RW: Measurement of electric conductivity of dental cement. III. Effect of increased contact area and thickness; values for resin, calcium hydroxide, zinc oxide–eugenol, *J Dent Res* 34:597, 1955.

Powers JM, Capp JA, Craig RG: Abrasion of temporary filling materials, *Mich Dent Assoc J* 56:281, 1974.

Powers JM, Craig RG: A review of the composition and properties of endodontic filling materials, *Mich Dent Assoc J* 61:523, 1979.

Powers JM, Farah JW, Craig RG: Modulus of elasticity and strength properties of dental cements, *J Am Dent Assoc* 92:588, 1976.

Richter WA, Ueno H: Clinical evaluation of dental cement durability, *J Prosthet Dent* 33:294, 1975.

Smith DC: Dental cements: current status and future prospects, *Dent Clin North Am* 27:763, 1983.

Tanizaki K, Inoue K: Effect of tannin-fluoride preparation on the reduction of secondary caries, *J Osaka Univ Dent Sch* 19:129, 1979.

Vermilyea S, Powers JM, Craig RG: Rotational viscometry of a zinc phosphate and a zinc polyacrylate cement, *J Dent Res* 56:762, 1977.

Walls AW, McCabe JF, Murray JJ: An erosion test for dental cements, *J Dent Res* 64:1100, 1985.

Watts DC, Smith R: Thermal diffusion in some polyelectrolyte dental cements: the effects of powder/liquid ratio, *J Oral Rehabil* 11:285, 1984.

Wilson AD: The chemistry of dental cements, *Chem Soc Rev* 7:265, 1978.

Zinc Phosphate Cements

Cameron JC, Charbeneau GT, Craig RG: Some properties of dental cements of specific importance to the cementation of orthodontic bands, *Angle Orthod* 33:233, 1963.

Crisp S, Jennings MA, Wilson AD: A study of temperature changes occurring in the setting dental cements, *J Oral Rehabil* 5:139, 1978.

Davidson HD: Effect of zinc oxyphosphate cement upon the enamel following placement of orthodontic bands, *Am J Orthod* 42:792, 1956.

Kendziar GM, Leinfelder KF, Hershey HG: The effect of cold temperature mixing on the properties of zinc phosphate cement, *Angle Orthod* 46:345, 1976.

Mitchem JC, Gronas DG: Clinical evaluation of cement solubility, *J Prosthet Dent* 40:453, 1978.

Muhler JC (Indiana Univ Foundation, Bloomington, Ind): Dental cement. Canadian Patent 912,026 (Cl 6-36), Oct 17, 1972; Appl July 20, 1970, 23 pp.

Servais GE, Cartz L: Structure of zinc phosphate dental cement, *J Dent Res* 50:613, 1971.

Williams JD, Swartz ML, Phillips RW: Retention of orthodontic bands as influenced by the cementing media, *Angle Orthod* 35:278, 1965.

Wilson AD: Specification test for the solubility and disintegration of dental cements: a critical evaluation, *J Dent Res* 55:721, 1976.

Zinc Oxide–Eugenol Cements

Brauer GM: A review of zinc oxide–eugenol type filling materials and cements, *Rev Belg Med Dent* 20:323, 1965.

Brauer GM, McLaughlin R, Huget EF: Aluminum oxide as a reinforcing agent for zinc oxide–eugenol-*o*-ethoxybenzoic acid cements, *J Dent Res* 47:622, 1968.

Civjan S, Brauer GM: Clinical behavior of *o*-ethoxybenzoic acid-eugenol-oxide cements, *J Dent Res* 44:80, 1965.

Civjan S, Brauer GM: Physical properties of cements, based on zinc oxide, hydrogenated rosin, *o*-ethoxybenzoic acid, and eugenol, *J Dent Res* 43:281, 1964.

Civjan S, Huget EF, Wolfhard G, Waddell LS: Characterization of zinc oxide–eugenol cements reinforced with acrylic resin, *J Dent Res* 51:107, 1972.

El-Tahawi HM, Craig RG: Thermal analysis of zinc oxide–eugenol cements during setting, *J Dent Res* 50:430, 1971.

Gilson TD, Myers GE: Clinical studies of dental cements. I. Five zinc oxide–eugenol cements, *J Dent Res* 47:737, 1968.

Gilson TD, Myers GE: Clinical studies of dental cements. II. Further investigation of two zinc oxide–eugenol cements for temporary restorations, *J Dent Res* 48:366, 1969.

Gilson TD, Myers GE: Clinical studies of dental cements. III. Seven zinc oxide–eugenol cements used for temporarily cementing completed restorations, *J Dent Res* 49:14, 1970.

Gilson TD, Myers GE: Clinical studies of dental cements. IV. A preliminary study of a zinc oxide–eugenol cement for final cementation, *J Dent Res* 49:75, 1970.

Grieve AR: Sealing properties of cements used in root filling, *Br Dent J* 132:19, 1972.

Grossman LI: Physical properties of root canal cements, *J Endodont* 2:166, 1976.

Harvey W, Petch NJ: Acceleration of the setting of zinc oxide cements, *Br Dent J* 80:1, 1946.

Higginbotham TL: A comparative study of the physical properties of five commonly used root canal sealers, *Oral Surg, Oral Med, Oral Pathol* 24:89, 1967.

McComb D, Smith DC: Comparison of physical properties of polycarboxylate-based and conventional root canal sealers, *J Endodont* 2:228, 1976.

Molnar EJ, Skinner EW: Study of zinc oxide-rosin cements. I. Some variables which affect the hardening time, *J Am Dent Assoc* 29:744, 1942.

Nielsen TH: Sealing ability of chelate root filling cements. Part I. Device for measuring linear changes of setting chelate cements, *J Endodont* 6:731, 1980.

Powers JM, Craig RG: A review of the composition and properties of endodontic filling materials, *Mich Dent Assoc J* 61:523, 1979.

Silvey RG, Myers GE: Clinical studies of dental cements. V. Recall evaluation of restorations cemented with a zinc oxide–eugenol cement and a zinc phosphate cement, *J Dent Res* 55:289, 1976.

Silvey RG, Myers GE: Clinical studies of dental cements. VI. A study of zinc phosphate, EBA reinforced zinc oxide–eugenol and polyacrylic acid cements as luting agents in fixed prostheses, *J Dent Res* 56:1215, 1977.

Silvey RG, Myers GE: Clinical studies of dental cements. VII. A study of bridge retainers luted with three different dental cements, *J Dent Res* 57:703, 1978.

Vermilyea SG, Huget EF, DeSimon LB: Extrusion rheometry of fluid materials, *J Dent Res* 58:1691, 1979.

Wilson AD, Mesley RJ: Chemical nature of cementing matrixes of cements formed from zinc oxide and 2-ethoxy benzoic acid-eugenol liquids, *J Dent Res* 53:146, 1974.

Zinc Polyacrylate Cements

Ady AB, Fairhurst CW: Bond strength of two types of cements to gold casting alloy, *J Prosthet Dent* 29:217, 1973.

Bertenshaw BW, Combe EC: Studies on polycarboxylate and related cements. I. Analysis of cement liquids, *J Dent* 1:13, 1972.

Bertenshaw BW, Combe EC: Studies on polycarboxylate and related cements. II. Analysis of cement powders, *J Dent* 1:65, 1972.

Brännström M, Nyborg H: Pulpal reaction to polycarboxylate and zinc phosphate cements used with inlays in deep cavity preparations, *J Am Dent Assoc* 94:308, 1977.

Chamberlain BB, Powers JM: Physical and mechanical properties of three zinc polyacrylate dental cements, *Mich Dent Assoc J* 58:494, 1976.

Crisp S, Lewis BG, Wilson AD: Zinc polycarboxylate cements: a chemical study of erosion and its relationship to molecular structure, *J Dent Res* 55:299, 1976.

Crisp S, Prosser HJ, Wilson AD: An infra-red spectroscopic study of cement formation between metal oxides and aqueous solutions of poly(acrylic acid), *J Mater Sci* 11:36, 1976.

Jendresen MD, Trowbridge HO: Biological and physical properties of a zinc polycarboxylate cement, *J Prosthet Dent* 28:264, 1972.

Jurecic A (Pennwalt Corporation): Acrylic acid copolymers in dental cements, *Canadian Pat* 909,414, Sept 5, 1972.

McLean JW: Polycarboxylate cements–five year's experience in general practice, *Br Dent J* 132:9, 1972.

Mizrahi E, Smith DC: Direct cementation of orthodontic brackets to dental enamel, *Br Dent J* 127:371, 1969.

Mizrahi E, Smith DC: The bond strength of a zinc polycarboxylate cement, *Br Dent J* 127:410, 1969.

Oilo G: Linear dimensional changes during setting of two polycarboxylate cements, *J Oral Rehabil* 3:161, 1976.

Plant CB: The effect of polycarboxylate cement on the dental pulp–a study, *Br Dent J* 129:424, 1970.

Powers JM, Johnson ZG, Craig RG: Physical and mechanical properties of zinc polyacrylate dental cements, *J Am Dent Assoc* 88:380, 1974.

Smith DC: A new dental cement, *Br Dent J* 125:381, 1968.

Truelove EL, Mitchell DG, Phillips RW: Biologic evaluation of a carboxylate cement, *J Dent Res* 50:166, 1971.

Glass Ionomer and Hybrid Ionomer Cements

Barry TI, Clinton DJ, Wilson AD: The structure of a glass-ionomer cement and its relationship to the setting process, *J Dent Res* 58:1072, 1979.

Berry EA III: The clinical uses of glass ionomer cements. In Hardin JF: Clark's clinical dentistry, vol 4, Philadelphia, 1993, Lippincott.

Berry EA III, Powers JM: Bond strength of glass ionomers to coronal and radicular dentin, *Oper Dent* 19:122, 1994.

Council on Dental Materials, Instruments, and Equipment: Reported sensitivity to glass ionomer luting cements, *J Am Dent Assoc* 109:476, 1984.

Crisp S, Kent BE, Lewis BG, Ferner AJ, Wilson AD: Glass ionomer cement formulations. II. The synthesis of novel polycarboxylic acids, *J Dent Res* 59:1055, 1980.

Crisp S, Lewis BG, Wilson AD: Characterization of glass-ionomer cements. 1. Long term hardness and compressive strength, *J Dent* 4:162, 1976.

Crisp S, Lewis BG, Wilson AD: Characterization of glass-ionomer cements. 5. The effect of the tartaric acid concentration in the liquid component, *J Dent* 7:304, 1979.

Crisp S, Lewis BG, Wilson AD: Characterization of glass-ionomer cements. 6. A study of erosion and water absorption in both neutral and acidic media, *J Dent* 8:68, 1980.

Crisp S, Pringuer MA, Wardleworth D, Wilson AD: Reactions in glass ionomer cements. II. An infrared spectroscopic study, *J Dent Res* 53:1414, 1974.

Crisp S, Wilson AD: Reactions in glass ionomer cements. I. Decomposition of the powder, *J Dent Res* 53:1408, 1974.

Crisp S, Wilson AD: Reactions in glass ionomer cements. III. The precipitation reaction, *J Dent Res* 53:1420, 1974.

Dahl BL, Tronstad L: Biological tests of an experimental glass ionomer (silicopolyacrylate) cement, *J Oral Rehabil* 3:19, 1976.

Finger W: Evaluation of glass ionomer luting cements, *Scand J Dent Res* 91:143, 1983.

Fitzgerald M, Heys RJ, Heys DR, Charbeneau GT: An evaluation of a glass ionomer luting agent: bacterial leakage, *J Am Dent Assoc* 114:783, 1987.

Forss H: Release of fluoride and other elements from light-cured glass ionomers in neutral and acidic conditions, *J Dent Res* 72:1257, 1993.

Forsten L: Fluoride release from a glass ionomer cement, *Scand J Dent Res* 85:503, 1977.

Friedl K-H, Powers JM, Hiller K-A: Influence of different factors on bond strength of hybrid ionomers, *Oper Dent* 20:74, 1995.

Hunt PR, editor: *Glass ionomers: the next generation,* Proceedings of the 2nd International Symposium on Glass Ionomers. Philadelphia, 1994.

Johnson GH, Herbert AH, Powers JM: Changes in properties of glass-ionomer luting cements with time, *Oper Dent* 13:191, 1988.

Kawahara H, Imanishi Y, Oshima H: Biological evaluation on glass ionomer cement, *J Dent Res* 58:1080, 1979.

Maldonado A, Swartz ML, Phillips RW: An in vitro study of certain properties of a glass ionomer cement, *J Am Dent Assoc* 96:785, 1978.

McComb D: Retention of castings with glass ionomer cement, *J Prosthet Dent* 48:285, 1982.

Mitra SB, Li MY, Culler SR: Setting reaction of Vitrebond light cure glass-ionomer liner/base. In Watts DC, Setcos JC: Proceedings of the Conference on Setting Mechanisms of Dental Materials, Transactions of the Academy of Dental Materials 5:2, 1992.

Negm MM, Beech DR, Grant AA: An evaluation of mechanical and adhesive properties of polycarboxylate and glass ionomer cements, *J Oral Rehabil* 9:161, 1982.

Nicholson JW: The setting of glass-polyalkenoate ("glass-ionomer") cements. In Watts DC, Setcos JC: Proceedings of the Conference on Setting Mechanisms of Dental Materials, Transactions of the Academy of Dental Materials 5:2, 1992.

Oilo G: Bond strength of new ionomer cements to dentin, *Scand J Dent Res* 89:344, 1981.

Prosser HJ, Richards CP, Wilson AD: NMR spectroscopy of dental materials. II. The role of tartaric acid in glass-ionomer cements, *Biomed Mater Res J* 16:431, 1982.

Ryan MD, Powers JM, Johnson GH: Properties of glass ionomer luting cements, *Mich Dent Assoc J* 67:17, 1985.

Shalabi HS, Asmussen E, Jorgensen KD: Increased bonding of a glass-ionomer cement to dentin by means of FeCl$_3$, *Scand J Dent Res* 89:348, 1981.

Wilson AD: Resin-modified glass-ionomer cements, *Int J Prosthodont* 3:425, 1990.

Wilson AD, Crisp S, McLean JW: Experimental luting agents based on the glass ionomer cements, *Br Dent J* 142:117, 1977.

Wilson AD, Crisp S, Prosser HJ, Lewis BG, Merson SA: Aluminosilicate glasses for polyelectrolyte cements, *I&EC Prod Res & Develop* 19:263, 1980.

Resin Cements

Aksu MN, Powers JM, Lorey RE, Kollig JN: Variables affecting bond strength of resin-bonded bridge cements, *Dent Mater* 3:26, 1987.

Blackman R, Barghi N, Duke E: Influence of ceramic thickness on the polymerization of light-cured resin cement, *J Prosthet Dent* 63:295, 1990.

Blalock KA, Powers JM: Retention capacity of the bracket bases of new esthetic orthodontic brackets, *Am J Orthod Dentofac Orthop* 107:596, 1995.

Brännström M, Nyborg H: The presence of bacteria in cavities filled with silicate cement and composite resin materials, *Swed Dent J* 64:149, 1971.

Buzzitta VAM, Hallgren SE, Powers JM: Bond strength of orthodontic direct-bonding cement-bracket systems as studied *in vitro*, *Am J Orthod* 81:87, 1982.

Chan KC, Boyer DB: Curing light-activated composite cement through porcelain, *J Dent Res* 68:476, 1989.

Coleman RA: Dentin bonded post and cores: an *in vitro* failure analysis, Masters thesis, Ann Arbor, 1987, University of Michigan School of Dentistry.

de Pulido LG, Powers JM: Bond strength of orthodontic direct-bonding cement-plastic bracket systems *in vitro*, *Am J Orthod* 83:124, 1983.

Dickinson PT, Powers JM: Evaluation of fourteen direct-bonding orthodontic bases, *Am J Orthod* 78:630, 1980.

Evans LB, Powers JM: Factors affecting *in vitro* bond strength of no-mix orthodontic cements, *Am J Orthod* 87:508, 1985.

Faust JB, Grego GN, Fan PL, Powers JM: Penetration coefficient, tensile strength, and bond strength of thirteen direct bonding orthodontic cements, *Am J Orthod* 73:512, 1978.

Faust JB, Grego GN, Powers JM: Handling characteristics and cost of thirteen direct bonding orthodontic cements, *Mich Dent Assoc J* 60:419, 1978.

Howe DF, Denehy GE: Anterior fixed partial dentures utilizing the acid-etch technique and a cast metal framework, *J Prosthet Dent* 37:28, 1977.

Jenkins CBG: Etch-retained anterior pontics, a 4-year study, *Br Dent J* 144:206, 1978.

Jordan RE, Suzuki M, Sills PS, Gratton DR, Gwinnet JA: Temporary fixed partial dentures fabricated by means of the acid-etch resin technique: a report of 86 cases followed for up to three years, *J Am Dent Assoc* 96:994, 1978.

Lambert PM, Moore DL, Elletson HH: *In vitro* retentive strength of fixed bridges constructed with acrylic pontics and an ultraviolet-light-polymerized resin, *J Am Dent Assoc* 92:740, 1976.

Lee H, Swartz ML: Evaluation of a composite resin crown and bridge luting agent, *J Dent Res* 51:756, 1972.

Livaditis GJ: Cast metal resin-bonded retainers for posterior teeth, *J Am Dent Assoc* 101:926, 1980.

Livaditis GJ, Thompson VP: Etched castings: an improved retentive mechanism for resin-bonded retainers, *J Prosthet Dent* 47:52, 1982.

Maijer R, Smith DC: Variables influencing the bond strength of metal orthodontic bracket bases, *Am J Orthod* 79:20, 1981.

O'Keefe K, Powers JM: Light-cured resin cements for cementation of esthetic restorations, *J Esthet Dent* 2:129, 1990.

O'Keefe K, Powers JM, McGuckin RS, Pierpont, HP: *In vitro* bond strength of silica-coated metal posts in roots of teeth, *Int J Prosthodont* 5:373, 1992.

Powers JM: Adhesive resin cements, *Shigaku* 79:1140, 1991.

Rabchinsky DS, Powers JM: Color stability and stain resistance of direct-bonding orthodontic cements, *Am J Orthod* 76:170, 1979.

Reynolds IR, von Fraunhofer JA: Direct bonding of orthodontic attachments to the teeth: the relation of adhesive bond strength to gauze mesh size, *Br J Orthod* 3:91, 1976.

Rochette AL: Attachment of a splint to enamel of lower anterior teeth, *J Prosthet Dent* 30:418, 1973.

Schouboe PJ, Paffenbarger GC, Sweeney WT: Resin cements and posterior type direct filling resins, *J Am Dent Assoc* 52:584, 1956.

Siomka LV, Powers JM: In vitro bond strength of treated direct-bonding metal bases, *Am J Orthod* 88:133, 1985.

Tate WH, DeSchepper EJ, Powers JM: Bond strength of resin cements to a hybrid composite, *Am J Dent* 6:195, 1993.

Wright WL, Powers JM: *In vitro* tensile bond strength of reconditioned brackets, *Am J Orthod* 87:247, 1985.

Zachrisson BU, Brobakken BO: Clinical comparison of direct versus indirect bonding with different bracket types and adhesives, *Am J Orthod* 74:62, 1978.

Cavity Varnishes, Liners, and Bases

Bryant RW, Wing G: A simulated clinical appraisal of base materials for amalgam restorations, *Aust Dent J* 21:322, 1976.

Chong WF, Swartz ML, Phillips RW: Displacement of cement bases by amalgam condensation, *J Am Dent Assoc* 74:97, 1967.

Farah JW, Hood JAA, Craig RG: Effects of cement bases on the stresses in amalgam restorations, *J Dent Res* 54:10, 1975.

Farah JW, Powers JM, Dennison JB, Craig RG, Spencer J: Effects of cement bases on the stresses and deflections in composite restorations, *J Dent Res* 55:115, 1976.

Fisher FJ: The effect of three proprietary lining materials on micro-organisms in carious dentin, *Br Dent J* 143:231, 1977.

Going RE: Status report on cement bases, cavity liners, varnishes, primers, and cleansers, *J Am Dent Assoc* 85:654, 1972.

Gordon SM: Gum copal solution for cavity lining and varnish, *J Am Dent Assoc* 23:2374, 1936.

Gourley JM, Rose DE: Comparison of three cavity base materials under amalgam restorations, *J Can Dent Assoc* 38:406, 1972.

Hyde DG: Physical properties of root canal sealers containing calcium hydroxide, Masters thesis, Ann Arbor, 1986, University of Michigan School of Dentistry.

Leinfelder KF: Changing restorative traditions: the use of bases and liners, *J Am Dent Assoc* 125:65, 1994.

McComb D: Comparison of physical properties of commercial calcium hydroxide lining cements, *J Am Dent Assoc* 107:610, 1983.

McComb D, Ericson D: Antimicrobial action of new, proprietary lining cements, *J Dent Res* 66:1025, 1987.

Plant GC, Wilson HJ: Early strengths of lining materials, *Br Dent J* 129:269, 1970.

Söremark R, Hedin M, Rojmyr R: Studies on incorporation of fluoride in a cavity liner (varnish), *Odontol Revy* 20:189, 1969.

Swartz ML, Phillips RW, Norman RD, Niblack BF: Role of cavity varnishes and bases in the penetration of cement constituents through tooth structure, *J Prosthet Dent* 16:963, 1966.

9 Amalgam

An amalgam is an alloy of mercury with one or more other metals. Dental amalgam is produced by mixing liquid mercury with solid particles of an alloy of silver, tin, copper, and sometimes zinc, palladium, indium, and selenium. This combination of solid metals is known as the amalgam alloy. It is important to differentiate between dental amalgam and the amalgam alloy that is commercially produced and marketed as small filings, spheroid particles, or a combination of these, suitable for mixing with liquid mercury to produce the dental amalgam.

The freshly mixed mass of the amalgam alloy and liquid mercury developed by the dentist has a plasticity that permits it to be conveniently packed or condensed into a prepared tooth cavity. A dental amalgam restoration results. Such amalgam restorations usually are limited to the replacement of tooth tissue in posterior teeth because of their silvery gray metallic appearance. Dental amalgam has been used as an occlusal restoration for small lesions; for mesial-occlusal (MO), distal-occlusal (DO), or mesial-occlusal-distal (MOD) restorations; or in combination with metallic retentive pins for crown restorations. Dental amalgam restorations are reasonably easy to insert, are not overly technic-sensitive, maintain anatomical form, have reasonably adequate resistance to fracture, prevent marginal leakage after a period of time in the mouth, and have a relatively long service life.

The drawbacks of dental amalgams are that their color does not match tooth structure, they are more brittle and less tough than desirable, they are subject to corrosion and galvanic action, they eventually show marginal breakdown, and they can not be bonded to tooth structure as well as desired, and thus, although they fill the space where tooth structure was removed, they do not restore the strength of the clinical crown.

In this chapter the composition and morphology of the different dental amalgams are presented, followed by a discussion of low- and high-copper amalgams, the chemical reactions occurring during amalgamation, and the resultant microstructures. Various physical and mechanical properties are covered in the next section, as well as the factors related to the manipulation of amalgam. Finally, mercury toxicity and potential biological effects of amalgam are presented.

■ DENTAL AMALGAM ALLOYS

Composition and Morphology

ANSI/ADA Specification No. 1 for amalgam alloy includes a requirement for composition. This specification does not state precisely what the composition of alloys shall be; rather, it permits some variation in composition. The chemical composition must consist essentially of silver and tin. Copper, zinc, gold, palladium, indium, selenium, or mercury may be included in lesser amounts. Metals such as palladium, gold, and indium in smaller quantities and copper in larger quantities have been included to alter the corrosion resistance and certain mechanical properties of the finished amalgam mass. These and other elements may be included, provided that the manufacturer submits the composition of the alloy, together with adequate clinical and biological data, to the American Dental Association Council on Scientific Affairs to show that the alloy is safe to use in the mouth as directed.

Alloys with more than 0.01% zinc are classified as zinc containing, and those with less than 0.01%, as nonzinc alloys. Zinc has been included in amalgam alloys as an aid in manufacturing by helping to

TABLE 9-1   Approximate Composition of Low- and High-Copper Amalgam Alloys

| Alloy | Particle Shape | Element, wt % | | | | | |
		Ag	Sn	Cu	Zn	In	Pd
Low copper	Irregular or spherical	63-70	26-28	2-5	0-2	0	0
High copper							
Admixed regular	Irregular	40-70	26-30	2-30	0-2	0	0
	Spherical	40-65	0-30	20-40	0-1	0	0-1
Admixed unicomposition	Irregular	52-53	17-18	29-30	0	0	0.3
	Spherical	52-53	17-18	29-30	0	0	0.3
Unicompositional	Spherical	40-60	22-30	13-30	0	0-5	0-1

produce clean, sound castings of the ingots. However, improved manufacturing procedures have resulted in the elimination of zinc in most alloys.

The approximate composition of commercial amalgam alloys is shown in Table 9-1, along with the shape of the particles. The alloys are broadly classified as low-copper alloys (5% or less copper) and high-copper alloys (13% to 30% copper). Particles are (1) irregularly shaped, (2) microspheres of various sizes, or (3) a combination of the two. Scanning electron micrographs of the particles are presented in Fig. 9-1. The low-copper alloys are either irregular or spherical. Both morphologies contain silver and tin in the ratio approximating the intermetallic compound Ag_3Sn. High-copper alloys contain either all spherical particles of the same composition (unicompositional) or a mixture of irregular and spherical particles of different or the same composition (admixed).

When the particles have different compositions the admixed alloys are made by mixing particles of silver and tin with particles of silver and copper. The silver-tin particle is usually irregular, whereas the silver-copper particle is usually spherical in shape. The composition of the silver-tin particles in most commercial alloys is the same as that of the low-copper alloys. Different manufacturers, however, have somewhat different compositions for the silver-copper particle. The compositional ranges of the spherical silver-copper particles are shown in Table 9-1. The admixed regular alloy contains 33% to 60% spherical particles that have a composition close to the eutectic composition of Ag_3Cu_2 (see Fig. 5-16); the balance are irregular particles.

Like the admixed alloy, the unicompositional alloys have higher copper contents than the conventional lathe-cut or spherical low-copper alloys, but all the particles are spherical, as seen in Fig. 9-1. The silver content of the unicompositional alloys varies from 40% to 60%, and the copper content varies from 13% to 30%, with small variations in the tin content.

A high-copper admixed alloy is also available, in which both spherical and irregular particles have the same composition and the copper content is between 29 and 30%. High-copper alloys are less frequently supplied as unicompositional, irregular particles. The lathe-cut, high-copper alloys contain more than 23% copper.

Interest has increased in admixed amalgams containing 10-15% In in the mercury. The addition of In to Hg decreases the amount of Hg needed, decreases the Hg vapor during and after setting, and increases the wetting. These amalgams had low creep and lower early compressive strengths, but higher final strengths than comparable amalgams without indium. It is proposed that the lower levels of Hg vapor is due to oxides of In formed at the surface or the lower amount of Hg used in the mix.

It is estimated that over 90% of the dental amalgams currently placed are high-copper alloys. Of the high-copper alloys more admixed are used than spherical types with fewer irregularly shaped or lathe-cut types being selected. A high-copper alloy is selected to obtain a restoration with high early strength, low creep, good corrosion resistance, and good resistance to marginal fracture.

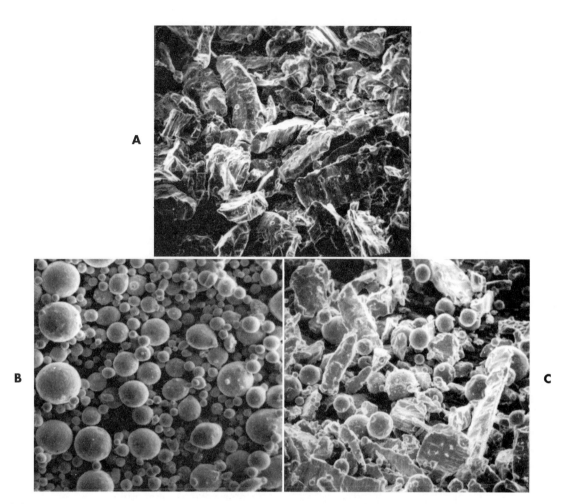

Fig. 9-1 Scanning electron micrographs of lathe-cut **A**, spherical **B**, and admixed **C**, amalgam alloys.

In general, alloy composition; particle size, shape, and distribution; and heat treatment control the characteristic properties of the amalgam.

Production

Irregular particles

To produce lathe-cut alloys, ingredient metals are heated, with protection from oxidation, until melted and then poured into a mold to form an ingot. The ingot is cooled relatively slowly with the formation of mainly Ag_3Sn (γ) and some Cu_3Sn (ϵ), Cu_6Sn_5 (η') and Ag_4Sn (β). After the ingot is completely cooled, it is heated for various periods of time (frequently 6 to 8 hours) at 400° C to produce a more homogeneous distribution of Ag_3Sn. The ingot is

then reduced to filings by being cut on a lathe and ball milled. The particles are passed through a fine sieve and then are ball milled to form the proper particle size. The particles are typically 60 to 120 μm in length, 10 to 70 μm in width, and 10 to 35 μm in thickness. Most products are labeled as fine-cut. The particle size and shape of lathe-cut amalgam alloys are shown in Fig. 9-1, *A*.

In general, freshly cut alloys amalgamate and set more promptly than aged particles, and some aging of the alloy is desirable to improve the shelf life of the product. The aging is related to relief of stress in the particles produced during the cutting of the ingot. The alloy particles are aged by subjecting them to a controlled temperature of 60° to 100° C for 1 to 6 hours. Irregularly shaped high-copper particles are made by spraying the molten alloy into water under high pressure.

Spherical particles

Spherical particles of low- or high-copper alloys are produced when all the desired elements are melted together. In the molten stage the metallic ingredients form the desired alloy. The liquid alloy is then sprayed under high pressure of an inert gas through a fine crack in a crucible into a large chamber. Depending on the surface energy difference between the molten alloy and that of the gas used in the spraying process, the shape of the sprayed particles may be spherical or somewhat irregular, as shown in Fig. 9-1, *B*. In addition, as seen in Fig. 9-1, *B*, the size of the spheres varies from 2 to 43 μm.

Silver-Tin Alloy

Because two of the principal ingredients in the amalgam alloy are silver and tin, it is appropriate to consider the binary system and the equilibrium phase diagram for these two metals, as shown in Fig. 9-2.

The most important feature in this diagram concerning the silver-tin alloy is that, when an alloy containing approximately 27% tin is slowly cooled below a temperature of 480° C, an intermetallic compound (Ag_3Sn), known also as the gamma (γ) phase, is produced. This Ag_3Sn compound is an important ingredient in the silver amalgam alloy and combines with mercury to produce a dental amalgam of desired mechanical properties and handling. This silver-tin compound is formed only over a narrow composition range. The silver content for such an alloy would be approximately 73%. Practically, the tin content is held between 26% and 30%, and the remainder of the alloy consists of silver, copper, and zinc. If the concentration of tin is less than 26%, the beta one (β$_1$) phase, which is a solid solution of silver and mercury, forms. In one product 5% tin is replaced by 5% indium, whereas another product contains less than 1% palladium. Addition of this small amount of palladium enhances the mechanical properties and corrosion resistance. The replacement of silver by an equal amount of copper produces a copper-tin compound (Cu_3Sn).

In general, larger (>30%) or smaller (<26%) quantities of tin in the alloy are detrimental to the final properties of the amalgam. The reason for this unfavorable shift in properties is generally considered to that the amount of Ag_3Sn is reduced as the percentage of tin is altered beyond the indicated limits. This is the basis for the alloy compositions of current products with acceptable properties, all being within rather narrow limits.

Silver-tin amalgam alloys compounded to produce largely Ag_3Sn react favorably with mercury to produce only slight dimensional setting changes when properly manipulated. The strength of the amalgam mass is greater from the Ag_3Sn compound than from an excess of tin. In addition, the setting time is shortened by an increase in silver content. Creep resistance is also superior when an alloy of Ag_3Sn is used rather than one with higher tin content.

■ AMALGAMATION PROCESSES

Low-Copper Alloys

The amalgam alloy is intimately mixed with liquid mercury to wet the surface of the particles so that the reaction between liquid mercury and alloy can proceed at a reasonable rate. This mixing is called trituration. During this process, mercury diffuses into the γ phase of the alloy particles and begins to react with the silver and tin portions of the particles, forming various compounds, predominantly silver-mercury and tin-mercury compounds, which depend on the exact composition of the alloy. The silver-mercury compound is Ag_2Hg_3 and is known as the gamma one (γ$_1$) phase, and the tin-mercury compound is $Sn_{7.8}Hg$ and is known as the gamma two (γ$_2$) phase. However, the silver-tin, silver-mercury, and tin-mercury phases are not pure. For example, Ag_3Sn always contains some copper and occasionally small amounts of zinc. The Ag_2Hg_3 dissolves small amounts (1% to 3%) of tin and Cu_6Sn_5 (η′), and similarly Cu_6Sn_5 could dissolve various elements present. Therefore γ, γ$_1$, and γ$_2$ are better descriptives of these three phases formed in dental amalgam than are the pure compounds.

While crystals of the γ$_1$ and γ$_2$ phases are being formed, the amalgam is relatively soft and easily condensable and carvable. As time progresses, more crystals of γ$_1$ and γ$_2$ are formed; the amalgam becomes

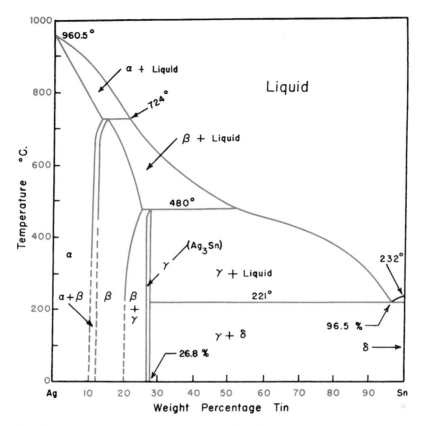

Fig. 9-2 Silver-tin phase diagram. (Adapted from Murphy AJ: *Inst Metals J* 35:107, 1926.)

harder and stronger, and it is no longer condensable or carvable. The lapse of time between the end of the trituration and when the amalgam hardens and no longer becomes workable is called working time.

The amount of liquid mercury used to amalgamate the alloy particles is not sufficient to react with the particles completely. Therefore the set mass of amalgam contains unreacted particles. About 27% of the original Ag_3Sn compound remains as unreacted particles. A simplified reaction of a low-copper amalgam alloy with mercury can be summarized in the following manner:

$$Ag_3Sn(\gamma) + Hg(l) \rightarrow Ag_2Hg_3(\gamma_1) + Sn_{7.8}Hg(\gamma_2) +$$
$$\text{excess} \qquad\qquad Ag_3Sn(\gamma) \text{ unreacted}$$

The dominating phase in a well-condensed, low-copper dental amalgam is the Ag_2Hg_3 (γ_1) phase, which is about 54% to 56% by volume. The percentages of the γ and the γ_2 phases are 27% to 35% and 11% to 13%, respectively.

High-Copper Alloys

The main difference between the low- and the high-copper alloys is not merely the percentage of copper but the effect that the higher copper content has on the amalgam reaction. The copper in these alloys is in either the silver-copper eutectic or Cu_3Sn form. The proper amount of copper causes most, if not all, of the γ_2 phase to be eliminated within a few hours after its formation or prevents its formation entirely. This phase is the weakest and most corrodible phase in the amalgam and causes shorter serviceability of amalgam restorations. Therefore high-copper amalgams tend to have superior physical and mechanical properties.

Reaction of mercury in an admixed high-copper alloy

During trituration, mercury diffuses into the amalgam particles and dissolves. The solubility of mercury in silver, tin, and copper differs considerably. A

1-mg amount of mercury dissolves in copper at the same time and temperature as 10 and 170 mg of mercury dissolves in silver and tin, respectively. Therefore particles composed mainly of silver and tin dissolve almost all the mercury, and very little mercury is dissolved by the silver-copper eutectic particles. The mercury dissolved in the silver-tin particles reacts as in low-copper alloys and forms the γ_1 and γ_2 phases, leaving some silver-tin particles unreacted. In a relatively short time, however, the newly formed γ_2 phase ($Sn_{7.8}Hg$) around the silver-tin particles reacts with silver-copper particles, forming Cu_6Sn_5, the eta' (η') phase of the copper-tin system, along with some of the γ_1 phase (Ag_2Hg_3) around the silver-copper particles. The amalgamation reaction may be simplified as follows:

$$Ag_3Sn(\gamma) + Ag\text{-}Cu \text{ (eutectic)} + Hg(l) \rightarrow Ag_2Hg_3(\gamma_1) +$$
$$Sn_{7.8}Hg(\gamma_2) + Ag_3Sn(\gamma) \text{ unreacted} +$$
$$Ag\text{-}Cu \text{ (eutectic) unreacted}$$

and later

$$Sn_{7.8}Hg(\gamma_2) + Ag\text{-}Cu \text{ (eutectic)} \longrightarrow Cu_6Sn_5(\eta') + Ag_2Hg_3(\gamma_1)$$

Reaction of mercury in a unicompositional alloy

In unicompositional alloys the difference in solubility of mercury in tin, silver, and copper also plays an important role. Because the solubility of mercury in tin is 170 times more than in copper and 17 times more than in silver, much more mercury dissolves and reacts with tin than with copper or silver. Thus tin in the periphery of the particle is depleted by the formation of the γ_2 phase, whereas the percentage of copper increases as a result of the limited reaction with mercury. As a result, particles of unicompositional alloys in the very early stages of setting are surrounded by γ_1 and γ_2 phases, whereas the periphery of a unicompositional alloy becomes an alloy of silver and copper. As with the admixed type of alloy, the γ_2 phase reacts with the silver-copper phase, forming Cu_6Sn_5 (η') and more Ag_2Hg_3 (γ_1).

The difference in the elimination of the γ_2 phase in an admixed and unicompositional alloy is that, in the admixed type, the γ_2 forms around the silver-tin particles and is eliminated around the silver-copper particles. In unicompositional alloys the particles at the beginning of the reaction function like silver-tin particles of the admixed type, providing proper working time and ease of manipulation. Later the same particles function like the silver-copper particles of the admixed type, eliminating the γ_2 phase.

The unicompositional particle is composed of a very fine distribution of Ag_3Sn (γ) and Cu_3Sn (ε). The overall simplified reaction with Hg is

$$Ag_3Sn(\gamma) + Cu_3Sn(\varepsilon) + Hg(l) \longrightarrow Cu_6Sn_5(\eta') + Ag_2Hg_3(\gamma_1)$$

Thus the reaction of mercury with either the high-copper admixed or the unicompositional alloys results in a final reaction, with Cu_6Sn_5 (η') being produced rather than $Sn_{7.8}Hg$ (γ_2).

In some high-copper alloys, there may be residual γ_2, less than 1%. Note that there is no definitive proof that the γ_2 phase ever forms, even temporarily. By the time electron microprobe analyses can be performed, the reaction will have reached equilibrium, and the final reaction products of η' and γ_1 will have already formed.

Microstructure of Amalgam

In dental applications the amount of liquid mercury used to amalgamate with the alloy particles is less than that required to complete the reaction. Thus the set amalgam mass consists of unreacted particles surrounded by a matrix of the reaction products. The reaction is principally a surface reaction, and the matrix bonds the unreacted particles together. The initial diffusion and reaction of mercury and alloy are relatively rapid, and the mass changes rapidly from a plastic consistency to a hard mass. Completion of the reaction may take several days to several weeks, which is reflected by the change in mechanical properties over this time.

The microstructures of set amalgam of the low-copper, lathe-cut, and spherical types are shown in Fig. 9-3. The outlines of the unreacted alloy particles (γ) are visible (*A*). The γ_1 and γ_2 phases in the matrix are identified by the letters *B* and *C,* respectively. Voids in each of the two samples are identified by the letter *D.* After the completion of the solid-state reaction in the high-copper admixed and unicompositional alloys, the microstructures show no γ_2 phase (Fig. 9-4).

■ PROPERTIES OF AMALGAM

Important properties for dental amalgam include dimensional changes, (compressive) strength, creep,

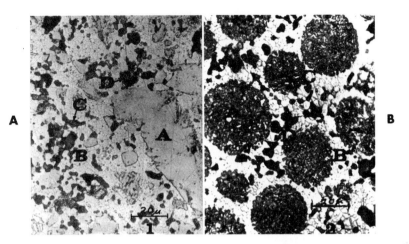

Fig. 9-3 Microstructure of set dental amalgam, etched with iodine etch. **A,** Lathe-cut particles: *A,* unreacted original particle, γ; *B,* γ$_1$; *C,* γ$_2$; *D,* void. **B,** Spherical alloy particles: *A,* original particle; *B,* γ$_1$; *C,* γ$_2$; *D,* void. (From Allen FC, Asgar K, Peyton FA: *J Dent Res* 44:1002, 1965.)

and corrosion resistance. These properties may be explained, in part, by the composition, microstructure, and manipulation of the amalgam.

ANSI/ADA Specification No. 1 for Amalgam Alloy

ANSI/ADA Specification No. 1 for amalgam alloy contains requirements that aid significantly to control the qualities of dental amalgam. The specification lists three physical properties as a measure of quality of the amalgam: creep, compressive strength, and dimensional change. When a cylindrical specimen is 7 days old, a 36 MPa stress is applied in a 37° C environment. Creep is measured between 1 and 4 hours of stressing. The maximum allowable creep is 3%. The minimum allowable compressive strength 1 hour after setting, when a cylindrical specimen is compressed at a rate of 0.25 mm/minute, is 80 MPa. The dimensional change between 5 minutes and 24 hours must fall within the range of ±20 μm/cm.

Physical and Mechanical Properties

Compressive strength

Resistance to compression forces is the most favorable strength characteristic of amalgam. Because amalgam is strongest in compression and much weaker in tension and shear, the prepared cavity design should maximize the compression forces in service and to minimize tension or shear forces. The early compressive strengths (after 1 hour of setting) for several low- and high-copper alloys are listed in Table 9-2. The percent mercury used in preparing the samples is also listed; the lathe-cut alloy requires the greatest amount of mercury, and the unicompositional alloy the least. Notice that amalgams are viscoelastic and the compressive strength is a function of the rate of loading. In general, the higher the rate of loading, the higher the compressive strength, although some studies have shown that at very high strain rates, compressive strength may decrease. As a result, when comparing the compressive strength of amalgam samples, it is imperative that they be tested at the same rate of loading.

When subjected to a rapid application of stress either in tension or in compression, a dental amalgam does not exhibit significant deformation or elongation and, as a result, functions as a brittle material. Therefore a sudden application of excessive forces to amalgam tends to fracture the amalgam restoration.

The high-copper unicompositional materials have the highest early compressive strengths of more than 250 MPa at 1 hour. The compressive strength at 1 hour was lowest for lathe-cut alloy (45 MPa), followed by one of the low-copper spherical alloys (88 MPa), and then two low-copper spherical alloys and the high-copper admixed alloy (118 to 141 MPa).

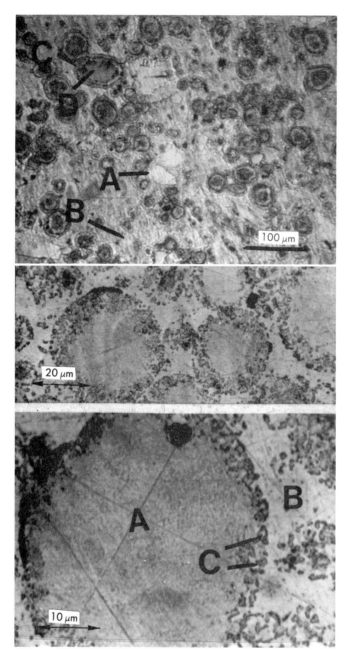

Fig. 9-4 Microstructure of high-copper admixed (*top*) and spherical unicompositional (*middle* and *bottom*) alloys. *Top, A* is an unreacted portion of γ; *B* is the γ_1 phase; *C* is the reaction zone around the Ag-Cu eutectic particle; *D* is an unreacted portion of a Ag-Cu particle. *Bottom, A* is an unreacted portion of a spherical unicompositional Ag-Sn-Cu particle; *B* is the γ_1 phase; *C* is the reaction zone around an original particle.

TABLE 9-2 Compressive Strength and Creep of Amalgams

Product	Mercury in Mix (%)	1-hr Compressive Strength (MPa) (0.5 mm/min)	7-Day Compressive Strength (MPa)		Creep (%)
			0.2 mm/min	0.05 mm/min	
LOW-COPPER ALLOYS					
Fine-cut					
Caulk 20th Century	53.7	45	302	227	6.3
Micro Cut					
Spherical					
Caulk Spherical	46.2	141	366	289	1.5
Kerr Spheraloy	48.5	88	380	299	1.3
Shofu Spherical	48.0	132	364	305	0.50
HIGH-COPPER ALLOYS					
Admixed					
Dispersalloy	50.0	118	387	340	0.45
Unicompositional					
Sybraloy	46.0	252	455	452	0.05
Tytin	43.0	292	516	443	0.09

Adapted from Malhotra ML, Asgar K: *J Am Dent Assoc* 96:446, 1978.

TABLE 9-3   Tensile Strength and Dimensional Change of Amalgams

Product	Tensile Strength at 0.5 mm/min, MPa		Dimensional Change (µm/cm)
	15 min	7 days	
LOW-COPPER ALLOYS			
Fine-cut			
Caulk 20th Century	3.2	51	−19.7
Micro Cut			
Spherical			
Caulk Spherical	4.7	55	−10.6
Kerr Spheraloy	3.2	55	−14.8
Shofu Spherical	4.6	58	−9.6
HIGH-COPPER ALLOYS			
Admixed			
Dispersalloy	3.0	43	−1.9
Unicompositional			
Sybraloy	8.5	49	−8.8
Tytin	8.1	56	−8.1

Adapted from Malhotra ML, Asgar K: *J Am Dent Assoc* 96:447, 1978.

These data indicate that only some of the older lathe-cut alloys would not meet the requirement for compressive strength at 1 hour of ANSI/ADA Specification No. 1. High values for early compressive strength are an advantage for an amalgam because they reduce the possibility of fracture by prematurely high contact stresses from the patient before the final strength is reached. The compressive strengths at 7 days, or the final strengths, again are highest for the high-copper unicompositional alloys, with only modest differences in the other alloys.

Tensile strength

The tensile strengths of various amalgams after 15 minutes and 7 days are listed in Table 9-3. The tensile strengths at 7 days for both non-γ_2 and γ_2-containing alloys are about the same. The tensile strengths are only a fraction of their compressive strengths; therefore cavity designs should be constructed to reduce tensile stresses resulting from biting forces.

The tensile strengths at 15 minutes for the high-copper unicompositional alloys are 75% to 175% higher than for the other alloys. However, no correlation exists between the tensile strengths at 15 minutes and 7 days. The high early tensile strengths of the high-copper unicompositional alloys are important because they resist fracture by premature biting stresses better than other amalgams.

Transverse strength

These values are sometimes referred to as the modulus of rupture, and because amalgams are brittle materials they can withstand little deformation during transverse strength testing. The main factors related to the high deformations are (1) the slow rates of load application, (2) high creep of the specific amalgam, and (3) higher temperature of testing. Thus high copper amalgams with low creep, should be supported by bases with high moduli in order to minimize deformation and transverse failure.

Strength of various phases

The relative strengths of the different amalgam phases are important. By studying the initiation and propagation of a crack in a set amalgam, the relative strength of the different phases can be observed. Fig. 9-5 shows the propagation of a crack in a dental amalgam specimen. It is possible to view the crack initiation and propagation of an amalgam specimen under a conventional metallographical

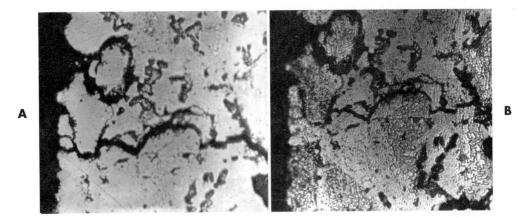

Fig. 9-5 Propagation of a crack in a dental amalgam. **A,** Unetched. **B,** After etching. (From Asgar K, Sutfin L: *J Dent Res* 44:985, 1965.)

microscope with a strain viewer. The propagation of the crack can be halted, and the specimen etched for the identification of the various phases. Results of such studies have led to the following ranking, from strongest to weakest, of the different phases of a set low-copper amalgam: Ag_3Sn (γ), the silver-mercury phase (γ_1), the tin-mercury phase (γ_2), and the voids.

Silver-mercury and tin-mercury act as a matrix to hold the unreacted amalgam alloy together. When relatively smaller amounts of silver-mercury and tin-mercury phases form, up to a certain minimum required for bonding together of the unreacted particles, a set amalgam is stronger. When a higher percentage of mercury is left in the final mass, it reacts with more of the amalgam alloy, producing larger amounts of silver-mercury and tin-mercury phases and leaving relatively smaller amounts of unreacted particles. The result is a weaker mass. Therefore the effect of various manipulative conditions can be explained in this manner. In high-copper amalgams, there is preferential crack propagation through the γ_1 phase and around copper-containing particles.

Elastic modulus

When the elastic modulus is determined at low rates of loading, such as 0.025 to 0.125 mm/min, values in the range of 11 to 20 GPa are obtained. High-copper alloys tend to be stiffer than low-copper alloys. If the rate of loading is increased so that the viscoelastic property does not significantly influence the elastic modulus, values of approximately 62 GPa have been obtained.

Creep

The viscoelastic properties of amalgam are also reflected by the creep or permanent deformation under static loads. Under a continued application of force in compression, an amalgam shows a continued deformation, even after the mass has completely set. Amalgam has no tendency for work hardening or for resisting deformation more effectively after the mass has been deformed, as may be experienced with the cast gold alloys.

Values for creep are determined in an instrument similar to that shown in Fig. 9-6. A cylindrical sample is placed in the position indicated by the arrow 7 days after preparation. A static stress of 36 MPa is applied by the spring. The change in length of the sample is determined at 37° ± 0.3° C by a calibrated differential transformer the output of which is recorded on a chart. The change in length between 1 hour after placement of the static stress and 4 hours after placement is used to calculate the percentage creep.

Creep values for various amalgams are listed in Table 9-2. The highest value of 6.3% was found for the low-copper cut alloy, and the lowest values (0.05% to 0.09%) were determined for the high-copper unicompositional spherical alloys. The high-copper admixed alloy and one of the low-copper alloys had slightly higher creep values of 0.45% to

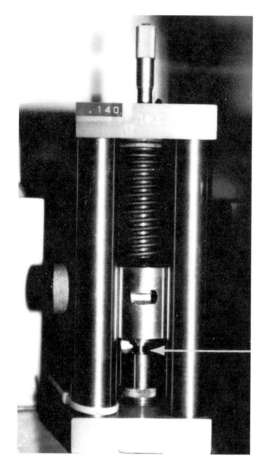

Fig. 9-6 An instrument for measuring creep of amalgam. Arrow points to specimen.

0.50%, and the remaining two low-copper spherical alloys had values of 1.3% to 1.5%. Creep data have been fit to both logarithmic and exponential relations.

Multiple regression analyses of creep data have shown that the most influential variables were volume percentage of the η' phase, grain size of the γ_1 phase, volume percentage of the γ and ε phases, number of very small η' crystals (less than 1.5 μm)/mm, and weight percentage of mercury. All of these values correlate negatively with creep, except weight percentage of mercury. When γ_1 has a concentration of tin greater than 1%, creep is controlled more by the distribution of tin and tin-mercury intergranular precipitates than by grain size. Following aging at oral temperature for 6 months, amalgam exhibits a decrease in creep. This decrease

in creep is related to β_1 formation and not to changes in either γ_1 grain size or composition.

A direct relationship exists between γ_2 content and a high incidence of marginal fracture of amalgam restorations. In addition, there is a general relationship between low static creep values and low marginal fracture in clinical service, which may be explained by the fact that the time to rupture under a constant load is inversely proportional to creep rate. Amalgams having higher compressive strengths at 7 days, determined at slow rates of loading, have demonstrated better marginal integrity. In general, amalgams having both low values of creep and high 7-day compressive strength at slow rates of loading have better clinical performance.

Note that the low creep values of high-copper amalgams increase the brittleness of the amalgam and decrease the relief of stresses at contact areas under load. As a result, a high-modulus base under a high-copper amalgam is essential to minimize deformation and the development of tensile stresses at the amalgam-cement base interface.

Dimensional change

The dimensional change during the setting of amalgam is one of its most characteristic properties. Current amalgams mixed with mechanical amalgamators have dimensional changes that are usually negative. The initial contraction at short times (the first 20 minutes) is believed to be associated with the solution of mercury in the alloy particles. After this period an expansion occurs, although the total change remains negative, which is believed to be a result of the reaction of mercury with silver and tin and the formation of the intermetallic compounds. The dimensions become nearly constant after 6 to 8 hours, and thus the values after 24 hours are final values. The only exception to this statement is the excessive delayed dimensional change resulting from contamination of a zinc-containing alloy with water during trituration or condensation.

The dimensional change may be determined with an instrument such as the one shown in Fig. 9-7. The amalgam specimens identified by the arrows are placed in position 5 minutes after setting, and the probe is placed on top of them. The probe is mechanically attached to a differential transformer, and the electrical output is used to determine the expansion or

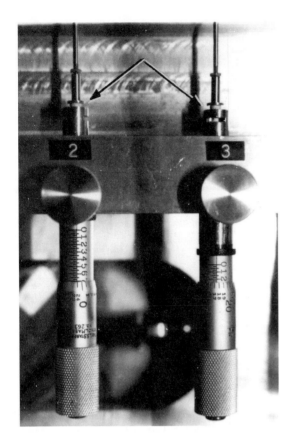

Fig. 9-7 An instrument for measuring dimensional change of amalgam. Arrows point to amalgam specimens.

contraction. The change in length can be determined continuously, although ANSI/ADA Specification No. 1 requires only the value at 24 hours.

The dimensional changes in micrometers per centimeter for the various alloys are listed in Table 9-3. The largest dimensional change of –19.7 μm/cm occurred with the low-copper, lathe-cut alloy, and the lowest change of –1.9 μm/cm was for the high-copper admixed alloy. The remainder of the alloys consisted of a group with values ranging from –8.8 to –14.8 μm/cm. All the amalgams meet the requirements of ANSI/ADA Specification No. 1 of ±20 μm/cm. Notice that the ranking of the dimensional change does not correlate with any of the other mechanical properties. The dimensional change is susceptible to influence from various manipulative factors, especially final mercury content. Higher mercury content results in less shrinkage but also in lower mechanical strength.

Some question remains concerning the significance of dimensional change with respect to clinical success. The belief was that if amalgam expanded during hardening, leakage around the margins of restorations would be eliminated. With current alloys and proper technics of trituration, however, most alloys show some shrinkage. Evidently the detrimental effect of shrinkage of amalgam occurs when the amalgam mass shrinks more than 50 μm/cm. ANSI/ADA Specification No. 1 for dental amalgam allows up to 20 μm/cm shrinkage, and no correlation of clinical success with the magnitude of the shrinkage determined in the laboratory has been shown. Furthermore, the expansion of an amalgam mass may seem to have a beneficial effect for one-surface restorations such as class 1 and 5 types but offers hardly any advantage when class 2 and 6 types of restorations are considered. The expanded amalgam around the cervical areas of class 2 and 6 restorations would have to pull away from the preparation, and it may have as undesirable an effect as the shrinking of amalgams for one-surface restorations.

Corrosion

In general, corrosion is the destructive attack of a metal by chemical or electrochemical reaction with its environment. Excessive corrosion can lead to increased porosity, reduced marginal integrity, loss of strength, and the release of metallic products into the oral environment.

The following compounds have been identified on dental amalgams in patients: SnO, SnO_2, $Sn_4(OH)_6Cl_2$, Cu_2O, $CuCl_2 \cdot 3Cu(OH)_2$, $CuCl$ as well as $CuSCN$ and $AgSCN$.

Because of their different chemical compositions, the different phases of an amalgam have different corrosion potentials. Electrochemical measurements on pure phases have shown that the Ag_2Hg_3 phase has the highest corrosion resistance, followed by Ag_3Sn, Ag_3Cu_2, Cu_3Sn, Cu_6Sn_5, and $Sn_{7-8}Hg$. However, the order of corrosion resistance assigned is true only if these phases are pure and they are not in the pure state in dental amalgam.

The presence of small amounts of tin, silver, and copper that may dissolve in various amalgam phases has a great influence on their corrosion resistance. The γ_1 phase has a composition close to Ag_2Hg_3

with 1% to 3% of dissolved tin. The higher the tin concentration of Ag_2Hg_3, the lower its corrosion resistance. In general, the tin content of the γ_1 phase is higher for low-copper alloys than for high-copper alloys. The presence of a relatively high percentage of tin in low-copper alloys reduces the corrosion resistance of their γ_1 phase so that it is lower than their γ phase. This is not true for high-copper alloys. The average depth of corrosion for most amalgam alloys is 100 to 500 μm.

In the low-copper amalgam system, the most corrodible phase is the tin-mercury, or γ_2 phase. Even though a relatively small portion (11% to 13%) of the amalgam mass consists of the γ_2 phase, in time and in an oral environment the structure of such an amalgam will contain a higher percentage of corroded phase. On the other hand, neither the γ nor the γ_1 phase is corroded as easily. Studies have shown that corrosion of the γ_2 phase occurs throughout the restoration, because it is a network structure. Corrosion results in the formation of tin oxychloride from the tin in the γ_2 and also liberates mercury, as shown in the following equation:

$$Sn_{7.8}Hg + \frac{1}{2}O_2 + H_2O + Cl^- \longrightarrow Sn_4(OH)_6Cl_2 + Hg$$

The reaction of the liberated mercury with unreacted γ can produce additional γ_1 and γ_2. It is proposed that the dissolution of the tin oxide or tin chloride and the production of additional γ_1 and γ_2 result in porosity and lower strength.

The high-copper admixed and unicompositional alloys do not have any γ_2 phase in the final set mass. The η' phase formed with high-copper alloys is not an interconnected phase such as the γ_2 phase, and it has better corrosion resistance. However, η' is the least corrosion-resistant phase in high-copper amalgams, and a corrosion product, $CuCl_2 \cdot 3Cu(OH)_2$, has been associated with storage of amalgams in synthetic saliva, as shown below.

$$Cu_6Sn_5 + \frac{1}{2}O_2 + H_2O + Cl^- \longrightarrow CuCl_2 \cdot 3Cu(OH)_2 + SnO$$

Phosphate buffer solutions inhibit the corrosion process; thus saliva may provide some protection of dental amalgams from corrosion.

A study of amalgams that had been in service for 2 to 25 years revealed that the bulk elemental compositions were similar to newly prepared amalgams, except for the presence of a small amount of chloride and other contaminants. The compositions of the phases were also similar to new amalgams, except for internal amalgamation of the γ particles. The distribution of phases in the clinically aged amalgams, however, differed from that of new amalgams. The low-copper amalgams had decreased amounts of γ, γ_1, and γ_2 and increased β_1 and tin-chloride. High-copper admixed amalgams had decreased γ, increased β_1, and enlarged reaction rings of γ_1 and η'. There was also evidence of a conversion of γ_1 to β_1 and γ_2 to η'.

Note that the processes of corrosion and wear are frequently coupled and that wear can lower the corrosion potential and increase the corrosion rate by an order of magnitude.

Fig. 9-8 compares an amalgam restoration on the distal portion of a tooth prepared from a low-copper spherical alloy with one on the mesial portion prepared from high-copper admixed alloy. The restorations have been in service for 3 years, and the higher marginal fracture, presumably resulting from the corrosion of the γ_2 phase of the low-copper amalgam, is readily apparent.

Surface tarnish of low-copper amalgams is more associated with γ than γ_1, whereas in high-copper amalgams surface tarnish is related to the copper-rich phases, η' and silver-copper eutectic.

Properties of Mercury

ANSI/ADA Specification No. 6 for dental mercury requires that the mercury has a clean reflecting surface that is free from a surface film when agitated in air. It should have no visible evidence of surface contamination and contain less than 0.02% non-volatile residue. Mercury that complies with the requirements of the United States Pharmacopeia (USP) also meets requirements for purity in ANSI/ADA Specification No. 6. Mercury amalgamates with small amounts of many metals and is contaminated by sulfur gases in the atmosphere, which combine with the mercury to form sulfides. Small quantities of these foreign materials in the mercury destroy its bright, mirrorlike surface and can be readily detected by visual inspection.

Mercury, which has a freezing point of –38.87° C, is the only metal that remains in the liquid state at room temperatures. It combines readily to form

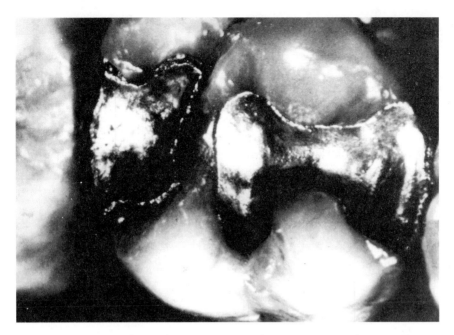

Fig. 9-8 Amalgam restoration from a low-copper spherical alloy (*left*) and an amalgam from a high-copper admixed alloy (*right*) after 3 years of service. (Courtesy Charbeneau GT, Ann Arbor, 1979, University of Michigan School of Dentistry.)

an amalgam with several metals such as gold, silver, copper, tin, and zinc, but does not combine under ordinary conditions with such metals as nickel, chromium, molybdenum, cobalt, and iron.

Mercury boils at 356.9° C, and, if pure, has a significant vapor pressure at room temperature. Extended inhalation can result in mercury poisoning. Globules dropped on a surface roll about freely without leaving a tail and retain their globular form. This tendency to form globules is related to the high surface tension of liquid mercury, which is 465 dynes/cm at 20° C, as compared with 72.8 dynes/cm for water. Mercury with a very high degree of purity exhibits a slight tarnish after a short time because impurities contaminate the metal and produce a dull surface appearance. Impurities in mercury can reduce the rate at which it combines with the silver alloy.

■ MANIPULATION OF AMALGAM

Selection of Alloy

The selection of an alloy involves a number of factors, including particle size, particle shape, and composition, particularly as it relates to the elimina-

tion of the γ_2 phase and the presence or absence of zinc. It is estimated that over 90% of the dental amalgams currently placed are high-copper alloys. The majority of the alloys selected are spherical-unicompositional or admixed types with the admixed being favored slightly. A high-copper alloy is selected because a restoration with no γ_2, high early strength, low creep, good corrosion resistance, and good resistance to marginal fracture results.

Finer particle sizes are used for low-copper, irregular alloys because of improved properties and enhanced clinical convenience. Finer particles produce a smoother surface during carving and finishing. The clinical manipulation of dental amalgam alloys is influenced to a modest extent by the shape of the particles. Lathe-cut alloys exhibit rough, irregular surfaces having a large area-to-volume ratio to react with mercury, and generally require nearly 50% or more mercury to obtain adequate plasticity during trituration. Spherical alloys are smoother, consist of various sizes of spheres (2 to 43 μm), which is important in packing, have more regular surfaces with a lower area-to-volume ratio, and generally require less mercury for trituration and suitable plasticity development. Mercury concentrations as low as 42% permit acceptable handling characteristics with certain products.

The lathe-cut and spherical alloys react differently to condensation forces. These differences result from frictional forces within the amalgam mass that offer higher resistance to the face of the condenser in lathe-cut alloys than in spherical alloys. Carving the excess amalgam from the overfilled cavity to restore morphological and functional anatomy presents further differences.

Because of improved manufacturing, few products contain zinc because the contamination of a zinc-containing alloy by moisture may result in excessive dimensional change. If an alloy contains more than 0.01% zinc, the package must carry a printed precaution that the amalgam made from the material will show excessive corrosion and expansion if moisture is introduced during mixing and condensation.

Proportions of Alloy to Mercury

Correct proportioning of alloy and mercury is essential for forming a suitable mass of amalgam for placement in a prepared cavity. Some alloys require mercury-alloy ratios in excess of 1:1 whereas others use ratios of less than 1:1, with the percentage of mercury varying from 43-54%. Automatic mechanical dispensers for alloy and mercury have been used in the past and are described in previous editions of this textbook. With the recommendation for "no touch" procedures for handling mercury and amalgam, capsules with preproportioned amounts of alloy and mercury have been substituted for mercury and alloy dispensers. The correct amounts of alloy and mercury are kept separated in the capsule by a membrane as shown in the sketch in Fig. 9-9. Just prior to trituration of the mix the membrane is ruptured by compression of the capsule or is automatically activated during trituration. Various manufacturers' amalgam alloys with their corresponding capsules are shown in Fig. 9-10. Some capsules contain a plastic pestle in the shape of a disk or rod as illustrated in the disassembled capsules in Fig. 9-11. In order to prevent any escape of mercury from the friction-fitted capsule during trituration some capsules are hermetically sealed and in this instance the mercury is contained in a small plastic film packet that ruptures during mixing.

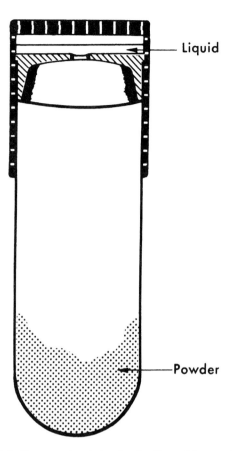

Fig. 9-9 Cross-sectional sketch of a disposable capsule containing amalgam alloy and mercury.

Size of mix

Manufacturers commonly supply capsules containing 400, 600, or 800 mg of alloy and the appropriate amount of Hg. The capsules containing different weights of alloy are color coded for ease of identification. Clinical concensus is that these amounts are sufficient for most restorations. It is usually suggested that if larger amounts are required that several smaller mixes be made at staggered times so the consistency of the mixed amalgam remains reasonably constant during the preparation of the restoration. However capsules containing 1200 mg of alloy are available if a large amount of amalgam is needed for producing an amalgam core on a severely broken-down tooth.

Mixing of Amalgam

Trituration of amalgam alloy and mercury is done with a mechanical mixing device called an

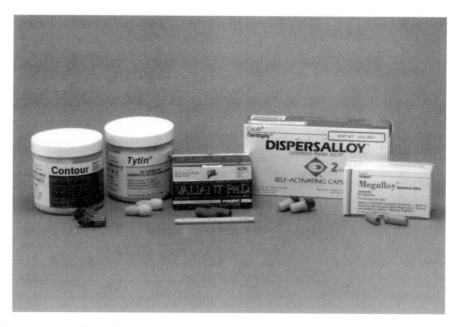

Fig. 9-10 Various amalgam alloys with their corresponding capsules. Note that Tytin and Megalloy are spherical alloys, and Dispersalloy, Contour, and Valiant Ph D are admixed alloys. (From Craig RG, O'Brien WJ, Powers JM: *Dental Materials: properties and manipulation,* ed 6, St Louis, 1996, Mosby.)

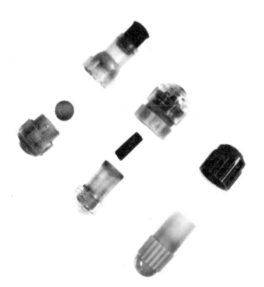

Fig. 9-11 Types of capsules with and without pestles.

amalgamator. Two recent amalgamators are shown in Fig. 9-12. They have controls for the speed and the time of trituration. The amalgamator shown on the left has a slot on the lower right for the insertion of plastic cards. There is a separate card for each size mix and insertion of the card automatically sets the correct mixing time and speed. Each of the amalgamators has a housing that is placed over the capsule area during trituration to confine any mercury lost from the capsule during mixing.

The capsule holder is attached to a motor that rotates the holder and capsule eccentrically. The trituration may be accomplished simply by the agitation of the alloy particles and mercury or the manufacturer may have included a plastic pestle to aid in the mixing.

Spherical or irregular low-copper alloys may be triturated at low speed (low energy), but most high-copper alloys require high speed (high energy). Mechanical amalgamators show some variation in speed with the amount of alloy and mercury in the capsules and this can be adjusted for by changing the time or speed. The trituration work is a combination of the time and speed of mixing. Time of amalgamation is the easiest factor to vary; however, it should be emphasized that variations of 2 to 3 seconds of mixing time may be enough to produce an amalgam that is considered to be under- or overmixed.

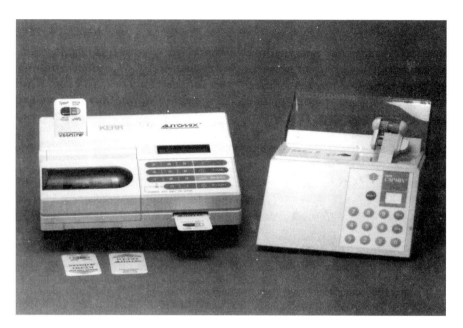

Fig. 9-12 Mechanical amalgamators for triturating amalgam. Note that both amalgamators have housings that are closed over the area of the capsules to confine any mercury that may inadvertantly leak from the capsule during trituration. (From Craig RG, O'Brien WJ, Powers JM: *Dental Materials: properties and manipulation,* ed 6, St Louis, 1996, Mosby.)

Low-, medium-, and high-speed amalgamators operate at about 32-3400, 37-3800, and 40-4400 cycles per minute at correct live voltage. However, an amalgamator set at low speed of 3300 cpm may actually be operating at 3000 cpm with a decrease in line voltage from 120 to 100 volts, and undermixed amalgams may result. This problem can be avoided by installing a voltage regulator between the line plug and the amalgamator. Using a parameter called the coherence time (t_c), defined as the minimum mixing time required for an amalgam to form a single coherent pellet, it has been found that the compressive strength, dimensional change, and creep are optimized if mixing is carried out for a time of $5t_c$. The value of t_c can be determined experimentally for a particular amalgam alloy, size of mix, and speed of the amalgamator. However, most packages of amalgam alloys will contain recommendations for times and speeds for a variety of amalgamators and these guidelines should be followed.

With the introduction of disposable capsules containing predispensed amounts of amalgam alloy and mercury, the mercury and alloy dispensers have become absolute as have reusable capsules.

However their selection and use are described in the ninth and earlier editions of this textbook.

Undermix, normal mix, and overmix

Undermixing, normal mixing, or overmixing can result from variations in the condition of trituration of the alloy and mercury. The three mixes have a different appearance and respond differently to subsequent manipulation. The undermixed amalgam appears dull and crumbly, the normal mix appears shiny and separates in a single mass from the capsule, and the overmixed amalgam appears soupy and tends to stick to the inside of the capsule. Examples of these mixes are shown in Fig. 9-13. The three types of mixes have characteristically different mechanical properties of dimensional change, strength, and creep. These three conditions can be developed from variations in the mixing variables described earlier. Therefore the type of mix contributes to the success or failure of the amalgam restoration.

Not all types of alloys respond in the same manner to overtrituration and undertrituration. Spherical and lathe-cut alloys respond differently.

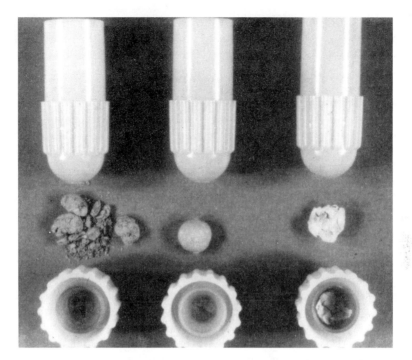

Fig. 9-13 Undermixed amalgam, *left;* normal mix, *center,* overmixed amalgam, *right.* (Courtesy Dr. K Asgar, University of Michigan School of Dentistry, Ann Arbor, Mich.) (From Craig RG, O'Brien WJ, Powers JM: *Dental Materials: properties and manipulation,* ed. 6, St Louis, 1996, Mosby.)

The effect of overtrituration and undertrituration of amalgam on working time, dimensional change, compressive and tensile strengths, and creep is summarized as follows.

Working time. Working time of all types of amalgam, spherical or irregular, decreases with overtrituration. High- or low-copper alloys respond alike.

Dimensional change. Overtrituration results in slightly higher contraction for all types of alloys. High- and low-copper alloys show the same effect.

Compressive and tensile strengths. Both compressive and tensile strengths of irregular-shaped alloys increase by overtrituration. However, this is not true for spherical alloys. Compressive and tensile strengths of spherical alloys are greatest at normal trituration time. Both overtrituration and undertrituration reduce compressive and tensile strengths. The admixed high-copper alloys consist of both shapes of particles and behave like spherical alloys; normal trituration times produce the highest strength values with overtrituration resulting in significant decreases in strength.

Creep. Overtrituration increases creep, and undertrituration lowers it. As mentioned earlier in this chapter, two properties that are closely related to the clinical behavior of alloys are low creep and high compressive strength. By overtriturating irregular amalgams, a higher compressive strength can be obtained, which is beneficial. However, the amalgam has a higher creep, a property that is not desirable. If there is doubt about the correct trituration time, a slightly overtriturated amalgam is better than a slightly undertriturated one. This suggestion is particularly true for high-copper alloys.

Some manufacturers recommend alteration of the trituration time to obtain a longer or shorter working time. Alteration of the trituration time does change the working time of amalgam, but it also affects other properties. When amalgam is triturated for shorter-than-normal times, mercury does not completely wet the outer surface of amalgam particles. As a result, mercury does not react with the amalgam alloy over the entire surface of the particle. The mass remains soft for a longer period of time, producing an amalgam with a longer working time. Such an amalgam mass contains excessive amounts of porosity, has lower strength, and possesses poorer corrosion resistance.

Overtrituration reduces working time, causing the reaction rate to increase because the amalgamated mass becomes hot. When amalgams with longer or shorter working times are desired, one should use amalgam alloys that are designed to react faster or slower and not attempt to achieve the change by altering the trituration time.

Condensation of Amalgam

During condensation, adaptation of the amalgam mass to the cavity walls is accomplished and the operator controls the amount of mercury that will remain in the finished restoration, which in turn influences the dimensional change, creep, and compressive strength. In general, the more mercury left in the mass after condensation, the weaker the alloy. With irregularly shaped alloys, in which a higher percentage of mercury is used initially, the operator should remove as much mercury as possible during condensation by using as great a force as possible on the condenser. With spherical alloys, the initial mercury is lower, and it is not necessary to remove as much mercury as for the irregularly shaped alloys; however, increasing the condensation pressure from 3 to 7 MPa results in a significant increase in compressive strength. Further increase in condensation pressure to 14 MPa does not result in additional compressive strength.

Hand or mechanical condensation

A large number of instruments designed for hand condensation of amalgam have been available to the dental profession for many years. The instruments and the technic for their use have been described in textbooks of operative dentistry.

In general, a suitable instrument for hand condensation of amalgam would be shaped so that the operator could readily grasp it and exert a force of condensation by appropriately placing one finger on a finger rest of the instrument. Hand instruments that do not permit a convenient grasping may inhibit proper condensation practices and mercury removal. In many instances, circular condenser tips may prove adequate, whereas in other cavity areas and design,

the triangular, oval, crescent, or other shape of tip may be effective. In general, a condenser tip that is too small in cross section tends to be ineffective in condensing a reasonable quantity of amalgam. The size of the condenser tip and the direction and magnitude of the force placed on the condenser also depend on the type of amalgam alloy selected.

With irregularly shaped alloys, one should use condensers with a relatively small tip, 1 to 2 mm, and apply high condensation forces in a vertical direction. During condensation, as much mercury-rich mass as possible should be removed from the restoration.

When condensers with small tips are used with high condensation forces on spherical amalgams, the particles tend to roll over one another, the tip penetrates the amalgam, and the mass does not adapt well to the cavity walls. With spherical alloys one should use condensers with larger tips, almost as large as the cavity permits. For example, at the cervical margin of a class 2 preparation with a small opening, a condenser with a very small tip should be used. As the cavity is filled and the opening toward the occlusal surface becomes larger, condensers with larger tips should be used. Because of the spherical shape of the particles, a lateral direction of condensation provides better adaptation of amalgam to cavity walls than of condensation toward the pulpal floor. With high-copper spherical amalgams, a vertical and lateral direction of condensation with vibration is recommended.

Small-to-medium diameter condensers are advocated with admixed high-copper alloys with a medium-to-high force and vertical and lateral directions of condensation.

Many mechanical devices are available for condensing amalgam. These devices are more popular and more useful for condensing irregularily shaped alloys when high condensation forces are required. With the development of spherical alloys, the need for mechanical condensers was eliminated. Ultrasonic condensers are not recommended because during condensation they increase the mercury vapor level to values above the safety standards for mercury in the dental office.

Effect of delay in condensation

It is important that an amalgam be condensed into the tooth cavity promptly after the mercury and alloy are suitably mixed. Delay of the condensation operation permits the amalgam to set partially before being transferred to the cavity, which in turn makes it impossible to remove the mercury effectively during condensation. As a result, an amalgam mass that has remained uncondensed for any period of time will contain more mercury than one that is condensed promptly. The resulting amalgam with the additional mercury content will show less strength in compression and higher creep. Delay in the condensation operation reduces the plasticity of the mix, and amalgams with reduced plasticity do not adapt well to the cavity walls. In a large restoration involving considerable time to place the amalgam mass, condensation of the final portions of amalgam becomes a problem. In such cases, it is preferable to make two smaller mixes of amalgam rather than one excessively large mix and not to use the amalgam if more than 3 or 4 minutes have elapsed from the time of initial mixing.

Mercury content of amalgam restorations

Amalgam restorations containing greater amounts of mercury in the set mass demonstrate less favorable clinical characteristics. Having more mercury in the set amalgam produces a greater amount of Ag_2Hg_3 and $Sn_{7-8}Hg$, the γ_1 and γ_2 phases, thereby leaving less unreacted Ag_3Sn, the γ phase. As discussed earlier, both γ_1 and γ_2 have lower strength than the γ phase. Therefore when amalgam specimens are subjected to compressive stress, those containing increasing quantities of mercury exhibit decreasing strength values. The compressive strength decreases 1% for each 1% increase in mercury above 60%.

The mercury content of an amalgam restoration is not uniform throughout. Higher concentrations of mercury are located around the margins of the restoration. As a result, cavities should be overfilled and then carved back to minimize this problem. When using alloys that require higher mercury-to-alloy ratios, as much mercury as possible should be removed from the amalgamated mass. Note that the maximum allowable amount of mercury remaining in a hardened amalgam mass depends on the original mercury-to-alloy ratio. In other words, for alloys requiring high mercury-to-alloy ratios for trituration, 50% mercury in the hardened amalgam might be

acceptable; however, for alloys needing low mercury-to-alloy ratios for trituration, 50% mercury in the set amalgam would be detrimental.

Although the lower mercury-to-alloy ratios currently being used are favorable regarding the total quantity of mercury in the set mass, remember that condensation forces alter mercury content within the restoration. Because condensation brings mercury to the surface of the amalgam mass, such "plashy" material should be periodically removed when filling the cavity to prevent trapping high mercury concentrations within the restoration. Overfilling of the cavity is carried out for the same reason—to remove the amalgam that contains higher mercury content from the restoration contour.

When alloys that permit lower mercury-to-alloy ratios are used to obtain a plastic mass suitable for condensation, the operator should expect a lesser volume of excess mercury to be brought to the surface for removal than was observed with older materials.

Moisture contamination during insertion

Moisture contamination during the mixing and condensing operations is the factor that may produce excessive expansion. There is no evidence, however, that the presence of moisture on the surface will cause any serious damage once the condensation operation is completed and the restoration is finished, except for trimming and polishing.

Because moisture in the saliva is a potential source of contamination for the amalgam, the tooth cavity must remain dry and the amalgam must be free from contamination with saliva. Technics and procedures in operative dentistry provide for such a dry field of operation, and these technics should be followed faithfully. In the past the presence of saliva on the amalgam during condensation probably was a true source of excessive delayed expansion and other poor qualities in the restoration.

Moisture contamination of a zinc-containing amalgam mass from any source results in an excessive delayed expansion of several hundred micrometers per centimeter after the restoration has been placed in the tooth for several hours or days. This excessive expansion results from the decomposition of moisture. The trapped hydrogen gas in the amalgam restoration continues to be developed until sufficient force is produced to cause the excessive expansion. This decomposition of moisture results from the presence of zinc in the amalgam alloy and can be overcome by the use of nonzinc alloys.

Factors Related to Finishing Amalgam Restorations

When an amalgam restoration has been properly placed, with adequate condensation, and the excess mercury has been removed from the final surface layer of the restoration, it will be sufficiently hardened within a few minutes to permit careful carving. If the restoration is not well condensed, it will not harden promptly, and the carving operation must be delayed. Usually the amalgam is sufficiently well set and hardened that carving with sharp instruments can be started almost immediately after condensation.

Burnishing, or rubbing the newly condensed amalgam with a metal instrument having a broad surface contact, can be employed to smooth the surface, thereby making the amalgram more susceptible to finishing and polishing. Burnishing can produce a tenfold reduction in surface roughness.

If final finishing and polishing are to be done at a second appointment, the restoration should be left undisturbed for a period of at least 24 hours. The patient should be cautioned that the freshly inserted restoration is relatively weak and that heavy biting forces should be avoided for a few hours after the time of insertion. Occlusal contacts must be carefully established. However, current all-spherical high-copper alloys have a much higher early strength than other types and can withstand biting forces sooner than earlier amalgams. One-hour compressive strengths of spherical high-copper alloys are about twice as high as high-copper admixed types and are comparable with those of low-copper alloys at 6 to 7 hours.

High-copper amalgams with high early strengths can be finished at the first appointment. After condensation the surface is burnished and carved for clear definition of the margins, and all excess amalgam is removed. A creamy paste of triple-x silex and water is applied gently with an unwebbed rubber cup and a slow-speed handpiece. Light pressure should be applied for no more than 30 seconds per surface, and polishing should be directed from the center toward the margins of the restoration.

This early finishing begins 8 to 10 minutes after the start of trituration, depending on the particular alloy. Results of a 3-year clinical study have shown that restorations polished 8 minutes after trituration and those polished after 24 hours had no difference in longevity. Also, as time in the mouth increased, it became difficult to determine which method had been used to finish the restoration. The 24-hour polishing procedure used in the study was that normally used for polishing amalgam restorations. The procedure used for the 8-minute polish was different; no polishing bur was used, and the amalgam was carved carefully. Because the 24-hour polishing technic requires a second appointment, many restorations go without polishing. The main advantage of the 8-minute polishing technic is the elimination of the second appointment. This technic is limited to those amalgams that have high early compressive strengths.

A well-finished and well-polished restoration will retain its surface appearance and be easier to keep clean than one that is poorly finished. This belief relates to the fact that a rough surface on the restoration contains microscopic pits in which acids and small food particles from the mouth accumulate. These tend to encourage galvanic action on the surface of the restoration to develop a tarnish and perhaps even a corroded appearance.

The final polish at a second appointment is developed through a series of final finishing and polishing steps after a careful carving operation (Table 9-4). This final polish is accomplished through a sequence of operations that includes the use of fine stones and abrasive disks or strips. To develop the final polish, a rotating soft brush is used to apply a suitable polishing agent, such as extrafine silex, followed by a thin slurry of tin oxide.

During the final polishing operation, the restoration should remain moist to avoid overheating from the use of dry polishing surfaces. Because the amalgam is weak in tension and shear resistance, it should not be drawn over the margin by burnishing or drawing operations that tend to produce extensions that subsequently will be fractured from the amalgam mass. To avoid such overextensions, all recommended operative practices should be followed faithfully.

TABLE 9-4   Average Surface Roughness of Dental Amalgam Produced by Various Methods of Instrumentation

Method of Instrumentation	Average Surface Roughness (μm)	Method of Instrumentation	Average Surface Roughness (μm)
Carved	4.62*	*Rotating Polish Instruments–cont'd*	
Carved and immediately smoothened	0.36*	B.S. Rubber cup with Amalgloss	0.28
Condensed against uncontoured matrix band	0.61	No. 11 soft Robinson Brush	
		with flour of pumice	0.31
Dental tape used immediately on above	1.92	with extrafine silex	0.18
		with tin oxide	0.15
Rotating Finishing Instruments		Robinson soft cup brush	
S.S. White Green stone	0.64-1.02*	with flour of pumice	0.20
Finishing bur	0.46-0.64*	with Caulk Zircate	0.18
Moore's Adalox Coarse (wet)	1.19	with extrafine silex	0.18*
Medium (wet)	0.74	with tin oxide	0.10*
Fine (wet)	0.81		
Moore's Waterproof Fine (wet)	0.59*	*Interproximal Finishing Strips*	
Moore's Medium Sand	1.22	R and R Medium Cuttle	1.02
Fine Sand	0.76	Fine Cuttle	0.69
Medium Cuttle	0.53	Extrafine Cuttle	0.31
Fine Cuttle	0.30	Moyco "Evenwet" Medium	
Dedeco "Interprox" wheel	0.23	Cuttle (wet)	0.69
		Fine Cuttle (wet)	0.61
Rotating Polishing Instruments		Extrafine Sand (wet)	0.31*
No. 11 soft Robinson Brush, with Mynol Proph Paste	0.41	Above + Dentotape (J and J) with extrafine silex	0.23
B.S. Rubber polishing cup with Mynol Paste	0.38	Extrafine Sand + Dentotape with tin oxide	0.15
No. 11 soft Robinson Brush with Amalgloss	0.28	Extrafine Sand + Dentotape with silex + tin oxide	0.10*

From Charbeneau GT: *Mich Dent Assoc J* 47:320, 1965.
*Suggested sequence for finishing and polishing an occlusoproximal amalgam restoration.

Bonding of Amalgam

Although amalgam has been a highly successful restorative material when used as an intracoronal restoration it does not restore the strength of the clinical crown to its original strength. Pins of various types have been used with amalgam to increase retention of the restoration, but they do not reinforce the amalgam and increase its strength.

With the development of adhesive systems for dental composites came the opportunity to attempt to bond amalgams to tooth structure. Adhesive plastics containing 4-META, an acronym for 4-methacryloxyethyl trimellitate anhydride (see Chapter 10), have been the most successful products. Shear bond strengths of amalgam to dentin as high as 10 MPa have been reported using these adhesives. Comparable values for the shear bond strength of microfilled composites to dentin using these same adhesives have been 20-22 MPa. The fracture resistance of teeth restored with amalgam-bonded MOD restorations was more than twice those containing unbonded amalgams. Also, in spite of the lower shear strength of amalgam bonded to dentin test samples compared to composites, the fracture strength of MODs in teeth restored with bonded amalgams was as high as for composites although neither were as high (45-80%) as values for the intact tooth. As expected amalgam bonded MODs having narrow preparations had higher strengths than those with wide preparations. Other studies showed the retention of amalgam-bonded MODs with proximal boxes was as great as pin-retained amalgams. In addition, amalgam-bonded restorations decreased marginal leakage in Class V restorations compared to unbonded amalgams. Finally, the plastic bonding agents for amalgam have not been successful in increasing the amalgam-to-amalgam bond strength in the repair of amalgam restorations. Thus at this stage of development, adhesive bonding of amalgam restorations to tooth structures is an improvement over nonbonded amalgams.

■ MERCURY TOXICITY

Amalgams have been used for 150 years and about 200 million amalgams are inserted each year in the United States and Europe. Therefore amalgam use has a substantial history, although periodically, concern arises about the biocompatibility of amalgam. Allergic reactions to mercury in amalgam restorations do occur, albeit infrequently. This is not surprising because there is no material that 100% of the population is immune to 100% of the time. However, such allergic responses usually disappear in a few days or if not on removal of the amalgam, and aside from varying reports of mercury accumulation, no other local or systemic effects from mercury contained in dental amalgam have been demonstrated. If amalgam is used correctly, biocompatibility should not be a problem.

Even in their passive condition, metals are not inert. Both *in vitro* and *in vivo* experiments have established that there is a passive dissolution from all metals. Linked to the issues of dissolution, corrosion, and potential allergic response and toxicity are eight questions:
1. Is any material released into the mouth?
2. What material is released?
3. What is the form of the released material?
4. How much material is released?
5. In what subsequent reactions do the released products get involved?
6. What percentage of the released products is excreted and what percentage is retained?
7. Where does the retained percentage accumulate?
8. What biological response(s) will result from the retained fraction?

Therefore any analysis of the literature and discussion of mercury toxicity, namely in amalgams, must continually refer to these eight questions, particularly questions 3 and 4, relating to the dosage and form of the mercury to which the body is exposed.

Sources of Mercury

In addressing these eight questions, the source(s) of the potential toxins must be evaluated. Exposure to mercury can occur from many different sources, including diet, water, air, and occupational exposure (Table 9-5). The World Health Organization (WHO) has estimated that eating seafood once a week raises urine mercury levels to 5 to 20 $\mu g/L$, two to eight times the level of exposure from amalgam (1 $\mu g/L$ = 1 mg/m^3 = 1 part per billion [ppb]). Thus the amount of mercury vapor released from amalgam is less than that received from eating many common fish. It has been estimated that a patient with 9 amalgam occlusal surfaces will inhale only 1.7 mg of mercury per day, which is about 1% of the amount inhaled in a work place 8 hours a day, 5 days a week with the level allowed by OSHA (50 mg Hg/m^3 of air). Blood and urine mercury levels are easily influenced by other factors and cannot often be directly linked to amalgam. In general, elemental mercury from amalgam seems to make only a small contribution to the total body burden of mercury. On the basis of epidemiological studies, blood and serum mercury levels correlate highly with occupational exposure and diet, whereas urine mercury relates to amalgam burden. Urine mercury levels relate to methods of condensation and ventilation more than to the amalgam per se.

Forms of Mercury

Mercury has many forms, including organic and inorganic compounds. The most toxic organic compounds are methyl and ethyl mercury, and the next most toxic form is mercury vapor. The least toxic forms of mercury are the inorganic compounds. Liquid mercury reacts with silver to form an inorganic silver-mercury compound via a metallic bond. Reports of people and animals being poisoned by

TABLE 9-5 Estimated Daily Intake of Mercury

Source	μg Hg Vapor	μg Inorganic Hg	μg Methyl Hg
Atmosphere	0.12	0.038	0.034
Drinking water	–	0.05	–
Food, fish	0.94	–	3.76
Food, nonfish	–	20.00	–

eating food high in mercury are traced to the contamination of these foods by methyl mercury.

Mercury vapor is released, in minute quantities, during all procedures involving amalgam, including mixing, setting, polishing, and removal. Mercury vapor has also been reported to be released during mastication and drinking hot beverages. The amount of mercury on amalgam surfaces has correlated with the quantity of mercury used during trituration. However, measuring the flow and flow rate is difficult and not precise, especially when working with a small area such as the mouth. Furthermore, ambient mercury must be considered especially if such readings are taken in a dentist's office. With good ventilation mercury levels return to background levels in 10-20 minutes after placing an amalgam, and a charcoal filter system decreases levels 25% during the operative procedure. Fresh amalgams release more mercury than 2-year-old amalgams even with a *Strep. mutans* biofilm and it has been shown that most oral organisms can grow in dental plaque containing 2 μg of mercury. Under normal conditions amalgam is covered by saliva, tending to reduce vapor pressure. Amalgams can also be constrained with a sealant resin for the first several days after insertion. Addition of indium (8% to 14%) also decreases the vapor pressure.

Concentrations of Mercury

The Occupational Safety and Health Administration (OSHA) has set a Threshold Limit Value (TLV) of 0.05 mg/m^3 as the maximum amount of mercury vapor allowed in the workplace. Nearly all dental offices worldwide comply with this standard. As an example of the factor of safety in this boundary, the fetuses of pregnant rats exposed to atmospheres with mercury concentrations of 2 mg/m^3 showed no ill effects. Fetuses exposed to mercury concentrations of 5 mg/m^3, or 40 times the allowable concentration, were stillborn. The lowest dose of mercury that illicits a toxic reaction is 3 to 7 μg/kg body weight. Paresthesia (tingling of extremities) occurs at about 500 μg/kg of body weight, followed by ataxia at 1000 μg/kg of body weight, joint pain at 2000 μg/kg of body weight and hearing loss and death at 4000 μg/kg of body weight. Therefore these values are much greater in magnitude than the exposure to mercury from amalgam or from a normal diet.

Mercury in urine

The body cannot retain metallic mercury and therefore passes it through the urine. By using radioactive mercury in amalgams, it is possible to monitor the mercury levels in urine caused only by dental amalgams. One study showed that urine mercury levels peak at 2.54 μg/L 4 days after placing amalgams, and after 7 days return to zero. On removal of amalgam, urine mercury levels reach a maximum value of 4 μg/L and return to zero after a week. Although mercury is readily cleared in both cases, peak urine levels of mercury are nearly twice as great when amalgam is removed rather than inserted. The same is true for mercury vapor, with higher levels recorded on removal of an amalgam than on insertion. Other studies, using more sensitive technics such as atomic absorption spectroscopy, show conflicting findings. There are reports demonstrating both no increase in urine mercury levels as well as higher levels. Even in those cases in which urine mercury is elevated, the concentrations are still less than 1 μg/L.

As a comparison, consider the WHO estimate that eating seafood once a week will raise urine mercury to 5 to 20 μg/L, or two to eight times the level of exposure from amalgam determined in the study just cited. Neurological changes are not detected until urine mercury levels exceed 500 μg/L, nearly 170 times the peak levels found on insertion of an amalgam.

Mercury in blood

The maximum allowable level of mercury in the blood is 3 μg/L. Several studies have shown that freshly placed amalgam restorations elevate blood mercury levels to 1 to 2 μg/L. Removal of amalgam decreases blood mercury levels, with a half time of approximately 1 to 2 months for elimination of mercury. However, as with urine mercury levels, there is first an increase of around 1.5 μg/L, which decreases in about 3 days. One study monitored blood mercury levels for a year and even showed that patients with amalgams had lower average blood mercury level (0.6 μg/L) than patients without amalgams (0.8 μg/L). Presumably the blood mercury level is easily influenced by other factors and therefore cannot be explicitly related to amalgam. Evidently a relationship exists between plasma and urine mercury levels.

Another study showed that patients with and without amalgams do not differ in the mean number or percentage of lymphocytes. Some studies have shown the blood mercury levels of dentists to be normal, whereas others report an increase. For those studies that indicate higher blood mercury levels in dentists, results have varied regarding any correlation between mercury concentration and number of amalgams placed. Elevated blood mercury levels may relate to mercury spills in the office, a factor that can easily be controlled. Both blood and serum mercury levels seem to correlate best with occupational exposure and not with the number of amalgams or length of time with amalgams in place.

Release of corrosion products

Mercury release into various media, including water, saline, buffered citric and phosphoric acid, and synthetic saliva, has been measured by a number of technics, such as atomic emission spectroscopy and atomic absorption spectroscopy. Ion release tends to be greatest in the first 1 to 24 hours after trituration. Once the amalgam is fully set, ionic dissolution is very low. This reduction in ion flux with time probably results from a combination of the chemical reaction progressing further and the forma-

tion of a passive surface film. In general, low-copper alloys release more ions than high-copper alloys because of their inferior corrosion resistance. Greater amounts of mercury and silver are released from unpolished specimens than from polished specimens.

The effect of electrolytic concentration on corrosion has been compared for conventional and high-copper admixed alloys following storage for 4 months. The main corrosion products were tin compounds at the surface of the amalgams. Low-copper amalgam showed surface corrosion only, whereas subsurface corrosion occurred with high-copper amalgam, especially following immersion in an NaCl solution without phosphate. For low-copper amalgam the release of elements decreased with time, possibly indicating passivation. For high-copper amalgam the release of elements increased with time, except for copper and tin in a solution with a high concentration of phosphate, indicating that phosphate inhibits corrosion of the copper-tin phases. Other studies have revealed a tendency for tin and copper to be preferentially released from amalgam. Presumably tin release originates from surface corrosion, whereas copper release results from subsurface corrosion. Stronger galvanic influences enhance copper release and, to a lesser extent, zinc release. Tin tends to provide a passive layer and to suppress the dissolution of mercury. It is suspected that indium functions similarly. In zinc-free alloys, the tin oxide is mercury depleted.

Another recent study has shown that following 1 week of aging in 0.9% NaCl solution at 37° C, the amount of mercury released from γ_1 was 14 to 60 times that released from amalgam and 5 times that released from β_1. The γ_2 phase released the least amount of mercury.

Are Amalgams Poisonous?

Allergic reactions to mercury in amalgam restorations occur infrequently, although there are case reports of allergic contact dermatitis, gingivitis, stomatitis, and remote cutaneous reactions. Such responses usually disappear on removal of the amalgam. Other local or systemic effects from mercury contained in dental amalgam have not been demonstrated. No well-conducted scientific study has conclusively shown that dental amalgam produces any ill effects.

Random reports of various diseases, such as multiple sclerosis, cannot unequivocally link the diseases to amalgams and therefore must be interpreted with caution. Reports of multiple sclerosis patients being instantly cured when amalgam is removed cannot be upheld scientifically. Because a week must pass for all mercury to be cleared by the body, an instantaneous recovery after removing the potential source of the mercury is unlikely.

Local reactions

In patients with oral lesions near amalgam sites, positive patch tests have been reported. However, the appropriate patch test has still not been determined, and many of the materials used for patch testing contain excessive concentrations of mercury. There are also reports of inflammatory reactions of the dentin and pulp, similar to the reactions to many other restorative materials. Mercury has been found in the lysosomes of macrophages and fibroblasts in some patients with lesions. Inflammation can usually be alleviated with a cavity liner. With the increased use of more corrosion-resistant amalgams, the volume of corrosion products and subsequent reactions are reduced.

Macrophages play an important role in the removal of foreign particulate matter from tissue. A number of cell culture studies have assessed the potential cytotoxicity of amalgam and its constituents. Unreacted mercury or copper leaching out from high-copper alloys has usually been the constituent leading to adverse responses. An *in vitro* study of the effects of particulate amalgams and their individual phases on macrophages showed that all particles except the γ_2 are effectively phagocytized by macrophages. Cell damage was seen in treated cultures exposed to particulate γ_1.

Systemic reactions

Implantation studies have shown that amalgam is reasonably well tolerated by soft and hard tissue. In a rabbit muscle implantation model, biological reactions to amalgams were found to depend on the time of implantation. All amalgams were strongly toxic 1 hour after setting. After 7 days, only high-copper amalgam showed any reaction.

In another series of studies, low- and high-copper amalgam powders and various phases of amalgam were implanted subcutaneously in guinea pigs. The result was a mild, early inflammatory response in which particles were taken up by macrophages and giant cells. After 1.5 to 3 months, chronic granulomas developed. With low-copper amalgam, early changes occurred in the intracellular material, associated with the rapid degradation of the γ_2 phase. Later, intracellular particles from both low- and high-copper amalgam underwent progressive degradation, producing fine secondary particles containing silver and tin, which were distributed throughout the lesions and gave rise to macroscopic tattooing of the skin. Secondary material and small, degrading primary particles from both types of amalgam were detected in the submandibular lymph nodes.

Elevated mercury levels were detected in the blood, bile, kidneys, liver, spleen, and lungs, with the highest concentrations found in the renal cortex. Mercury was excreted in the urine and feces. Mercury levels in the blood, liver, renal cortex, and feces were lower with the high-copper amalgam.

Black, refractile particulate deposits approximately 1 to 3 μm in diameter were found in the cytoplasm and nuclei of kidney cells. The ratio of nuclear to cytoplasmic deposits was higher in animals receiving high-copper amalgam. The cytoplasmic deposits consisted of collections of fine particles within lysosomes. Both lysosomal and nuclear deposits contained mercury and selenium, which were present in the animals' diet at low levels. Neither this study nor others have demonstrated any changes in biochemical function of any of the laden organs.

Subcutaneous implantation of only the powdered γ_2 phase led to a limited initial release of mercury from extracellular material. Thereafter, chronic granulomas developed around the implants, and particles degraded slowly in macrophages and giant cells. Fine secondary particles containing tin were produced. Subcutaneous implantation of only the powdered γ_1 phase induced a severe initial tissue response, and the majority of the material was extruded from the healing wounds. This process was accompanied by the release of significant amounts of mercury that appeared in the body organs and excreta. The small numbers of particles remaining in the tissues underwent a slow degradation in macrophages and giant cells in chronic granulomas. Minute secondary particles containing silver and sulphur were deposited in the tissues and gave rise to macroscopic tattooing of the skin above the implants.

In another study, primates received occlusal amalgam fillings or maxillary bone implants of amalgam for 1 year. Amalgam fillings caused deposition of mercury in the spinal ganglia, anterior pituitary, adrenal, medulla, liver, kidneys, lungs, and intestinal lymph glands. Maxillary amalgam implants released mercury into the same organs except for the liver, lungs, and intestinal lymph glands. Organs from control animals were devoid of precipitate.

Note that studies on powders probably overestimate the amount of breakdown products, and therefore biological response because the surface area of powders can be 5 to 10 times the surface area of a solid component. It must also be emphasized that any reaction to amalgam, whether in cell culture, local tissue response, or systemic response, does not necessarily imply a reaction to mercury. Such reactions could be in response to some other constituent of the amalgam or corrosion product. For example, *in vitro* cell culture testing, which measured fibroblasts affected by various elements and phases of amalgams, has shown that pure copper and zinc show greater cytotoxicity than pure silver and mercury. Pure tin has not been shown to be cytotoxic (Fig. 9-14). The γ_1 phase is moderately cytotoxic. Cytotoxicity is decreased by the addition of 1.5% and 5% tin (Fig. 9-15). However, the addition of

1.5% zinc to γ_1 containing 1.5% tin increases cytotoxicity to the same level as that of pure zinc. Whenever zinc is present, higher cytotoxicity is revealed. High-copper amalgams show the same cytotoxicity as a zinc-free, low-copper amalgam. The addition of selenium does not reduce amalgam cytotoxicity, and excessive additions of selenium increase cytotoxicity. The cytotoxicity of amalgams decreases after 24 hours, possibly from the combined effects of surface oxidation and further amalgamation. The results of this study suggest that the major contributor to the cytotoxicity of amalgam alloy powders is probably copper, whereas that for amalgam is zinc.

Risks to Dentists and Office Personnel

Of the two groups of people, (i.e., patients and dental office personnel) potentially at risk to mercury exposure, the dental office personnel are at greater risk to mercury vapor and therefore mercury toxicity. The blood mercury levels of dentists have been shown to be normal. However, no adverse body responses appear when the following recommendations in mercury hygiene are practiced:

1. Store mercury in unbreakable, tightly sealed containers.
2. To confine and facilitate the recovery of spilled mercury or amalgam, perform all operations involving mercury over areas that have impervious and suitably lipped surfaces.

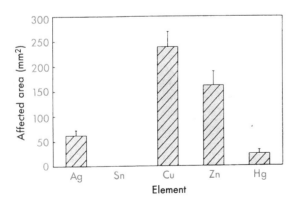

Fig. 9-14 Quantitative representation of the affected areas of fibroblasts, which reveals the magnitude of cytotoxicity of amalgam elements. Standard deviations are represented by bars. (From Kaga M, Seale NS, Hanawa T, Ferracane JL, Waite DE, Okabe T: Cytotoxicity of amalgams, alloys, and their elements and phases, *Dent Mater* 7:68, 1991.)

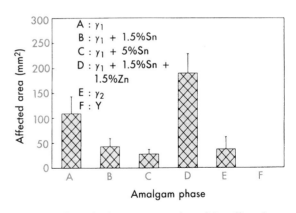

Fig. 9-15 Quantitative representation of the affected areas of fibroblasts, which reveals the magnitude of cytotoxicity of amalgam phases. Standard deviations are represented by bars. (From Kaga M, Seale NS, Hanawa T, Ferracane JL, Waite DE, Okabe T: Cytotoxicity of amalgams, alloys, and their elements and phases, *Dent Mater* 7:68, 1991.)

3. Clean up any spilled mercury immediately. Droplets may be picked up with narrow-bore tubing connected (via a wash-bottle trap) to the low-volume aspirator of the dental unit.
4. Use tightly closed capsules during amalgamation.
5. Use a no-touch technic for handling the amalgam.
6. Salvage all amalgam scrap and store it under water that contains sodium thiosulfate (photographic fixer is convenient).
7. Work in well-ventilated spaces.
8. Avoid carpeting dental operatories because decontamination of carpeting is very difficult.
9. Eliminate the use of mercury-containing solutions.
10. Avoid heating mercury or amalgam.
11. Use water spray and suction when grinding dental amalgam.
12. Use conventional dental amalgam condensing procedures, manual and mechanical, but do not use ultrasonic amalgam condensers.
13. Perform yearly mercury determinations on all personnel regularly employed in dental offices.
14. Periodically determine mercury vapor levels in operatories.
15. Alert all personnel who handle mercury, especially during training or indoctrination periods, of the potential hazard of mercury vapor and the necessity for observing good mercury and amalgam hygiene practices.

SELECTED PROBLEMS

Problem 1. An amalgam mix is difficult to remove from the capsule and appears excessively wet. What can be done to obtain a better mix?

Solution a. The most frequent cause is related to overtrituration. Trituration time should be decreased by 1 or 2 seconds, and the mix should then be tested for plasticity.

Solution b. The speed of trituration may have been too fast and a slower speed should be selected for the next mix. Remember that the work of trituration is important in obtaining a normal mix and that the work is a function of the speed and the time of trituration; increasing either increases the work of trituration.

Problem 2. Mixes of amalgam are consistently on the dry side and lack plasticity during condensation. What can cause a dry mix to occur, and how can it be corrected?

Solution a. In contrast to the previous case, a dry mix is frequently caused by undertrituration. Several mixes should be made at increased trituration times (an additional 1 to 2 seconds), and each one should be tested for plasticity. Listen for significant sound changes during trituration; the pestle can become wedged for the first few seconds, and the work-energy during that time is lost. Another choice would be to use a higher speed on the amalgamator.

Solution b. A dry mix can result from loss of mercury from the capsule during trituration. The two portions of most predispensed capsules are held together by a friction fit and occasionally some mercury can leak out during mixing. Check the inside of the housing covering the capsule area for small droplets of mercury, which also may appear like dust. If mercury is found, follow the cleanup procedures listed in the text at the end of this chapter. Changing to a hermetically sealed type of capsule is suggested if the problem persists.

Problem 3. When larger restorative procedures are performed with amalgam, the amalgam is difficult to carve and seems to set before an adequate carving can be completed. What can cause this problem?

Solution a. The working time of an alloy can be influenced by the specific composition or particle size of an alloy and by the aging treatment during manufacturing. If the working characteristics of a particular alloy appear to change from those previously experienced, the cause may be an alteration made by the manufacturer. On the other hand, if the faster reaction rate occurs at initial trials with a new or unfamiliar alloy, this may simply indicate that the alloy has a short setting time and is unsuitable for use by certain operators or with specific technics.

Solution b. The two most common manipulative variables that can accelerate the reaction and make carving difficult are overtrituration and decreased mercury/alloy ratios. An overtriturated mix is recognizable by its shiny and very wet appearance and by its high initial plasticity. A low mercury/alloy ratio appears quite dry during condensation and presents difficulty in handling.

Solution c. The increased rate of the reaction may be compensated for by making several smaller mixes as material is used. Do not try to complete large restorations from a single mix or continue to use a mix after it has exceeded the usable range for plasticity. Also, the technic should be evaluated; most carving problems can be remedied by obtaining assistance and improving operator speed.

Problem 4. When trying a new alloy, some amalgams may appear dry and brittle at the carving stage and tend to break away in large increments rather than carving smoothly. What can cause this problem?

Solution a. A check should be made with a stopwatch to determine the point after initiating the mix at which this brittleness or loss of plasticity is first noticed. Prolonged condensation involves working the material beyond its limit of plasticity, and the loss of cohesiveness between increments complicates carving. Delayed condensation, in which there is a short, unavoidable interruption during the procedure, can also result in working the material after significant matrix has formed, causing the structure to break down. The result is a weak, friable surface that will not carve smoothly. It is very important to condense and carve an alloy in one continuous operation and within the time framework of the setting reaction for the alloy being used.

Solution b. The setting or working time of the alloy could be too short for the particular procedure being performed. Newer alloys appear to be faster setting and somewhat less consistent with respect to working time. The causes for a shortened setting time or an increased reaction rate are reviewed in the preceding problem.

Solution c. In certain instances a lack of condensation force can result in a restoration with a large number of air voids or poor cohesion between increments. Frequently this occurs when the cavity preparation is not confining and an unstable matrix technic is used. It can also occur when moisture contamination interferes with cohesion between increments.

Problem 5. What factors are related to excessive tarnish and corrosion that appear several years after placement?

Solution a. A high residual mercury level in the final restoration can lead to increased corrosion as a result of an increase in the tin-mercury (γ_2) phase. This mercury can result from a mercury/alloy ratio that is too high in the initial mix or from inadequate condensation to remove excessive mercury.

Solution b. Patients on a high-sulfur diet or dietary supplement show increased tarnish on amalgam restorations. A well-polished surface is the best preventive measure to minimize tarnishing.

Solution c. Surface texture is also important in preventing corrosion. Small scratches and exposed voids develop concentration cells, with saliva as the electrolyte. Thus corrosion weakens the amalgam in critical areas such as the margin interface and begins the breakdown process. One of the major advantages of polishing amalgam surfaces to a smooth texture is that polishing minimizes the effects of corrosion and thus enhances clinical performance.

Solution d. Galvanic action can also develop in the mouth when two dissimilar metals come into contact. The most frequent occurrence of this is when gold and amalgam are placed in adjacent teeth. The effects can be seen in the darkened corrosion products appearing on the surface of the amalgam. This does not occur in every mouth, and the severity may relate to salivary composition and its function as an electrolyte.

Solution e. Moisture contamination during condensation causes air voids to develop throughout the mass of the restoration and corrosion to progress at a faster rate.

Problem 6. As amalgam restorations wear, the marginal integrity is usually the first area to show signs of failure. Small increments of either amalgam or unsupported enamel fracture, and crevices develop, thus leading to increased leakage and eventual secondary caries. What factors contribute to marginal deterioration of this type?

Solution a. Initially, every margin of a preparation should be examined for potential areas of enamel failure. Unsupported enamel rods and undercut walls are potential sites for fracture when subjected to occlusal forces. All cavosurface margins should be smooth-flowing curves and be free of unsupported enamel. Cavity walls should meet the external surface of the tooth at a 90-degree angle to provide optimum support for the tooth and sufficient bulk in the amalgam to resist fracture along the margin.

Solution b. Carving of the amalgam should be continuous with existing tooth form and should provide an accurate adaptation to the exposed cavity margin. Thin overextensions of amalgam beyond the margins and onto enamel can fracture readily into the bulk of amalgam and leave a crevice.

Solution c. Inadequate condensation of the amalgam in areas adjacent to the margins, especially in the areas of occlusal overpacking, causes a high residual mercury level to remain at the margin interface. The excessive γ_2 phase in that area leads to an increase in flow and corrosion and a decrease in strength that predisposes the restoration to fracture.

Solution d. Use of an alloy with a higher creep value, such as a microcut, results in evidence of early marginal fractures when subjected to occlusal function. The high-copper content alloys have less creep and demonstrate more durable marginal adaptation.

Problem 7. Small interproximal restorations often fail by fracturing across the occlusal isthmus. How can this type of failure be avoided?

Solution a. The major cause of gross fracture of amalgam restorations is usually found in the design of the cavity preparation. Sufficient bulk of material must be provided to support occlusal forces. This can best be accomplished by keeping the isthmus narrow and providing adequate cavity depth; however, on occasion the reverse might be necessary to avoid pulpal involvement. The axiopulpal line angle should be rounded to reduce stress concentration in that area.

Solution b. Occlusal contacts should be adjusted to avoid excessive contact on the marginal ridge. A torquing action places the isthmus under tension and results in fracture sooner.

Solution c. A smaller condenser must be used in the isthmus area so that adequate condensation can be accomplished. Inadequately condensed amalgam results in a weakening of the area and a predisposition to fracture.

Solution d. If enough dentin is removed during cavity preparation to require the placement of a cement base, a sufficiently rigid material must be selected for use. Zinc phosphate cement is the best material having a high enough modulus to minimize deflection of the amalgam. Other dental cements, particularly zinc oxide–eugenol types, have low moduli and under occlusal function allow too much deflection and brittle failure is likely to occur in the amalgam. The axiopulpal line angle is a critical area and should be reconstructed in a supporting base of zinc phosphate cement.

Problem 8. A high-copper, fast-setting amalgam could not be finished by the early polishing procedure until 20 minutes after amalgamation, and a satisfactory finish could not be obtained. What was the cause, and what would be the proper clinical procedure at this point?

Solution a. For amalgams of this type to be polished at the first appointment, finishing should be started 8 to 10 minutes after trituration, depending on the alloy. If the finishing is delayed until 20 minutes after trituration, the setting of the amalgam has proceeded too far, and strength of the alloy is too great to complete the finishing with triple-x silex and water. If the finishing is delayed too long, attempts at early finishing should be stopped, and final finishing should be done in the standard manner at a second appointment.

Problem 9. A spherical amalgam mix was condensed with a 2-mm diameter condenser in order to obtain a high condensation pressure and a well-condensed restoration. However, a low-strength amalgam restoration and failure resulted. Why?

Solution a. Spherical alloys when triturated with mercury do not resist small condenser tips well and allow them to penetrate the mass and thus reduce the condensation pressure. Larger-diameter tip condensers should be used that do not penetrate the mass as readily thus allowing higher pressures and better condensation. These amalgams appear to condense easily and there is a tendency to use less than desired condensation force. For optimum strength a condensation pressure of 7 MPa should be used.

Problem 10. Why should scrap amalgam be stored in a sodium thiosulfate solution such as photographic fixer rather than just water?

Solution a. Any mercury vapor released will react with the thiosulfate ions and lower the vapor pressure of mercury to levels below instrument detection of 0.01mg/m^3.

If scrap amalgam is stored over only water the amount of mercury in the air above the water increases with the log of time.

Problem 11. What assurances can you give a patient to dispell fears of mercury toxicity from dental amalgams?

Solution a. Except for the rare allergic reaction there is no scientific documentation of local or systemic effects of dental amalgams.

Patients with 9 occlusal surfaces of amalgam will inhale less than 1% of the mercury that a person would inhale in a workplace having a level allowed by OSHA.

Mercury ingested is eliminated through feces and urine.

The daily intake of mercury from air, water, and food exceeds that from dental amalgams.

■ REFERENCES

Abraham JE, Svare EW: The effect of dental amalgam restorations on blood mercury levels, *J Dent Res* 63:71, 1984.

Allan FC, Asgar K, Peyton FA: Microstructure of dental amalgam, *J Dent Res* 44:1002, 1965.

Asgar K: Amalgam alloy with a single composition behavior similar to Dispersalloy, *J Dent Res* 53:60, 1974.

Asgar K, Sutfin L: Brittle fracture of dental amalgam, *J Dent Res* 44:977, 1965.

Bakir F, Damluji SF, Amin-Zaki L, Murtadha M, Khalidi A, Al-Rawi NY, Tikriti S, Dhohir HI, Clarkson TW, Smith JC, Doherty RA: Methyl mercury poisoning in Iraq, *Science* 181:230, 1973.

Baran G, O'Brien WJ: Wetting of amalgam alloys by mercury, *J Am Dent Assoc* 94:898, 1977.

Barkmeier WW, Gendusa NJ, Thurmond JW, Triolo PT Jr: Laboratory evaluation of Amalgambond and Amalgambond Plus, *Am J Dent* 7:239, 1994.

Berlin MH, Clarkston TW, Friberg LT, Mangos L, Nordberg GF, Radford EP, Ramel C, Skerufaring S, Thruhaut R, Vostal J, Korbodovr J, Nielsenkadsk F: Maximum allowable concentrations of mercury vapor in air, *Lakartidningen* 64:3628, 1967.

Birke G, Johnels AG, Plantin L-O, Sjöstrand B, Westmark T: Hg i livsmedel (3): Metylkvicksilverförgiftning genom förtaring av fisk? [Hg in food (3): Methyl mercury poisoning through eating fish?] *Lakartidningen* 64:3628, 1967.

Bolewska J, Holmstrup P, Moller-Madsen B, Kenrad B, Danscher G: Amalgam-associated mercury accumulations in normal oral mucosa, oral mucosal lesions of lichen planus and contact lesions associated with amalgam, *J Oral Pathol Med* 19:19, 1990.

Boyer DB, Edie JW: Composition of clinically aged amalgam restorations, *Dent Mater* 6:146, 1990.

Boyer DB, Roth L: Fracture resistance of teeth with bonded amalgams, *Am J Dent* 7:91, 1994.

Brockhurst PJ, Culnane JT: Organization of the mixing time of dental amalgam using coherence time, *Aust Dent J* 32:28, 1987.

Brown IH, Maiolo C, Miller DR: Variation in condensation pressure during clinical packing of amalgam restorations, *Am J Dent* 6:255, 1993.

Brown IH, Miller DR: Alloy particle shape and sensitivity of high-copper amalgams to manipulative variables, *Am J Dent* 6:248, 1993.

Brune D: Corrosion of amalgams, *Scand J Dent Res* 89:506, 1981.

Bryant RW: γ_2 Phase in conventional dental amalgams—discrete clumps or continuous network? a review, *Aust Dent J* 29:163, 1984.

Burglund A: Estimation of the daily dose of intra-oral mercury vapor inhaled after release from dental amalgam, *J Dent Res* 69:1646, 1990.

Burrows D: Hypersensitivity to mercury, nickel and chromium in relation to dental materials, *Int Dent J* 36:30, 1986.

Chang SB, Siew C, Gruninger SE: Factors affecting blood mercury concentrations in practicing dentists, *J Dent Res* 71:66, 1992.

Chew CL, Soh G, Lee AS, Yeoh TS: Comparison of release of mercury from three dental amalgams, *Dent Mater* 5:244, 1989.

Consumer Reports: The mercury in your mouth 56(5):316, 1991.

Corpron R, Straffon L, Dennison J, Carron S, Asgar K: Clinical evaluation of amalgams polished immediately after insertion: 5-year results, *J Dent Res* 63:178, 1984.

Council on Dental Materials and Devices: Recommendations in mercury hygiene, *J Am Dent Assoc* 92:1217, 1976.

Council on Dental Materials, Instruments, and Equipment. Addendum to American National Standards Institute/American Dental Association, Specification No. 1 for alloy for dental amalgam, *J Am Dent Assoc* 100:246, 1980.

Council on Dental Materials, Instruments, and Equipment: Safety of dental amalgam, *J Am Dent Assoc* 106:519, 1983.

Cox SW, Eley BM: Further investigations of the soft tissue reaction to the gamma 1 phase (Ag_2Hg_3) of dental amalgam, including measurements of mercury release and redistribution, *Biomaterials* 8:296, 1987.

Cox SW, Eley BM: Further investigations of the soft tissue reaction to the gamma 2 phase ($Sn_{7-8}Hg$) of dental amalgam, including measurements of mercury release and redistribution, *Biomaterials* 8:301, 1987.

Cox SW, Eley BM: Mercury release, distribution and excretion from subcutaneously implanted conventional and high-copper amalgam powders in the guinea pig, *Arch Oral Biol* 32:257, 1987.

Cox SW, Eley BM: Microscopy and x-ray microanalysis of subcutaneously implanted conventional and high-copper dental amalgam powders in the guinea pig, *Arch Oral Biol* 32:265, 1987.

Cox SW, Eley BM: The release, tissue distribution and excretion of mercury from experimental amalgam tattoos, *Br J Exp Pathol* 67:925, 1986.

Craig RG: Biocompatibility of mercury derivatives, *Dent Mater* 2:91, 1986.

Danscher G, Horsted-Bindslev P, Rungby J: Traces of mercury in organs from primates with amalgam fillings, *Exp Mol Pathol* 52:291, 1990.

Edgren BN, Denehy GE: Microleakage of amalgam restorations using Amalgambond and Copalite, *Am J Dent* 5:296, 1992.

Eley BM, Cox SW: The development of mercury- and selenium-containing deposits in the kidneys following implantation of dental amalgams in guinea pigs, *Br J Exp Pathol* 67:937, 1986.

Eley BM, Cox SW: Renal cortical mercury levels associated with experimental amalgam tattoos: effects of particle size and amount of implanted material, *Biomaterials* 8:401, 1987.

Farah JW, Hood JAA, Craig RG: Effects of cement bases on the stresses in amalgam restorations, *J Dent Res* 54:10, 1975.

Farah JW, Powers JM, editors: Dental amalgam and mercury, *The Dental Advisor* 8(2):1, 1991.

Farah JW, Powers JM, editors: High copper amalgams, *The Dental Advisor* 4(2):1, 1987.

Ferracane JL, Engle JH, Okabe T, Mitchem JC: Reduction in operatory mercury levels after contamination or amalgam removal, *Am J Dent* 7:103, 1994.

Fischer GM, Stewart GP, Panelli J: Amalgam retention using pins, boxes, and Amalgambond, *Am J Dent* 6:173, 1993.

Gottlieb EW, Retief DH, Bradley EL: Microleakage of conventional and high copper amalgam restorations, *J Prosthet Dent* 53:355, 1985.

Gronka PA, Bobkoskie RL, Tomchick GJ, Bach F, Rakow AB: Mercury vapor exposures in dental offices, *J Am Dent Assoc* 81:923, 1970.

Guthrow CE, Johnson CB, Lawless KB: Corrosion of dental amalgam and its component phases, *J Dent Res* 46:1372, 1967.

Haikel Y, Gasser P, Salek P, Voegel JC: Exposure to mercury vapor during setting, removing, and polishing amalgam restorations, *J Biomed Mater Res* 24:1551, 1990.

Heintze U, Edwardsson S, Derand T, Birkhed D: Methylation of mercury from dental amalgam and mercuric chloride by oral streptococci *in vitro*, *Scand J Dent Res* 91:150, 1983.

Hero H: On creep mechanisms in amalgam, *J Dent Res* 62:44, 1983.

Holland GA, Asgar K: Some effects of the phases of amalgam induced by corrosion, *J Dent Res* 53:1245, 1974.

Ianzano JA, Mastrodomenico J, Gwinnett AJ: Strength of amalgam restorations bonded with Amalgambond, *Am J Dent* 6:10, 1993.

Jensen SJ, Jørgensen KD: Dimensional and phase changes of dental amalgam, *Scand J Dent Res* 93:351, 1985.

Johansson C, Moberg LE: Area ratio effects on metal ion release from amalgam in contact with gold, *Scand J Dent Res* 99:246, 1991.

Johnson GH, Bales DJ, Powell LV: Clinical evaluation of high-copper dental amalgams with and without admixed indium, *Am J Dent* 5:39, 1992.

Johnson GH, Powell LV: Effect of admixed indium on properties of a dispersed phase high-copper dental amalgam, *Dent Mater* 8:366, 1992.

Jørgensen KD: The mechanism of marginal fracture of amalgam fillings, *Acta Odont Scand* 23:347, 1965.

Jørgensen KD, Esbensen AL, Borring-Moller G: The effect of porosity and mercury content upon the strength of silver amalgam, *Acta Odont Scand* 24:535, 1966.

Jørgensen KD, Wakumoto S: Occlusal amalgam fillings; marginal defects and secondary caries, *Odont Tskr* 76:43, 1968.

Kaaber S: Allergy to dental materials with special reference to the use of amalgam and polymethylmethacrylate, *Int Dent J* 40:359, 1990.

Kaga, M, Seale NS, Hanawa T, Ferracane, JL, Okabe T: Cytotoxicity of amalgams, *J Dent Res* 67:1221, 1988.

Kaga M, Seale NS, Hanawa T, Ferracane JL, Waite DE, Okabe T: Cytotoxicity of amalgams, alloys, and their elements and phases, *Dent Mater* 7:68, 1991.

Katz JL, Grenoble DE: A composite model of the elastic behavior of dental amalgam, *J Biomed Mater Res* 5:515, 1971.

Kawakami M, Staninec M, Imazato S, Torii M, Tsuchitani Y: Shear bond strength of amalgam adhesives to dentin, *Am J Dent* 7:53, 1994.

Kuntz WD: Maternal and cord blood background mercury level, *Am J Obstet Gynecol* 143:440, 1982.

Kurland LT, Faro SN, Siedler H: Minamata disease, *World Neurol* 1:370, 1960.

Laine J, Kalimo K, Forssell H, Happonen RP: Resolution of oral lichenoid lesions after replacement of amalgam restorations in patients allergic to mercury compounds, *Br J Dermatol* 126:10, 1992.

Langolf GD, Chaffin DB, Henderson R, Whittle HP: Evaluation of workers exposed to elemental mercury using quantitative test of tremor and neuromuscular function, *Am Ind Hyg Assoc J* 39:976, 1978.

Langworth S, Elinder CG, Gothe CJ, Vesterberg O: Biological monitoring of environmental and occupational exposure to mercury, *Int Arch Occup Environ Health* 63:161, 1991.

Leinfelder KF: Dental amalgam alloys, *Curr Opin Dent* 1:214, 1991.

Lloyd CH, Adamson M: Fracture toughness (KlC) of amalgam, *J Oral Rehabil* 12:59, 1985.

Lyttle HA, Bowden GH: The level of mercury in human dental plaque an interaction *in vitro* between biofilms of *Streptococcus mutans* and dental amalgam, *J Dent Res* 72:1320, 1993.

Lyttle HA, Bowden GH: The resistance and adaptation of selected oral bacteria to mercury and its impact on their growth, *J Dent Res* 72:1325, 1993.

Mackert JR Jr: Dental amalgam and mercury, *J Am Dent Assoc* 122:54, 1991.

Mackert JR Jr, Leffell MS, Wagner DA, Powell BJ: Lymphocyte levels in subjects with and without amalgam restorations, *J Am Dent Assoc* 122:49, 1991.

Mahler DB: Amalgam, International State-of-the-Art Conference on Restorative Dental Materials, Bethesda, Md, 1986.

Mahler DB: Slow compressive strength of amalgam, *J Dent Res* 51:1394, 1972.

Mahler DB, Adey JD: Factors influencing the creep of dental amalgam, *J Dent Res* 70:1394, 1991.

Mahler DB, Adey JD, Marantz RL: Creep versus microstructure of gamma 2 containing amalgams, *J Dent Res* 56:1493, 1977.

Mahler DB, Adey JD, Marek M: Creep and corrosion of amalgam, *J Dent Res* 61:33, 1982.

Mahler DB, Adey JD, Marshall SJ: Effect of time at 37 degrees C on the creep and metallurgical characteristics of amalgam, *J Dent Res* 66:1146, 1987.

Mahler DB, Marantz RL, Engle JH: A predictive model for the clinical marginal fracture of amalgam, *J Dent Res* 59:1420, 1980.

Mahler DB, Nelson LW: Factors affecting the marginal leakage of amalgam, *J Am Dent Assoc* 108:50, 1984.

Mahler DB, Terkla LG, van Eysden J, Reisbick MH: Marginal fracture vs mechanical properties of amalgam, *J Dent Res* 49:1452, 1970.

Mahler DB, van Eysden J, Terkla LG: Relationship of creep to marginal fracture of amalgam, *J Dent Res* 54:183, 1975.

Malhotra ML, Asgar K: Physical properties of dental silver-tin amalgams with high and low copper contents, *J Am Dent Assoc* 96:444, 1978.

Mandel ID: Amalgam hazards: an assessment of research, *J Am Dent Assoc* 122:62, 1991.

Marek M: Acceleration of corrosion of dental amalgam by abrasion, *J Dent Res* 63:1010, 1984.

Marek M: Corrosion test for dental amalgam, *J Dent Res* 59:63, 1980.

Marek M: The effect of the electrode potential on the release of mercury from dental amalgam, *J Dent Res* 72:1315, 1993.

Marek M: The release of mercury from dental amalgam: the mechanism and *in vitro* testing, *J Dent Res* 69:1167, 1990.

Marek M, Hockman RF, Okabe T: *In vitro* corrosion of dental amalgam phases, *J Biomed Mater Res* 10:789, 1976.

Marshall SJ, Lin JHC, Marshall GW: Cu_2O and $CuCl_2 \cdot 3Cu(OH)_2$ corrosion products on copper rich dental amalgams, *J Biomed Mater Res* 16:81, 1982.

Mateer RS, Reitz CD: Galvanic degradation of amalgam restorations, *J Dent Res* 51:1546, 1972.

McCabe JF, Carrick TE: Dynamic creep of dental amalgam as a function of stress and number of applied cycles, *J Dent Res* 66:1346, 1987.

Meletis EI, Gibbs CA, Lian K: New dynamic corrosion test for dental materials, *Dent Mater* 5:411, 1989.

Miller JM, Chaffin DB, Smith RG: Subclinical psychomotor and neuromuscular changes exposed to inorganic mercury, *Am Ind Hyg Assoc J* 36(10):725, 1975.

Moberg LE, Johansson C: Release of corrosion products from amalgam in phosphate containing solutions, *Scand J Dent Res* 99:431, 1991.

Molin M, Marklund S, Bergman B, Bergman M, Stenman E: Plasma-selenium, glutathione peroxidase in erythrocytes and mercury in plasma in patients allegedly subject to oral galvanism, *Scand J Dent Res* 95:328, 1987.

Molin M, Marklund S, Bergman B, Nilsson B: Mercury, selenium, and glutathione peroxidase in dental personnel, *Acta Odontol Scand* 47:383, 1989.

Mueller HJ, Bapna MS: Copper- , indium- , tin- , and calcium-fluoride admixed amalgams: release rates and selected properties, *Dent Mater* 6:256, 1990.

Nuckles DB, Draughn RA, Smith TI: Evaluation of an adhesive system for amalgam repair: bond strength and porosity, *Quint Internat* 25:829, 1994.

O'Brien WJ, Greener EH, Mahler DB: Dental amalgam. In Reese JA and Valega TM, editors: *Restorative dental materials: an overview,* London, 1985, Quintessence.

Ogura H, Miyagawa Y, Nakamura K: Creep and rupture of dental amalgam under bending stress, *Dent Mater J* 8:65, 1989.

Okabe T, Ferracane J, Cooper C, Matsumoto H, Wagner M: Dissolution of mercury from amalgam into saline solution, *J Dent Res* 66:33, 1987.

Okabe T, Yomashita T, Nakajima H, Berglund A, Zhao L, Guo I, Ferracane JL: Reduced mercury vapor release from dental amalgams prepared with binary Hg-In liquid alloys, *J Dent Res* 73:1711, 1994.

Olsson S, Bergman M: Daily dose calculations from measurements of intro-oral mercury vapor, *J Dent Res* 71:414, 1992.

Olsson S, Berhlund A, Bergman M: Release of elements due to electrochemical corrosion of dental amalgam, *J Dent Res* 73:33, 1994.

Olstad ML, Holland RI, Pettersen AH: Effect of placement of amalgam restorations on urinary mercury concentration, *J Dent Res* 69:1607, 1990.

Osborne JW, Gale EN: Failure at the margin of amalgams as affected by cavity width, tooth position, and alloy selection, *J Dent Res* 60:681, 1981.

Ott KH, Vogler J, Kroncke A, Schaller KH, Valentin H, Weltle D: Mercury concentrations in blood and urine before and after placement of non-gamma 2 amalgam fillings, *Dtsch Zahnarztl Z* 44:551, 1989.

Palaghias G: The role of phosphate and carbonic acid-bicarbonate buffers in the corrosion processes of the oral cavity, *Dent Mater* 1:139, 1985.

Pierce P, Thompson JF, Likosky WH, Nickey LN, Barthel WF, Hinman AR: Alkyl mercury poisoning in humans, *J Am Med Assoc* 220:1439, 1972.

Powell LV, Johnson GH, Bales DJ: Effect of admixed indium on mercury vapor release from dental amalgam, *J Dent Res* 68:1231, 1989.

Powers JM, Farah JW: Apparent modulus of elasticity of dental amalgams, *J Dent Res* 54:902, 1975.

Rao GS, Radchenko V, Tong YS: Reproductive effects of elemental mercury vapor in pregnant wistar rats, Annual Session Program, American Association for Dental Research Abstracts, Cincinnati, 232, 1983.

Ryge G, Telford RF, Fairhurst CW: Strength and phase formation of dental amalgam, *J Dent Res* 36:986, 1957.

Sarkar NK, Eyer CS: The microstructural basis of creep of gamma 1 in dental amalgam, *J Oral Rehabil* 14:27, 1987.

Sarkar NK, Park JR: Mechanism of improved corrosion resistance of Zn-containing dental amalgams, *J Dent Res* 67:1312, 1988.

Scarlett JM, Gutenmann WH, Lisk DJ: A study of mercury in the hair of dentists and dental-related professionals in 1985 and subcohort comparison of 1972 and 1985 mercury hair levels, *J Toxicol Environ Health* 25:373, 1988.

Schmalz G, Schmalz C: Toxicity tests on dental filling materials, *Int Dent J* 31:185, 1981.

Skare I, Engqvist A: Urinary mercury clearance of dental personnel after a long-term intermission in occupational exposure, *Swed Dent J* 14:255, 1990.

Snapp KR, Boyer DB, Peterson LC, Svare CW: The contribution of dental amalgam to mercury in blood, *J Dent Res* 68:780, 1989.

Staninec M: Retention of amalgam restorations: undercuts versus bonding, *Quint Internat* 20:347, 1989.

Staninec M, Holt M: Bonding of amalgam to tooth structure: tensile, adhesion and microleakage tests, *J Prosthet Dent* 59:397, 1988.

Syrjanen S, Hensten-Pettersen A, Nilner K: *In vitro* testing of dental materials by means of macrophage cultures. II. Effects of particulate dental amalgams and their constituent phases on cultured macrophages, *J Biomed Mater Res* 20:1125, 1986.

Takaku S: Studies of mercury concentration in saliva with particular reference to mercury dissolution from dental amalgam into saliva, *Gakho Shikwa* 82:285, 1982.

Veron C, Hildebrand HF, Martin P: Dental amalgams and allergy, *J Biol Buccale* 14:83, 1986.

von Mayenburg J, Rakoski J, Szliska C: Patch testing with amalgam at various concentrations, *Contact Dermatitis* 24:266, 1991.

Wing G, Ryge G: Setting reactions of spherical-particle amalgam, *J Dent Res* 44:1325, 1965.

Young FA Jr, Johnson LB: Strength of mercury-tin phase in dental amalgam *J Dent Res* 46:457, 1967.

Zardiackas LD, Anderson L Jr: Crack propagation in conventional and high copper dental amalgam as a function of strain rate, *Biomaterials* 7:259, 1986.

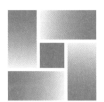

10 *Direct Esthetic Restorative Materials*

Tooth-colored restorative materials have increasingly been used to replace missing tooth structure and to modify tooth color and contour, thus enhancing facial esthetics. Direct esthetic materials discussed in this chapter include diacrylate composite resins, pit and fissure sealants, and glass ionomer restorative materials. Although sealants are used for preventive purposes, their chemistry and composition are related to the resin restoratives, and therefore are appropriate in this discussion.

Historically, silicate restoratives were developed first, followed by acrylic resins, then composite resins and sealants, and finally the glass ionomers. Silicates were introduced in 1871 and were prepared from a silicate powder base that included alumina-silica glass and a phosphoric acid liquid. The etched glasses were bound together with a gel matrix that was extremely sensitive to moisture and became very soluble in oral fluids. The main advantage to silicates as a direct esthetic restorative was the slow but sustained fluoride release from the glass fluxes, which provided an anticariogenic feature. The biological response to silicates was poor, and pulpal protection was required to minimize inflammation. Early clinical failure was noted readily and was most frequently related to dissolution in oral fluids, loss of translucency, surface crazing, and a lack of adequate mechanical properties. These deficiencies caused the demise of these materials.

Acrylic restorative resins were unfilled, low molecular weight polymers and lacked the reinforcement provided by the ceramic filler particles used in the composite resin systems. The acrylic restorations were less susceptible to fracture, less soluble in oral fluids, and more color stable than were the silicate materials. The acrylic polymers did not have high resistance to abrasion, but could be augmented readily as they wore down. They were frequently used with metal pins to provide retention for larger restorations. The initial color of a resin restoration matched tooth color closely, and multiple shades could be used to provide characterization. Early clinical failure of these materials was related directly to dimensional instability. High polymerization shrinkage and thermal dimensional changes, approximately 10 times greater than tooth structure, caused an interfacial gap to form along margins of the restoration. Oral fluids leaked into these gaps, resulting in unsightly stains and often recurrent caries.

■ COMPOSITE RESTORATIVE RESINS

The development of composites or filled resin restorative materials has resulted in higher mechanical properties, lower thermal coefficient of expansion, lower dimensional change on setting, and higher resistance to abrasion, thereby improving clinical performance. Later development of adhesive bonding systems for composites to tooth structure has also improved the quality of composite restorations.

Composites were initially developed for anterior class 3 to 5 restorations, in which esthetics were crucial, and for class 1 restorations, in which moderate occlusal stresses occur; however, modifications of materials and technics have extended their application to class 2 posterior restorations.

Composition and Chemical Reaction

The organic polymer matrix in most filled resin systems is either an aromatic or urethane diacrylate oligomer. These oligomers are viscous, and the viscosity is reduced to a useful clinical level by the

$$CH_2=C-C-O-CH_2CH_2-O-CH_2CH_2-O-CH_2CH_2-O-C-C=CH_2$$

addition of a diluent monomer such as triethylene glycol dimethacrylate shown above.

The basic chemistry and general setting reactions for the free radical–addition polymerization involved are presented in Chapter 6. The polymerization reaction can be chemically initiated (autocured) with a peroxide initiator and an amine accelerator, or it can be photoinitiated with a beam of visible blue light (460 nm) in the presence of a light-sensitive absorber such as camphoroquinone and an accelerator such as aliphatic amine. A few products use a combination of chemical and photoinitiation to carry out the polymerization reaction. The polymerized resin is highly cross-linked because of the presence of the difunctional carbon-carbon double bonds.

The degree of polymerization varies, depending on whether it is in the bulk or in the air-inhibited layer of the restoration, or according to the distance the material is from the light and the length of the exposure for the light-activated composite. The percentage of the double bonds that react may vary from 35% to 80%. The degree of polymerization has been increased by postcuring at elevated temperatures (e.g., 7 minutes at 120° C); however, for this to be possible the clinical technic must be changed from a direct insertion procedure to a direct or indirect inlay technic, in which the inlay is attached to the tooth with a composite cement.

The dispersed inorganic phase may consist of several inorganic materials such as quartz, borosilicate glass, lithium aluminum silicate, barium aluminum silicate, strontium or zinc glass, or colloidal silica. When sufficient amounts of the heavy elements are present, the final composite can be opaque to x-rays, a characteristic that is helpful in making a postoperative diagnosis.

The inorganic phase is treated with an organosilane before being mixed with the unreacted low molecular weight polymer (oligomer). The organosilane contains functional groups, such as methoxy, which hydrolyze and react with the inorganic filler as well as unsaturated organic groups that react with the oligomer during polymerization. These organosilanes are called coupling agents because they form a bond between the inorganic and organic phases of the composite.

Filler

A helpful method of classifying dental composites is by the particle size, shape, and distribution of filler. Historically, early composites contained large (20 to 30 μm) spherical particles, followed by products containing large irregularly shaped particles, very small or microfine particles (0.04 to 0.2 μm), fine particles (0.5 to 3 μm), distribution of fine particles, and finally blends (hybrids) containing mostly fine particles with some microfine particles. Currently composites may be classified as fine, microfine, or hybrid products.

Fine-particle composites contain irregularly shaped glass or quartz particles of fairly uniform diameter or consist of a distribution of two or more sizes of fine particles, which permits more efficient packing and allows the smaller particles to fill the spaces between the larger particles. Fine-particle composites may contain 60% to 70% by volume of filler, which, depending on the density of the filler, translates into 77% to 88% by weight of filler in the composite. Most manufacturers report filler concentration in weight percent (wt%). A micrograph of a typical fine-particle filler is shown in Fig. 10-1, *A*.

Microfine composites contain very high surface area silica (100 to 300 m^2/g) having particle diameters of 0.04 to 0.2 μm. Because of the high surface area, only 25% by volume or 38% by weight can be added to the oligomer to keep the consistency of the paste sufficiently low for clinical applications. Fillers consisting of microfine silica in polymerized oligomers are prepared and ground into particles 10 to 20 μm in diameter. These reinforced fillers may be added to the oligomer in concentrations so that the inorganic content can be increased to 32% to 50% by volume or about 50% to 60% by weight. A variation of this modification is used in which most of the filler is reinforced filler, with smaller amounts of microfine silica added to the oligomer. When

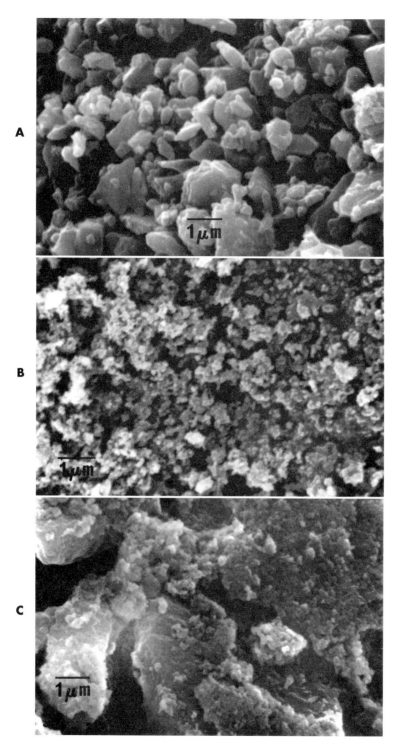

Fig. 10-1 Scanning electron micrographs of types of filler. **A,** Fine inorganic filler; **B,** microfine silica filler; **C,** microfine silica in organic polymer filler.

comparing the filler concentrations of microfilled and fine-particle composites, care should be taken because manufacturers frequently report the filler content as a percentage of the reinforced filler, which contains more organic than inorganic material. A typical microfine silica filler is shown in Fig. 10-1, *B,* and a reinforced filler containing microfine silica is shown in Fig. 10-1, *C.*

Hybrid composites may be bimodal or trimodal blends of fine or microfine filler (5% to 15%) in which the smaller particles fit into the space between the large particles. Hybrid composites may contain inorganic filler concentrations of up to 70% by volume and still possess a workable clinical consistency. The general trend for most products has been hybrid composites.

Idealized schematic cross-sectional sketches of fine, microfine, and hybrid composites are shown in Fig. 10-2. The filler particles are surrounded by polymer, however no attempt was made to have the volume percentage of fillers accurate. Also in a real cross section of a fine particle composite it would appear that there was a wider range of particle sizes than actually were present because the section would not necessarily pass through the major diameter of each particle.

Oligomers

The two most common general classes of oligomers that have been used in dental composites are Bis-GMA and urethane dimethacrylate (UDMA). These oligomers were described in Chapter 6. The oligomers are similar in that they contain reactive carbon double bonds at each end that can undergo addition polymerization. The vis-

cosity of the oligomers, especially Bis-GMA, is so high that diluents must be added so that a clinical consistency can be reached when they are compounded with the filler. Low molecular weight compounds with difunctional carbon double bonds, usually triethylene glycol dimethacrylate (TEGMA), are added by the manufacturer to reduce and control the viscosity of the compounded composite. A few products use both Bis-GMA and UDMA oligomers.

Coupling agents

For a composite to have successful properties, a good bond must form between the inorganic filler and the organic oligomer during setting. Bonding is accomplished by the manufacturer treating the surface of the filler with a coupling agent before mixing it with the oligomer. The most common coupling agents are organic silicon compounds called silanes. A typical silane is shown below.

$$CH_2{=}C-\overset{\displaystyle O}{\overset{\displaystyle \|}{C}}-O-CH_2CH_2CH_2-\underset{\displaystyle OCH_3}{\overset{\displaystyle OCH_3}{Si}}-OCH_3$$

3-methacryloxypropyltrimethoxysilane

During the deposition of the silane on the filler the methoxy groups hydrolyze to hydroxy groups that react with adsorbed moisture or –OH groups on the filler. They can also condense with –OH groups on an adjacent hydrolyzed silane to form a homopolymer film on the surface of the filler. During the setting reaction of the oligomer, the carbon double bonds of the silane react with the

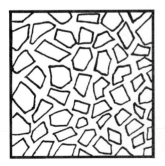
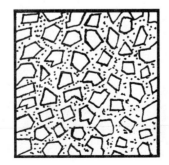
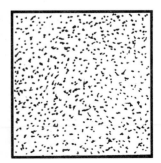

Fig. 10-2 Schematic sketch of cross section of fine *left,* hybrid, *center,* and microfine, *right,* composite. (From Craig RG, O'Brien WJ, Powers JM: *Dental materials: properties and manipulation,* ed 6, St Louis, 1996, Mosby.)

$$n\mathrm{CH_3O - Si - OCH_3} \rightarrow n\mathrm{HO - Si - OH} \rightarrow \ldots - \mathrm{Si - O - Si - O - Si -} \ldots$$

oligomer, thus forming a bond from the filler through the coupling agent to the polymer matrix (see the schematic sketch above). This coupling reaction binds the filler and the oligomer so that when a stress is applied to a composite, the stress can be transferred from one strong filler particle to another through the rather low-strength polymer. As a result, the strength of the composite is intermediate to that of the filler and the polymer separately.

Initiators and accelerators

Polymerization of composites is achieved by chemical or visible light activation, with the latter being more common. Chemical activation is accomplished by an organic amine reacting with an organic peroxide to produce free radicals, which in turn attack the carbon double bonds, causing polymerization. Because carbon double bonds are present at each end of the oligomer and diluent, the polymer is highly cross-linked. The amine and peroxide react at room temperature so that before reaction the composite consists of two pastes, one con-taining the amine and, the other, the peroxide. Once the two pastes are mixed, the polymerization reaction proceeds rapidly. The reaction is described in Chapter 6, and an example of a two-paste system is shown in Fig. 10-3.

Light activation is accomplished with blue light of about 460 nm, which is absorbed usually by camphoroquinone added by the manufacturer in amounts varying from 0.2% to 1.0%. The reaction is accelerated by the presence of an organic amine containing a carbon double bond (see Chapter 6). The camphoroquinone and the amine are stable in the presence of the oligomer at room temperature, as long as the composite is not exposed to blue light. The light-activated composites are supplied completely compounded in opaque containers by the manufacturer, an example of which is shown in Fig. 10-4 where five shades are packaged in screw-type syringes.

Pigments

Inorganic oxides are usually added in small amounts to provide shades that match the majority of

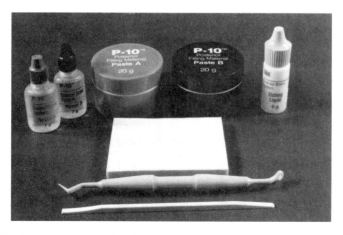

Fig. 10-3 Chemically initiated two-paste composite. (From Craig RG, O'Brien WJ, Powers JM: *Dental materials: properties and manipulation,* ed 6, St Louis, 1996, Mosby.)

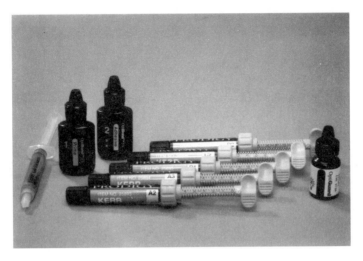

Fig. 10-4 Single-paste visible light-initiated composite.

tooth shades. Five or more common shades are supplied that range from yellow to gray (see Fig. 10-4). For shades outside this range, manufacturers supply a universal shade and highly pigmented composites (tints) that can be blended to match shades outside the normal range.

Packaging of Composites

Composites were initially introduced as two-paste systems; however, single-paste systems using photoinitiation currently are more common.

Two-paste system

Equal volumes of the two pastes are dispensed by estimation onto a treated paper pad for mixing. An error as high as 30% in the estimation will not result in significant differences in the properties of the set material. Depending on the viscosities of the pastes, they may require stirring before they are used to eliminate settling of the inorganic phase.

The two-paste systems are always chemically activated, and working time from the initiation of mixing is critical. A freshly mixed composite must be inserted quickly, and a bulk cure is obtained. Bulk curing requires that blending shades or adding tints for color characterization be done by adding the colorant to the base paste before mixing it with the catalyst paste. Although bulk curing of a chemically activated system results in a uniform degree of polymerization except for an air-inhibited layer, it also

results in the greatest amount of internal shrinkage and bonding stress at the enamel margin. The advantages of photoinitiation have resulted in a sharp decline in the use of the chemically activated composites, except for the development of a core buildup around retentive pins.

Single-paste systems for photoinitiation

Polymerization of single-paste systems is initiated by visible blue light. An incandescent light is used that emits a beam of blue light (approximately 460 nm). Appropriate filtering at the light source eliminates any stray ultraviolet radiation (Fig. 10-5). The radiation beam is transmitted to the tooth surface by a quartz rod curved to provide clinical access, by a flexible bundle of quartz fibers attached to a fiber-optic handpiece, or by a liquid-filled transmission tube. A number of studies have measured the intensity of the various light sources and the peak of the spectral distribution of the emitted beam. The peak wavelength appears to vary among light sources from about 450 to 490 nm (Fig. 10-6). The intensity measurements are not easily correlated for these studies but appear to vary within a range of 200% to 300%. The absorption spectrum for 0.5 wt% of camphoroquinone has a maximum at 470 nm and therefore could react more readily in response to different light sources. A decrease in line voltage of 6% shows a corresponding reduction in output of about 25% in intensity in some lamps, but only 10% in lamps with voltage regulators in their circuitry. In general, the output from the various lamps decreases with continuous use and the intensity is not uniform for all areas of the light tip, being greatest at the center. Also, the intensity of the light decreases with distance from the source nearly linearly to the log of the intensity/distance. Although the intensity is important with respect to the depth

of cure, it has been shown for some products that a three-fold difference in intensity had only a 15% difference in the depth of cure.

The storage life of photoinitiated resins in opaque syringes is approximately 12 months at room temperature, but it can be significantly prolonged by storage at refrigerator temperatures. The paste is quite viscous and should not require stirring

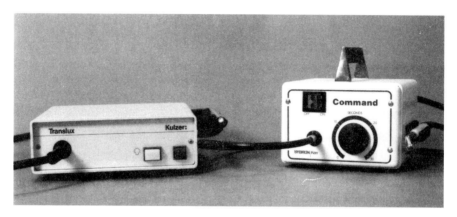

Fig. 10-5 Visible light sources for photoinitiation of composition.

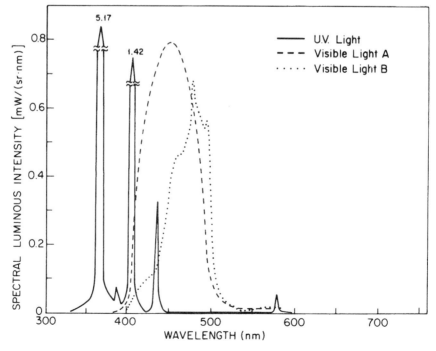

Fig. 10-6 Wavelength versus intensity for two visible lights compared with an ultraviolet light. (Adapted from O'Brien WJ, Yee J Jr, Dennison JB, Johnston WM, Stefanski R, Yee WJ, Fanian F: *J Am Dent Assoc* 106:839, 1983.)

to maintain uniform filler particle distribution (Fig. 10-7). Because no mixing is required, incorporation of air is minimized and a more void-free restoration should result. Small increments can be taken from the paper pad and packed into the cavity preparation using instruments such as those shown at the bottom of Fig. 10-3. The composite can be placed in a syringe and then injected into the cavity preparation. Single-paste composites are also supplied as compules such as those shown in Fig. 10-8. Compules are available in various shades, identified by removable colored coded tips, that match shade guides (Fig. 10-8). The compules are placed in a syringe, the tip is removed, and the composite is injected into the cavity preparation. One advantage offered by photoinitiated resins is a prolonged working time that can be controlled by the operator and modified according to clinical requirements. Composites that have been extruded onto a paper pad polymerize when exposed to sufficient light from fluorescent lamps or chairside lamps. Fluorescent lights labeled "gold" can be substituted, and they provide unlimited working time for single-paste composites.

A controlled setting time allows for the individual polymerization of small increments of composite,

thus permitting the use of multiple shades of composite within a single restoration and accommodating for polymerization shrinkage within each increment as opposed to the total shrinkage in a bulk

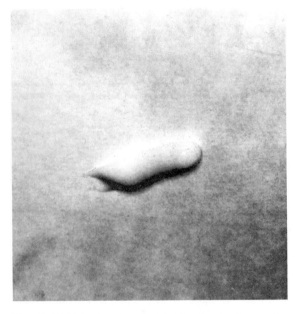

Fig. 10-7 High-viscosity, photoinitiated resin dispensed on a paper pad.

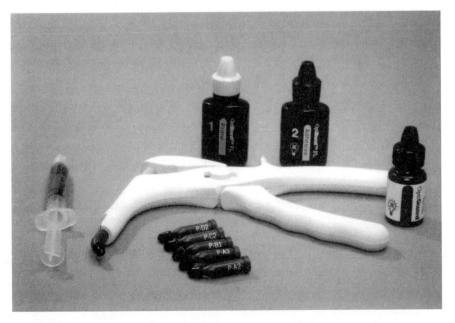

Fig. 10-8 Single-paste composite supplied in compules of various shades with the injection syringe.

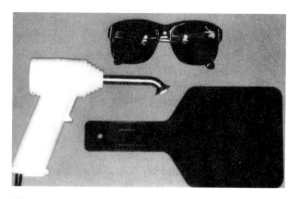

Fig. 10-9 Eye protection devices that can be used when a polymerizing visible light device is used. *Top to bottom:* glasses, an instrument shield, and a flat plate.

cure method. The setting time of photoinitiated material and the depth of cure within a given mass depend on the intensity and penetration of the light beam. A material with a low absorption coefficient cures to the greatest depth. The presence of ultraviolet absorbers for color stabilization, fluorescent dyes for clinical esthetics, or excessive initiator concentration has a detrimental effect on completeness of cure and causes some variation among commercial products. Although there is minimal potential for radiation damage to surrounding soft tissue inadvertently exposed to visible light, caution must be used to prevent retinal damage to the eye by observing the light beam for any length of time during clinical use. A number of devices are marketed to filter the visible light beam so that the operator can directly observe the curing procedure. These are eyeglasses, flat shields that can be held over the field of vision, and curved shields that attach directly to the handpiece delivering the light beam (Fig. 10-9).

■ PROPERTIES OF DIRECT RESTORATIVE COMPOSITES

Setting and Working Times

The setting times for chemically activated composite resins range from 3 to 5 minutes. These short setting times have been accomplished by controlling the concentration of initiator and accelerator.

For the composite systems, both exothermic curves and rheological measurements have been made to estimate clinically usable working and final

setting times. The changes in viscosity that occur in chemically activated composites during the setting procedure are related to the resin matrix and are not influenced by the particle size or volume fraction of the inorganic filler. The rate at which viscosity increases appears to be related less to the filler than to initiator concentration, diluent type and content, and the basic polymer backbone specific to individual commercial products.

Setting time for the photoinitiated composites cannot be measured in terms of viscosity change. Initiation of the reaction is related specifically to the application of the light beam to the material, and approximately 75% of the polymerization takes place during the first 10 minutes. The curing reaction continues for a period of 24 hours. All the available unsaturated carbon-carbon bonds do not react, and studies report that about 25% remain unreacted in the bulk of the restoration. If the surface of the restoration is not protected from air by a transparent matrix, inhibition of polymerization occurs, and the number of unreacted carbon double bonds may be as high as 75% in the tacky surface layer. Although the restoration can be finished with abrasives and is functional after 10 minutes, the optimum physical properties are not reached until about 24 hours after the reaction is initiated.

For most composites that are initiated by visible light, there is a critical time period after dispensing of the paste onto a paper pad during which fresh composite flows against tooth structure at an optimum level. Within 60 to 90 seconds after exposure to ambient light, the surface of the composite seems to lose its capability to flow readily against tooth structure, and further work with the material becomes difficult.

Polymerization Shrinkage

The volumetric polymerization shrinkage of typical fine-particle and microfine composites is listed in Table 10-1. Values for hybrids are not listed because of the wide variation in fillers, but properties are slightly less than fine composites or are intermediate to fine and microfine composites. The free volumetric polymerization shrinkage is a direct function of the amount of oligomer and diluent, and thus the fine-particle composites shrink only 1% to 1.7% compared with the microfine composites of 2% to

TABLE 10-1   Properties of Fine and Microfine Composites

Property	Fine Composites	Microfine Composites
Polymerization shrinkage (%)	1.0-1.7	2-3
Thermal coefficient of expansion (/° C)	$25\text{-}38 \times 10^{-6}$	$55\text{-}68 \times 10^{-6}$
Thermal conductivity (cal/sec/cm^2[° C/cm])	$25\text{-}30 \times 10^{-4}$	$12\text{-}15 \times 10^{-4}$
Water sorption (mg/cm^2)	0.3-0.6	1.2-2.2
Elastic modulus (MPa)	9000-10,000	3000-5000
Compression strength (MPa)	200-340	230-290
Tensile strength, diametral (MPa)	34-62	26-33
Hardness, Knoop (kg/mm^2)	55-80	22-36
Bond strength to etched enamel (MPa)	24	20
Bond strength to dentin (MPa)	5-24	10-17
Clinical wear μm/yr	85-100	25-60
Radiopacity (mm Al)*	2.7-5.7	–

*If advertised as a radiopaque. Enamel is 4.0 and dentin is 2.5 mm.

3%. This shrinkage creates polymerization stresses as high as 130 kg/cm^2 between the composite and the cavity of the tooth. These stresses severely strain the interfacial bond between the composite and the tooth, leading to a very small gap that can allow marginal leakage of saliva. This stress can exceed the tensile resistance of enamel and result in stress cracking and enamel fractures along the interfaces. The potential for this type of failure is even greater with the microfine composites, in which there is a much higher volume percent of polymer present, and polymerization shrinkage is greater. The net effect of setting contraction can be reduced by incremental addition of a photoinitiated material and polymerization of each increment independently, which allows for some contraction within each increment before successive additions.

Thermal Properties

The thermal expansion coefficients of composites are listed in Table 10-1. The values for composites are considerably less than the average of values for the polymer matrix and the inorganic phase separately; thus the addition of 50% by volume of inorganic phase is more effective in reducing the thermal coefficient of expansion than would be anticipated. The values more closely approach those for dentin (8.3 $\times 10^{-6}$/° C) and enamel (11.4 $\times 10^{-6}$/° C) than has been possible with previous unfilled resin restorative materials. The higher values for the microfine com-

posites are related mostly to the greater amount of polymer present. Certain glasses may be more effective in reducing the effect of thermal change than are others, and some resins have more than one type of filler to compensate for differential rates. The hybrids exhibit slightly greater thermal dimensional changes than the fine composites, but the difference is small and should not be clinically significant.

The difference between the thermal coefficient of expansion of composites and teeth, combined with the gap from polymerization shrinkage, allows for the percolation of oral fluids. When a tooth containing a composite is chilled, the restoration tends to contract more than the surrounding tooth structure, which enlarges the space between the two and allows greater oral fluid penetration. When the tooth is warmed or the temperature returns to body conditions, the space is diminished, and the oral fluid is forced out of the space between the tooth and the restoration (percolation).

Thermal stresses place an additional strain on the acid-etched bond, which further compounds the detrimental effect of the polymerization shrinkage. Thermal changes are also cyclic in nature, and although the entire restoration may never reach thermal equilibrium during the application of either hot or cold stimuli, the cyclic effect can lead to material fatigue and early bond failure. This condition is particularly true with microfine composites, which have a coefficient of expansion greater than fine composites.

The thermal conductivity of fine composites is greater than microfine products because of the higher conductivity of the inorganic fillers compared with the polymer matrix. However, for highly transient temperatures, the composites do not change temperature as fast as tooth structures, and this difference does not present a clinical problem.

Water Sorption

The water sorption values for composites are listed in Table 10-1. Water sorption of microfine composites is greater than that for fine composites, as well as hybrids, because of the higher volume fraction of polymer. The quality and stability of the silane coupling agent are important in minimizing the deterioration of the bond between the filler and polymer and the amount of water sorption. It has been postulated that water sorption is not all detrimental and that the corresponding expansion associated with the uptake of water from oral fluids could counteract some setting contraction. In the measurement of hygroscopic expansion starting 15 minutes after the initial polymerization, most resins required 7 days to reach equilibrium and about 4 days to show the majority of expansion. The fine composites have lower values of water sorption (0.3 to 0.6 mg/cm^2) than the microfine composites (1.2 to 2.2 mg/cm^2) and therefore exhibit less expansion when exposed to water.

Solubility

The water solubility of composites varies from 0.01 to 0.06 mg/cm^2. Adequate exposure to the light source is critical in photoinitiated composites. Inadequate polymerization can readily occur at a depth from the surface if insufficient light penetrates. Inadequately polymerized resin has greater water sorption and solubility, possibly manifested clinically with early color instability.

However, during the storage of fine composites in water, the leaching of inorganic ions can be detected, and such ions are associated with a breakdown in interfacial bonding. Silicon leaches into the water bath in the greatest quantity (15 to 17 µg/ml) during the first 30 days of storage and decreases with time of exposure. The microfine composites leach silicon more slowly and with a 100% increase in amount during the second 30-day period (14.2 µg/ml). Boron, barium, strontium, and lead, which are pre-sent in glass fillers, are leached to various degrees (6 to 19 µg/ml) from the various resin-filler systems. The breakdown and leakage can be contributing factors to the low resistance to wear and abrasion that is so common to composite resins, especially when used in posterior teeth.

Mechanical Properties

The compressive strengths of composite materials are listed in Table 10-1. The compressive strengths of the microfine composites are less than those of fine composites. The modulus of elasticity for fine composites (9000 to $10,000$ MPa) is two to three times the value for microfine composites (3000 to 5000 MPa). For comparison, the modulus of elasticity is $62,000$ MPa for amalgam, $18,600$ MPa for dentin, and $82,700$ MPa for enamel.

The tensile strengths of the microfine composites (26 to 33 MPa) are only about half those of fine composites (34 to 62 MPa), but this may be related to the diametral method of testing. When samples are tested in true tension, a more significant difference appears with the microfine composites functioning more like the unfilled polymers. The higher values for the fine composites reflect the higher volume fraction of the high-strength, brittle, inorganic dispersed phase and the transfer of stress given by the more ductile polymer matrix.

Although not reported for dental composites, the strain at rupture and the toughness of composites are lower than those for the unfilled polymers. For example, the elongation at rupture of an industrial composite containing 50% by volume of inorganic phase was only 20% of the value obtained for the unfilled polymer. For this reason fine composites are more brittle than unfilled polymers, and microfine composites are less brittle than the fine composites.

The Knoop hardness of composites is low (see Table 10-1) compared with values of 343 kg/mm^2 for human enamel, and 110 kg/mm^2 for dental amalgam.

The Knoop hardness of the fine composites and hybrids (55 to 80 kg/mm^2) is somewhat greater than similar values for the microfine composites (23 to 36 kg/mm^2), which reflects the hardness and volume fraction of filler particles. These values indicate a moderate resistance to indentation under functional stresses for the more highly filled materials, but this difference does not appear to be a major factor in resisting functional wear. A microhardness measurement such as Knoop can be misleading on composites with larger-size filler particles, in which the small indentation could be made solely on the organic or the inorganic phase. However, with most current products, filler particle sizes have become much smaller, and the microhardness values appear more reliable.

The clinical wear rates of composites are listed in Table 10-1 with occlusal loss of height reported in μm/year. Note that the microfine composites were more resistant to wear than the fine composites. Clinical wear of hybrid composites is in the same range as microfine with values from 20 to 65 μm/year.

Wear of composites is a complex phenomenon involving abrasion, attrition, and erosion and as a result no single mechanical property has been predictive of clinical wear. However, it has been shown that proper application of coupling agents is essential and that wear resistance is reduced to half when no silane treatment was used on the inorganic phase. Increasing the volume fraction of filler is also important in increasing wear resistance. However, microfilled composites with lower volume fraction of fillers have better clinical wear resistance than composites with larger filler particles at higher volume fraction of filler; some laboratory wear tests show the opposite effect. This discrepancy possibly may be explained by noting that although the microfilled composites have lower volume fraction of filler than fine composites, there are more filler particles per volume in the microfilled composites. Thus a wear crack can propogate only a short distance before being blunted by another filler particle.

It has also been shown clinically that subsurface and internal voids result in accelerated wear, which is reasonable because they serve as stress concentration when the restoration is placed under chewing forces. Therefore photoinitiated composites are potentially more wear resistant because no mixing is required and restorations should be more free of voids. Inadequate cure of composites also decreases wear resistance and microfilled composites require longer exposure to curing lights because the filler disperses the light and results in shorter depth of penetration of the light. Curing the microfilled composite in layers can assure adequate depth of penetration of the light.

Radiopacity

Early composites were characteristically radiolucent because the filler was quartz, and a clinical evaluation was conducted either by direct observation or by transillumination. Later composites included glasses having atoms with high atomic numbers, such as barium, strontium, and zirconium. The typical fillers, such as quartz, lithium aluminum glasses, and silica, are not radiopaque and must be blended with other fillers to produce a radiopaque composite. Even at their highest volume fraction of filler, the amount of radiopacity seen in composites is noticeably less than that exhibited by a metallic restorative like amalgam (Fig. 10-10). The microfine composites are being marketed with some degree of radiopacity by the incorporation of very finely divided heavy metal glass particles, but the degree of radiopacity imparted is barely sufficient to aid in diagnosis. Aluminum is used as a standard reference for radiopacity. A 2-mm thickness of dentin is equivalent in radiopacity to 2.5 mm of aluminum, and enamel is equivalent to 4 mm of aluminum. To be effective a material should exceed the radiopacity of enamel, but international standards accept radiopacity equivalent to 2 mm of aluminum. Amalgam has a radiopacity greater than 10 mm of aluminum, which exceeds all the composite materials available.

Depth of Cure (Photoinitiated Resins)

Maximum intensity of the light radiation beam is concentrated near the surface of a photoinitiated

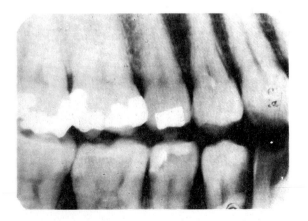

Fig. 10-10 A dental radiograph illustrating the radiopacity of posterior composite resins (mandibular) and amalgam (maxillary) restorations.

composite. As the light penetrates into the material, it is scattered and reflected and loses intensity. A number of factors influence the degree of polymerization at given depths from the surface after photoinitiation. The concentration of photoinitiator or light absorber in the composite must be such that it will react at the proper wavelength and be present in sufficient concentration. The filler content and particle size are critical to dispersion of the light beam. For this reason, microfine composites with smaller and more numerous particles scatter more light than fine composites with larger and fewer glass particles, and longer exposure times are needed to obtain adequate depth of cure.

The light intensity at the resin surface is a critical factor in completeness of cure both at the surface and within the material. The tip of the light source must be held within 1 mm of the surface to gain optimum penetration. The shade of the resin is critical because the more opaque shades reduce light transmission and cure only to minimal depths. A standard exposure time using most visible lights is 20 seconds. In general, this is sufficient to cure a light shade of resin to a depth of 2 or 2.5 mm. A 40-second exposure improves the degree of cure at all depths, but it is required to obtain sufficient cure with the darker shades. Application of the light beam through 1 mm or less thickness of tooth structure produces a sufficient cure at shallower depths, but the hardness values obtained are not so consistent at given depths. The light beam does not spread sufficiently beyond the diameter of the tip at the emitting surface; therefore it is necessary to "step" the light across the surface of large restorations so that the entire surface receives a complete exposure. Larger tips have been manufactured for placement on most lamps. However, as the light beam is distributed over a larger surface area, the intensity at a given point is reduced. It is therefore expedient to use a longer exposure time of up to 60 seconds when larger emitting tips are used.

A practical test can be developed to evaluate the effective depth of cure of a specific light source on a photoinitiated composite. A small section of 5 to 10 mm is cut from a clear straw and placed on a glass slide. The section is then packed with unpolymerized composite and leveled at the top. The light is applied directly to the top surface for 20 to 40 seconds according to the operator's technic. The straw is cut off, and the uncured composite is scraped from the bottom of the sample with a sharp knife. The length of the apparently cured sample is measured and divided in half to estimate the effective depth of cure in the system.

Bond Formation to Tooth Structure

Enamel

The adhesion values of composites to etched enamel are listed in Table 10-1 as between 20 and 24 MPa. The adhesion is principally a result of mechanical retention of the polymer matrix or bonding agent into the rough etched surface of enamel, and the failure can occur within the composite, reflecting relative tensile strengths. Bonds that are formed between a low-viscosity polymer bonding agent and an enamel surface are primarily mechanical and depend on the penetration of the resin into irregularities on the enamel surface. To obtain an optimum bond strength, the surface must be conditioned with an etching solution, frequently 35% to 50% phosphoric acid. The etched enamel surface has an increased surface area for bonding, a higher surface energy to enhance wetting, and demineralized porous rod ends into which the resin can penetrate (Fig. 10-11) and produce mechanical tags as shown in Fig. 10-12. Adequate bonding to enamel depends on a dry etched surface that must be kept isolated from moisture and salivary mucoproteins. In many years of clinical testing, the acid-etched bond to enamel has proved successful as the major retentive factor in restoring anterior teeth with composite resin and in sealing pits and fissures from the ingress of decay-producing bacteria.

Dentin

Research on dentin bonding agents has focused on attachment between the mineral or collagen portions of dentin and composites. A variety of systems have been marketed with claims of chemical attachment to dentin; however, the prevailing belief is that the bonding mechanism is primarily the result of micromechanical retention resulting from good wetting and penetration of the bonding agent into dentin. However, acid etching of dentin, similar to that done on enamel, is not recommended because dentinal tubules extend to the pulp chamber and contain tissue fluid. Attachment to dentin requires

50 % PHOSPHORIC ACID (REAGENT)

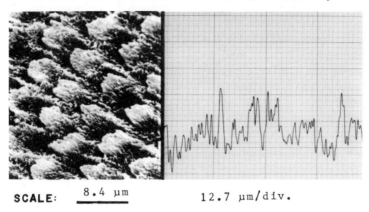

SCALE: 8.4 µm   12.7 µm/div.

Fig. 10-11 Demineralized enamel rods showing porous ends and roughness profile of the surface.

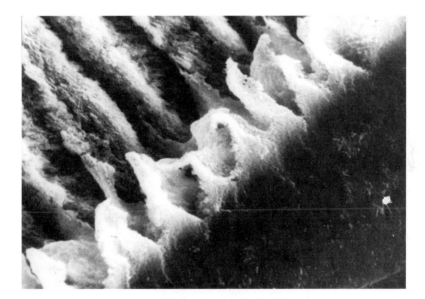

Fig. 10-12 Mechanical tags of composite that penetrated into etched enamel.

removal of the smear layer resulting from cavity preparation, consisting of hydroxyapatite and partially denatured collagen, and decalcification of intertubular dentin to a depth of 1-5 µm. The objective is to remove the smear layer and etch the intertubular dentin but leave the dentin tubules plugged with debris (like the smear layer). The morphology of dentin varies with location and bonding varies from regions of high tubule density to sclerotic areas.

Bonding agents usually consist of a bifunctional monomer with hydrophilic groups to improve wetting to dentin and hydrophobic groups to polymerize with the composite. The bonding agent may be polymerized separately from the composite to minimize shrinkage stresses if both are polymerized at the same time. As shown in Table 10-1 considerable variation exists among reported bond strengths but agreement does exist that the bond strength to dentin is less than that to enamel. It also has been shown the dentin bonding agents work well on enamel and thus two separate bonding agents are not necessary.

Regardless of the system selected, the following conditions are essential: (1) isolation of the bonding surface, (2) maintenance of a clean surface, (3) correct application of bonding agent, (4) use of a protective liner for deep restorations, (5) use of mechanical retention in the cavity design when no enamel is available for retention from etching.

Dentin bonding agents can be classified as: (1) polyurethanes (PUs); (2) organic phosphonates (OPs); (3) mellitic anhydrides plus methyl methacrylate (4-META); (4) hydroxyethyl methacrylates plus glutaraldehyde (HEMA + GA); (5) ferric oxalate plus the reaction product of *N*-phenyl or tolyl glycine and glycidyl methacrylate (NPG-GMA) plus the reaction product of pyromellitic dianhydride and 2-hydroxyethyl methacrylate (PMDM); (6) hydroxyethylmethacrylate/Bis-GMA plus a maleic acid etchant (HEMA/Bis-GMA); and (7) biphenyl dimethacrylate (BPDM).

The urethane-bonding type is formed by the reaction of a polyol and a diisocyanate such as

Polyol   **Diisocyanate**

The object is for the diisocyanate to react with the polyol and the $-OH$ or $-NH_2$ groups in the dentin mineral or organic components. The composite can then bond to the polyurethane.

The phosphonate-bonding types may or may not be halogenated and are typical of

or

The claim is that the phosphate end reacts with calcium in hydroxyapatite and the carbon-carbon double bond at the other end reacts with the composite.

The mellitic anhydride type is dissolved in methyl methacrylate and is typical of the following, frequently referred to as 4-META.

The objective is for the anhydride to hydrolyze to a diacid with $-OH$ groups on the surface of dentin and to function like an acrylic acid, and for the carbon-carbon double bond to react with the composite.

The hydroxyethyl methacrylate (35%) plus glutaraldehyde (5%) consists of

HEMA   **Glutaraldehyde**

The objective is for the glutaraldehyde to react with an amino group in the organic portion of dentin and also to react with HEMA, which in turn will react with the composite through the carbon-carbon double bond. The surface of dentin coated with the gluteraldehyde-HEMA was examined 30 seconds after contact using an atomic force microscope, and dentin tubules were not observed and the dentinal surface was covered by a solid, bumpy layer.

The ferric oxalate NTG-GMA/PMDM system consists of three components:

$$Fe_2(C_2O_4)_3 \cdot 6H_2O,$$

and

$$CH_2{=}\overset{\overset{\displaystyle CH_3}{|}}{C}{-}\overset{\overset{\displaystyle }{\underset{\underset{\displaystyle O}{\|}}{C}}}{}{-}O{-}CH_2CH_2{-}O{-}\overset{\overset{\displaystyle }{\underset{\underset{\displaystyle O}{\|}}{C}}}{}{-}$$

$$HO{-}\overset{\overset{\displaystyle O}{\|}}{C}$$
(benzene ring with substituents)
$$\overset{\overset{\displaystyle O}{\|}}{C}{-}O{-}CH_2CH_2{-}O{-}\overset{\overset{\displaystyle CH_3}{|}}{\underset{\underset{\displaystyle O}{\|}}{C}}{-}C{=}CH_2.$$

The ferric oxalate removes the smear layer from the dentin and serves as a mordant, while the NTG-GMA and PMDM bond to the dentin and contain carbon-carbon double bonds to react with the composite. Several variations of this concept have been used substituting *N*-tolyl glycine for *N*-phenyl glycine and using other primer systems such as dilute nitric acid or phosphoric acid. An adhesive containing HEMA and a Bis-GMA is photocured onto a dentin surface that has been primed with an aqueous acidic solution of HEMA and maleic acid. This system was based on producing a graded layer between the hydrophilic dentin and the hydrophobic composite. A modification of this system uses a 10% maleic acid etchant and a primer consisting of an aqueous solution of HEMA and polyalkenoic acid copolymer. This and other recent systems produce bonds that are not sensitive to being placed on moist dentin as opposed to dry dentin.

Another dentin bonding system uses aqueous organic acid solutions containing aluminum salts as a conditioning liquid and a bonding solution of mono and polyfunctional methacrylic acid.

A biphenyl dimethacrylate (BPDM), containing carboxylic acid groups, is a dentin bonding agent similar to PMDM and has the following structural formula,

TABLE 10-2   Shear Bond Strengths and Marginal Gap Sizes between Dentin and Composite

Bonding Agent Type	Shear Bond Strength (MPa)	Gap Size for 4-mm Diameter Restoration (μm)
PU	3	–
OP	4	10
4-META	14	4
HEMA + GA	17	2
NTG-GMA/ PMDM	14	8
HEMA/ Bis-GMA	24	–
BPDM	28	–

Bond strengths of these systems usually are measured in shear after the composite is attached. The literature is difficult to interpret because a rather wide range of bond strengths has been reported for the same type of dentin bonding agent. Best estimates of the published shear bond strengths for the various types of bonding agents are listed in Table 10-2.

The minimum bond strength needed to overcome the polymerization shrinkage of a typical composite has been estimated for restorations of various sizes, and as expected, larger restorations resulted in larger gap sizes. The gap sizes for a 4-mm diameter restoration for four of the systems are also given in Table 10-2. These data suggest that a dentin bonding agent should have a tensile or shear bond strength of at least 17.6 MPa to eliminate a gap at the margin of a 4-mm diameter restoration. Because the gap size is a function of the size of the restoration, it can be reduced by polymerizing the composite in layers.

These bonding agents have been tested on human enamel, and in all instances the values are substantially higher or equal to those against dentin. As a result, these materials are used in bonding composites to enamel in combination with acid etching.

$$CH_2{=}\overset{\overset{\displaystyle CH_3}{|}}{C}{-}\overset{\underset{\underset{\displaystyle O}{\|}}{C}}{}{-}O{-}CH_2CH_2{-}O{-}\overset{\underset{\underset{\displaystyle O}{\|}}{C}}{}\ \text{(biphenyl with }HO{-}\overset{\overset{\displaystyle O}{\|}}{C}\text{ and }\overset{\overset{\displaystyle O}{\|}}{C}{-}OH)\ \overset{\underset{\underset{\displaystyle O}{\|}}{C}}{}{-}O{-}CH_2CH_2{-}O{-}\overset{\overset{\displaystyle CH_3}{|}}{\underset{\underset{\displaystyle O}{\|}}{C}}{-}C{=}CH_2.$$

Biocompatibility studies have demonstrated that dentin bonding agents showed no or slight pulp reactions in animals and no or slight inflammation of human pulp when a thin layer of dentin was present. The surface treatments on dentin are designed to remove the smear layer produced by cavity preparation but to leave the dentinal tubules plugged, thus minimizing any pulpal reaction.

Studies of the leakage of saliva around the margins of restorations treated with dentin bonding agents demonstrated some decrease in leakage *in vitro* compared with controls. Even when combined clinically with the acid etching and bonding to adjacent enamel, the dentin bond appears insufficiently maintained to fully support functional tensile and shear stresses. After 3 years of controlled evaluation, less than 75% of nonprepared cervical restorations were retained with a dentin bonding agent alone. When the resin was bonded to etched enamel along the occlusal margin, retention improved to approximately 90% over the same 3-year period, but penetrating margin discoloration was evident in greater than 30% of the retained restorations. The dentin-polymer interface exposed along cervical margins appears the most vulnerable to hydrolytic breakdown and the development of fluid leakage.

Significant advances in dentin bonding agents show that recent systems can produce bonds between dentin and composites equal to bonds between enamel and composites, however bond strengths should not be interpreted to mean that marginal leakage is eliminated. In general, increased dentin bonding has resulted in reduced marginal leakage, but has not eliminated it. Also, it has been shown that bond strengths decrease significantly in the oral environment. Thus presently bond strengths are not sufficient to change cavity design to nonretentive preparations. Finally, the evidence suggests that bonding with newer dentin adhesives containing hydrophilic and hydrophobic groups results mainly from microetching of the surface resulting in a demineralized zone that is penetrated by the adhesive rather than from chemical bonding.

Biocompatibility

Histological studies of the effect of chemically activated acrylic resins on the dental pulp indicate a reaction comparable with that of zinc phosphate cement; therefore cavity liners are recommended. Although they produce a less severe inflammatory reaction of the pulp, composite resins are also potential irritants and require the use of calcium hydroxide or glass ionomer cavity liners. The reaction noted in most histopathological studies is moderate in degree and usually reversible. The acid etchant appears to open the dentinal tubules and, although not apparently harmful in itself, permits a greater penetration of the low-viscosity bonding agent with potentially irritating low molecular weight monomers. The protection should be placed specifically over areas of exposed dentin where tubules are most likely to communicate directly with the pulp. Many current etchants remove the smear layer but leave the tubules plugged, thus reducing penetration of components of the composite to the pulp. The components most likely to penetrate to the pulp are the low molecular weight dimethacrylates such as TEGDMA. Eugenol is an inhibitor for the polymerization reaction, and composites should not be placed directly on zinc oxide–eugenol bases. Fluorides have been added to composites to produce some anticariogenic effect.

Color

The color and blending of shades for the clinical match of esthetic restorations are vitally important and should be given greater consideration by the dental practitioner. The characteristics of color are discussed in Chapter 3, and these principles can be applied specifically to composite resins for determining appropriate shades for clinical use. The universal shade varies greatly in color among currently marketed products. The ranges obtained by both spectrophotometric and visual observations are shown in Table 10-3 as analyzed initially after setting and then after 300 hours of accelerated aging. All materials were in the yellow range for hue, both initially and after aging. However, a shift in hue was noticed for some materials after 10 hours, some to yellow-red and others to yellow-green, but the change was neutralized with time. The luminous reflectance showed a general decrease with exposure, but no change was noted in value or dominant wavelength. A general intensification of chroma and rise in excitation purity resulted from weathering. Translucency is a characteristic that gives a vital

TABLE 10-3   Variation in Color Characteristics for the Universal Shades of Composite Resin

Characteristic	Initial	After Weathering for 300 hr
Spectrophotometric*		
Luminous reflectance	51.6-78.9	49.1-71.7
Dominant wavelength (nm)	575.9-579.6	575.9-579.3
Excitation purity	0.16-0.31	0.25-0.37
Visual observation (Munsell)*		
Hue (Y)	2.5-5.0	2.5-5.0
Value	7.0-8.5	7.0-8.0
Chroma	2-4	3-5

*Samples evaluated on a white background.

appearance to an esthetic restoration. The graph in Fig. 10-13 illustrates the increase in opacity, as demonstrated by contrast ratio, with an increase in sample thickness.

In clinical studies a change in color was observed in anterior composite restorations over a 3-year period (Table 10-4). Although they were still visually in the same hue, there was a significant decrease in value (darkening) and an increase in chroma (saturation of color). Change of color and loss of shade match with surrounding tooth structure are perhaps the most frequent reasons for replacement of restorations. Stress cracks within the polymer matrix and partial debonding of the filler to the resin as a result of hydrolysis tend to increase opacity and alter the appearance. Discoloration can also occur through the effect of ultraviolet radiation from daylight and result from water exchange within the polymer matrix and its interaction with unreacted polymer sites and unused initiator or accelerator.

Material Selection

In the current market, little variation is found in physical properties among specific groups of composites. Most products fall into one of three major categories: fine, microfine, or hybrid composites. Fine-particle composites and hybrids are chosen primarily for their high mechanical properties and

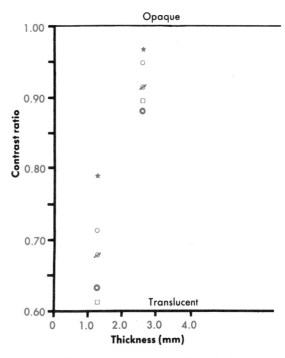

Fig. 10-13 Change in contrast ratio for typical restorative resins with increasing sample thickness. One material (*) is an unfilled acrylic; the other four are composites.

TABLE 10-4   Change in Color for Clinical Restorations Using the Munsell System (Means)

Time of Observation	Autocured (Mean)
VALUE	
Insertion	7.6
6 mo	7.6
12 mo	7.4
24 mo	7.4
36 mo	7.3
CHROMA	
Insertion	2.2
6 mo	2.2
12 mo	2.2
24 mo	2.5
36 mo	3.0

rigidity. They provide the most support in stress-bearing areas such as large restorations involving one or both incisal angles. They are more opaque and can be shaded readily to match basic tooth shades or to cover stained enamel. Microfine composites, on the other hand, are selected primarily because they are more translucent and provide optimum esthetics as a thin veneer over normal tooth enamel. Higher in polymer content, microfine composites are more ductile and less subject to brittle failure. Handling characteristics also are important factors, and such variables as working time, setting time, viscosity, color, radiopacity, and cost merit full consideration.

■ MANIPULATION AND HANDLING CHARACTERISTICS

Composites

Composites are supplied as two pastes or a single paste. The paste-paste systems are chemically initiated and possess an infinite depth of cure. The single-paste systems are photoinitiated, with more optimum handling characteristics, but they do not have an infinite depth of cure. Dual-cure systems are also available where polymerization is both chemical- and photoinitiated. The use of chemically initiated composites is mainly reserved for the preparation of cores with most restorative work using photoinitiated composites.

Two-paste system

Equal quantities of the two pastes are dispensed onto a mixing pad with a disposable plastic spatula. The spatulas have blades on both ends, and one end should be used to dispense one paste, and the other end, the second paste. This precaution prevents contamination of the two pastes and hardening of the pastes in the jars. The two pastes are mixed thoroughly and quickly, which usually requires 20 to 30 seconds. A metal spatula should not be used for fine-particle composites because the fillers are sufficiently hard to abrade some of the metal off the spatula and incorporate it into the mix, which alters the shade and discolors the composite restoration. The filler particles should be uniformly distributed in each paste, but, especially in a warm environment, the particles may settle within the oligomer. Therefore each paste should be stirred periodically to ensure adequate filler distribution. Settling of the filler can be avoided and shelf life can be prolonged if the pastes are refrigerated when stored for

extended periods. Only small increments of each paste should be placed on the mixing pad, sufficient to place only one restoration at a time.

Insertion

Enamel bonding agents consist of the oligomer diluted with lower molecular weight monomers to form a low-viscosity liquid that can be applied directly over etched enamel. The bonding agent should readily wet the enamel surface and penetrate the irregularities to form retentive mechanical tags of resin from 15 to 50 μm in length (see Fig. 10-12). Dentin bonding agents can also be used as a substitute. A composite can then be placed while the bonding agent is still fluid, and the two resins will polymerize together. More frequently light-activated bonding agents are polymerized before placing the composite to ensure complete curing of the tag layer and improve bonding to dentin. The air-inhibited polymer on the surface of the polymerized material bonds with the first layer of composite restorative material and cures when covered.

The mixed two-paste composite will have a working time of 1 to 1.5 minutes and a setting time of 3 to 5 minutes. It may be inserted into the cavity preparation by several methods, depending on the viscosity of the particular product. It may be packed into the cavity preparation with a variety of instruments made of plastics that do not adhere to the mixed composite. If the viscosity of the mix is not too high, it can be injected from a syringe into the cavity preparation, which reduces the incorporation of voids in the restoration and facilitates placement of the composite into the areas of retention. The cavity preparation is slightly overfilled, and a matrix is immediately placed into position and held firmly for about 2 minutes. The matrix is removed 3.5 to 4 minutes after the start of the mix, and after 2 to 6 additional minutes the composite is sufficiently hard for finishing to begin.

Single-paste system

Single-paste systems are the most frequently used composites and they are initiated by visible light and have a shelf life of up to 1 year. Care must be exercised to dispense only small increments of material from the syringe and to avoid exposure of the material at the end of the syringe to sunlight by replacing the cap immediately. Unused composite should never be returned to the syringe or kept for future use. Storage should be in a cool and dry environment to maintain shelf life for all composites. The limitations encountered in these materials are penetration of the light beam and depth of cure (2.5 mm maximum for most lights). In deep cavities or large restorations, increments of paste may build restoration contour by use of the air-inhibited surface layer to secure chemical bonding between increments.

Insertion of a photoinitiated resin should capitalize on the strengths of the system. Shade matching should never be achieved by mixing two viscous pastes together, but can be effectively accomplished by layering. The darker shade or the shade with the most intense chroma should be placed first and then overlaid with the lighter or more translucent shade. If material sticks to the placement instrument, a small amount of uncured bonding agent can serve as a lubricant. After each increment is contoured, it should be exposed to the light beam and exposed for a longer period of time (up to 60 seconds) when darker or more opaque shades are used. With an extended working time, the restorations can be contoured before light activation; thus the finishing requirements are reduced.

Finishing

The objectives in finishing composite resin restorations are important and are directed toward obtaining a positive gingival tissue response. Proper finishing procedures should establish (1) a smooth surface texture that will reflect light in a similar manner to adjacent tooth enamel, (2) a restoration contour that is physiologically acceptable to supporting tissues, (3) an occlusal relationship that minimizes applied stress in all functional mandibular movements, (4) proper margin adaptation of the resin at the cavosurface margin, and (5) a general contour that is in harmony with tooth form and promotes esthetics. Development of optimum restoration contour and surface texture minimizes plaque retention and decreases stain accumulation, while facilitating the removal of plaque in a daily oral hygiene program.

Finishing is accomplished by initial gross reduction with carbide finishing burs, Green Stones, or coarse aluminum oxide disks. Final finishing is accomplished with fine silicon carbide, aluminum oxide disks, or White Arkansas Stones. Finishing procedures usually can be started 5 minutes after mixing or photoinitiation.

A glossy surface is obtained when the composite sets against the matrix and no finishing is done, but unfortunately finishing is almost always required clinically. As finishing takes place, small voids incorporated during the insertion of the material may be exposed, and they can collect unsightly stains. It has been found that chemically initiated composites have more marginal defects than photoinitiated composites. The degrees of roughness created by a variety of finishing instruments can be compared in Table 10-5. The fine-particle composites have almost as smooth a surface texture as the microfine composites. Clinically, a slight difference in surface texture appears between the fine and hybrid composites and the microfine composites, with the latter maintaining a glossy surface and the former exhibiting a satin or slightly granular texture. However, clinical studies have not detected any advantage of the microfine composites with respect to gingival health, marginal adaptation, or caries. With all three types of composites the degree of gingivitis increases with time, and recurrent caries is the major reason for replacement.

TABLE 10-5 Surface Roughness of Fine, Hybrid, and Microfine Composites Finished with Various Abrasives

Finishing Agent	Roughness (μm)	
	Fine and Hybrid	Microfine
Mylar matrix	0.12	0.09
Abrasive disks		
Coarse	2.02	1.87
Medium	0.6	0.71
Fine	0.3	0.25
Superfine	0.11	0.09
Carbide finishing bur	0.65	—
Diamond stones		
Medium grit	1.41	—
Superfine grit	0.67	—
Polishing paste	0.1	0.1

Modified from Herrgott AML, Ziemiecki TL, Dennison JB: *J Am Dent Assoc* 119:729, 1989.

A successively finer texture is developed with the sequential application of disks with finer grits. The coarsest disk is used for the gross reduction of excess composite and the development of contour. The sequence of finer disks produces a smoother surface texture and refined marginal adaptation. Heavy contours or anatomical morphology, particularly on posterior restorations, can be established with diamond stones or carbide finishing burs applied usually at ultraspeed. Diamond abrasives are manufactured in varying grits and should be applied sequentially with a water spray to reduce frictional heat. Both 12- and 30-blade carbide finishing burs can be used to develop restricted areas of anatomical contour and should be applied cautiously to avoid chipping the composite.

When repairing a large composite resin restoration, the bond between freshly mixed composite and previously set material is less than the bulk strength of the composite. The potential for success in bonding an increment of fresh composite resin to previously set material is best if applied at the same appointment and before the set surface has been contaminated with finishing debris or salivary fluids. Once contamination has occurred or the original composite has fully set for a 24-hour period, the surface should be roughened mechanically to expose fresh composite. The surface should be acid etched to clean the glass filler particles in fine and hybrid composites, and a layer of bonding agent should be applied. This agent should be allowed to soak in well before curing, and then the repair resin can be applied over the bonding agent. The tensile strength of such a repair bond is about 75% of the original value but appears to hold up well clinically.

Effects of Tooth Bleaching Agents

Bleaching agents containing 10% carbamide peroxide were used to treat polished surfaces of microfilled and hybrid composites over a period of four weeks, and slight changes in the surfaces were observed. Microcracks appeared on the surface of microfilled composite and slight roughening of the hybrid composite was observed in scanning electron micrographs. Knoop microhardness measurements showed that the bleaching treatment resulted in some softening of the surface (5-13 KHNs).

■ EXTENDED APPLICATIONS FOR COMPOSITES

Modifications have been made in the oligomer formulation and in the type and amount of filler used to produce specific products with specialized applications. The following are major areas in which composites are used in clinical dentistry other than for the direct restoration of lost tooth structure in anterior teeth. Some of these applications have been very successful clinically, whereas others have only limited value but represent the most conservative treatment available at the present time. Much research is in progress to develop new products that will meet specific esthetic demands of the dental profession, particularly in the area of an amalgam substitute.

Anterior Veneers

The application of anterior cosmetic veneers to mask hypoplasia or tooth discoloration has become an integral part of dental practice. Composites can be placed in a thin layer over etched enamel and can be sculptured to provide enhanced tooth form or esthetics. Lower viscosity composites suitable for direct application against etched enamel have been developed, usually of a chemically activated type to be placed in a bulk manner with a confined tooth form used as a matrix. Such a technic is difficult to control, usually results in air void entrapment, and demands excessive finishing. A variety of even lower viscosity composites (less than 20 wt% filler) have also been formulated, with opacifiers added in a variety of tooth-colored shades to block out severely stained enamel. Tinted composites with added color modifiers are also available in varied shades such as yellow, brown, blue, black, and pink to provide characterization for an anterior veneer. These shade modifiers are all photoinitiated and, although they require additional exposure to light, can be cured as they are applied to gain the desired esthetic effect. By layering these composites either under or between applications of the composite restorative, lifelike color characteristics can be developed, the externally exposed composite has optimum physical properties, and the diluted stains are internally protected.

Labial veneers can also be made indirectly on a model with newer materials in which the degree of polymerization can be increased with higher-energy light sources, vacuum chambers, and applied heat. The prefabricated veneer is then luted to the etched tooth enamel surface with a lower viscosity composite cement. The weakest portion of the bonded interface is the bond between the precured composite veneer and the freshly applied composite cement. Unsightly leakage can occur at this interface, which periodically requires repair. Laboratory-fabricated composite veneers are more resistant to abrasion and are more color-stable than direct veneering composites.

Porcelain Bonding

Porcelain-bonding systems have been developed to lute indirect anterior veneers to etched enamel, as well as to place a composite restoration that replaces fractured porcelain (Fig. 10-14) and restores esthetics. Each of these systems contains a hydrolyzable silanating agent that provides a relatively weak bond to the ceramic surface. When broken porcelain is being repaired, the interface must be roughened to increase surface texture and to create some mechanical locking. In limited clinical studies, these restorations frequently lasted only short periods of time because they were generally in full incisal function. Those restorations sustaining the least use have the best prognosis for retention. Porcelain veneers can be bonded to enamel with similar technics and a low-viscosity composite cement. This procedure is more successful because a larger surface area of porcelain is available, and it is generally roughened by a hydrofluoric acid treatment during fabrication.

The entire porcelain veneer is also well supported against fracture by underlying enamel, but the interface at the margin is still subject to leakage, which would require repair with polymer.

Core Build-Up

Modifications have been made to alter the viscosity and the setting time of highly filled composites to formulate core materials that will closely adapt to pins and posts (Fig. 10-15). Core materials are usually chemically initiated so that they can be inserted with a syringe, enclosed in a metal or celluloid crown form or matrix, and cured in bulk. For this reason, these materials usually have a slightly prolonged working time (approaching 2 minutes) and a relatively quick "snap" set. Because core materials are highly filled composites, they provide optimum resistance to deflection forces and shear stresses. They should also be highly colored or opaque materials so that there will be a visible interface at the composite-tooth junction during final cavity preparation.

Posterior Restorations

A specific group of composites with improved properties has been developed for restoring posterior teeth with tooth-colored materials. Most composites are hybrids or blends with bimodal or trimodal filler distributions that increase filler content. Several microfine systems have also been improved for posterior use, but the resulting properties are still inferior to those of the fine composites. Table 10-6

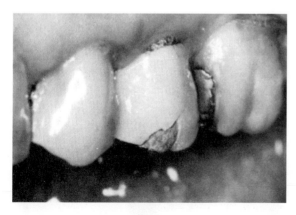

Fig. 10-14 A fractured porcelain-to-metal restoration that could be repaired with composite resin.

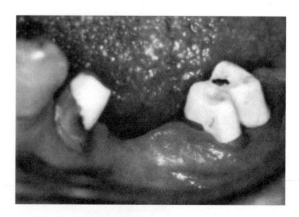

Fig. 10-15 A reconstructed composite resin core prepared for a cast metal crown.

indicates the degree of improvement seen in several of the critical properties related to failure of restorations. Microfine filler has been sintered into macrosized particles to improve wear resistance in at least one product. In another product a hydrophobic resin matrix has been used to reduce water sorption, with the hope that failure of the silane coupling agent will be reduced.

Composites for posterior applications contain heavy metal glass fillers to supply significant radiopacity, as discussed earlier in this chapter. They are also viscous to permit a certain degree of condensation during insertion and the development of anatomical form and contour. Posterior composites are used in conjunction with a glass ionomer cavity liner and a dentin bonding agent to secure the best possible bond to dentin. They are hard to finish because margins are not easy to recognize, and access can be difficult. Although a reasonably small occlusal restoration on a premolar or maxillary first molar can be successful for 5 to 6 years, there is ample opportunity for the marginal seal to fail and leakage to occur. The major mode of failure that occurs when composite resin is placed into posterior function is wear or loss of substance (Fig. 10-16), which limits the application in the posterior area or at least necessitates early replacement to sustain occlusal function.

The American Dental Association has recognized posterior composites as a distinct group of materials through an acceptance classification based on clinical performance. To be accepted a composite must be placed in a controlled clinical study and lose no more than 50 μm per year (100 μm after 2 years and 250 μm after 5 years). Evaluation is done indirectly on models taken at 6-month recalls, and the measurement is made of the deepest portion of exposed enamel margin (Fig. 10-17). Hybrid composites have been shown to lose 20-65 μm/year and microfilled composites 25-55 μm/year. A matter of uncertainty in the dental profession is whether a 250-μm loss of substance truly represents a clinically acceptable restoration that adequately supports occlusal function. Computer graphic tracings of a more quantitative nature indicate that the volume loss of material is greatest in localized areas of occlusal functional contact. For optimum results,

TABLE 10-6   Critical Physical Properties for a Posterior Composite Resin

Property	Value
Compressive strength (MPa)	250-320
Tensile strength (MPa)	35-40
Modulus of elasticity (MPa $\times 10^3$)	5-13
Thermal coefficient of expansion (/° C $\times 10^{-6}$)	15-30
Water sorption (mg/cm^2)	0.1-0.85

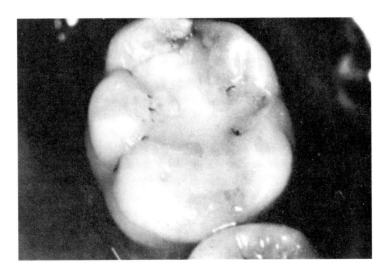

Fig. 10-16 A posterior composite resin restoration exhibiting excessive occlusal wear and marginal discoloration.

posterior composite resin restorations should be limited to class 1 and 2 cavities on premolars with minimal buccal-lingual extension and in which some occlusal support can be maintained on the natural tooth (Fig. 10-18).

The degree of polymerization of composites used in posterior applications can be increased by an indirect procedure in which the restoration is postcured at 125° C. In one procedure, the posterior composite is placed in a nonretentive preparation, removed after setting, postcured at 125° C, and then cemented to the tooth with a composite cement. This indirect procedure not only results in a composite restoration with a higher degree of polymerization with improved properties, but also reduces the shrinkage of the composite during polymerization to that of the shrinkage of the thin layer of the composite cement.

In a second procedure, an impression is taken of the cavity preparation in an addition silicone, and a die is made in this impression using an addition silicone putty or a fast-setting epoxy. The posterior composite restoration is formed in the die and after setting is postcured to improve the properties. The composite restoration is then cemented to the tooth using a composite cement. In addition to the previous advantages, this second procedure provides a better opportunity to develop proximal contacts.

Orthodontics

Lower viscosity–filled composites are also being used for the cementation of orthodontic brackets to the facial surfaces of both anterior and posterior teeth. The enamel is acid etched in the usual manner, and each bracket is applied directly to the surface in the desired position. The high-modulus fine composites resist stress better than unfilled or microfine composites, so most orthodontic composites are fine particle or hybrid composites. Long-term clinical results indicate that the bond is strong enough to support the forces to move anterior teeth and premolars. However, there is variable response to the increased torque set up in moving molars, and in those situations orthodontic bands are usually placed. Isolation is the key to success in any bonding procedure, but it is even more critical in this area where multiple units are being placed at one appointment.

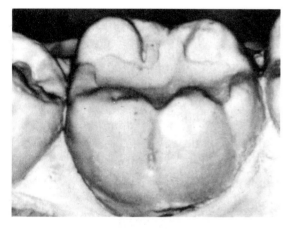

Fig. 10-17 A stone model of posterior composite resin restorations with exposed enamel walls at the margins.

■ PIT AND FISSURE SEALANTS

Pits and fissures in the occlusal surfaces of permanent teeth are particularly susceptible to decay, and fluoride treatments have been least effective in preventing caries in these areas. This susceptibility is related to the physical size and morphology of the individual pit or fissure, which can provide shelter for organisms and obstruct oral hygiene procedures. Cross-sectional views of typical fissure morphology, varying from a wide V shape to a bottleneck shape, are shown in Fig. 10-19. A technic termed *occlusal sealing* was introduced in 1965; this technic involved the use of methyl-2-cyanoacrylate, which was mixed

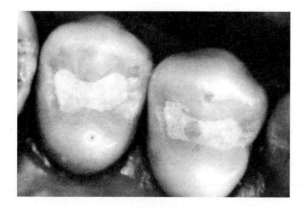

Fig. 10-18 An ideal conservative class 1 posterior composite resin restoration on a maxillary premolar with minimal buccal-lingual isthmus width.

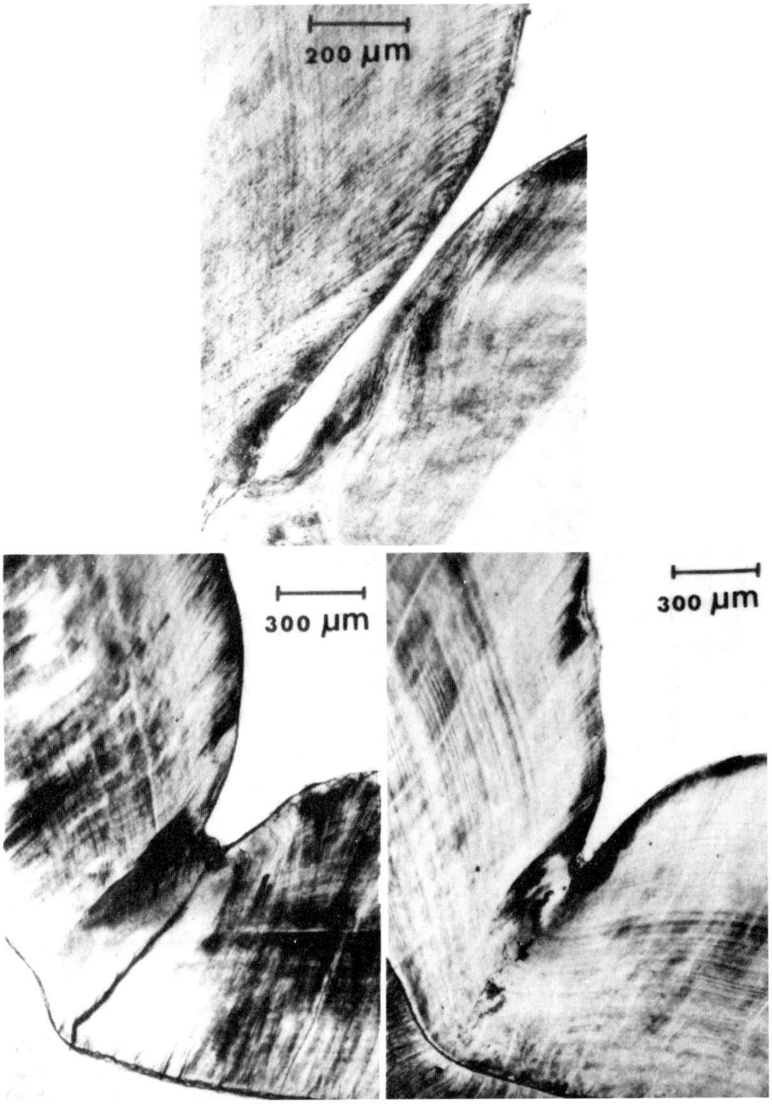

Fig. 10-19 Sections of teeth illustrating shapes of fissures. (From Gwinnett AJ: *J Am Soc Prevent Dent* 3:21, 1973.)

with poly(methyl methacrylate) and inorganic powder and then placed in the pits and fissures. The cyanoacrylate polymerized on exposure to moisture. Since that time the sealant systems that have been evaluated include the Bis-GMA resins (polymerized either by chemical means or by visible light), a polyurethane sealant containing inorganic fluoride compounds, and polyacrylate materials. Sealants have also been used with fluoride treatment, and a cyanoacrylate sealant has been used after fluoride treatment in an attempt to maintain a high surface concentration of fluoride for a longer period of time than is possible with the usual treatment.

Composition and Reactions

Bis-GMA resins

The full name for Bis-GMA is 2,2-bis[4(2-hydroxy-3-methacryloyloxy-propyloxy)-phenyl] propane. The chemistry of the Bis-GMA types is the same as that described for the composites. The principal difference is that the Bis-GMA sealants must be much more fluid to penetrate into the pits and fissures and also into the etched areas produced on the enamel, which provide for retention of the sealant. Three parts of the viscous Bis-GMA are mixed with one part of diluent such as methyl methacrylate (MMA) to obtain a reasonably low-viscosity sealant. The sealants photoinitiated by blue light are activated by the inclusion of a diketone and an aliphatic amine. The complete reactions for composites are given in Chapter 6. If the aperture of the emitting source is held 1 mm from the surface of the sealant, it should harden in 20 seconds. This control is particularly valuable when sealant is applied to very young patients or when cooperation is a problem.

Several Bis-GMA sealants that polymerize by an organic amine accelerator are available. The material is supplied as a two-component system: one component contains Bis-GMA and benzoyl peroxide initiator, and the other component contains Bis-GMA with 5% organic amine accelerator. The two components are usually dispensed as viscous drops onto a suitable mixing surface (e.g., dappen dish, paper pad), and after adequate mixing they are applied directly to the tooth surface. The polymerization is an addition reaction in response to the formation of radicals, although somewhat less cross-linked than those of the composite systems. The reaction is exothermic, but the clinical effect is minimal because the material is placed in limited bulk. The rate of reaction for all materials is sensitive to temperature, and the material would therefore set more quickly in the mouth than on the mixing surface.

During polymerization there is a surface layer of air inhibition that varies in depth with different commercial products. Sufficient material must be applied to completely coat all pits and fissures with a layer thick enough to ensure complete polymerization after removal of the tacky surface layer. Premature contamination with moisture during insertion and the early application of biting forces can disrupt the setting and affect its strength.

Properties

Reports of the physical properties of sealants have been scarce because sample preparation with such low-viscosity materials is difficult. The relationship between properties and clinical service is even

TABLE 10-7   Physical Properties of Bis-GMA Resin Sealants

Property	Unfilled Amine-Accelerated	Filled Amine-Accelerated
Compressive strength (MPa)	130	170
Tensile strength (MPa)	24	31
Modulus of elasticity (GPa)	2.1	5.2
Hardness, Knoop (kg/mm^2)	20	25
Water sorption at 7 days (mg/cm^2)	2.0	1.3

more speculative than for most restorative materials. Typical properties obtained for an unfilled sealant and a filled sealant are given in Table 10-7. With the addition of about 40% by weight of finely divided filler particles, as in the composite systems, all properties except tensile strength showed improvement. The samples were tested for tensile failure by the diametral method, and the high deformation before fracture affects the reliability of the data. The modulus of elasticity showed the most dramatic improvement, and the increased rigidity makes the filled material less subject to deflection under occlusal stress. Filler is also added with the hope of improving wear resistance and making the material more visible on clinical inspection.

Penetration studies on closed capillary tubes, which are somewhat analogous to pits and fissures, have indicated that a sealant will adapt more closely to the enamel surface if it possesses a high coefficient of penetration. Optimum penetration will occur when the sealant has a high surface tension and a low viscosity, thus permitting it to flow readily along the enamel surface. The surface energy is demonstrated by the contact angle of a drop of liquid on the enamel surface. A drop that spreads readily has a low contact angle and is indicative of a highly wetted surface that is most conducive to a strong bond. Polymer tags that form in direct apposition to the surface irregularities created by acid etching are responsible for the mechanical bond that retains the sealant to enamel. Functional durability of the sealant bond can be related to stresses induced by initial polymer shrinkage, thermal cycling, deflection under occlusal forces, water sorption, and abrasion, with total failure manifested by the clinical loss of material.

Manipulation

Enamel surface preparation

The penetration of any of the sealants to the bottom of the pit is important. The wettability of the enamel by the sealant is improved by etching, and some advocate the use of pretreatment with silanes in a volatile solvent. The problem of filling the fissure is real; air frequently is trapped in the bottom of the fissure, or the accumulation of debris at the base of the fissure prevents it from being completely filled, as shown in Fig. 10-20. Control of the viscosity of the sealant is important to obtain optimum results. The viscosity is important in the penetration of the etched areas of enamel to provide adequate retention of the sealant. Penetration of sealant, forming what have been called tags, to a depth of 25 to 50 μm is shown in Fig. 10-21.

The pit and fissure surface is preconditioned by etching for a specified time (1 minute is adequate for enamel with a normal mineral and fluoride content) with a solution or a gel of 35% to 50% phosphoric acid. The acid must be thoroughly flushed with water, and the area dried with warm air. Inadequate rinsing permits phosphate salts to remain on the surface as a contaminant interfering with bond formation. The etched surface should not be rubbed during either etching or drying because the roughness developed can easily be destroyed. Isolation of the site is imperative throughout the procedure so that optimum tag formation and clinical success can be gained. If salivary contamination occurs during the treatment, the surface should be rinsed and dried, and the acid etching repeated. On clinical inspection, acid-etched enamel should appear white and dull with an obviously rough texture. If this appearance is not uniform, a second minute of etching should be carried out. The etched area should extend beyond the anticipated area for sealant application to secure optimum bonding along the margin and reduce the potential for early leakage.

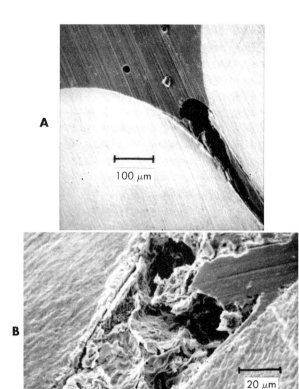

Fig. 10-20 Section showing a fissure incompletely filled with sealant as a result of air, **A,** and debris, **B.** (From Gwinnett AJ: *J Am Soc Prevent Dent* 3:21, 1973.)

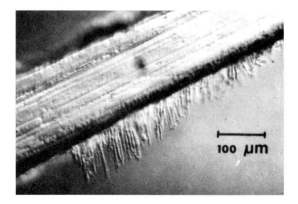

Fig. 10-21 Penetration of sealant into etched enamel; these tags are responsible for the bonding to enamel. (From Gwinnett AJ: *J Am Soc Prevent Dent* 3:21, 1973.)

Bis-GMA-amine–accelerated sealant

Several amine-accelerated sealants are marketed commercially, and all seem to have different handling characteristics and methods of application. All systems have two components, as described earlier, and must be dispensed onto a mixing surface. Because quantities are usually small, caution must be taken to include all material in the mixing and to use a gentle motion to minimize air incorporation. Air inclusions during mixing and insertion can be manifested clinically as surface voids, which can discolor and retain plaque. The sealant must be applied quickly after mixing to work during the optimum period of low viscosity and to ensure penetration. Depending on the viscosity of the sealant and the setting time, it may be best applied with a thin brush, a ball applicator, or a syringe. Manipulation late in the setting reaction can disrupt the polymerization and induce bond failure. The air-inhibited surface layer should be wiped away after a 3- to 5-minute wait, and the coating carefully inspected for voids and areas of incomplete coverage. Defects can be covered at this time by repeating the entire reapplication procedure, including the acid etch, and reapplying the sealant only to those areas indicated.

Bis-GMA-light–accelerated sealant

Bis-GMA-light–accelerated sealant is supplied in a light-tight container and should be usable for a 12-month period. The sealant is applied to the pit and fissure area with a ball-tipped applicator, and when polymerization is desired, the end of the light source is held 1 to 2 mm from the surface. The sealant is exposed to light for 20 seconds. The advantage in using a light-accelerated sealant is that the working time can be completely controlled by the operator and integrated with patient behavior. Also, the material sets quickly, and treatment need not be prolonged as when an amine-accelerated material polymerizes.

Clinical Studies of Sealants

The following three pieces of information have been proposed as necessary in the evaluation of any clinical study on sealants: a statistical test of the significance; the net gain as a result of treatment (when pairs of teeth are studied, the net gain is the number of pairs in which the treated tooth is sound and the untreated tooth is decayed minus the number of pairs in which the treated tooth is decayed and the untreated tooth is sound); and the percent of effectiveness (the net gain divided by the total number of carious controls expressed in percentage). Comparing the results obtained in different studies is difficult because not all studies have been analyzed in this manner, and variables are involved that relate to materials, technics, tooth selection, and evaluation criteria. The criteria most frequently selected for evaluation are the presence of sealant (retention), margin discoloration (early sign of leakage), and caries (effectiveness of caries reduction).

Many clinical studies have reportedly used Bis-GMA systems. A sealant accelerated by radiation demonstrated a retention rate of 42% and an effectiveness of 35% in caries reduction after 5 years. In a similar study a filled resin sealant showed a retention rate of 53% and a clinical effectiveness of 54% after 4 years. Early results involving a quicker-setting unfilled resin sealant with very good penetration showed a retention rate of 80% and an effectiveness of 69% after 3 years. In another study an attempt was made to compare sealant treatment with amalgam restorations on contralateral teeth. It was found that operating time for placement of a chemically accelerated sealant was about half (6 minutes) that used to place an amalgam restoration (14 minutes). The teeth were maintained caries free for a 5-year period by reapplication of the sealant when indicated by clinical reexamination. The highest retreatment rate occurred at 6 months (18%) and then diminished as time progressed, but at each recall period at least two teeth (approximately 4%) required reapplication.

Current evidence indicates that sealants should not be used (1) on relatively flat occlusal surfaces where pits and fissures are not well defined, (2) on teeth with many proximal lesions, (3) on teeth that have been free of caries for a number of years, or (4) on teeth of a patient who does not maintain good oral hygiene or who does not seek regular professional dental examinations.

■ GLASS IONOMERS

Composition and Reaction

Glass ionomers set by a hardening reaction between an ion-leachable calcium aluminum fluorosilicate glass powder and polymers and copolymers of acrylic or maleic acid. The polymer acid may be dissolved in water containing tartaric acid, which is mixed with the glass powder. Freeze-dried polymer acid may be blended with the glass powder, which is mixed with a water solution of tartaric acid, or freeze-dried polymer acid and tartaric acid may be blended with the glass powder, which is mixed with water. In each system, hydrated protons from the polymer acid attack the surface of the glass particles, releasing Al^{+3} and Ca^{+2} ions. Metallic salt bridges are formed between the polymer acids, and a cross-linked gel matrix is formed as the initial set of the mix develops. Excess glass powder is always present so that the reaction products bind the unreacted portion of the glass together. During the initial setting reaction, calcium ions are more rapidly bound to the polyacrylate chains, whereas a more prolonged and permanent set occurs as the trivalent aluminum ion-exchange enters the reaction and strengthens the cross-linking effect. A similar chelation reaction can take place between the setting ionomer mix and calcium on the surface of tooth structure, resulting in an adhesive bond that can be used in tooth restoration.

Properties

The handling characteristics and physical properties of ionomers can be varied significantly by altering the glass composition or polyacid formulations. Specific modifications made in the particle size or the molecular weight, concentration, and viscosity of the liquid can be used to adjust the working time, the setting time, the optical properties, and various mechanical properties that are necessary in clinical application. Some typical values are given in Table 10-8 to compare the physical properties of a glass ionomer with similar properties for a zinc polyacrylate material. The properties for a glass ionomer restorative are similar to those of a zinc polyacrylate cement, except that they have higher compressive strength and modulus. As a restorative material, the major weaknesses of the glass ionomer are a lack of translucency, although recent products have translu-

TABLE 10-8   Physical Properties of a Glass Ionomer and a Zinc Polyacrylate Material

Property	Glass Ionomer	Zinc Polyacrylate
Setting time (min)	4	6
Compressive strength (MPa)	150	70
Tensile strength (MPa)	15	12
Modulus of elasticity (MPa)	20,000	4000
Solubility (%)	0.4	0.1
Bond strength to dentin (MPa)	4	3-4
Bond strength to enamel (MPa)	5	–

cencies matching tooth structure, and a matte surface texture. The flux used in fusion of the glass contains fluoride and has an anticariogenic effect on adjacent tooth structure. It should be emphasized that the mechanical properties increase for at least a week after setting.

Clinical Application

Glass ionomers are used for class 3 and 5 restorations and can restore cervical abrasions and erosion lesions without cavity preparation.

A product marketed as an aqueous solution of polyacrylic acid and a glass powder is shown in Fig. 10-22, *A*. For all hand-spatulated mixes, the powder-to-liquid ratio is critical, and the mixing is done by quickly adding two equal increments of powder. Spatulation is done on a treated mixing pad and should be completed within 30 seconds. The smear layer should be partially removed from the dentin surface with a 15% to 25% solution of polyacrylic acid, which is thoroughly rinsed after 15 to 20 seconds. The tooth surface should not be desiccated but should be moist. Freshly mixed material can be put directly onto the tooth surface with a placement instrument or loaded into a syringe for application. The working time must not be exceeded during manipulation, or the bond to the dentin may be disrupted. Once the surface gloss disappears and a satin sheen is evident (approximately 90 seconds), the materials should be covered with a protective

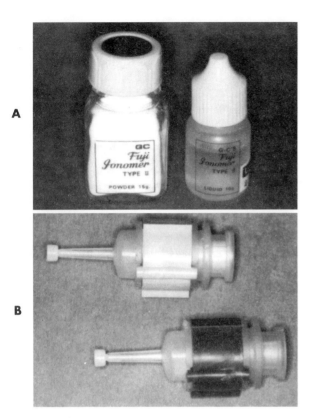

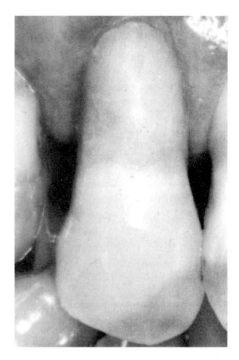

Fig. 10-23 Glass ionomer restoration showing crazing.

Fig. 10-22 Glass ionomer restorative materials marketed as, **A,** a powder/liquid system or **B,** a precapsulated system for mechanical mixing.

coating to preserve it from dehydration or early contact with moisture. Such coatings as cocoa butter, a special thickened varnish, or a light-cured resin bonding agent are all acceptable. For best results, initial finishing should be minimal, and final finishing should be delayed at least 24 hours until the gel matrix is more completely set. The use of a cement glaze on the set glass ionomer has been shown to protect the surface from a storage media of pH4 lactic acid under conditions of thermal cycling.

An alternative type of glass ionomer material involves anhydrous polymaleic acid included with a glass powder that is mixed with a water solution containing tartaric acid. The reaction rate within the matrix is faster with this material, and finishing can be accomplished after 10 to 15 minutes. This anhydrous material is very sensitive to moisture uptake because the first stage of the reaction involves solution of the polyacid. It is therefore dispensed in a premeasured capsule (Fig. 10-22, *B*), which must be activated and mechanically mixed in an amalgamator. Working time is slightly longer, and consistency is more reliable with this method of mixing.

Cervical restorations of glass ionomer are always somewhat sensitive to dehydration, which can cause crazing, loss of translucency, and sometimes partial loss of material (Fig. 10-23). Clinically, solubility and abrasion do not appear to present problems or lead to early failure. Surface texture is noticeably rougher than that of composites, but in a controlled study, this did not produce increased signs of inflammation in adjacent gingiva. Cases of postoperative sensitivity have been reported, and biocompatibility studies of cultured pulp cells have demonstrated differences among products, with the best showing only slight cytotoxicity, and others showing moderate reactions. Therefore a thin coating of a calcium hydroxide liner should be applied to those areas of the preparation closest to the pulp.

For the construction of cores, glass ionomer can be reinforced and made radiopaque by adding metal. In one current product the alloy is sintered into the glass, and the "cermet" particles are mixed with the polyacid liquid either on a paper pad or in a predispensed capsule. In another product amalgam alloy filings are mixed with the glass powder before spatulation with the liquid. Metal-reinforced ionomer cores can be placed quickly, provide some bond to dentin, adapt well to pins and posts, release fluoride, and can be reduced after 5 to 10 minutes to prepare for a cast gold restoration. However, they are not strong enough to be indefinitely retained in the mouth without metal coverage.

A third variety of glass ionomer is a lower viscosity lining material used primarily for pulpal protection under composites. The ionomer is impermeable to the acid etchant and the oligomer and develops only a mild, reversible pulpal reaction. The ionomer liner bonds to underlying dentin, and the etched glass ionomer surface is a good bonding substrate for the composite. This "sandwich" procedure is particularly applicable to cervical and posterior composite restorations.

A fourth type is the resin-modified glass ionomer. These materials are indicated for class 3 and 5 restorations, cervical erosion or abrasion lesions, root caries lesions, and temporary repair of fractured teeth. This type is a hybrid of the traditional glass ionomer reaction and the chemical and/or photoinitiation of the polymerization of HEMA (hydroxyethyl methacrylate). When photoinitiation alone is used the products have been referred to as dual-cure materials, and when both chemical and photoinitiation is used they have been called triple-cure materials. The HEMA is present in the liquid, which also contains polyacrylic acid containing some pendant methacrylate groups and tartaric acid. When the powder (containing the glass, which may be modified to provide radiopacity) and liquid are mixed, the usual glass ionomer acid-base reaction starts, as does the polymerization of the HEMA if chemical initiators are present. If the material uses a light curing system only the HEMA polymerizes after exposure to blue light (470 nm). In either case, the initial set is a result of the polymerization of HEMA, which forms a matrix that is strengthened by the slower acid-base reaction. The setting time of the photoinitiated resin-reinformed glass ionomer is about 20 seconds compared to about 4 minutes for the standard glass ionomer. The compressive strength of the resin-reinforced glass ionomers is approximately the same as for the standard glass ionomer, but the diametral tensile and transverse strengths of the resin-reinforced glass ionomers are about double. Also, the bond to enamel and dentin is approximately double for the resin-modified glass ionomer. Both the resin-reinforced and standard glass ionomer materials release fluoride rapidly for the first week followed by a gradual decrease in rate of release up to six months. Finally a slow but steady release has been measured for three years and this release should continue. Regardless of the type of glass ionomer they release fluoride better than composite formulated to contain fluorides.

Glass ionomer is a clinically successful restorative material with extremely technic-sensitive properties. It is used as a restorative in areas not exposed to occlusal function, as a cavity liner for pulpal protection and dentin bonding, as a core material to support cast metal or ceramic restorations, and as a luting agent for certain castings.

SELECTED PROBLEMS

Problem 1. In the selection of a composite for use in placing a large class 4 restoration, what are several advantages of a photoinitiated system?

Solution. Contour can be more adequately achieved through incremental addition; fewer air voids should be incorporated because mixing of two pastes is not necessary; shade development can more readily be accomplished through the increments of different-colored composites; and less excess material should exist after insertion and curing of the restoration, thus finishing should be facilitated.

Problem 2. An extensive posterior core buildup is required on a lower molar. What are the reasons that a chemically activated composite is the material of choice?

Solution. Uniform curing takes place under a crown form, lower viscosity resin adapts better to pins or posts, and opaque-colored composites can be used to differentiate core from tooth structure during crown preparation.

Problem 3. When small air voids appear on the surface of a photoinitiated composite restoration during finishing, what are the causative manipulative factors?

Solution. The problem may be caused by exposing the dispensed composite to operatory light before incremental insertion, extended working of each increment to the point that voids are incorporated between layers, mixing of increments of two different shades of pastes on a pad before insertion, or excessive use of alcohol as a lubricant on the insertion instrument.

Problem 4. Is there reason to expect that a large class 4 restoration will be more color stable when a photoinitiated composite is used instead of a chemically activated composite? Why?

Solution. Yes. A chemically activated composite contains an aromatic amine accelerator that breaks down more readily when exposed to ultraviolet light than the aliphatic amine in a photoinitiated system does.

Problem 5. When a thin composite anterior veneer is being placed to modify tooth color, what are the advantages of a microfine composite?

Solution. The advantages are the following: greater translucency improves vitality in the final shade; smoother surface texture provides a glossy surface with light-reflective patterns similar to enamel; and in a thin layer supported by the bond to enamel, high physical and mechanical properties are not as important as in a free-standing class 4 restoration.

Problem 6. In polymerizing a large photoinitiated composite resin restoration, what manipulative variables can be controlled to improve the depth of cure?

Solution. The following variables can be controlled: the exposure time of the light can be increased for darker shades and thicker increments (beyond 2 mm); the light source can be maintained within 1 mm of the resin surface; and the light wand can be drawn across the resin surface in steps, with multiple exposures ensuring uniformity of cure.

Problem 7. In selecting a composite for a large, class 4 anterior restoration with significant incisal function, what are the enhanced properties found in a fine-particle or hybrid composite that make it the material of choice?

Solution. The properties are greater strength and elastic modulus, lower polymerization shrinkage, lower thermal coefficient of expansion, lower water sorption, and greater wear resistance.

Problem 8. In the clinical evaluation of a 2-year-old composite restoration, penetrating marginal discoloration is often noted. What factors contribute to this bond failure?

Solution. Contributing factors are residual stress from polymerization shrinkage, fatigue stresses on the bond from thermal cycling, contamination at the bond site during material insertion, deflection stress at the restoration margins caused by intermittent functional loading of the restoration, and hydrolytic breakdown of the bond at the tooth interface (particularly if it is dentin).

Problem 9. When repairing an anterior veneer restoration with a small area of severe marginal leakage, the discolored composite is removed, and the deficient area is rebonded with new material. What is the character of the bond between old cured composite and new?

Solution. The bond is micromechanical and is formed against the roughened surface of cut composite. It

is a weak chemical bond formed between exposed unreacted bonds in the old material and the new bonding agent, has less cohesive strength than the original composite, and is more durable if an adjacent fresh enamel area can also be prepared by acid etching.

Problem 10. In assessing the use of composites in posterior teeth, what are the factors that currently contribute to early wear and failure?

Solution. These factors are the loss of substance as a result of deterioration of the silane-coupling agent bonding the filler particles to the matrix, excessive polymerization shrinkage from the relatively large volume of such restorations, stress crack propagation across filler-polymer interfaces, and low abrasion resistance of a relatively large volume of polymer matrix.

Problem 11. In the selection of a material as a pit and fissure sealant, what are the characteristics of a filled resin sealant?

Solution. The characteristics are better physical properties and improved abrasion resistance (but with occlusal prematurities that should be adjusted after insertion); a slightly higher viscosity than an unfilled sealant, but a much lower viscosity than a composite; and better control in application procedures.

Problem 12. In the selection of a sealant material, what are the characteristics of an unfilled resin sealant?

Solution. The characteristics are lower viscosity, less wear resistance but with occlusal prematurities that will wear down readily, and less control in application procedures.

Problem 13. Postoperative evaluation of a freshly placed sealant revealed subsurface air voids, some communicating with the external surface. What manipulative variables can be controlled to minimize this problem?

Solution. The problem can be minimized by control of the following variables: avoid mixing or stirring the sealant if at all possible after it is dispensed for application, or use a photoinitiated resin; avoid using a brush for application, which tends to carry excess material and incorporate air; use a ball-tipped applicator, which permits the application of smaller increments of material to specific sites on the tooth surface with only minimal manipulation of the setting sealant; avoid moisture contamination during application because it can produce subsurface voids after equilibrium is reached through water sorption; avoid using a material beyond its shelf life or one that has been stored in a warm environment because the increase in viscosity results in air entrapment during application; and avoid applying the sealant to a nonwettable or inadequately etched enamel surface.

Problem 14. Six months after sealant application, a first molar was clinically evaluated at recall and found to have no sealant present. What are the possible causes for this early failure?

Solution a. One cause might be inadequately prepared enamel surface, possibly caused by (1) failure to remove pellicle and debris from the surface during preoperative prophylaxis cleaning, (2) inadequate acid etching by using concentrated or diluted etchant, exposure to etchant for insufficient time, or the presence of acid-resistant enamel with a high fluoride composition, (3) insufficient rinsing of the acid etchant solution or gel, leaving contaminating salts present to reduce surface energy, (4) moisture or salivary contamination during sealant application, and (5) contamination of the etched enamel site by oil or by water in the compressed air used for drying.

Solution b. A second causative factor might be inadequately cured photoinitiated sealant, possibly caused by (1) the light wand held too high above the tooth surface, (2) failure to make multiple light applications to completely expose the entire surface, (3) inadequate exposure time to the light source, (4) use of a sealant that has previously been exposed to light or has been used beyond its shelf life, and (5) use of an opaque or deeply colored sealant without increasing the exposure time.

Problem 15. At recall evaluations, sealants may have an orangish-brown stain along specific marginal areas, which is indicative of bond failure and marginal leakage. What are the causative factors for this failure?

Solution. The causative factors are inadequate enamel preparation at the failure site or contamination of the etched enamel, overextension of sealant beyond the periphery of adequately etched enamel, and functional occlusal forces placed directly over thin extensions of sealant that produce stresses that exceed the bond strength of sealant to enamel.

Problem 16. In selecting a glass ionomer material for use in restorative dental procedures, can one material be used for all purposes by simply adjusting the powder/liquid ratio to control viscosity?

Solution. No, for the following reasons: viscosity is better controlled by use of polyacrylic acids that are prepolymerized to specific polymer chain lengths; powder/liquid ratios are specific to particular acid chain lengths and could adversely affect physical properties if adjusted improperly; setting and working times are related to powder-liquid ratios and prepolymer chain lengths and could be inadvertently reduced below levels of clinical acceptability.

Problem 17. In restoring a nonretentive cervical deficiency without cavity preparation, what manipulation variables could directly influence clinical retention?

Solution. The manipulative variables are inadequately removing the smear layer with a dilute polyacrylic acid liquid; working the material beyond the stage in which gloss is lost from the surface, which could disrupt bond formation to dentin; excessively drying or dehydrating the material immediately after placement, which could result in loss of the chemical bond to dentin and thus necessitate the application of a protective varnish or resin coating; and prematurely exposing it to moisture immediately after placement, which can cause leaching of critical elements from the matrix.

Problem 18. What are the characteristics of a glass ionomer lining cement that make it suitable for pulpal protection beneath composite resin restorations?

Solution. The characteristics are as follows: they are impermeable to the penetration of acid etchant or bonding resin; they bond to dentin, which decreases the potential for microleakage; they are biologically acceptable to pulpal tissue when greater than 0.5 mm of dentin is present; and the liner can be acid etched after 5 minutes to create a mechanical bond with the resin bonding agent of the restoration.

Problem 19. What is the primary indication for use of a glass ionomer as a complete restorative material? Why?

Solution. The primary indicator is the restoration of lesions involving either cervical enamel or root caries because of bonding to dentin. Glass ionomers leach fluoride into the immediate oral environment and are anticariogenic.

Problem 20. What are the clinical advantages of a metal-reinforced glass ionomer for construction of a core in the restoration of extensively destroyed teeth with cast gold crowns?

Solution. The advantages are bond formation to dentin, leaching of fluoride, radiopacity, higher-strength and elastic modulus, early strength that permits quick reduction in cavity preparation, and color that permits easy discrimination of core from tooth structure during cavity preparation.

■ REFERENCES

Resins and Composites

Asmussen E: Clinical relevance of physical, chemical, and bonding properties of composite resins, *Oper Dent* 10:61, 1985.

Bailey SJ, Swift EJ Jr: Effects of home bleaching products on composite resins, *Quint Int* 23:489, 1992.

Berry EA III, von der Lehr WN, Herrin HK: Dentin surface treatments for the removal of the smear layer: an SEM study, *J Am Dent Assoc* 115:65, 1987.

Blankenau RJ, Kelsey WP, Cavel WT, Blankenau P: Wavelength and intensity of seven systems for visible light-curing composite resins: a comparison study, *J Am Dent Assoc* 106:471, 1983.

Boyer DB, Chan KC, Reinhardt JW: Build-up and repair of light-cured composites: bond strength, *J Dent Res* 63:1241, 1984.

Braem M, Finger W, Van Doren VE, Lambrechts P, Vanherle G: Mechanical properties and filler fraction of dental composites, *Dent Mater* 5:346, 1989.

Burke FJT, McCaughey AD: The four generations of dentin bonding, *Am J Dent* 8:88, 1995.

Cook WD: Spectral distributions of dental photopolymerization sources, *J Dent Res* 61:1436, 1982.

Council on Dental Materials, Instruments, and Equipment: Posterior composite resins: an update, *J Am Dent Assoc* 113:950, 1986.

Council on Dental Materials, Instruments, and Equipment: Visible light-cured composites and activating units, *J Am Dent Assoc* 110:100, 1985.

Craig RG: Chemistry, composition, and properties of composite resins, *Dent Clin North Am* 25:219, 1981.

Cross M, Douglas WH, Fields RP: The relationship between filler loading and particle-size distribution in composite resin technology, *J Dent Res* 62:850, 1983.

Dennison JB, Powers JM, Koran A: Color of dental restorative resins, *J Dent Res* 57:557, 1978.

DeWald J, Ferracane JL: A comparison of four modes of evaluating depth of cure of light-activated composites, *J Dent Res* 66:727, 1987.

Dietschi D, Holy J: A clinical trial of four light-curing posterior composite resins: two-year report, *Quint Int* 21:965, 1990.

Eldiway M, Powers JM, George LA: Mechanical properties of direct and post-cured composites, *Am J Dent* 6:222, 1993.

Fan PL, Edahl A, Leung RL, Stanford JW: Alternative interpretations of water sorption values of composite resins, *J Dent Res* 64:74, 1985.

Fan PL, Wozniak WT, Reyes WD, Stanford JW: Irradiance of visible light-curing units and voltage variation effects, *J Am Dent Assoc* 115:442, 1987.

Farah JW, Powers JM, editors: Anterior and posterior composites, *Dent Advis* 8(4):1, 1991.

Farah JW, Powers JM, editors: Composites, *Dent Advis* 11(3):1, 1994.

Farah JW, Powers JM, editors: Dentin bonding agents, *Dent Advis* 12(2):1, 1995.

Ferracane JL: Elution of leachable components from composites, *J Oral Rehabil* 21:441, 1994.

Ferracane JL, Moser JB, Greener EH: Rheology of composite restoratives, *J Dent Res* 60:1678, 1981.

Gerzina TM, Hume WR: Effect of dentine on release of TEGDMA from resin composite *in vitro*, *J Oral Rehabil* 21:463, 1994.

Gwinnett AJ, Yu S: Effect of long-term water storage on dentin bonding, *Am J Dent* 7:109, 1994.

Hanks CT, Craig RG, Diehl ML, Pashley DH: Cytotoxicity of dental composites and other dental materials in a new *in vitro* device, *J Oral Path* 17:396, 1988.

Hanks CT, Strawn SE, Wataha JC, Craig RG: Cytotoxic effects of composite resin components on cultured mammalian fibroblasts, *J Dent Res* 70:1450, 1991.

Hanks CT, Wataha JC, Parsell RR, Strawn SE: Permeability of biological and synthetic molecules through dentine, *J Oral Rehabil* 21:475, 1994.

Harrington E, Wilson HJ: Determination of radiation energy emitted by light activation, *J Oral Rehabil* 22:377, 1995.

Herrgott AML, Ziemiecki TL, Dennison JB: An evaluation of different composite systems finished with various abrasives, *J Am Dent Assoc* 119:729, 1989.

Heymann HO, Bayne SC: Current concepts in dentin bonding: focusing on dentinal adhesion factors, *J Am Dent Assoc* 124:34, 1993.

Hinoura K, Moore BK, Phillips RW: Tensile bond strength between glass ionomer cements and composite resins, *J Am Dent Assoc* 114:167, 1987.

Hirasawa T, Hirano S, Hirabayashi S, Harashima I, Aizawa M: Initial dimensional change of composites in dry and wet conditions, *J Dent Res* 62:28, 1983.

Inohoshi S, Willems G, Van Meerbeek B, Lambrechts P, Braem M, Vanherle G: Dual-cure luting composites, Part I filler particle distribution, *J Oral Rehabil* 20:133, 1993.

International Symposium on Adhesives in Dentistry, *Oper Dent,* Suppl 5, 1992.

Johnson GH, Bales DJ, Gordon GE, Powell LV: Clinical performance of posterior composite resin restorations, *Quint Internat* 23:705, 1992.

Johnson GH, Gordon GE, Bales DJ: Postoperative sensitivity associated with posterior composite and amalgam restorations, *Oper Dent* 13(2):66, 1988.

Johnson GH, Powell LV, Gordon GE: Dentin bonding systems: a review of current products and techniques, *J Am Dent Assoc* 122:34, 1991.

Jones DW: Composite restorative materials, *J Canad Dent Assoc* 56:851, 1990.

Kalachandra S: Influence of fillers on the water sorption of composites, *Dent Mater* 5:283, 1989.

Kim K-H, Park J-H, Imai Y, Kishi T: Fracture toughness and acoustic emission behavior of dental composite resins, *Engin Fract Mech* 40:811, 1991.

Letzel H: Survival rates and reasons for failure of posterior composite restorations in multicentre clinical trial, *J Dent* 17:S10, 1989.

Leung RL, Fan PL, Johnston WM: Post-irradiation polymerization of visible light-activated composite resin, *J Dent Res* 62:363, 1983.

McInnes-Ledoux PM, Zinck JH, Weinberg R: The effectiveness of opaquer and color-modifier materials: a laboratory study, *J Am Dent Assoc* 114:205, 1987.

Mitchem JC, Gronas DG: The continued in vivo evaluation of the wear of restorative resins, *J Am Dent Assoc* 111:961, 1985.

Munksgaard EC, Hansen EK, Asmussen E: Effect of five adhesives on adaptation of resin in dentin cavities, *Scand J Dent Res* 92:544, 1984.

Neo JC, Denehy GE, Boyer DB: Effects of polymerization techniques on uniformity of cure of large-diameter, photoinitiated composite resin restorations, *J Am Dent Assoc* 113:905, 1986.

Oysaed H, Ruyter IE: Water sorption and filler characteristics of composites for use in posterior teeth, *J Dent Res* 65:1315, 1986.

Pallav P, DeGee AJ, Davidson CL, Erickson RL, Glasspoole EA: The influence of admixing microfiller to small-particle composite resin on wear, tensile strength, hardness, and surface roughness, *J Dent Res* 68:489, 1989.

Pameijer CH, Stanley HR: Pulp reaction to a dentin bonding agent, *Am J Dent* 8:138, 1995.

Papadogianis Y, Boyer DB, Lakes RS: Creep of posterior dental composites, *J Biomed Mater Res* 19:85, 1985.

Pashley DH, Ciucchi B, Sano H, Horner JA: Permability of dentin to adhesive agents, *Quint Internat* 24:618, 1993.

Powers JM, Dennison JB, Koran A: Color stability of restorative resins under accelerated aging, *J Dent Res* 57:964, 1978.

Powers JM, Dennison JB, Lepeak PJ: Parameters that affect the color of direct restorative resins, *J Dent Res* 57:876, 1978.

Powers JM, Fan PL, Hostetler RW: Properties of Class V restorative materials, *J Mich State Dent Assoc* 63:275, 1981.

Powers JM, Hostetler RW, Dennison JB: Thermal expansion of composite resins and sealants, *J Dent Res* 58:584, 1979.

Pratten DH and Johnson GH: An evaluation of finishing instruments for an anterior and a posterior composite, *J Prosthet Dent* 60:154, 1988.

Rathbun MA, Craig RG, Hanks CT, Filisko FE: Cytotoxicity of a BIS-GMA dental composite before and after leaching in organic solvents, *J Biomed Mater Res* 25:443, 1991.

Satrom KD, Morris MA, Crigger LP: Potential retinal hazards of visible light photopolymerization units, *J Dent Res* 66:731, 1987.

Schweikl H, Schmalz G, Bey B: Mutagenicity of dentin bonding agents, *J Biomed Mater Res* 28:1061, 1994.

Simonsen RJ, editor: Posterior composite resin symposium, *Quint Internat* 18:515, 1987.

Soderholm K-J: Leaking of fillers in dental composites, *J Dent Res* 62:126, 1983.

Soderholm K-J, Zigan M, Ragan M, Fischlschweiger W, Bergman M: Hydrolytic degradation of dental composites, *J Dent Res* 63:1248, 1984.

Stanford CM, Fan PL, Schoenfeld CM, Knoeppel R, Stanford JW: Radiopacity of light-cured posterior composite resins, *J Am Dent Assoc* 115:722, 1987.

Stoddard JW, Johnson GH: An evaluation of polishing agents for composite resins, *J Prosthet Dent* 65:491, 1991.

Suh BI, Ferber C, Baez R: Optimization of hybrid composite properties, *J Esthetic Dent* 2:44, 1990.

Tirtha R, Fan PL, Dennison JB, Powers JM: *In vitro* depth of cure of photo-activated composites, *J Dent Res* 61:1184, 1982.

Van Dijken JWV: A clinical evaluation of anterior conventional, microfiller, and hybrid composite resin fillings—a 6-year follow-up study, *Acta Odontol Scand* 44:357, 1986.

Van Dijken JWV, Ruyter IE, Holland RI: Porosity in posterior composite resins, *Scand J Dent Res* 94:471, 1986.

Van Dijken JWV, Sjöström S, Wing K: The effect of different types of composite resin fillings on marginal gingiva, *J Clin Periodont* 14:185, 1987.

Vanherle G, Smith DC: *Posterior composite resin dental restorative materials,* The Netherlands, 1985, Peter Szule (Minnesota Mining and Mfg Co.).

Von Meerbeek B, Peumans M, Verschueren M, Gladys S, Braem M, Lambrechts P, Vanherle G: Clinical status of ten dentin adhesive systems, *J Dent Res* 73:1690, 1994.

Wataha JC, Hanks CT, Strawn SE, Fat JC: Cytotoxicity of components of resin and other dental restorative materials, *J Oral Rehabil* 21:453, 1994.

Wathen WF, editor: Esthetic dentistry—a new direction, *J Am Dent Assoc* (Spec Iss) Dec:7–E, 1987.

Watts DC, Haywood CM, Smith R: Thermal diffusion through composite restorative materials, *Br Dent J* 154:101, 1983.

Wendt SL Jr: The effect of heat used as a secondary cure upon the physical properties of three composite resins. I. Diametral tensile strength, compressive strength, and a marginal dimensional stability, *Quint Int* 18:265, 1987.

Wendt SL Jr: Microleakage and cusp fracture resistance of heat-treated composite resin inlays, *Am J Dent* 4:10, 1991.

Wendt SL Jr, Leinfilder KF: The clinical evaluation of heat-treated composite resin inlays, *J Am Dent Assoc* 120:177, 1990.

Pit and Fissure Sealants

Buonocore MG: Adhesive sealing of pits and fissures for caries prevention, with use of ultraviolet light, *J Am Dent Assoc* 80:324, 1970.

Charbeneau GT, Dennison JB: Clinical success and potential failure after single application of a pit and fissure sealant: a four-year report, *J Am Dent Assoc* 98:559, 1979.

Consensus development conference statement on dental sealants in the prevention of tooth decay, National Institutes of Health, *J Am Dent Assoc* 108:233, 1984.

Council on Dental Research, American Dental Association: Cost-effectiveness of sealants in private practice and standards for use in prepaid dental care, *J Am Dent Assoc* 110:103, 1985.

Dennison JB, Powers JM: Physical properties of pit and fissure sealants (annot), *J Dent Res* 58:1430, 1979.

Dennison JB, Straffon LH, Corpron RE, Charbeneau GT: A clinical comparison of sealant and amalgam in the treatment of pits and fissures. I. Clinical performance after 18 months, *Pediat Dent* 2:167, 1980.

Dennison JB, Straffon LH, Corpron RE, Charbeneau GT: A clinical comparison of sealant and amalgam in the treatment of pits and fissures. II. Clinical application and maintenance during an 18 month period, *Pediat Dent* 2:176, 1980.

Garcia-Godoy F, Gwinnett AJ: Penetration of acid solution and gel in occlusal fissures, *J Am Dent Assoc* 114:809, 1987.

Handleman SL, Buonocore MG, Heseck DJ: A preliminary report on the effect of fissure sealant on bacteria in dental caries, *J Prosthet Dent* 27:390, 1972.

Horowitz HS, Heifetz SB, Poulsen S: Retention and effectiveness of a single application of an adhesive sealant in preventing occlusal caries: final report after five years of a study in Kalispell, Montana, *J Am Dent Assoc* 95:1133, 1977.

Mertz-Fairhurst EJ, Fairhurst CW, Williams JE, Della-Giustina VE, Brooks JD: A comparative clinical study of two pit and fissure sealants: seven year results in Augusta, Ga, *J Am Dent Assoc* 109:252, 1984.

Myers CL, Rossi F, Cartz F: Adhesive taglike extensions into acid-etched tooth enamel, *J Dent Res* 53:435, 1974.

O'Brien WJ, Fan PL, Apostolidis A: Penetrativity of sealants and glazes, *Oper Dent* 3:51, 1978.

Pahlavan A, Dennison JB, Charbeneau GT: Penetration of restorative resins into acid-etched human enamel, *J Am Dent Assoc* 93:1170, 1976.

Ripa LW: Occlusal sealing: rationale of the technique and historical review, *J Am Soc Prevent Dent* 3:32, 1973.

Silverstone LM: Fissure sealants, *Caries Res* 8:2, 1974.

Straffon LH, Dennison JB, More FG: Three-year evaluation of sealant: effect of isolation on efficacy, *J Am Dent Assoc* 110:714, 1985.

Taylor CL, Gwinnett AJ: A study of the penetration of sealants into pits and fissures, *J Am Dent Assoc* 87:1181, 1973.

Glass Ionomers

Aboush YEY, Jenkins CBG: An evaluation of the bonding of glass-ionomer restoratives to dentin and enamel, *Br Dent J* 161:179, 1986.

Bapna MS, Mueller HJ: Leaching from glass ionomer cements, *J Oral Rehabil* 21:577, 1994.

Berry EA III, Powers JM: Bond strength of glass ionomers to coronal and radicular dentin, *Oper Dent* 19:122, 1994.

Braundau HE, Ziemiecki TZ, Charbeneau GT: Restoration of cervical contours on nonprepared teeth using glass ionomer cement: a 4 1/2 year report, *J Am Dent Assoc* 104:782, 1984.

Council on Dental Materials, Instruments, and Equipment: Using glass ionomers, *J Am Dent Assoc* 121:181, 1990.

Croll TP: Glass ionomers in esthetic dentistry, *J Am Dent Assoc* 123:51, 1992.

Croll TP: Visible light-hardened glass-ionomer cement base/liner as an interim restorative material, *Quint Internat* 22:137, 1991.

Croll TP, Killian CM: Restoration of Class II carious lesions in primary molars using light-hardened glass-ionomer-resin cement, *Quint Internat* 24:561, 1993.

Earl MSA, Hume WR, Mount GJ: Effect of varnishes and other surface treatments on water movement across the glass-ionomer cement surface, *Aust Dent J* 30:298, 1985.

Farah JW, Powers JM, editors: Glass ionomers, *Dent Advis* 7(2):1, 1990.

Farah JW, Powers JM, editors: Posts, pins and cores, *Dent Advis* 10(1):8, 1993.

Forss H: Release of fluoride and other elements from light-cured glass ionomer in neutral and acidic conditions, *J Dent Res* 72:1257, 1993.

Garcia R, Caffesse RG, Charbeneau GT: Gingival tissue response to restoration of deficient cervical contours using a glass-ionomer material, a 12-month report, *J Prosthet Dent* 46:393, 1981.

Heys RJ, Fitzgerald M, Heys DR, Charbeneau GT: An evaluation of a glass ionomer luting agent: pulpal histological response, *J Am Dent Assoc* 114:607, 1987.

Hinoura K, Miyayaki M, Onose H: Dentin bond strength of light-cured glass-ionomer cements, *J Dent Res* 70:1542, 1991.

Hotta M, Hirukawa H, Aono M: The effect of glaze on restorative glass-ionomer cements: evaluation of environmental durability in lactic acid solution, *J Oral Rehabil* 22:685, 1995.

Kent BE, Lewis BG, Wilson AD: The properties of a glass ionomer cement, *Br Dent J* 135:322, 1973.

Knibbs PJ, Plant CG: A clinical assessment of an anhydrous glass-ionomer cement, *Br Dent J* 161:99, 1986.

Maldonado A, Swartz ML, Phillips RW: An in vitro study of certain properties of a glass ionomer cement, *J Am Dent Assoc* 96:785, 1978.

McLean JW, Wilson AD: The clinical development of the glass-ionomer cements, *Aust Dent J* 22:31, 1977.

Mount GJ: The role of glass ionomer cements in esthetic dentistry: a review, *Esthet Dent Update* 4:7, 1993.

Müller J, Brucker G, Kraft E, Hörz W: Reaction of cultured pulp cells to eight different cements based on glass ionomers, *Dent Mater* 6:172, 1990.

Reisbick MH: Working qualities of glass-ionomer cements, *J Prosthet Dent* 46:525, 1981.

Saito S: Clinical studies on glass ionomer, *Int J Dent Med* 6:2, 1977.

Sidhu S, Watson TF: Resin-modified glass ionomer materials: a status report for the American Journal of Dentistry, *Am J Dent* 8:59, 1995.

Wilson AD, Prosser HJ, Powis DM: Mechanism of adhesion of polyelectrolyte cements to hydroxyapatite, *J Dent Res* 62:590, 1983.

11 *Impression Materials*

Impression materials are used to register or reproduce the form and relationship of the teeth and oral tissues. Hydrocolloids and synthetic rubbers are among the materials most commonly used to make impressions of various areas of the dental arch, whereas zinc oxide–eugenol and modeling compound are used less frequently. Each of these classes of materials has certain advantages and disadvantages. An understanding of the physical characteristics and the limitations of each material is necessary for its successful use in clinical dentistry.

■ PURPOSE OF IMPRESSION MATERIALS

Impression materials are used to make an accurate replica of the oral tissues. The area involved may vary from a single tooth to the whole dentition, or an impression may be made of an edentulous mouth. The impression gives a negative reproduction of the tissues, and by filling it with dental stone or other model material, a positive cast is made that can be removed after the model material has set. An impression and a stone cast made from it are shown in Fig. 11-1. Casts of the mouth are used in the fabrication of restorations and prostheses and in an evaluation of the dentition when orthodontic, occlusal, or other problems are involved.

Usually the impression material is carried to the mouth in a plastic condition in a tray and applied to the area under treatment. When the impression material has set, it is removed from the mouth with the tray. The cast is made by filling the impression with dental stone or other model material. Sometimes the impression is electroformed with copper or silver to make a metal cast or model. The accuracy, detail, and quality of this final replica are of greatest importance. When the positive reproduction takes the form of the tissues of the upper or lower jaw and serves for the construction of denture bases or other such restorations, it is described as a cast. The positive reproduction of the form of a prepared tooth constitutes a die for the preparation of inlays or bridge structures. When a positive likeness of the arch or certain teeth is reproduced for orthodontic treatment, it is sometimes described as a model, although the term *cast* is proper. On other occasions and in other branches of dentistry, these three terms are used interchangeably. Sometimes impression materials are used to duplicate a cast or model that has been formed when more than one positive reproduction is required. Such impression materials are referred to as duplicating materials.

Examples of typical impression trays are shown in Fig. 11-2. The tray is placed so that the material is brought into contact with the oral tissues and held without movement until the impression material has set. The tray with the impression material is then removed from the mouth, and the impression is ready for making a positive replica. The details of both the clinical impression technic and the production of the cast vary with each impression material and are described in appropriate textbooks.

■ DESIRABLE QUALITIES

Contact with living tissues in the mouth and the needs of clinical procedures dictate critical requirements for the physical properties of dental impression materials. No impression material fulfills all these requirements, and the selection of the material best suited for a particular clinical situation and technic rests with the dentist. The desirable

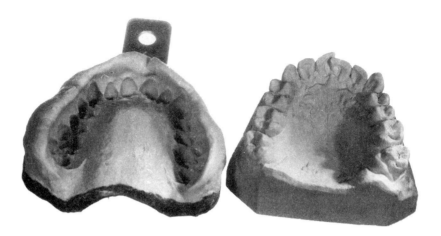

Fig. 11-1 An alginate impression and a stone cast removed from the impression.

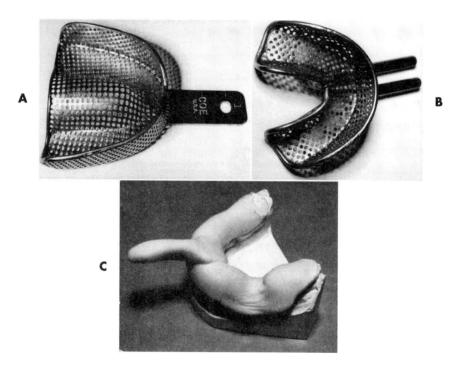

Fig. 11-2 Three types of impression trays. **A,** Perforated metal tray for use with the alginate hydrocolloid impression materials. **B,** Water-cooled metal tray for the agar hydrocolloid impression materials; water enters tubes on the occlusal surface of the tray through one of the projecting tubes and is conveyed away through the other projecting tube. **C,** Custom acrylic tray on a study cast for a rubber impression material.

properties of an impression can be summarized briefly as follows:

1. A pleasant odor, taste, and esthetic color
2. Freedom from toxic or irritant constituents
3. Adequate shelf life for requirements of storage and distribution
4. Economically commensurate with the results obtained
5. Easy to use with the minimum of equipment
6. Setting characteristics that meet clinical requirements
7. Satisfactory consistency and texture
8. Readily wets oral tissues
9. Elastic properties with freedom from permanent deformation after strain
10. Adequate strength so that it will not break or tear on removal from the mouth
11. Dimensional stability over temperature and humidity ranges normally met in clinical and laboratory procedures for a period long enough to permit the production of a cast or die
12. Compatibility with cast and die materials
13. Accuracy in clinical use
14. Readily disinfected without loss of accuracy
15. No release of gas during the setting of the impression or cast and die materials

■ TYPES OF IMPRESSION MATERIALS

The elastic impression materials, alginate hydrocolloid, agar hydrocolloid, and the rubber materials, are perhaps the most widely used today, and the properties of these are examined first. The zinc oxide–eugenol materials, gypsum, and compound impression materials are discussed later in this chapter.

ALGINATE HYDROCOLLOIDS

Dental alginate impression materials change from the sol phase to the gel phase because of a chemical reaction. Once gelation is completed, the material cannot be reliquefied to a sol. These hydrocolloids are called irreversible to distinguish them from the agar reversible hydrocolloids to be described later. They have become widely used to take study impressions for orthodontic and other purposes and, to a limited extent, have been applied in inlay, crown, and bridge procedures.

The alginate impression products have good elastic properties and compare well with the agar materials. Preparation for use requires only the mixing of measured quantities of powder and water. The resulting paste flows well and registers fine surface detail accurately. Casts are made by pouring dental plasters, stone, or investment into the impression, and no separating medium is necessary. The powder is supplied in bulk containers along with suitable measures for dispensing the correct quantities of powder and water. It is also available in small sealed packets containing a quantity suitable for one impression and ready for mixing with a measured quantity of water. Both these methods of packaging, together with the measuring devices supplied by the manufacturer, are shown in Fig. 11-3.

Composition and Chemistry

Alginic acid is prepared from a marine plant and is a linear polymer of anhydro-β-D-mannuronic acid of high molecular weight. Its chemical structure is shown on the next page.

The potassium and sodium salts of alginic acid have properties that make them suitable for compounding a dental impression material. Solutions of these soluble salts, when reacted with a calcium salt, produce an insoluble elastic gel, and the nature of this reaction is as follows in the case of the commonly used potassium salt:

Potassium alginate +

Calcium sulfate dihydrate $\xrightarrow{\text{(+ Water)}}$ Calcium alginate gel +

Potassium sulfate

In an alginate impression compound the soluble alginate and the calcium sulfate dihydrate are both included in the powder, and as the powder is mixed with water, the sparingly soluble calcium sulfate dihydrate dissolves and reacts with the potassium alginate to produce calcium alginate. The calcium alginate is insoluble in water, and its formation causes the mixed material to gel. This reaction is irreversible, and it is not possible to convert the calcium alginate to a sol after it has set.

To meet the critical requirements of a dental impression material, this reaction must be controlled to attain desirable properties of consistency, working

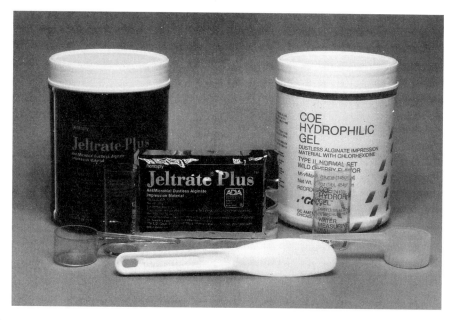

Alginic acid

x = 180 to 930, or a molecular weight of 32,000 to 200,000

Fig. 11-3 Alginate impression products: in bulk in a can with a scoop for measuring powder, a measuring cylinder for water, and a preweighed alginate in a foil package. Both of these products are dustless and contain disinfection agents. (From Craig RG, O'Brien WJ, Powers JM: *Dental materials: properties and manipulation,* ed 6, St Louis, 1996, Mosby.)

time, setting time, strength, elastic quality, and smooth, hard surfaces on gypsum casts. These requirements are achieved by adding agents to control the rate of the reaction, to develop strength and elasticity in the gel, and to counteract the delaying effect that the alginate has on the setting of gypsum products. The use of suitable fillers in correct quantities produces a consistency that is suitable for clinical technics.

The composition and function of ingredients in a typical alginate impression material are shown in Table 11-1. When water is mixed with the alginate powder, the calcium ions from the sparingly soluble calcium sulfate dihydrate react with phosphate ions from the sodium phosphate to form insoluble calcium phosphate. Calcium phosphate is formed

rather than calcium alginate because it has a lower solubility; thus the sodium phosphate is called a retarder and provides working time for the mixed alginate. After the phosphate ions are depleted, the calcium ions react with the soluble alginate to form the insoluble calcium alginate, which together with water forms the irreversible gel.

The manufacturers adjust the concentration of sodium phosphate to produce what are called regular- and fast-set alginates. They also adjust the concentration of filler to control the flexibility of the set impression material from what is called soft-set to hard-set. Although alginate impressions are usually made in a tray, injection types are also available that are much more fluid after mixing and more flexible after setting. The alginate powder is finely divided, and con-

TABLE 11-1 Ingredients in an Alginate Impression Powder and Their Functions

Ingredient	Weight (%)	Function
Potassium alginate	18	To dissolve in water and react with calcium ions
Calcium sulfate dihydrate	14	To react with potassium alginate to form an insoluble calcium alginate gel
Potassium sulfate, potassium zinc fluoride, silicates, or borates	10	To counteract the inhibiting effect of the hydrocolloid on the setting of gypsum, giving a high-quality surface to the die
Sodium phosphate	2	To react preferentially with calcium ions to provide working time before gelation
Diatomaceous earth or silicate powder	56	To control the consistency of the mixed alginate and the flexibility of the set impression
Organic glycols	Small	To make the powder dustless
Wintergreen, peppermint, anise	Trace	To produce a pleasant taste
Pigments	Trace	To provide color
Disinfectants (e.g., quaternary ammonium salts and chlorhexidine)	1-2	To help in the disinfection of viable organisms

siderable dust may be involved during dispensing. The dimensions of 10% to 15% of the siliceous dust particles are similar to asbestos fibers that produce fibrogenesis and carcinogenesis; therefore inhalation of the dust should be avoided. Coating the powder with a glycol results in a dustless alginate, and no detectable levels of dust have been measured at the operator level for the dustless products. Alginates containing disinfectants reduce the viable organisms by up to 90%; however, additional disinfection by solutions or sprays should be carried out.

Proportioning and Mixing

The proportioning of the powder and water before mixing is critical to obtaining consistent results. Changes in the water/powder ratio will alter the consistency and setting times of the mixed material and also the strength and quality of the impression. Usually the manufacturers provide suitable containers for proportioning the powder and water by volume, and these are sufficiently accurate for clinical use.

The mixing time for regular alginate is 1 minute, and it should be measured, because both undermixing and overmixing are detrimental to the strength of the set impression. Fast-set alginates should be mixed with water for 45 seconds. The powder and water are best mixed in a rubber bowl with an alginate spatula or a spatula of the type used for mixing plaster and stone.

Properties

Some typical properties of alginate used as a tray type of impression material are listed in Table 11-2 along with comparable values for agar impression material, which are discussed in the next major section.

Working time

The fast-set materials have working times of 1.25 to 2 minutes, whereas time of the regular-set materials may be as long as 4.5 minutes but more frequently is about 3 minutes. With a mixing time of 45 seconds for the fast-set types, 30 to 75 seconds of working time remain before the impression needs to be completely seated. For the regular-set materials a mixing time of 60 seconds leaves 2 to 3.5 minutes of working time for materials that set at 3.5 to 5 minutes. In either situation the mixed alginate must be loaded into the tray, and the impression made promptly.

Setting time

Setting times range from 1 to 5 minutes. The ANSI/ADA Specification requires that it be at least that listed by the manufacturer and at least 15 seconds longer than the stated working time. Lengthening the setting time is better accomplished by reducing the temperature of the water used with the mix than by reducing the proportion of powder

TABLE 11-2   Typical Properties of Alginate and Agar Hydrocolloid Tray Type of Impression Materials

	Working Time (min)	Setting Time (min)	Gelation (° C)	Recovery from Deformation* (%)	Flexibility[†] (%)	Compressive Strength[‡] (g/cm^2)	Tear Strength[§] (g/cm)
Alginate	1.25-4.5	1.5-5.0	–	98.2	8-15	5000-9000	380-700
Agar	–	–	37-45	99.0	4-15	8000	800-900

*At 10% compression for 30 sec.
[†]At a stress of 1000 g/cm^2.
[‡]At a loading rate of 10 kg/min.
[§]ASTM Tear Die C at 25 cm/min.

and water. Reducing the ratio of powder to water reduces the strength and accuracy of the alginate. Selecting an alginate with a different setting time should also be considered rather than changing the water/powder ratio.

The setting reaction is a typical chemical reaction, and the rate can be approximately doubled by a temperature increase of 10° C. However, using water that is cooler than 18° C or warmer than 24° C is not advisable. The clinical setting time is detected by a loss of surface tackiness. If possible, the impression should be left in place 2 to 3 minutes after the loss of tackiness because the tear strength and resistance to permanent deformation increase significantly during this period.

Permanent deformation

A typical alginate impression is compressed about 10% in areas of undercuts during removal. The actual magnitude depends on the extent of the undercuts and the space between the tray and the teeth. The ANSI/ADA Specification requires that the recovery from deformation be more than 95% (or a permanent deformation of less than 5%) when the material is compressed 20% for 5 seconds at the time it would normally be removed from the mouth. As indicated in Table 11-2, a typical value for recovery from deformation is 98.2%. The corresponding permanent deformation is 1.8%.

The permanent deformation, indicated as percent compression set, is a function of the percent compression, the time under compression, and the time after removal of the compressive load, as illustrated in Fig. 11-4. Note that the permanent deformation is a time-dependent property. Lower permanent deformation

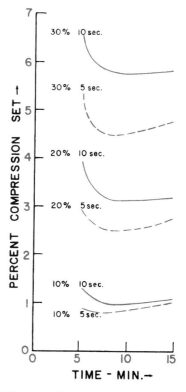

Fig. 11-4 Variation of compression set with time of an alginate impression material at strains of 10%, 20%, and 30% applied for 5 and 10 seconds. (Adapted from Wilson HJ: *Br Dent J* 121:466, 1966.)

(higher accuracy) occurs (1) when the percent compression is lower, (2) when the impression is under compression a shorter time, and (3) when the recovery time is longer, up to about 8 minutes after the release of the load. Clinically these factors translate

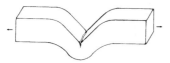

Fig. 11-5 Sketch of tear strength specimen with load applied in the directions of the arrows; the specimen tears at the V notch.

into requirements for a reasonable bulk of alginate between the tray and the teeth and a rapid or snap removal of the impression. The usual procedures followed to produce a gypsum model provide adequate time for any recovery that might occur.

Flexibility

The ANSI/ADA Specification permits a range of 5% to 20% at a stress of 1000 g/cm^2, and most alginates have a typical value of 14%. However, some of the hard-set materials have values from 5% to 8%. A reasonable amount of flexibility is required for ease of removal of the impression.

Strength

The compressive and tear strengths of alginates are listed in Table 11-2. Both of these properties are time dependent, with higher values obtained at higher rates of loading. The compressive strengths range from 5000 to 9000 g/cm^2. The ANSI/ADA Specification requires that certified products have a compressive strength of at least 3570 g/cm^2. The tear strengths vary from 380 to 700 g/cm, and this property is probably more important than the compressive strength. The tear strength is a measure of the force-to-thickness ratio needed to initiate and continue tearing and is frequently determined on a specimen of the shape shown in Fig. 11-5. Tearing occurs in the thin sections of the impression, and the probability of tearing decreases with increasing rates of removal. The effect of loading rate on the tear strength of several alginates is shown in Fig. 11-6. Values for tray materials range from 3.8 to 4.8 N/cm at 2 cm/min to 6 to 7 N/cm at 50 cm/min. The lower tear strength at corresponding rates for the syringe materials reflects the decreased alginate in the syringe material.

Compatibility with gypsum

The selection of an alginate-gypsum combination that produces good surface quality and detail is

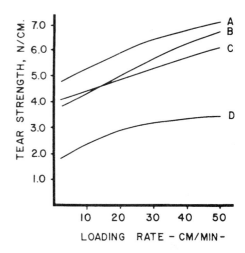

Fig. 11-6 Tear strength of alginate impression materials as a function of rate of loading; materials *A, B,* and *C* are designed to be used in a tray; *D* is a syringe material. (Adapted from MacPherson GW, Craig RG, Peyton FA: *J Dent Res* 46:717, 1967.)

highly important. The surface quality and ability of alginate-gypsum combinations to reproduce fine V-shaped grooves are shown in Fig. 11-7, *A* and *B*. A model plaster was poured against an alginate in Fig. 11-7, *A,* and dental stone was poured against the same alginate in Fig. 11-7, *B*. The finest groove was 0.025 mm wide in each instance. The combination in Fig. 11-7, *B,* was not as compatible as the one in Fig. 11-7, *A,* with respect to either surface quality or detail. For purposes of comparison, in Fig. 11-7, *C,* the same dental stone used in Fig. 11-7, *B,* was poured against polysulfide rubber.

The impression first must be rinsed well in cold water to remove saliva and any blood, and then disinfected. Next, all free surface water should be removed before preparing a gypsum model. Saliva and blood interfere with the setting of gypsum, and if free water accumulates, it tends to collect in the deeper parts of the impression and dilute the model material, yielding a soft, chalky surface. The excess surface water has been removed when the reflective surface becomes dull. If the alginate impression is stored for a half hour or more before preparing the model, it should be rinsed with cool water to remove any exudate on the surface caused by syneresis of the alginate gel because it will retard the setting of the gypsum.

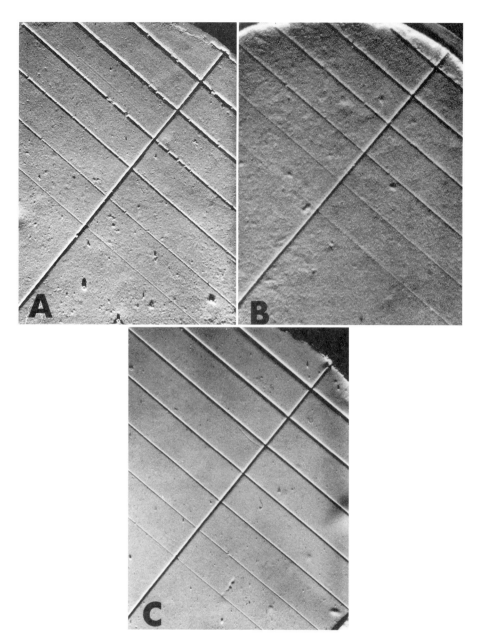

Fig. 11-7 Surface quality and reproduction of **A,** model plaster poured against alginate, **B,** dental stone poured against the same alginate, and **C,** the same dental stone poured against polysulfide rubber. It should be emphasized that another alginate with the same plaster and stone could yield opposite results. (From Craig RG, MacPherson GW: Ann Arbor, 1965, University of Michigan School of Dentistry.)

The set gypsum model should not remain in contact with the alginate impression for periods of several hours because contact of the slightly soluble calcium sulfate dihydrate with the alginate gel containing a great deal of water is detrimental to the surface quality of the model.

Dimensional stability

Alginate impressions lose water by evaporation and shrink on standing in air. Impressions left on the bench for as short a time as 30 minutes may become inaccurate enough to require remaking the impression. Even if the impression stored for more than 30 minutes in air is immersed in water, it is not feasible to determine when the correct amount of water has been absorbed, and in any case the previous dimensions would not be reproduced. For maximum accuracy the model material should be poured into the alginate impression as soon as possible. If for some reason the models cannot be prepared directly, the impressions should be stored in 100% relative humidity in a plastic bag or wrapped in a damp (but not wringing-wet) paper towel.

Storage of alginate impressions in 100% relative humidity is satisfactory for some materials for periods up to 2 hours, as indicated in Fig. 11-8 for material A. Materials C and D should not be stored in 100% relative humidity even for short periods.

Disinfection

Disinfection of impressions is a concern due to viral diseases such as hepatitis B, acquired immune deficiency syndrome, and herpes simplex because the viruses may be transferred to gypsum models and present a risk to dental laboratory and operating personnel.

Although many alginate powders now contain disinfection agents, disinfection of impressions is still recommended. The effect of disinfection in 1% sodium hypochlorite or 2% potentiated glutaraldehyde solutions on accuracy and surface quality has been measured after 10- to 30-minute immersion. Statistically significant dimensional changes were observed; however, the changes were 0.1%, and the quality of the surface was not impaired. Such changes would be insignificant for clinical applications such as the preparation of study models and working casts. The effect of disinfection on agar impression

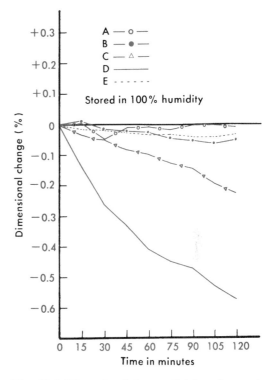

Fig. 11-8 Dimensional change of alginate impression materials stored in 100% relative humidity. (From Craig RG, MacPherson GW: Ann Arbor, 1965, University of Michigan School of Dentistry.)

materials has not been reported, but, considering the similarity of the two hydrocolloids, similar recommendations are reasonable.

AGAR HYDROCOLLOIDS

The agar hydrocolloid impression materials are compounded from reversible agar gels. When heated, they liquefy or go into the sol state, and on cooling they return to the gel state. Because this process can be repeated, a gel of this type is described as reversible, in contrast to the irreversible alginate gels.

The preparation of agar hydrocolloid for clinical use requires careful control and moderately expensive apparatus. Many dentists prefer a metal die for inlay and crown laboratory procedures, and no practical method has been developed to make a metal die from an agar or alginate impression. Agar impressions are dimensionally unstable on standing; thus models should be made as soon as possible after the impression is taken. The registration of the cervical areas of prepared teeth has presented difficulties when they are below the soft tissues of the gingiva. However, modern technics of tissue control have largely eliminated this problem. Complaints sometimes arise from patients as a result of thermal shock to the teeth, producing pain and discomfort. This situation can arise from either the heat from the impression material when introduced into the mouth or the comparatively low temperatures attained during cooling of the impression to obtain a set gel.

Provided that the agar type of impression material is used carefully with an understanding of its physical properties, it is an excellent elastic impression material of high accuracy and registers fine detail.

Chemical Ingredients

The main active constituent of a reversible hydrocolloid impression product is agar, often known commercially as agar-agar, which is a sulfuric ester of a galactan complex, having a complex structural formula, as shown below. This material forms a colloid with water, which liquefies between 71° and 100° C and sets to a gel again between 30° and 50° C, varying with the concentration of the agar.

A typical composition and the functions of the various ingredients are listed in Table 11-3. The material described is a tray type and is considerably stiffer at the time of making the impression compared to a syringe type. The agar content is reduced in the syringe type of material so that it is much

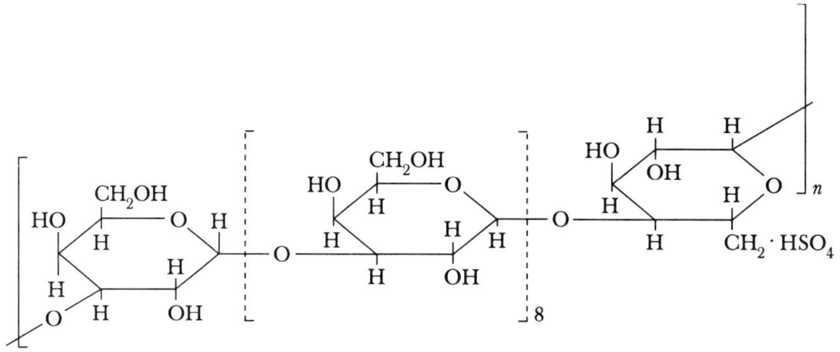

Agar

n = about 90, or for dental grade agar a molecular weight of about 150,000

TABLE 11-3 Typical Composition of Agar Impression Material and the Function of the Components

Ingredient	Weight (%)	Function
Agar	12.5	To provide the dispersed phase of the sol and the continuous fibril structure of the gel
Potassium sulfate	1.7	To counteract the inhibiting effect of borax and agar on the setting of gypsum model material
Borax	0.2	To produce intermolecular attraction in order to improve the strength of the gel
Alkyl benzoate	0.1	To prevent the growth of mold in the impression material during storage
Water	85.5	To provide the continuous phase in the sol and the second continuous phase in the gel; the amount controls the flow properties of the sol and the physical properties of the gel
Color and flavors	Trace	To improve the appearance and taste

Adapted from Preble B: US Patent No. 2,234,383, March 11, 1941.

more fluid at the time of injection than the tray material at the time of insertion.

Critical Factors of Manipulation

Clinically, the dental products can be liquefied conveniently by immersion in boiling water, usually 8 to 12 minutes, according to the bulk of material. Thin, small containers of agar gel liquefy more quickly than larger quantities. Usually the product is in a metal, plastic, or other type of disposable tube, and the whole tube is completely immersed in boiling water.

If the material is prepared as just described and then not used and allowed to cool, it may be reliquefied by immersion in boiling water. Often the time required to liquefy a second time will be longer, and an additional 2 to 4 minutes should be allowed each time the material is reliquefied. The set material may be firmer each time the material is boiled, and when this change in physical properties occurs, the number of times a product can be reboiled is limited. The exact number of times varies with each product, but four times is a safe maximum. If the material is to be used immediately after boiling, the tube is immersed in water at 43° to 49° C, and the tube is manipulated to ensure even cooling. The tube is then opened, and a tray is filled. The filled tray is finally tempered for a minimum of 2 minutes in water at 46° C ± 1°. Before the tray is placed in the mouth, a thin layer of material that has been in direct contact with the water in the bath is removed with a suitable instrument.

When the material is liquefied, it can be stored for several hours and kept ready for use by immersing the container in water at 63° to 66° C. When needed, the material is taken from the storage bath and placed immediately in a warmed tray. The filled tray is then tempered at 46° C ± 1° for a minumum of 2 minutes before it is inserted into the mouth. Tempering is necessary to cool the material to a temperature that is compatible with the oral tissues, and this also serves to develop a heavier consistency in the material.

A slightly more fluid agar material is made for use in injection syringes for inlay, crown, and bridge impressions. The increased fluidity is achieved by a decrease in the agar and an increase in the water content. Usually this material is supplied in small cylinders of the correct size to fit the syringe. The syringe, loaded with a cylinder, is placed in boiling water for 10 minutes and then stored at 63° C until needed. No tempering is required before use, and the syringe is taken from the storage bath, and the agar injected directly into the tooth preparation. The thin strand of material passing down the needle rapidly cools to a temperature compatible with the oral tissues. These procedures may vary from one product to another, and the manufacturer's directions should be followed carefully.

Convenient water heaters are available that provide three compartments: the first, in which water can be boiled to liquefy the material; the second, which can be adjusted to maintain a suitable temperature for storage; and the third, which is set to a temperature suitable as a tempering bath. One type of hydrocolloid heater is shown in Fig. 11-9. The temperatures of the storage and tempering baths should be checked daily with a thermometer to ensure that the dial settings have not been moved accidentally or that some other factor has not changed the bath temperature.

After the impression is placed in the mouth, the agar is cooled to obtain a set condition. Tap water is circulated for a minimum of 5 minutes around tubes built into a special type of hydrocolloid tray (Fig. 11-9). The temperature of this water should not be lower than 13° C. If the cooling water is at a higher temperature, a proportionately longer time is

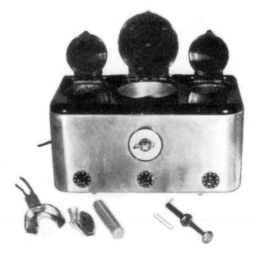

Fig. 11-9 A hydrocolloid heating and conditioning bath for boiling, storing, and tempering agar hydrocolloid, and tray and syringe materials and armamentarium.

required for the agar to set. If water cooler than 13° C is used, there is the danger that rapid gelling will be accompanied by the development of internal stresses that may be released subsequently to cause distortion of the impression.

When exposed to air, the agar hydrocolloids lose moisture and shrink. To obtain the greatest accuracy, agar impressions should be immediately poured in the appropriate stone. If a delay is necessary, they should be stored for the shortest possible time, preferably not more than 1 hour, in 100% relative humidity, or they may be wrapped in a damp towel for short intervals.

After the initial setting of the stone, the gypsum model and impression should be stored in a humidor to prevent drying and shrinkage of the impression before removal of the model.

Properties

Typical properties of the tray type of agar impression materials are listed in Table 11-2.

Gelation temperature

After boiling for 8 minutes, the material should be fluid enough to be extruded from the container. After tempering, the sol should be homogeneous and should set to a gel between 37° and 45° C when cooled, as required by ANSI/ADA Specification No. 11 for dental agar impression material.

Permanent deformation

Permanent deformation is determined in the same manner as for alginates and at the time the material is removed from the mouth. The ANSI/ADA Specification requires that the recovery from deformation be greater than 96.5% (permanent deformation be less than 3.5%) after the material is compressed 20% for 1 second. Most tray types of agar impression materials readily meet this requirement with recovery values of about 99%. However, a reasonable thickness of impression material should be present between the tray and the undercut areas so that compressions higher than 10% do not occur because higher compression results in higher permanent deformation. As for alginates, the magnitude of the permanent deformation depends on the time under compression, and impressions should be removed rapidly.

Flexibility

The ANSI/ADA Specification requirement for flexibility allows a range of 4% to 15%, and most agar impression materials meet this requirement. Materials with low flexibility can be accommodated in areas of undercuts by providing somewhat more space for the impression material so that it is subjected to a lower percentage of compression during removal.

Strength

The compressive strength of a typical agar impression material is 8000 g/cm^2. The tear strength of agar impression materials is about 800-900 g/cm, which is higher than the ANSI/ADA Specification requirement of 765 g/cm. Because agar impressions are viscoelastic, the strength properties are time dependent, and higher compressive and tear strengths occur at higher rates of loading. These properties again emphasize the importance of removing the impressions with a snap because such a procedure minimizes the chances of rupture or tearing of the impression.

Compatibility with gypsum

Not all agar impression materials are equally compatible with all gypsum products, and the manufacturer's suggestions should be followed. The ANSI/ADA specification requires manufacturers to list compatible model materials. Agar impression materials are more compatible with gypsum model materials than alginates. The impression should be washed of saliva and any trace of blood, which retard the setting of gypsum. After the impression is rinsed with water and disinfected, the excess liquid should be carefully blown from the impression with an air syringe, to avoid dehydrating the surface of the agar impression.

If the agar impression must be stored in a humidor, it should be rinsed with cool water to remove any exudate formed from syneresis before pouring up the gypsum model.

Dimensional stability

When stored in air, agar gels lose water and contract. The extent varies from product to product, as shown in Fig. 11-10. After 1 hour in air one product shrank only 0.15%, whereas another product shrank about 1%. Replacing the agar in water resulted in

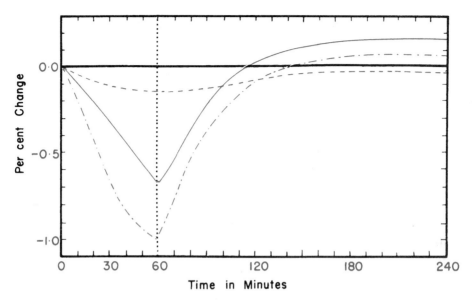

Fig. 11-10 Curves showing shrinkage of three agar hydrocolloids exposed to air over a period of 1 hour and subsequent expansion when immersed in water. (Adapted from Skinner EW, Cooper EN, Beck FE: *J Am Dent Assoc* 40:196, 1950.)

absorption and swelling. After an hour the materials had almost retained their original dimensions, although one was 0.05% larger, and two were 0.1% smaller. Continued storage in water resulted in continued swelling.

As with alginate impressions, agar impressions are best stored in 100% relative humidity if the gypsum models cannot be prepared immediately. Even in 100% humidity they can be stored for only limited times, such as 1 hour, without shrinkage of the impression material caused by syneresis. The best procedure is to pour up the impression immediately after removing, rinsing, disinfecting, and superficial drying.

The suggestions for disinfection of alginates should be followed with agar impressions.

Agar-Alginate Combination Impressions

The equipment needed for taking an agar impression can be minimized with an agar-alginate, syringe-tray combination impression. In this procedure a syringe type of agar in a cartridge is heated in boiling water for 6 minutes and stored in a 65° C water bath 10 minutes before use. Several products and a simple heater are shown in Fig. 11-11. The tray alginate of the regular set type is mixed and placed in a tray. The agar is injected around the preparation,

and the mixed alginate is promptly seated on top of the agar. The alginate sets in about 3 minutes, and the agar gels within this time as a result of being cooled by the alginate. During the setting of the alginate and gelling of the agar a bond forms between them. The impression may be removed in about 4 minutes. Cross sections of impressions of a laboratory model are shown in Fig. 11-12. The surface of the impression is in agar that is backed by the alginate. The same precautions used in preparing stone models in alginate or agar impressions should be observed.

Some combinations of agar and alginate bond together better than others, with tensile bond strengths ranging from 600 to 1100 g/cm². Values at the high end of the range resulted in cohesive failure of the agar, whereas those at the low end produced adhesive failure between the agar and alginate. Therefore following the manufacturer's suggestions for appropriate combinations is important.

The accuracy of the agar-alginate impressions was determined with a laboratory model shown in Fig. 11-13. Impressions were taken, and models were poured in high-strength stone. The accuracy of (1) the interpreparation distance, (2) the buccolingual diameter, and (3) the preparation height of the models was measured and compared to values

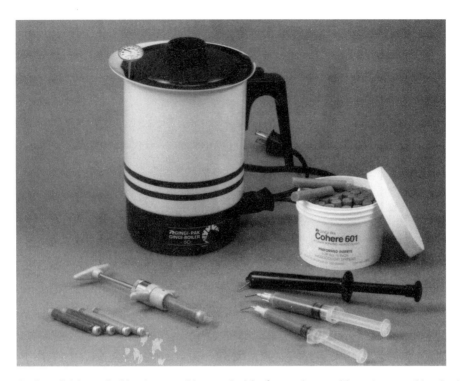

Fig. 11-11 Agar hydrocolloid supplied in glass cartridges and sticks for use in reusable syringes and in plastic disposable syringes, plus a simple heater for liquefying and storing agar for the agar-alginate combination technic. (From Craig RG, O'Brien WJ, Powers JM: *Dental materials: properties and manipulation,* ed 6, St Louis, 1996, Mosby.)

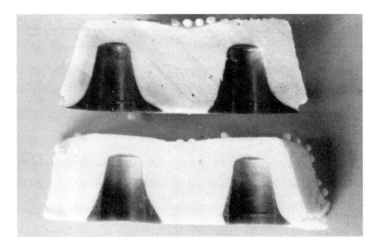

Fig. 11-12 Cross section of agar-alginate combination impressions showing thickness of the agar in various positions.

obtained with polysulfide, condensation silicone, polyether, and addition silicone impression materials. These values are listed in Table 11-4. Except for the interpreparation distance, the agar-alginate system had the same order of accuracy as the rubber impression materials.

In summary the advantage of the agar-alginate combination impression compared with the agar system alone is the simplification of the heating equipment, the elimination of water-cooled impression trays, and the overall simplification of the procedure. In addition, the agar is more compatible with gypsum model materials than alginates, making them useful for crown and bridge impressions, the accuracy is acceptable, and the cost of the materials is low.

Duplicating Impression Materials

In preparing partial dentures, a duplicate should be made of the plaster or stone cast of the patient's mouth. This duplicate is required for two reasons: (1) the cast on which the wax pattern of the metal framework is to be formed must be made from a

refractory investment because it must withstand the casting temperatures required for gold or base metal alloys and (2) the original cast is needed for checking the accuracy of the metal framework and for processing the plastic portion of the partial denture.

A duplicate refractory cast is obtained by making an impression of the original cast in an elastic duplicating material. The most common duplicating materials are agar hydrocolloid compounds. Their composition is quite similar to the agar impression compounds, but a greater proportion of water is used with the duplicating compounds. For example, an impression compound may be diluted with as much as one to three times its weight of water and used as a duplicating compound.

The agar duplicating materials have many advantages. They are reversible, and the material may be reused a number of times. This is particularly important in duplication procedures, because 200 to 400 ml of the material may be needed for each duplication. The agar duplicating materials may be continuously stored in the sol state at 54° to 66° C and used when needed without converting the material from the gel to the sol state each time it is required. After a duplication procedure, the gel is chopped up and reheated until in the sol condition and added to the material being stored at 54° to 66° C. This procedure may be repeated about 20 times before it is discarded. Of prime importance is that the agar duplicating materials have adequate strength and elastic properties to duplicate undercut areas. The accuracy of the agar duplication compounds is also quite satisfactory if proper technics are followed.

The disadvantages of agar duplicating materials are similar to those of agar impression compounds. The set material is a gel and therefore is subject to

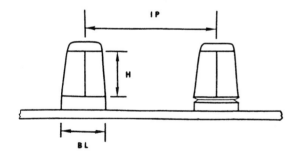

Fig. 11-13 Sketch of the model used to determine the accuracy of impressions.

TABLE 11-4 Percent Deviations of Models Prepared with Various Impression Materials and the Master Die

Location	Impression Type				
	Agar-Alginate	Polysulfide	Condensation Silicone	Polyether	Addition Silicone
Interpreparation	+0.20	+0.05	−0.03	−0.02	0.00
Buccolingual diameter	+0.32	+0.04	+0.03	−0.14	+0.22
Height	−0.22	−0.23	−0.25	−0.17	−0.03

Adapted from Johnson GH, Craig RG: *J Prosthet Dent* 55:1, 1986.

dimensional changes if stored in air or water. Generally, the best storage condition is 100% relative humidity. The best procedure is to pour the duplicate refractory cast as soon as possible. The agar is a polysaccharide and gradually hydrolyzes at the storage temperatures. Accompanying this hydrolysis is a loss of elasticity and strength, which eventually renders the agar duplicating material useless. While in use the duplicating material is contaminated by components of the stone, investment, hardening solutions, separators, and others. Indications are that some of these components accelerate the degradation of the agar.

Other types of materials such as alginate hydrocolloids, reversible plastic gels, and silicone and polyether rubber have been used as duplicating materials. Obviously the major objection to the alginate type is that the material is irreversible. However, its use does not require heating and storage equipment as the reversible agar and plastic duplicating compounds do. The reversible plastic gel is a polyvinylchloride gel that is quite fluid at 99° to 104° C. The main advantages of this material are the high-strength properties and the high chemical stability, which permit a large number of duplications before replacement. Silicones and polyethers that set to a rubber at room temperatures are examples of the nonreversible nonaqueous type. The principal problem with them has been their cost, and numerous technics have been developed to use minimum amounts in a duplicating procedure. At present, agar duplicating materials are the most common type used in dental laboratories.

Properties

ANSI/ADA Specification No. 20 for dental duplicating materials includes two types, thermoreversible and nonreversible. Within these two types are the hydrocolloid and nonaqueous classes.

The specification requires these materials to be free from foreign agents and impurities and to be suitable for taking impressions of plaster, stone, or investment casts of the oral tissues.

Pouring temperature and the temperature of gel formation are defined for the thermoreversible products. Working and setting times are specified for the nonreversible materials. Compatibility with at least one type of investment and the ability to reproduce detail satisfactorily are required. The duplicating material may be compatible with a silicate- or phosphate-bonded investment but not with a gypsum-bonded investment. A single agar duplicating material was poured up in *A,* a silicate-bonded investment; *B,* a phosphate-bonded investment; and *C,* a gypsum-bonded investment. The surface reproduction and detail are shown in Fig. 11-14. High-quality surfaces were obtained with silicate- and phosphate-bonded investments, but a poor-quality surface was found with gypsum-bonded investment. This incompatibility is frequently caused by the addition of glycerin or glycols to the duplicating material to reduce the loss of water from the gel; these compounds interfere with the setting of the gypsum matrix.

Type I products are required to show no mold growth after inoculation under controlled conditions. Requirements for permanent deformation (or recovery from deformation), strain in compression, and resistance to tearing are described for each type and class, and the acceptable values and ranges are listed in Table 11-5. Aging tests are described, and permissible changes in physical properties defined. Packaging must include instructions that indicate the type of investment that can be used with the material and, for type I products, must also include (1) method of liquefying, (2) tempering or storing temperature, and (3) pouring temperature.

RUBBER IMPRESSION MATERIALS

Three major types of rubber impression materials are used to record dental impressions: polysulfides, silicones (polysiloxanes), and polyethers. The silicone type is subdivided into two classes, condensation and addition. The latter class has also been called vinyl polysiloxane.

Polysulfide impression materials are supplied in three consistencies: low (syringe or wash), medium (regular), and high (tray). Addition silicones are available in these three consistencies plus a putty (very high) type, whereas the condensation silicones are usually supplied in a low consistency and putty-like consistency. Polyether impression materials are supplied as a medium-consistency type plus a thinner or as a low and a high consistency. Addition silicones are also supplied as a single consistency product, sometimes called a monophase material, with sufficient shear thinning to be used as both a low- and a

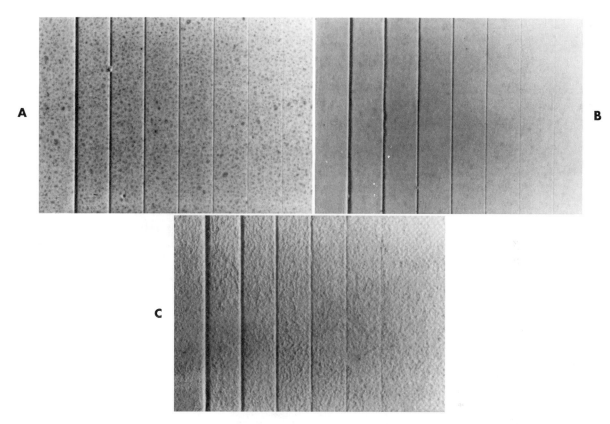

Fig. 11-14 Surface quality of **A,** silicate-bonded, **B,** phosphate-bonded, and **C,** gypsum-bonded investments formed against the same agar duplicating material. (From Craig RG, Dootz ER: Ann Arbor, 1965, University of Michigan School of Dentistry.)

TABLE 11-5   Specification Requirements of Some Properties of Dental Duplicating Materials

	Maximum Permanent Deformation (%)	Strain in Compression	Minimum Compressive Strength (g/cm²)		Minimum Resistance to Tear (g/cm)	
			Original	Aged	Original	Aged
TYPE I (THERMOREVERSIBLE)						
Class I (hydrocolloidal)	3	4-25	2200	2000	–	–
Class II (nonaqueous organic)	3	4-25	–	–	900	700
TYPE II (NONREVERSIBLE)						
Class I (hydrocolloidal)	3	4-25	2800	2600	–	–
Class II (nonaqueous organic)	3	4-25	–	–	900	700

high-consistency material. The low, medium, and high consistencies are supplied as two pastes labeled base and accelerator (catalyst). A few manufacturers of silicones supply the catalyst as a liquid. The very high consistency is supplied as a base putty and a catalyst putty (usually) or liquid.

The pastes are supplied in collapsible tubes, and usually equal lengths are dispensed on a paper pad for normal mixes, as shown in Fig. 11-15, *A*. Initial mixing is accomplished with a circular motion, as shown in Fig. 11-15, *B,* and final mixing to produce a mix free from streaks is done with broad strokes

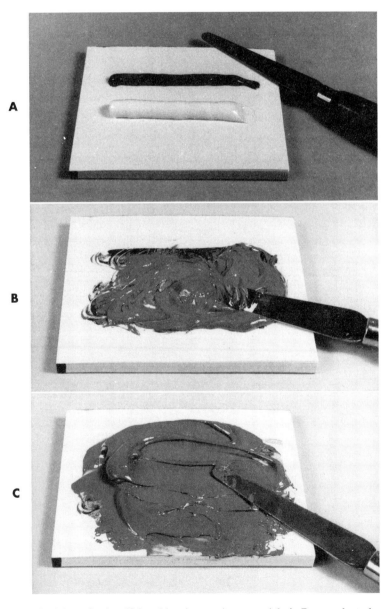

Fig. 11-15 Dispensing and mixing of polysulfide rubber impression material. **A,** Base and accelerator extruded onto a paper mixing pad. **B,** Initial mixing of base and accelerator. **C,** Final mixing of base and accelerator. (From Craig RG, O'Brien WJ, Powers JM: *Dental materials: properties and manipulation,* ed 6, St Louis, 1996, Mosby.)

of the spatula, as shown in Fig. 11-15, *C.* Mixing is readily accomplished in 45 seconds, although working with low-consistency material is easier than with high-consistency materials. When the catalyst is supplied as a liquid, a specified number of drops per unit length is indicated in the instructions, and mixing is accomplished in a manner similar to that of the two-paste systems.

The two-putty systems use scoops supplied by the manufacturer for dispensing and may be mixed with a heavy spatula or kneaded in the hands until free from streaks. The putty materials that have a liquid catalyst are initially mixed with a spatula until the catalyst is reasonably incorporated, and mixing is completed by hand.

Addition silicones of low to very high consistencies and a limited number of low-consistency polyethers are available in automatic mixing systems, an example of which is shown in Fig. 11-16. The base and catalyst are in separate cylinders of the cartridge. The cartridge is placed in a mixing gun with two plungers that are advanced by a rachet mechanism to extrude equal quantities of base and catalyst. The base and catalyst are forced through the static mixing tip shown assembled and disassembled in Fig. 11-16, *bottom.* The base and catalyst pastes are folded over each other many times as they are extruded, resulting in uniform mixes at the tip end.

The mixed material can be extruded directly into an injection syringe or into the impression tray. Intraoral delivery tips are available that can be screwed into the end of the static mixing tips as shown in Fig. 11-16, *bottom left,* and the mixed material can be injected into and around the cavity preparation. The tip can be removed, and additional mixed material can be extruded into the impression tray. The automixing systems have been shown to result in mixes with many fewer voids than hand mixes. Although for each mix the material left in the mixing tip is wasted, the average loss is only 1 to 2 ml depending on the manufacturer's tip, and three to four times this much is wasted in a hand mix as a result of overestimating the amount needed.

Impressions may be taken with only the medium-consistency material or with a combination of a high-consistency or puttylike consistency and a low-consistency material. A single-impression procedure may be used with the combination material in which the low-consistency material is injected into critical areas with a syringe and the high-consistency material is placed in a tray. When the tray containing the high material is placed in the area of the injected low-consistency material, the materials join, bond, and set together. After the materials have set, the tray and the impression are removed. An example of an impression for a bridge using this procedure is shown in Fig. 11-17.

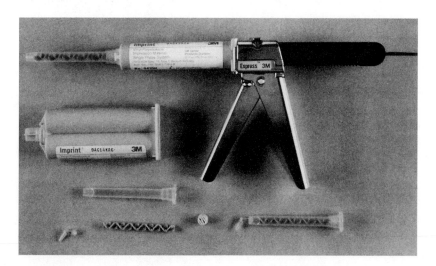

Fig. 11-16 Automixing system for addition silicone impression materials. *Left* and *top,* cartridges and the mixing gun with cartridge inserted and mixing tip attached; *bottom right,* static mixing tip with optional intra-oral delivery tip attached; *bottom left,* a disassembled mixing tip.

A double-impression procedure also may be used in which a preliminary impression is taken in high-consistency or puttylike-consistency material before cavity preparation. Space is provided for a low-consistency material by a variety of technics, and after cavity preparation a low-consistency material is

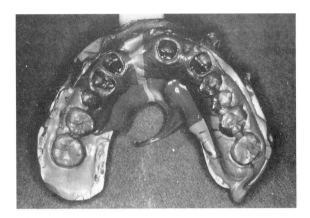

Fig. 11-17 A polysulfide impression of a maxillary anterior bridge case. Dark-colored material, low consistency rubber; light-colored material, high-consistency tray material. Note that the palate is omitted from the tray to facilitate removal of the impression.

syringed into the area, and the preliminary impression reinserted. The low- and high-consistency materials bond, and after the low-consistency material sets, the impression is removed. This is sometimes called a wash technic.

Composition and Reactions

This section describes the general composition and setting reactions of polysulfide, silicone, and polyether rubber impression materials, and the following section describes their physical properties, rather than presenting the information material by material. This approach permits a more direct comparison of the various types and their properties.

Polysulfides

Polysulfide impression materials are supplied as two pastes in collapsible tubes, one labeled "base" and the other labeled "accelerator" or "catalyst." Several products are shown in Fig. 11-18, and a typical list of ingredients and their concentration is given in Table 11-6. The polysulfide polymer has a molecular weight of 2000 to 4000 with terminal and pendant mercaptan groups (–SH). The terminal and pendant groups of adjacent molecules are oxidized by the accelerator

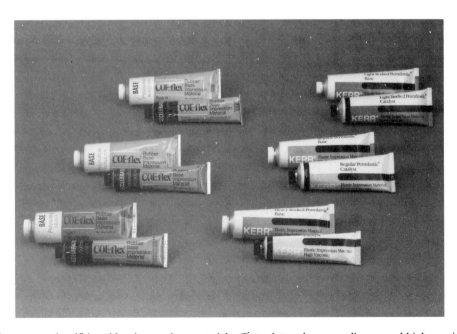

Fig. 11-18 Two-paste polysulfide rubber impression materials. *Top* to *bottom,* low- , medium- , and high-consistency types.
(From Craig RG, O'Brien WJ, Powers JM: *Dental materials: properties and manipulation,* ed 6, St Louis, 1996, Mosby.)

TABLE 11-6 Ingredients of a Typical Polysulfide Rubber Impression Material

Ingredient	Weight (%)
BASE	
Polysulfide polymer	80-85
Titanium dioxide, zinc sulfate, copper carbonate, or silica	16-18
ACCELERATOR	
Lead dioxide	60-68
Dibutyl or dioctyl phthalate	30-35
Sulfur	3
Other substances such as magnesium stearate and deodorants	2

to produce chain extension and cross-linking, respectively. This reaction can be represented diagrammatically as shown below. The reaction results in a rapid increase in molecular weight, and the mixed paste is converted to a rubber. The reaction is only slightly exothermic, with a typical increase in temperature of 3° to 4° C. Although the mixes set to a rubber in about 10 to 20 minutes, polymerization continues, and the properties change for a number of hours after the material sets. Cross-linking is used to reduce the permanent deformation (increase the recovery) of the set rubber under compression or extension during removal from the mouth.

The ingredients and their weight percent (wt%) may vary from one product to another. In general, the weight percent of the filler in the base paste increases from low to medium to high consistencies. The particle size of the fillers is about 0.3 µm. Although the most common active ingredient in the accelerator is lead dioxide, some magnesium oxide may also be present. Whitening agents cannot cover the dark color of the lead dioxide; thus these pastes are dark brown to gray-brown in color. Other oxidizing agents such as

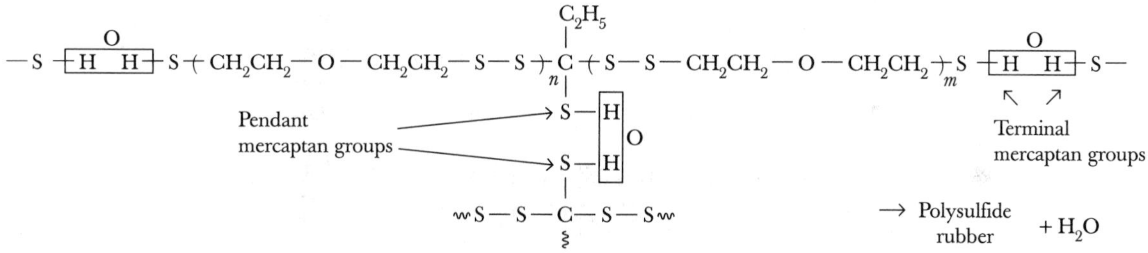
Pendant
mercaptan groups
Terminal
mercaptan groups
Polysulfide
rubber
+ H2O

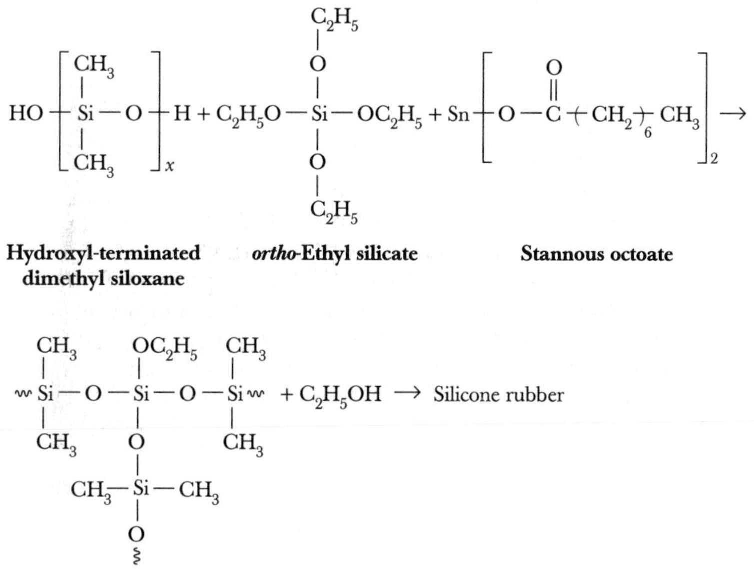
Hydroxyl-terminated
dimethyl siloxane
ortho-Ethyl silicate
Stannous octoate
+ C2H5OH
Silicone rubber

hydrated copper oxide, $Cu(OH)_2$, have been used as a substitute for lead dioxide, producing a green mix.

Silicones

Two types of silicones are used as rubber impression materials and are identified on the basis of their chemical reactions as condensation and addition types.

The condensation silicones are supplied as a base and an accelerator. The base contains a moderately low molecular weight silicone called a dimethyl siloxane, which has reactive terminal hydroxyl groups. Fillers may be copper carbonate or silica having particle sizes from 2 to 8 μm in concentrations from 35% to 75% for low consistencies to puttylike consistencies. The accelerator may be a liquid that consists of stannous octoate suspension and alkyl silicate, or it may be supplied as a paste by adding a thickening agent. The reaction proceeds as mentioned, producing a three-dimensional network rubber with the liberation of ethyl alcohol (shown below) and an exothermic temperature rise of about 1° C. The polymerization accompanied by the release of the by-product causes a shrinkage that is greater in the low consistency than in the puttylike consistency. In the product shown in Fig. 11-19, the shrinkage has been reduced by having only two reactive groups on the cross-linking agent, and thus only half the amount of by-product is formed. The accelerator does not have unlimited shelf life because the stannous octoate may oxidize and the ortho-ethyl silicate is not entirely stable in the presence of the tin ester.

The addition type is available in low, medium, heavy, and very heavy puttylike consistencies and is also a polysiloxane. In this instance the base contains a moderately low molecular weight polymer with silane ($-\underset{\underset{CH_3}{|}}{\overset{\overset{CH_3}{|}}{Si}}-H$) groups (more than 3 and frequently up to 10 per molecule) and filler. The accelerator (or catalyst) contains a moderately low molecular weight polymer with vinyl terminal groups plus filler and chloroplatinic acid catalyst. Unlike the condensation type, the addition reaction does not produce a low molecular weight by-product, as indicated in the reaction shown below, which is an ionic polymerization. A secondary reaction does occur if $-OH$ groups are present with the production of hydrogen gas. Several products contain finely divided palladium or platinum, which absorb the hydrogen. The manufacturer adds coloring agents to the accelerator and sometimes the base as an aid in evaluating the completion of mixing.

Silicone rubber impressions are hydrophobic; when mixes of gypsum products are poured into them, high-contact angles are formed, making the preparation of bubble-free models difficult. Surfactants have been added to addition silicones by some manufacturers, which reduce the contact angle, improve the wettability, and simplify the pouring of gypsum models. However, the addition of the surfactant makes the preparation of electroformed dies more difficult because the metallizing powder does not adhere as well to the surface of the hydrophilic addition silicone impression.

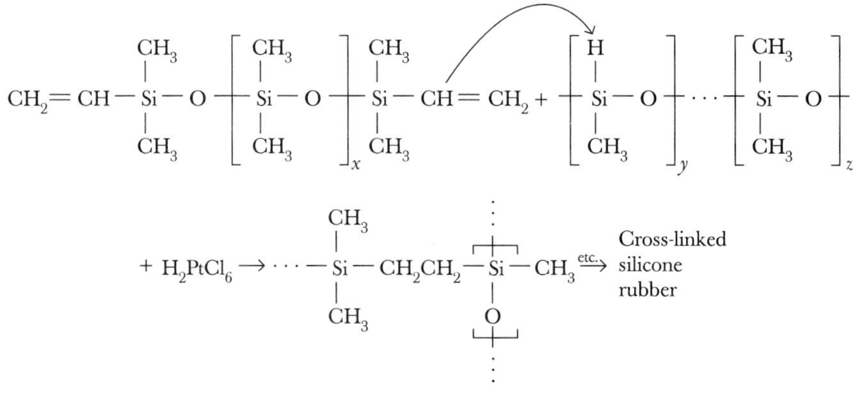

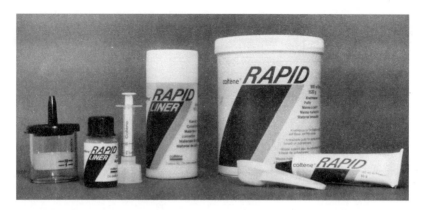

Fig. 11-19 Condensation silicone product having low consistencies and puttylike consistencies. The low-consistency wash and liquid accelerator are in the small container and bottle on the *left,* and the putty and paste accelerator are in the larger container and tube on the *right.* The liquid accelerator is dispensed with the syringe and mixed with the wash material in the container on the *left.* The putty is dispensed with the scoop.

A hydropholic addition silicone system is shown in Fig. 11-20, *A*; the system includes low-, medium-, and high-consistency materials in automix cartridges. Fig. 11-20, *B* shows a hydrophobic addition silicone of very high consistency available in an automix cartridge and as a two-putty system; note the larger diameter of the mixing tip to be used with the very high consistency material. The base and catalyst of the two putty system are mixed by hand. If the two putties are mixed by an operator wearing latex rubber gloves, the setting time is lengthened, and/or the material will not set. Sulfur compounds that are used in the vulcanization of latex rubber gloves can migrate to the surface on storage; during mixing of the two putties these compounds are incorporated and poison the platinum-containing catalyst, which results in retarded or no polymerization. Thorough washing of the gloves with detergent and water just before mixing sometimes minimizes this effect, and some brands of gloves interfere more with the setting than others. Vinyl gloves do not have such an effect.

A single viscosity hydrophilic addition silicone system is shown in Fig. 11-20, *C*. This product has been formulated to have enough shear thinning so that it can be used as both a syringe and a tray material (note that it is the material identified as *Hy* in Fig. 11-24). As illustrated, it is available as a two-paste system for hand mixing and in an automix cartridge for automatic mixing.

Polyethers

Polyethers usually are supplied as a medium-consistency type in a base and an accelerator tube. The base is a moderately low molecular weight polyether with ethylene imine rings as terminal groups. A silica filler is incorporated, as well as a plasticizer such as glycolether phthalate. The catalyst paste contains 2,5-dichlorobenzene sulfonate, as a cross-linking agent, along with a thickening agent. A separate tube contains a thinner that includes octyl phthalate and about 5% methyl cellulose as a thickening agent. Coloring agents may be added to base and accelerator as desired. A polyether system is also supplied as low- and high-viscosity types. Examples of polyether impression materials are shown in Fig. 11-21. The reaction in a simplified form is shown at the top of p. 306. The rubber is formed by cationic polymerization and opening of the imine rings. The backbone of the polymer is believed to be a copolymer of tetrahydrofuran and ethylene oxide. The setting reaction is slightly more exothermic than that of the other rubber impression materials, with a temperature rise of about 4° C.

Setting Properties

Typical values of the setting properties of rubber impression materials are presented in Table 11-7. The temperature rise in typical mixes of impression materials was pointed out in the previous section,

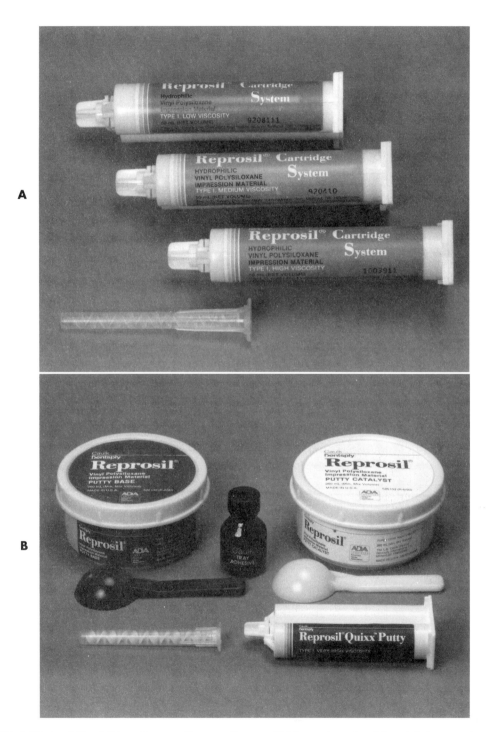

Fig. 11-20 A, Hydrophilic addition silicones of low, medium, and high consistencies, *left* to *right*, in automix cartridges. **B,** Hydrophobic addition silicones of very high consistency supplied as a two-putty system and in an automix cartridge; note the two scoops to dispense the putties and the tray adhesive.

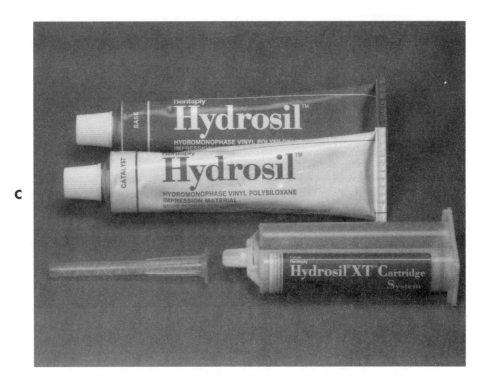

Fig. 11-20, cont'd. C, Single viscosity hydrophilic addition silicone supplied as a two-paste system and in an automix cartridge.

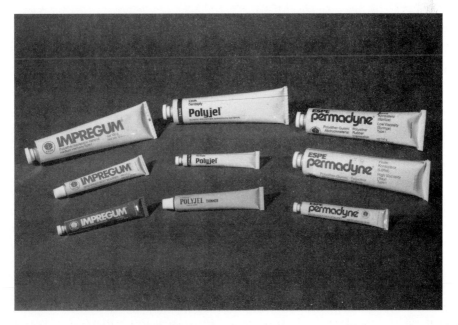

Fig. 11-21 Polyether impression materials. *Left* and *center,* medium-consistency type with base, catalyst, and thinner; *right,* low- and high-consistency types using the same catalyst.

TABLE 11-7   Setting Properties of Rubber Impression Materials

Material	Consistency	Temperature Rise (°C)	Viscosity 45 sec after Mixing (cp)	Working Time (min)	Setting Time (min)	Dimensional Change at 24 hr (%)
Polysulfides						
	Low	3.4	60,000	4-7	7-10	−0.40
	Medium		110,000	3-6	6-8	−0.45
	High		450,000	3-6	6-8	−0.44
Silicones						
Condensation	Low	1.1	70,000	2.5-4	6-8	−0.60
	Very high			2-2.5	3-6	−0.38
Addition	Low			2-4	4-6.5	−0.15
	Medium		150,000	2-4	4-6.5	−0.17
	High			2.5-4	4-6.5	−0.15
	Very high			1-4	3-5	−0.14
Polyethers						
	Low	4.2		2.5	4.5	−0.23
	Medium		130,000	2-3	3-4.5	−0.24
	Medium plus thinner			3-4	4-5.5	−0.23
	High			2.5	4.5	−0.19

but Table 11-7 illustrates that the temperature rise is small and of no clinical concern.

Viscosity

The viscosity of materials 45 seconds after mixing is listed in Table 11-7. As expected, the viscosity increases for the same type of material from low to high consistencies. The viscosity as a function of time after the start of mixing is shown in Fig. 11-22 for mixes stored at 25° C. The most rapid increase in viscosity with time occurred with the silicones and the polyether materials, with the latter increasing slightly more rapidly than the former. Attention must be paid to proper mixing times and times of insertion of the impression material into the mouth if the materials are to be used to their best advantage. For example, low-consistency polysulfide rubber injected or placed in the mouth at 5.5 minutes would have the same viscosity as medium-consistency polysulfide at 3 minutes. Similarly, a medium-consistency polysulfide at 4 minutes would have the same viscosity as a high-consistency material at 2 minutes.

A comparison of the viscosity of low-consistency polysulfide with alginate, zinc oxide–eugenol, and impression plaster is made in Fig. 11-23. The viscosity versus time curves were determined at 37° C. The alginate tray material had a higher viscosity than the low-consistency polysulfide, although the

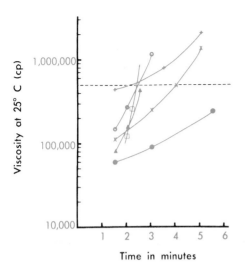

Fig. 11-22 Viscosity of rubber impression materials after mixing at 25° C. Polysulfide light, •; polysulfide regular, ×; polysulfide heavy, +; condensation silicone, ▲; addition silicone, ✪; polyether, ☐. (Adapted from Herfort TW, Gerberich WW, Macosko CW, Goodkind RJ: *J Prosthet Dent* 38:396, 1977.)

rate of increase in viscosity with time was less for the alginate material. Impression plaster had the lowest viscosity 1.5 minutes after starting the mix but the highest rate of increase in viscosity with time. The viscosity of the zinc oxide–eugenol materials was characterized by small increases with time. The paste-paste type had a constant viscosity with time up to 3.5 minutes; the powder-liquid type had a lower initial viscosity, with gradually increasing values up to 4.5 minutes.

The effect of shear rate (rotational speed of the viscometer) on the viscosity of single consistency (monophase) addition silicones is shown in Fig. 11-24. All products showed a decrease in viscosity with

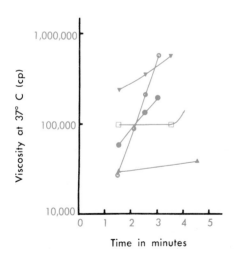

Fig. 11-23 Viscosity of various impression materials after mixing and storage at 37° C. Polysulfide light, •; zinc oxide–eugenol (powder-liquid), ▲; zinc oxide–eugenol (paste-paste), ☐; alginate (tray type), ▼; impression plaster, ✪. (Adapted from Koran A, Powers JM, Craig RG: *J Am Dent Assoc* 95:75, 1977.)

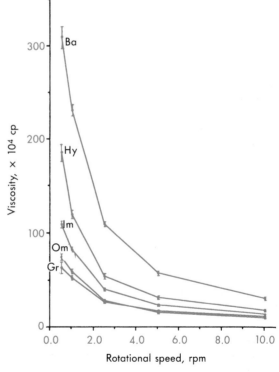

Fig. 11-24 Viscosity in centipoise as a function of shear rate (rotational speed of the viscometer) for five single consistency addition silicone impression materials. A rotational speed of 0.5 rpm would represent a shear rate comparable with that observed when placing the material in a tray, and a speed of 10 rpm would represent a shear rate comparable with that experienced when syringing the material. (From Kim KN, Craig RG, Koran A, III: *J Prosthet Dent* 67:794, 1992.)

increasing shear rate although the effect was much more pronounced for two products, Ba and Hy, with about an eightfold to elevenfold decrease from the lowest to the highest shear rate. The substantial decrease in viscosity at high shear stress, which is comparable with that during syringing, permits the use of a single mix of material with a portion to be used as a syringe material and another portion to be used as a tray material in the syringe-tray technic.

Working and setting times

The working and setting times of rubber impression materials are listed in Table 11-7. Polysulfides have the longest times, followed by silicones and polyethers. In general, for a given class of rubber impression material by a specific manufacturer the working and setting times decrease as the viscosity increases from low to high. The polyethers of low and medium viscosity have short working and setting times, which can be increased modestly by adding an equal length of thinner to the catalyst and base. Note that the working and setting times of the rubber impression materials are shortened by increases in temperature and humidity, and on hot humid days this effect should be considered in the clinical application of these materials.

The initial (or working) and final setting times can be determined fairly accurately by using a penetrometer with a needle and weight selected to suit these materials. The Vicat penetrometer, as shown in Fig. 11-25, with a 3-mm diameter needle and a total weight of 300 g, has been used by a number of investigators. A metal ring, 8 mm high and 16 mm in diameter, is filled with freshly mixed material and placed on the penetrometer base. The needle is applied to the surface of the rubber for 10 seconds, and a reading is taken. This is repeated every 30 seconds. The initial set is that time at which the needle no longer completely penetrates the specimen to the bottom of the ring. The final set is the time of the first of three identical nonmaximum penetration readings. When the material has set, the elasticity still allows penetration of the needle, but it is the same at each application. The final set is achieved at the time of the first reading.

Dimensional change on setting

The dimensional change between a die and the impression after 24 hours is listed in Table 11-7. The

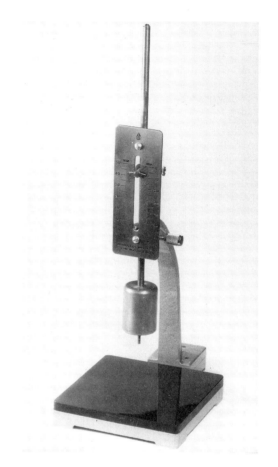

Fig. 11-25 Vicat penetrometer used to determine setting time of impression materials and other restorative materials.

condensation silicones have the largest dimensional change, about –0.6%. The shrinkage is a result of the evaporation of volatile by-products and the rearrangement of the bonds resulting from polymerization. The addition silicones have the smallest change, about –0.15%, followed by the polyethers at about –0.2% and the lead dioxide- and copper hydroxide-accelerated polysulfides at about –0.4%.

The rate of shrinkage of rubber impression materials is not uniform during the 24 hours after removal from the mouth. In general, about half of the shrinkage observed at 24 hours occurs during the first hour after removal, and for greatest accuracy the models and dies should be prepared promptly, although the rubber impression materials are much more stable in air than hydrocolloid products.

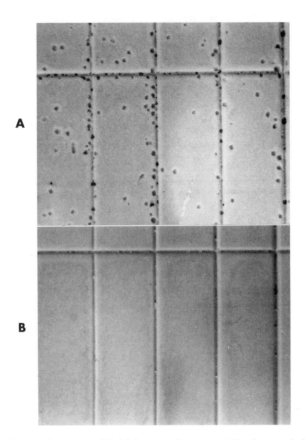

Fig. 11-26 Addition silicone impressions poured in high-strength stone at 15 minutes. **A,** Bubbles from release of hydrogen. **B,** No bubbles because palladium hydrogen absorber is included in the impression material.

Some addition silicone impression materials release hydrogen after setting, and to avoid bubbles, the gypsum models and dies should not be poured until after 1 to 2 hours, and epoxy dies should not be poured until the impression has stood overnight. The difference in the delay with gypsum and epoxy is that gypsum products have much shorter setting times than epoxy die materials. Some products contain a hydrogen absorber such as palladium, and gypsum and epoxy die materials can be poured against them as soon as practical. Examples of high-strength stone poured after 15 minutes against addition silicone with and without a hydrogen absorber are shown in Fig. 11-26.

The hydrophilic addition silicone materials are difficult to electroform because adherence of the metallizing powder to the surface of the impression is a problem. Polyether impressions should not be stored in water because they slowly absorb water and change dimensions. Nevertheless, accurate electroformed and gypsum dies can be prepared from polyether impressions.

Mechanical Properties

Typical mechanical properties of rubber impression materials are listed in Table 11-8. The permanent deformation (or recovery from deformation, which is 100% minus the permanent deformation), flow, and dimensional change are properties used in ANSI/ADA Specification No. 19 to classify elastomeric impression materials as Types I, II, or III. The requirements for these properties are given in Table 11-9. The rubber impression materials are further identified according to their viscosity as low, medium, high, and very high, as indicated in Table 11-10. The consistency diameter is used to classify the viscosity by measuring the diameter of the disk formed when 0.5 ml of mixed material is subjected to a 575-g weight at 1.5 minutes after

TABLE 11-8   Mechanical Properties of Rubber Impression Materials

Material	Consistency	Permanent Deformation (%)	Strain in Compression (%)	Flow (%)	Shore A Hardness	Tear Strength (g/cm)
Polysulfides						
	Low	3-4	14-17	0.5-2	20	2500-7000
	Medium	3-5	11-15	0.5-1	30	3000-7000
	High	3-6	9-12	0.5-1	35	–
Silicones						
Condensation	Low	1-2	4-9	0.05-0.1	15-30	2300-2600
	Very high	2-3	2-5	0.02-0.05	50-65	–
Addition	Low	0.05-0.4	3-6	0.01-0.03	35	1500-3000
	Medium	0.05-0.3	2-5	0.01-0.03	50	2200-3500
	High	0.1-0.3	2-3	0.01-0.03	60	2500-4300
	Very high	0.2-0.5	1-2	0.01-0.1	50-75	–
Polyethers						
	Low	1.5	3	0.03	35-40	1800
	Medium	1-2	2-3	0.02	35-60	2800-4800
	Medium plus thinner	2	6	0.04	30-50	2500
	High	2	3	0.02	40-50	3000

TABLE 11-9   Permanent Deformation, Flow, and Dimensional Change Requirements for Elastomeric Impression Materials

Type	Maximum Permanent Deformation (%)	Maximum Flow in Compression (%)	Maximum Dimensional Change in 24 hr (%)
I	2.5	0.5	−0.50
II	2.5	0.5	−1.00
III	5.5	2.0	−0.50

Adapted from ANSI/ADA Specification No. 19: *J Am Dent Assoc* 94:733, 1977.

mixing for 12 minutes. Because the setting times of rubber impression materials vary, the consistency diameter is affected not only by the viscosity but also by the setting time. The classification of a material by the consistency diameter may be different from that by a true viscosity measurement.

Permanent deformation

The order in which the permanent deformation of the rubber impression materials is listed in Table 11-8

and demonstrates that the addition silicones have the best recovery from deformation during removal from the mouth, followed by the condensation silicones and the polyethers, and then the polysulfides.

The trend is to report the percent recovery rather than the permanent deformation. Thus a material with a permanent deformation of 1% has a recovery from deformation of 99%.

Strain

The strain in compression under a stress of 1000 g/cm^2 is a measure of the flexibility of the material. Table 11-8 illustrates that in general, the low-consistency materials of each type are more flexible than the high-consistency rubber impressions. The polyethers containing thinner are more flexible than the regular material. Also, the silicones are stiffer than the polysulfides of comparable consistency, and the addition silicones are slightly stiffer than the condensation silicones.

Flow

The flow is measured on a cylindrical specimen 1 hour old, and the percent flow is determined 15 minutes after a load of 100 g is applied. As seen in

TABLE 11-10   Requirements by ANSI/ADA Specification No. 19 for the Various Viscosities of Rubber Impression Materials

Viscosity	Maximum Mixing Time (min)	Minimum Working Time (min)	Diameter of Consistency Disk (mm)	Strain in Compression (%)	Reproduction of Detail	
					Line Width in Impression (mm)	Line Width in Gypsum (mm)
Low	1	2	36-55	2.0-20	0.020	0.020
Medium	1	2	30-40	2.0-20	0.020	0.020
High	1	2	20-32	2.0-20	0.020	0.020
Very high	1	2	13-30	0.8-8.0	0.075	0.075

Adapted from ANSI/ADA Specification No. 19, approved March 30, 1982.

Table 11-8, the silicones and polyethers have the lowest values of flow, and the polysulfides have the highest values.

Typical rubber impression materials apparently have no difficulty meeting the mechanical property requirements of ANSI/ADA Specification No. 19. Although the hardness and the tear strengths of rubber impression materials are not mentioned in the specification, these are important properties, and they are also listed in Table 11-8.

Hardness

The Shore A hardness increases from low to high consistency. When two numbers are given, the first represents the hardness 1.5 minutes after removal from the mouth, and the second number is the hardness after 2 hours. The polysulfides and the low-, medium-, and high-viscosity addition silicones do not change hardness significantly with time, whereas the hardness of condensation silicones, of addition silicone putties, and of polyethers does increase with time. In addition, the hardness and the strain affect the force necessary for removal of the impression from the mouth. Low flexibility and high hardness can be compensated for clinically by producing more space for the impression material between the tray and the teeth.

Tear strength

The tear strength is important because it indicates the ability of a material to withstand tearing in thin interproximal areas. The tear strengths listed in Table 11-8 are a measure of the force needed to initiate and continue tearing a specimen of unit thickness. A few polysulfides have high tear strengths of 7000 g/cm, but the majority have lower values in the 2500 to 3000 g/cm range. As the consistency of the impression type increases, tear strength undergoes a small increase, but most of the values are between 2000 and 4000 g/cm. Values for very high consistency types are not listed because they are not important for these materials. Higher tear strengths for rubber impression materials are desirable, but compared with the values for hydrocolloid impression materials of 350 to 700 g/cm, they are a major improvement. Although polysulfides have high tear strengths, they also have high permanent deformation that may result in inaccurate impressions.

Detail reproduction

The requirements of the rubber impression materials are listed in Table 11-10. Except for the very high viscosity products, they all should reproduce a V-shaped groove and a 0.02-mm wide line in the rubber, and the rubber should be compatible with gypsum products so that the 0.02-mm line is transferred to gypsum die materials. Low-, medium-, and high-viscosity rubber impression materials have little difficulty in meeting this requirement.

Creep compliance

Rubber impression materials are viscoelastic, and their mechanical properties are time dependent. For example, the higher the rate of deformation, the higher the tear strength; and the longer the impressions are deformed, the higher the permanent deformation. As a result, plots of the creep compliance versus time describe the properties of these materials better than stress-strain curves. Creep compliance– time curves for low-consistency polysulfide, condensation silicone, addition silicone, and medium-consistency polyether are shown in Fig. 11-27. The initial creep compliance illustrates that the polysulfide is the most flexible and that the polyether is the least flexible. The flatness or parallelism of the curves with respect to the time axis indicates low permanent deformation and excellent recovery from deformation during the removal of an impression material; polysulfides have the poorest recovery from deformation, followed by the condensation silicone and then the addition silicone and polyether.

The recoverable viscoelastic quality of the materials is indicated by differences between the initial creep compliance and the creep compliance value obtained by extrapolation of the linear portion of the curve to zero time. As a result, the polysulfides have the greatest viscoelastic quality and require more time to recover the viscoelastic deformation,

followed by the condensation silicone, the polyether, and the addition silicone.

Wettability of Rubber Impression Materials

Wettability may be assessed by measuring the advancing contact angle of water on the surface of the set impression material. The advancing contact angles for rubber impression materials are listed in Table 11-11. The hydrophilic addition silicones and the polyethers were wetted the best, and the condensation silicones and hydrophobic addition silicones the least. The wettability was directly correlated to the ease of pouring high-strength stone models of an extremely critical die as shown in Table 11-11.

Disinfection of Rubber Impressions

A number of studies have been conducted on the effect of disinfecting rubber impression materials. The smallest dimensional changes were found for addition silicone impressions disinfected in acid-potentiated 2% glutaraldehyde, glutaraldehyde-

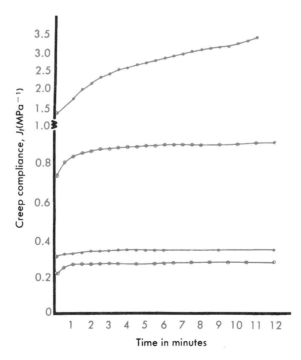

Fig. 11-27 Creep compliance of rubber impression materials at the time recommended for removal from the mouth. Curves from *top* to *bottom:* Polysulfide, condensation silicone, addition silicone, and polyether. (From Craig RG: *Mich Dent Assoc J* 59:259, 1977.)

containing phenol, chlorhexidine, and benzalkonium chloride, although the surface detail and accuracy of polysulfide impressions were satisfactory after disinfection in 2% glutaraldehyde. Polyethers do not appear to be suited for disinfection by immersion because of the water absorption; a spray of chlorine dioxide, however, has been found to minimize the imbibition of water.

Relationship of Properties and Clinical Application

Accuracy and the ability to record detail, as well as the ease of handling and the setting characteristics, are of prime importance in dental impressions.

The viscosity of silicones is lower than for the other rubber impression materials, which results in easier mixing. They have shorter working times than polysulfides but somewhat longer than polyethers. The single-mix materials have some advantage in that, as a result of shear thinning, they have low viscosities when mixed or syringed but higher viscosities when inserted in a tray. The time of placement of a rubber impression material is critical because the viscosity increases rapidly with time as a result of the polymerization reaction. If the material is placed after a rubbery consistency begins to develop, internal stresses induced in the impression are released after removal of the impression from the mouth, resulting in an inaccurate impression.

Thorough mixing is essential because portions of the mix could contain insufficient accelerator to polymerize thoroughly or may not set at the same rate as other portions of the impression. In this event removal of the impression would cause high permanent deformation and result in an inaccurate impression. Automixing systems produce mixes with fewer bubbles than hand mixing, resulting in a more bubble-free impression.

Polymerization of rubber impression materials continues after the material has set, and the mechanical properties improve with time. Removal too early may result in high permanent deformation; however, excessively long times in the mouth are unacceptable to the patient. The manufacturer usually recommends a minimum time for leaving the impression in the mouth, and this time is used for testing the materials according to ANSI/ADA Specification No. 19.

The dimensional changes on setting were the highest for the condensation silicones and polysulfides. The effect of these shrinkages can be compensated for by use of a double-impression technic with a high- and a low-consistency material, or with a putty- and a wash (low)–consistency material. In these instances a preliminary impression is taken in the high- or puttylike-consistency material, providing some space for the final impression in low-consistency material. The preliminary impression is removed, cavity preparation is accomplished, and the final impression is taken with the low-consistency material, using the preliminary impression as a tray. In this way the dimensional change in the high-consistency or putty-like consistency is negligible, and although the percent dimensional change of the low-consistency material is still large, the thickness is so small that the actual dimensional change is small. The double-impression technic is suitable for use with a stock impression tray because the preliminary impression serves as a custom tray. The syringe-tray technic in which two mixes are used and set at the same time should use a custom-made tray to provide a uniform thickness of impression material, which in turn produces a more accurate impression.

Clinical studies have shown that the viscosity of the impression material is the most important factor in producing impressions and dies with minimal bubbles and maximum detail. As a result, the syringe-tray technic produced superior clinical results in the reproduction of fine internal detail of proximal boxes or grooves.

The accuracy of the impression may be affected when the percentage of deformation and the time

TABLE 11-11   Wettability of Rubber Impression Materials

Material	Advancing Contact Angle of Water (deg)	Castability of High-Strength Dental Stone (%)
Polysulfide	82	44
Condensation silicone	98	30
Addition silicone		
Hydrophobic	98	30
Hydrophilic	53	72
Polyether	49	70

involved in removing the impression are increased. In both instances, increased permanent deformation results with the amount depending on the type of rubber impression material.

Because rubber impressions recover from deformation for a period after their removal, some increase in accuracy can be expected during this time. This effect is more noticeable with polysulfides than with the other impression materials. However, polymerization shrinkage is also occurring, and the overall accuracy is a combination of these two effects. Insignificant recovery from deformation occurs after 20 to 30 minutes; therefore dies should be prepared promptly after that time for greatest accuracy. Addition silicones that release hydrogen are an exception to this guide.

Second pours of gypsum products into rubber impressions produce dies that are not so accurate as the first because the rubber is deformed during the removal of the first die; however, they are usually sufficiently accurate to be used as a working die.

Rubber Impression Materials for Bite Registrations

Bite registrations used to articulate upper and lower models have often been taken in wax as is described in Chapter 13. However, the properties of waxes limit their accuracy because wax registrations (1) can be distorted upon removal, (2) may change dimensions by release of internal stresses depending on the storage condition, (3) have high flow properties, and (4) undergo large dimensional changes on cooling from mouth to room temperature.

Addition silicones and polyethers have been formulated for use as bite registration materials. Most of the products are addition silicones and most are supplied in automix cartridges. Properties of these bite registration materials are listed in Table 11-12. These materials are characterized by short working times and the length of time left in the mouth compared to typical rubber impression materials. They are also noted for their high stiffness, indicated by the low-percent strain in compression, and for their low flow and dimensional change even after 7 days. The property that distinguishes the addition silicones from the polyether is their lower dimensional change after removal; however, either is superior to the stability of waxes for taking bite registrations.

Recent Advances in Rubber Impression Materials

Automatic mixing systems have been developed for low- to very high consistency addition silicones and low-consistency polyethers. These systems consist of a double-barreled mixing gun that forces equal quantities of the base and the catalyst through a removable static mixing tip. The inside of the mixing tip contains a number of baffles that force the base and catalyst to be folded over and over on each other as they are extruded. These systems have the advantage of uniform dispensing and mixing of catalyst and base and fewer bubbles in the mixed and set material than in hand-spatulated mixes. Although about 1 ml of material is wasted in the tip with each mix, less material is wasted than in the standard mixing procedure, in which estimated equal lengths of catalyst and base are extruded onto a mixing pad.

More manufacturers are marketing hydrophilic addition silicone impression materials. Because most commercial laboratories prepare high-strength stone dies rather than electroforming these impressions, the difficulty in electroplating is of minimal concern. More

TABLE 11-12 Properties of Rubber Impression Materials Used for Taking Bite Registrations

Material	Mixing Type	Working Time (min)	Time in Mouth (mm)	Strain in Compression (%)	Flow (%)	Dimensional Change	
						1 Day (%)	7 Days (%)
Addition silicone	Automix	1.5-3.0	1.5-3.0	1.0-2.9	0.0-0.01	0.0 to −0.15	−0.04 to −0.20
Addition silicone	Handmix	1.4	2.5	0.92	0.0	−0.06	−0.08
Polyether	Handmix	2.1	3.0	1.97	0.0	−0.29	−0.32

addition silicones contain hydrogen absorbers so that dies can be poured as soon as desired, and more manufacturers are supplying addition silicones as single-viscosity (monophase) products with sufficient shear thinning qualities so they can be used as both a syringe and a tray material. The consistency of addition silicone impression materials has been modified, and they are frequently used as bite registration pastes. Also as described in Chapter 10, very high consistency addition silicones can be used to prepare dies on which indirect composite inlays are prepared.

ZINC OXIDE–EUGENOL IMPRESSION PASTES

The zinc oxide–eugenol impression pastes produce a rigid impression with a high degree of accuracy and good reproduction of surface detail. These materials have been used in the registration of the final impression and for stabilizing baseplates in bite registration.

The zinc oxide–eugenol products offer the following advantages as corrective impression pastes: (1) they adhere well to dried surfaces of compound, resin, and shellac bases; (2) they have sufficient resistance so that borders can be built up if the tray is slightly deficient in any area; (3) they are hard when set, and the resulting impression can be taken in and out of the mouth repeatedly, giving an opportunity to test for stability and tissue adaptation; (4) they allow adequate working time for unhurried border molding in the mouth; (5) they are accurate, register detail well, and are quite stable dimensionally; and (6) they require no separating medium before the cast is poured.

Nature and Composition

These materials are supplied as two pastes, which usually are supplied in collapsible metal tubes. One contains zinc oxide mixed with inert oils and other additives, and the other contains eugenol, accelerator, and additives with or without inert fillers. Recommended proportions of each paste are extruded onto a treated paper pad and thoroughly mixed. The setting time varies among products. A hard, brittle impression results with some products, whereas others produce a comparatively soft impression that will bend rather than fracture if deformed.

The composition of a typical zinc oxide–eugenol impression paste is as follows:

1. Base materials (mixed to a paste with inert oils)
   a. Zinc oxide 80%
   b. Inert oils 15%
2. Accelerators
   a. Oil of cloves or eugenol 15%
   b. Gum rosin and oils 65%
   c. Filler (talc or kaolin) 16%
   d. $MgCl_2$ accelerator and moisture 4%

Gum rosin is an important constituent and can be incorporated in either or both pastes. Rosin gives body and coherence to the mixed material and imparts thermoplastic properties to the set impression so that it can be softened in hot water for easy removal from the cast.

Magnesium chloride hastens the setting reaction to a time convenient for clinical impression procedures. The metallic salts of acetic, hydrochloric, and nitric acid also act as accelerators. Zinc oxide is mixed with inert oils such as mineral oil to form a paste, and the eugenol component may be mixed with an inert filler such as kaolin, talc, or diatomaceous earth to form a paste of suitable consistency.

Setting Reaction

Two molecules of eugenol react with one molecule of zinc oxide to form a chelate, zinc eugenolate, as shown on the next page. The methoxyl group ortho to a phenolic hydroxyl group permits the formation of two five-membered chelate rings with the zinc. If the zinc oxide powder is completely dehydrated before it is mixed with eugenol, the resulting paste will not harden. The presence of water is essential for the setting reaction. Zinc oxide with 2% water produces mixtures that require up to 24 hours to harden, whereas the presence of 5% water in the zinc oxide reduces the setting time to about 15 minutes.

Excess zinc oxide is always present, and the set impression consists of an amorphous zinc eugenolate matrix, which binds the unreacted zinc oxide together. Also available is an impression paste that uses zinc oxide and lauric acid rather than eugenol; the use of this material avoids the slight burning and stinging sensation of zinc oxide–eugenol impressions, as well as the taste and odor, and can be used on patients having an allergic reaction to eugenol.

Zinc eugenolate

Characteristic Properties

Zinc oxide–eugenol impression materials display numerous properties peculiar to this type of material and not shared by other compounds.

Proportioning and mixing

Usually an equal length of each paste is dispensed onto the mixing pad. Products have initial setting times from 2 to 4.5 minutes and final setting times from 2.5 to 6 minutes.

The paper pad and spatula required for mixing these pastes are shown in Fig. 11-28. A paper pad is used to avoid cleaning a glass mixing slab, to which the material adheres firmly. A stiff stainless steel spatula with an 8- to 10-cm blade and a large wooden or plastic handle is best for mixing the paste. Mixing is usually complete in 30 to 40 seconds when there are no colored streaks in the mix and a uniform consistency is obtained. After use, the spatula blade can be cleaned by warming in a flame until the rosin component softens, and the blade can be wiped clean with a paper towel. Solvents are available for cleaning the instruments. They consist mainly of naphtha, light cutting oils, or a similar substance blended with an aromatic oil.

Consistency of mix. Some pastes are quite fluid; others are buttery. A gradual change in consistency develops as the mixed material approaches a set condition. The paste slowly thickens until it reaches a point too stiff for clinical handling, and the time from the beginning of mix to this point is known as the working time, or initial set. The paste continues to harden, and when it is ready for removal from the mouth, the final set should have occurred.

Effect of temperature and humidity on setting

Zinc oxide–eugenol impression pastes set more quickly at higher temperatures and humidities. Products with a long setting time are usually more affected by changes of temperature and humidity than products with short setting times. Clinically this means that they set more promptly in the mouth than on the mixing pad and that hot, humid conditions in the office result in shorter working times.

Modification of the setting time

Adding a drop of water or alcohol when mixing speeds the set, and varying the ratio of the two component pastes may slow or speed the setting time, depending on the particular product. Addition of inert oils such as olive oil, mineral oil, or petrolatum during mixing slows the setting by diluting the accelerator. These variations affect not only the setting time but also the consistency, flow, and strength properties. The clinician will find it difficult to predict the exact effects produced by such additions, and the better plan is to select a product that gives the setting time and consistency required rather than to attempt to modify an unsuitable material.

Dimensional changes of impressions

Zinc oxide–eugenol impression materials shrink $\leq 0.1\%$ after 30 minutes. No significant further change occurs at 24 hours. Because they are used as corrective wash impressions, the stability of the tray must be considered as a possible source of distortion. A thin baseplate tray may warp on standing,

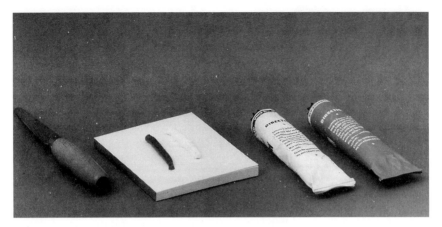

Fig. 11-28 Paper pads and spatula suitable for mixing impression materials of zinc oxide–eugenol type.

and as a result the zinc oxide–eugenol paste also may distort.

Hardness

The hardness is measured by noting the extent to which a loaded needle penetrates a small specimen of the set material. The hardness is expressed in terms of millimeters penetrated in a given time. Hardness values for six zinc oxide–eugenol impression pastes varied from 0.2 to 2.5 mm. These values were determined with a Krebs penetrometer in which the weight of the needle and its load was 100 g. The needle was applied to the surface of the specimen 30 minutes after mixing was started, and the amount of penetration noted 10 seconds later. Products with penetration values up to 0.5 mm are described as hard-set materials, whereas those with penetration values of 0.9 mm or more are soft-set products.

Pouring and separating the cast

Only gypsum products can be used to form casts from zinc oxide–eugenol impressions. The impression is rinsed well in cold water to remove any saliva or debris and is dried before a mix of plaster or stone is poured into it. No separating medium or surface-active agent is necessary. At least 1 hour is allowed for the stone to set before the impression is immersed into water at about 60° C for 5 to 10 minutes. This softens the impression, and it is removed from the cast with ease.

ANSI/ADA Specification No. 16 for Impression Paste–Zinc Oxide–Eugenol Type

ANSI/ADA Specification No. 16 describes the desirable properties for Type I hard and Type II soft impression materials. Consistency, initial and final setting times and penetration hardness tests are specified. The quality of the cast surface is determined by visual examination to check the absence of adhesion of paste to the cast or the reverse occurrence. The essential physical properties of the two types are listed in Table 11-13.

DENTAL IMPRESSION PLASTER

Dental impression plaster is rigid when set and its principal use is for mounting of casts on articulators or mixing with high-strength stone for study models; the rapid setting is an advantage in these applications.

Composition and Reactions

Impression plaster is mainly calcium sulfate hemihydrate, which when mixed with water reacts to become calcium sulfate dihydrate. The setting expansion is reduced to about 0.06% by the presence of additives such as potassium sulfate, chloride, or nitrate, which also function as accelerators for the reaction. Starch may be added to give a so-called soluble impression plaster, which facilitates its separation from model plaster or dental stone by softening when immersed in hot water.

TABLE 11-13   Physical Properties of Two Types of Zinc Oxide–Eugenol Impression Pastes

Type	Consistency		Initial Setting		Maximum Final Setting (min)	Penetration Hardness	
	Minimum (mm)	Maximum (mm)	Minimum (min)	Maximum (min)		Minimum (mm)	Maximum (mm)
I (hard)	30	50	3	6	10	–	0.5
II (soft)	20	45	3	6	15	0.8	1.5

Proportioning and Mixing

Impression plaster is mixed in a rubber bowl with a stiff, wide-bladed spatula. The recommended water/powder ratio should be used because variations affect the consistency and setting time of the mix and the strength of the set material. Increased proportions of water give a more fluid mix with a longer setting time and a weaker material.

The powder is sifted into the water and left undisturbed for 30 seconds, in which time the powder is wetted. The mass is then spatulated to achieve a homogeneous mass, which usually is 30 seconds or less. Excessive spatulation reduces the available working time.

Storage Problems

If impression plaster powder is stored in air under conditions of high relative humidity it will absorb water. This causes crystals of calcium sulfate dihydrate to form on the surface of the hemihydrate crystals. This causes a shortening of the setting time if the contamination is minimal or a lengthening if the contamination is extensive. However, if stored in an airtight container, impression plaster keeps for 1 or more years. The container lid must be replaced each time plaster is removed, and the tin must be located away from areas of high humidity, such as near a sterilizer or sink.

WAX AS AN IMPRESSION MATERIAL

Wax is used in some corrective impression technics in partial and complete denture prostheses. Impression waxes are available with a variety of softening temperatures, and these are further discussed in Chapter 13. Waxes with the lower softening points are used to register functional impressions. In these technics a thin layer of wax is applied to a denture base with occlusal bite rims and left in place in the mouth for a period of time. In this way the wax flows and adapts itself to the oral tissues under the influence of functional occlusion. Impression waxes with a higher softening point are used when necessary to extend the border of the denture base. The clinical technics for their use are adequately described in textbooks on prosthetic dentistry.

IMPRESSION COMPOUND

One of the oldest dental impression materials is impression compound. Tray compound has been largely replaced by acrylic tray materials, but impression compound is still used for border molding complete denture impressions and as a check on cavity preparations in the indirect inlay procedure. Undercuts in these preparations can be identified because the impression compound when cooled fractures on removal from an undercut area. Impression compounds are available in the form of sheets, sticks, cylinders, and cones; some examples are shown in Fig. 11-29. Impression compounds are thermoplastic materials and are softened to their working consistency by immersing in hot water or by warming over a flame. Compound impressions do not readily register fine surface detail. Some variation of the temperature at which softening takes place exists among different compounds, and they can be divided into high-fusing (tray) and low-fusing (impression) compounds.

Composition

Impression compound, shown in Table 11-14, is a mixture of thermoplastic resins and waxes, a filler,

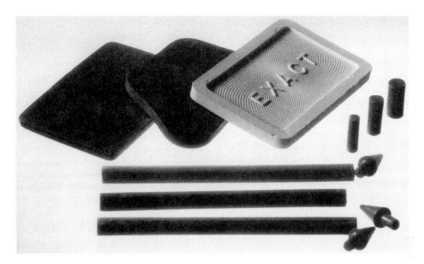

Fig. 11-29 Dental impression compound in the form of sheets, sticks, cylinders, and cones.

TABLE 11-14 Composition of an Impression Compound

Ingredient	Parts
Rosin	30
Copal resin	30
Carnauba wax	10
Stearic acid	5
Talc	75
Coloring agent	Appropriate amount

and a coloring agent. By varying the proportions of the various ingredients, compounds of differing physical properties can be made. The resins and waxes soften on heating and provide flow and cohesion, and the filler adds body and gives a suitable working consistency. Rouge produces a characteristic reddish brown color and it is the most common pigment.

Thermal Conductivity

The thermal conductivity of impression compounds is low. When immersed in hot water or heated over a flame, they soften on the outside rapidly, but time is required before the whole mass is softened throughout. When heating over a flame, care is needed to prevent the outside from being overheated and the more volatile components from

being vaporized or ignited. Prolonged immersion in hot water also leaches out the more soluble components and alters physical properties adversely.

The low thermal conductivity influences the cooling rate of these materials because the outside of a mass of compound hardens fairly rapidly, whereas the inner regions remain soft. Impressions must be given adequate time to cool completely before they are removed from the mouth.

Softening and Flow

The compounds should soften at a point just above mouth temperature and exhibit adequate flow to adapt closely to the tissues and register surface detail. They should harden at mouth temperature and exhibit a minimum of flow to reduce the danger of distortion on removal.

ANSI/ADA Specification No. 3 for dental impression compound lists the following criteria for flow qualities of the impression type: the flow at 37° C shall not be more than 6%, and the flow at 45° C shall not be less than 85%.

Sticks or small cones of compound are used for taking impressions of prepared restorations. These are usually softened when they are held some distance above a flame and are warmed carefully to avoid overheating the outside portion. The softened compound may be placed in a copper band, which has been adapted to the tooth and sealed in place by warming the band above the flame. Some operators then temper the compound by a brief immersion in water at a temperature just above the softening point of the compound.

Cooling

Impressions formed by placement of the softened compound into a suitable copper band for indirect inlay and crown technics are usually cooled in the mouth with water from a syringe. The water used for cooling should be within the range of 16° to 18° C because cold water is uncomfortable to the patient and tends to increase the internal stresses in the impression if cooling is too rapid. The exact time required for proper cooling varies with the size of the impression and the particular compound selected.

Effect of Wet Kneading

When the compound is softened in a water bath, kneading the material with the fingers is customary to improve the handling qualities. This wet kneading increases the flow of both the softened compound and the hardened impression and is believed to be caused by the incorporation of water in the compound, which acts as a plasticizer.

Wet kneading can modify the flow of the hardened compound to an extent that it exceeds the 6% permissible in the specification (Table 11-15). By kneading for 1 to 3 minutes, the flow of compounds may be more than doubled.

Clinically, excessive wet kneading can increase the flow qualities of the hardened material at mouth temperature to a point at which distortion may occur on removal. Once incorporated, the water

TABLE 11-15 Permissible Flow Values for Dental Compounds as Defined by ANSI/ADA Specification No. 3

Material	Flow	
	At 37° C	At 45° C
Type I (impression compound)	Less than 6%	More than 85%
Type II (tray compound)	Less than 2%	70%-85%

Adapted from Stanford JW, Paffenbarger GC, Sweeney WT: *J Am Dent Assoc* 51:56, 1955.

remains in the compound for long periods, and subsequent reheating with further kneading has a cumulative effect of increasing flow values.

Accuracy and Dimensional Stability

The optimum accuracy and dimensional stability of compound impressions can be ensured by carefully preparing and handling the material and attending to the details of the clinical technic in use. Softening the compound by a method that does not adversely affect its physical properties by overheating or prolonged heating is important. Equally important is that adequate flow is developed during softening to allow close adaptation to the tissues and a minimum of internal stresses in the impression. The tray, copper band, or other container used to convey the compound to the mouth must be strong, rigid and stable, and free from flexibility. In the mouth adequate cooling of the compound is essential to avoid distortion when the impression is removed. When the impression is obtained, the cast or die should be made as soon as possible to avoid inaccuracies caused by the release of stresses that produce warpage, which may occur on standing. One source of inaccuracy not within the control of the operator is the thermal contraction that the compound exhibits on cooling from mouth to room temperature.

Thermal Contraction

The linear contraction of an impression compound on cooling from mouth to room temperature is approximately 0.3%. This quality is inherent in the material and can result in inaccuracy unless it is recognized and adequate compensation is provided.

Tray Compounds

The special compounds for making impression trays are similar in composition and working qualities to the impression compounds, except that the temperature at which they soften is higher and the property of flow at mouth temperature is minimal. The ANSI/ADA Specification No. 3 requirements for tray compound are listed in Table 11-15. Tray compounds are used primarily to make individual trays for corrective wash impressions. The trays are made when softened tray compound is adapted to a study model and the border of the denture area is trimmed. Compound trays lack strength and dimensional stability; hence they have been replaced to a large extent by trays made in a similar manner from room temperature–curing acrylic resins.

ANSI/ADA Specification No. 3 for Dental Modeling Compound

Specification No. 3 has established certain limits for the desirable physical properties of both impression compound and tray compound. The impression compounds are required to be homogeneous and to show a smooth, glossy appearance after the surface has been passed through a flame. When trimmed with a sharp knife at room temperature, the cut margins must be firm and smooth. The manufacturer is required to indicate in the package the method of softening, the working temperature, and a curve or data showing the shrinkage of the compound from 40° to 20° C. Two physical tests are required by the specification. One is to test the percent flow at 37° C and at 45° C, and the other is to check the reproduction of the details of a test impression block. The acceptable values of percent flow for both impression and tray compound are shown in Table 11-15.

■ DIE, CAST, AND MODEL MATERIALS

Dental stones, plaster, electroformed silver and copper, epoxy resin, and casting investment are some of the materials used to make casts or dies from dental impressions. The selection of one of these is determined by the particular impression material in use and by the purpose for which the die or cast is to be used.

Impressions in agar or alginate hydrocolloid can be used only with a gypsum material, such as plaster, stone, or casting investment. Compound impressions, on the other hand, can be used to produce dies of plaster, stone, or electroformed copper. Various rubber impression materials can be used to prepare gypsum, electroformed or epoxy dies.

DESIRABLE QUALITIES OF A CAST OR DIE MATERIAL

Because the casts and dies are used in making appliances and restorations, accuracy and dimensional stability are of primary concern. Cast and die materials are required to reproduce an impression accurately and to remain dimensionally stable under normal conditions of use and storage. Such qualities as setting expansion, contraction, and dimensional variations in response to changes in temperature must be at a minimum. Not only should the cast be accurate, but it should also reproduce fine detail satisfactorily and have a smooth, hard surface. Such an accurate cast or die must also be strong and durable and withstand the subsequent manipulative procedures without abrasion of the surface or fracture. Qualities of strength, resistance to shearing forces or edge strength, and abrasion resistance are therefore important and are required in varying degrees, according to the purpose for which the cast or die is to be used. For example, a satisfactory study cast might be formed from dental model plaster in which these qualities are at a minimum because it will not be subjected to much stress in use. However, a rubber impression for indirect inlay production could be copper or silver formed to make a die in which these qualities are maximal to withstand the carving and finishing procedures that are a part of this technic.

Other less critical qualities are also of importance. The color of a cast or die can facilitate manipulative procedures such as waxing inlay patterns by presenting a contrast in color to the inlay wax. The ease with which the material can be adapted to the impression and the time required before the cast or die is ready for use are of considerable practical significance. A contrast in this respect is seen between dental stone, which can be easily vibrated into an impression, with the cast ready for use within an hour, and a copper die, which requires electroforming usually overnight.

DENTAL PLASTER AND STONE

The chemistry of dental plaster, stone, and high-strength stone and their physical properties are discussed in Chapter 12. These gypsum materials are used extensively to make casts and dies from dental impressions and can be used with any impression material. Stone casts are stronger and resist abrasion better than plaster casts and are used whenever a restoration or appliance is to be made on the cast. Plaster may be used for study casts, which are for record purposes only.

Hardening solutions, usually about 30% silica sols in water, are available to be mixed with stone. Increase in hardness of stone dies poured against impressions varies from 2% for silicones to 110% for polyether, with intermediate increases of 70% for agar and 20% for polysulfide. The dimensional change on setting of stones mixed with hardener is slightly greater than when mixes are made with water, +0.07% versus +0.05%. In most instances the abrasion or scraping resistance of mixes of stone made with hardening solutions is higher than comparable mixes made with water. A range of effects in the abrasion resistance of surface treatments of stone has been reported. Model and die sprays generally increase the resistance to scraping, although lubricants can decrease the resistance to scraping and the surface hardness.

High-strength dental stones make an excellent cast or die, readily reproduce the fine detail of a dental impression, and are ready for use after approximately 1 hour. The resulting cast is dimensionally stable over long periods of time and withstands most of the manipulative procedures involved in the production of appliances and restorations. However, procedures involving the bending, adapting, or finishing of metals can be accomplished only to a limited extent on high-strength stone dies and are better fulfilled on a metal die.

When wax patterns constructed on high-strength stone dies are to be removed, a separating agent or die lubricant is necessary to prevent the wax from adhering. Oils, liquid soap, detergents, and a number of commercial preparations can be used. Oils are generally to be avoided because some of them are wax solvents and soften the surface of the wax pattern, and in addition, oil on the surface of the wax increases the difficulty of painting the investment on the pattern in subsequent steps of the casting process. The lubricant is applied liberally to the high-strength stone die and allowed to soak in, and usually several applications can be made before any excess accumulates on the surface. The excess is blown off with an air blast before proceeding to make the wax pattern.

DIES FORMED BY THE ELECTRODEPOSITION OF METAL

Electroforming Impressions

The essential equipment for the electroforming of impressions to form indirect dies for inlay, crown, or bridge restorations are a source of direct electric current and an electrolyte. The electric current may be supplied by storage batteries, with a small variable resistance and an ammeter to indicate the energy in the system. Often the alternating current of 110V is converted to direct low-voltage current suitable for plating. In this case a transformer and rectifier with some fixed resistance are used, with the same variable resistance and ammeter described for storage-battery equipment. A small container for the electrolyte with inexpensive wire electrodes and a bar of pure copper or silver for the anode represent the necessary equipment.

A common electrolyte used for plating copper indirect dies is an acidic copper sulfate solution. Silver electrolytes contain silver cyanide in an alkaline solution. Because of the highly poisonous nature of cyanides and shipping restraints on the electrolytes, copper plating is more commonly used.

When solution of the copper sulfate occurs in the water, the salt dissociates to give cupric and sulfate ions. The positive copper ions are atoms that have lost electrons during dissociation. During electrolysis the positive ions are drawn to the negative electrode or cathode by electrostatic attraction. The negative sulfate (SO_4^-) ions have gained electrons and move toward the positive electrode or anode. Neutral or nondissociated molecules do not move under the influence of an electric field. Hence, if a nondissociated substance such as glucose is present in the electrolyte, it will inhibit only the migration of the copper or sulfate ions because the molecules are large but are not influenced by the electric current.

The anode is made of pure copper, and during electrolysis copper atoms give up two electrons ($2e$) and become Cu^{++} ions. The metallic copper of the anode therefore regenerates the solution as the plating process occurs with the removal of copper as the cathode. The Cu^{++} ion is attracted to the cathode (the impression), where it gains $2e$ and is deposited as metallic copper according to the equation $Cu^{++} + 2e \rightarrow Cu^0$. As long as there is free copper at the anode, the solution will maintain a constant composition.

The action at the electrodes may be summarized as the following equations:

Anode $Cu^0 - 2e \rightarrow Cu^{++}$
Cathode $Cu^{++} + 2e \rightarrow Cu^0$

Similar reactions occur in the electroforming of silver.

Anode $Ag^0 - e \rightarrow Ag^+$
Cathode $Ag^+ + e \rightarrow Ag^0$

Copper-Formed Dies

Metal dies can be made by copper-plating compound or silicone but not usually polysulfide impressions where silver-plating is preferred. Such a die is tough and has good strength characteristics, and metal inlays and restorations can be finished and polished satisfactorily on these dies.

A copper-forming apparatus suitable for dental use consists of a transformer and rectifier to reduce the voltage of the domestic supply and convert the alternating current (AC) to direct current (DC), which is needed for electroforming the impression. The low-voltage DC passes through a variable resistor, which is used to regulate the current and modify the rate at which metal is deposited, and a milliammeter, which indicates the current passing through the plating bath. A copper plate, which is attached to the anode, and the impression to be plated, which is at the cathode, are immersed in the electrolyte.

The copper plate becomes the anode and is made of electrolytically pure copper and is immersed in the plating solution so that the area of immersed copper is approximately equal to that of the impression to be plated. Copper anodes containing a trace of phosphorus are superior to pure copper.

The plating bath contains an acid solution of copper sulfate, and a number of formulas have been advocated. One acceptable example is given in Table 11-16.

TABLE 11-16 Composition of Solution for Copper-Forming Bath

Ingredient	Amount
Copper sulfate (crystals)	200 g
Sulfuric acid (concentrated)	30 ml
Phenolsulfonic acid	2 ml
Water (distilled)	1000 ml

The copper sulfate is the source of the copper, the sulfuric acid increases the conductivity of the solution, and the phenolsulfonic acid assists the penetration of copper ions to the deeper parts of an impression and improves the "throwing power" of the solution. Additives other than phenolsulfonic acid are suggested in formulas, of which dextrose, alcohol, phenol, and molasses are examples.

The surface of the impression is coated with a conductor of electricity before it is attached to the cathode lead wire.

When the impression is in compound, a colloidal dispersion of graphite is painted on the surface to be plated and allowed to dry before it is placed into the plating bath. When the impression is a silicone rubber, finely divided copper powder is brushed on the surface to be plated before placing the impression into the bath.

About 15 mA is a suitable current to start plating a single tooth impression. Once a thin layer of copper has covered the entire surface of the impression, the current can be increased to as much as two or three times the initial current. If too high a current setting is used, the copper deposit will be granular and friable in nature, and the die will be unsatisfactory. High-current densities also produce a heavier deposit on the areas of the impression nearest to the anode, and sometimes rapid plating results in a failure to adequately cover the deeper areas of an impression. Plating is allowed to proceed for 12 to 15 hours; overnight usually is a convenient period of time.

The quality of the deposit obtained with a freshly made plating solution often is not as good as that achieved when the solution has been in use a short time. Loss of water from evaporation should be replaced to maintain the correct concentration of the electrolyte. The sulfuric acid is slowly decomposed when the solution is in use, and the addition of a few milliliters of acid is required after a few weeks' use to maintain the quality of copper deposit. A sediment or sludge consisting mainly of fine particles of copper may sometimes accumulate on the floor of the bath, and then the solution should be filtered. When anodes containing a trace of phosphorus are used, the formation of sediment is considerably reduced.

In copper forming, the distance between the anode and the impression to be plated is important in relation to plating the deeper areas of an impression; the greater the anode-to-impression distance, the more even is the quantity of copper deposited over the impression and the more readily are the deep areas plated. About 6 inches is a suitable distance in practice; if the distance is shorter, there is a tendency for an excess of copper to be deposited on the more superficial areas of the impression, leaving the deeper areas inadequately plated.

The hydrophobic but not the hydrophilic addition silicone impression materials can be satisfactorily copper formed. The technic followed is as described in the previous paragraph; however, the impression surface is made conductive by the application of finely divided silver powder. The increased cost of silver and the increasing difficulties in obtaining cyanide silver plating solutions because of transport restrictions have resulted in the return to copper electroformed dies.

Silver-Formed Dies

With the advent of the polysulfide impression materials, silver forming was used as a method of making metal dies. Although it is possible to copper form polysulfide impression materials, consistent results are not always obtained, and the much easier procedure of silver forming lends itself to routine use. The alkaline silver baths used in silver forming soften the surface of impression compound, and silver forming cannot be used. Silicone and polyether impressions can also be silver formed. A pure silver anode is required, with a silver cyanide plating solution, of which the composition given in Table 11-17 is an example.

This solution is poisonous, and extreme care should be taken that the hands, workbench area, and clothing not become contaminated. This operation should not be used by inexperienced personnel.

TABLE 11-17 Composition of Solution for Silver-Forming Bath

Ingredient	Amount
Silver cyanide	36 g
Potassium cyanide	60 g
Potassium carbonate	45 g
Water (distilled)	1000 ml

The addition of acid to the solution produces hydrogen cyanide, an extremely poisonous gas, and for this reason copper-forming solutions should be kept far away, as any acid should be. The plating bath should have a cover that can be in place at all times to control evaporation and dissipation of fumes.

The impression is made conductive when the surface is brushed with powdered silver, which adheres well to rubber impressions. Alternatively, dispersions of silver powder in a volatile liquid vehicle are available, and they are painted on and allowed to dry.

A current setting of approximately 5 mA is suitable to start the plating of a single tooth impression. Once a layer of silver has been deposited over the surface, this current can be doubled or tripled. With larger impressions involving several teeth and the adjacent soft tissue areas, a current of approximately 10 mA/tooth is suitable for initial plating. Once the surface is covered with silver, the current can be doubled or tripled, and usually about 12 to 15 hours of plating produce a suitable thickness of silver.

Distilled water should be added to the electrolyte to replace any loss from evaporation, and the solution should be filtered from time to time. A polysulfide impression that has been silver formed is shown in Fig. 11-30, *A*. The model made from this silver-formed impression by pouring in of stone and removal of the impression after the stone has set is shown in Fig. 11-30, *B*.

Problems in metal-forming

There are the obvious effects of current failure either in the domestic power line or from some defect in the plating apparatus. However, even though the working apparatus is satisfactory, there are some problems related to the procedure itself that are sometimes puzzling.

Faulty conduction. The ammeter may show a current flowing, but the impression does not plate or plates irregularly or very slowly. This difficulty is caused by a short circuit through the electrolyte usually because of exposure of the conducting wire to the solution.

Exhausted solution. Plating is very slow, and the deposit is discolored. The solution should be discarded and replaced with a fresh solution. How long a solution lasts depends on the amount of usage and whether contamination occurs. A well-

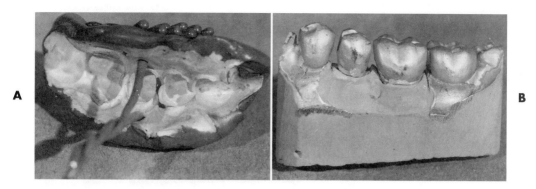

Fig. 11-30 **A,** Polysulfide impression showing connecting wires and layer of silver deposited by electroforming. **B,** Silver-formed model with stone base made from impression in **A.**

filtered solution protected from contamination and kept to correct concentration by adding distilled water when required gives the longest life. Cyanide solutions must be disposed of carefully.

Overconcentrated solution. Sometimes the ammeter reading drops rapidly to zero after the impression is placed in the bath. Resetting of the current regulator to establish the correct ammeter setting is followed by another drop of the ammeter reading to zero. This effect is caused by a too-concentrated solution. Adding the required amount of distilled water and rinsing the metal anode in distilled water solve the problem. An overconcentrated solution may also soften the surface of the rubber and discolor any stone areas of the cast.

Metal anode too small. An anode that is smaller in area than the impression or impressions to be plated leads to slow and irregular plating.

Friable metal deposit. If the metal deposit is granular and friable, although of correct color, the current setting is too high.

EPOXY DIE MATERIALS

Epoxy materials until recently were supplied in the form of a paste to which a liquid activator (amine) was added to initiate hardening. Because the activators are toxic, they should not come into contact with the skin while mixing and manipulating of the unset material. Shrinkage of 0.1% has occurred during hardening, which may take up to 24 hours. The hardened resin is more resistant to abrasion and stronger than a high-strength stone

die. The viscous paste is not so readily introduced into the details of a large impression as high-strength dental stone is, and a centrifugal casting machine has been developed to assist in the pouring of epoxy resins. Recently, fast-setting epoxy materials have been supplied in automixing systems similar to those described for automixing addition silicones and is shown in Fig. 11-31. The epoxy resin is in one cartridge, and the catalyst is in the other. Forcing the two pastes through the static mixing tip thoroughly mixes the epoxy material, which can be directly injected into a rubber impression. If desired a small intraoral delivery tip may be attached to the static mixing tip for injecting into detailed areas of the impression. The fast-setting epoxy hardens rapidly so that dies can be waxed up in a half-hour after injecting into the impression. Epoxy resins cannot be used with water-containing agar and alginate impression materials because the water retards the polymerization of the resin and thus are limited to use with rubber impression materials.

■ COMPARISON OF IMPRESSION AND DIE MATERIALS

High-strength stone dies may be from 0.35% larger than the master to 0.25% smaller than the master, depending on the location of the measurement and the impression material used. In general, occlusogingival (vertical) changes are greater than buccolingual or mesiodistal (horizontal) changes. The shrinkage of the impression material toward the surfaces of the tray in the horizontal direction

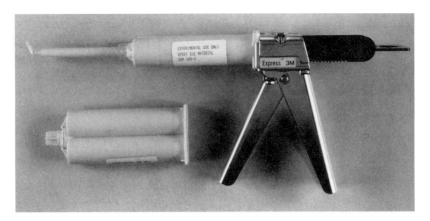

Fig. 11-31 Automix system for fast-setting epoxy die material.

usually results in dimensions larger than the master. In the vertical direction shrinkage is away from the free surface of the impression and toward the tray, and dimensions smaller than the master are obtained.

Invariably metal-formed dies show more vertical change than high-strength stone dies, with the differences being between 0.25% and 0.45%, depending on the impression materials, whereas the horizontal changes are not significantly different for the two die materials. The accuracy of the rubber impression materials is in the following order from best to worst, regardless of whether stone or metal dies are used: addition silicone, polyether, polysulfide, and condensation silicone.

The epoxy dies all exhibit some polymerization shrinkage, with values ranging from 0.1% to 0.3%, and as a result the dies are undersized.

The ability of an impression-die combination to reproduce surface detail does not rank the materials in the same order as the values for dimensional change do. If a release agent is not needed on the surface of the impression, epoxy dies reproduce detail the best (10 μm), followed by metal-formed dies (30 μm), and high-strength stone dies (170 μm). However, polysulfide impressions require the use of a release agent with epoxy dies, and their reproduction of detail is comparable to that obtained with high-strength stone. The silicone-epoxy combination produces the sharpest detail, although not all epoxy die materials are compatible with all silicone impression materials.

The resistance to abrasion and scraping should also be considered. Metal-formed dies have superior resistance to abrasion, epoxy dies have good resistance, and high-strength stone dies have the least resistance.

SELECTED PROBLEMS

Problem 1. A mix of alginate was made, and the setting time was shorter than previously experienced with this brand. The material was too stiff at the time of insertion to obtain adequate seating and surface detail. What factors should be considered in the correction of this difficulty?

Solution a. The most common cause for the shorter setting time is too high a temperature of the mix water. The setting reaction is a typical chemical reaction that is accelerated by increases in temperature; a 10° C increase in temperature almost doubles the rate of the reaction. In many operations a single water faucet is present with a mixing valve to control the temperature of the water. Gradual failure of the mixing valve can inadvertently result in the use of water substantially hotter than the 21° C usually recommended.

Solution b. The setting time can also be shortened by incorrect dispensing resulting in too high a powder-liquid ratio. If the alginate powder is not aerated before each dispensing, the weight of each scoop will be too high, because the apparent density of the powder is higher after standing compared with its density when it has been aerated. The increased amount of powder causes the setting or gelation time to be less than normally experienced.

Solution c. Aging of the alginate powder in a warm, humid atmosphere can affect the setting by reducing the effectiveness of the retarder, resulting in a shorter than normal setting time.

Problem 2. A mix of alginate was made, and it appeared thicker than normal. After the impression was taken, its surface seemed grainy and lacking in surface detail. What precautions should be taken to avoid this condition when the impression is retaken?

Solution. A thick consistency can result from lack of aeration of the powder before dispensing, as well as from an incorrect number of measures of powder or water. However, a thick, grainy mix can occur from inadequate mixing of the correct proportions of powder and water. Inadequate mixing may be caused by casual rather than vigorous spatulation or by not mixing for the full time recommended. Hot water used in combination with the two factors just mentioned accentuates the problem of thick, grainy mixes. If the next mix is carefully dispensed, the temperature of the water is checked, and the length of mixing is timed, a smooth, creamy consistency should result.

Problem 3. An alginate impression was taken of a patient with a fixed appliance, and tearing of the impression occurred in critical areas as a result of severely undercut areas. What can be done to improve the next impression, because alginate impressions are supposed to be elastic?

Solution. It is true that alginate impressions are flexible, although they are not entirely elastic (complete recovery) and have rather low resistance to tearing compared with rubber impression materials. Several precautions can be taken to improve the chances of an acceptable impression. The severely undercut areas can be blocked out, thus placing less stress on the alginate during removal. Recall that the strength of the alginate improves quite rapidly for 5 to 10 minutes after setting, and the impression can be left in the mouth a few extra minutes before removal. Also remember that the tear strength is a function of the rate of removal of the impression, and rapid rates enhance the chances of an acceptable impression. Finally, mixes with high powder-liquid ratios have higher tear strengths; however, the ratio must not be increased beyond the limit to obtain a smooth consistency that will record the surface detail desired.

Problem 4. An alginate impression is to be taken of a patient known to have a problem with gagging. What steps can be taken in materials management to reduce the problem and yet obtain a satisfactory impression?

Solution a. The viscosity of mixed alginates remains fairly constant until just before the setting time because the retardation reaction prevents the formation of the calcium alginate gel. When the working and setting times are known accurately, the insertion of the impression material into the mouth can be delayed until just before the end of the working time, while still allowing enough time to seat the impression. The impression then should be removed at the earliest possible time after it sets and yet has adequate properties. Thus the impression is in the mouth the shortest possible time.

Solution b. A fast-setting alginate can be selected that not only sets in a shorter time but has better mechanical properties in a shorter time than regular-setting material.

Solution c. Care should be taken during the loading of the maxillary impression tray to avoid excessive amounts of alginate in the posterior portion of the tray. The posterior part of the tray should be seated before the anterior portion with the patient's head in a position to avoid excess alginate flowing in a posterior direction on the palate.

Problem 5. The set alginate impression separated from the tray during removal from the mouth, resulting in distortion and tearing of the impression. What can be done to avoid this?

Solution. Two choices can be made. A change in the brand of alginate to one that adheres to the metal tray is one option. However, if a nonadhesive alginate is desired, a tray with perforations that provides mechanical retention should be selected.

Problem 6. An inaccurate model is obtained despite the use of the correct technic for mixing the alginate and the proper pouring procedure for the gypsum model. What possible factors might have resulted in the inaccurate impression?

Solution a. The tray selected may have been too small, thus providing too little alginate between the tray and the tissues. During the removal of the set alginate the percent compression may have been too high when the bulge of the tooth compressed the alginate in the undercut areas. This excessive compression results in higher than normal permanent deformation. The problem can be corrected by selecting a tray that provides about 5 mm of space between the tray and tissues. With the same amount of undercut the alginate is subjected to lower percent compression, and lower permanent deformation results.

Solution b. A second possible cause of the problem could be the premature removal of the impression. The permanent deformation of the impression on removal decreases with the time after setting. Therefore premature removal of the impression, even though the material is no longer tacky, can be the cause of excessive permanent deformation of the impression in undercut areas.

Solution c. A third possible cause of the inaccurate impression might be too slow a rate of removal of the set impression material. With everything else being equal, a slow rate of removal of the impression rather than a snap removal results in higher than normal amounts of permanent deformation.

Solution d. A fourth reason for the difficulty might be overextension of the alginate to areas not supported by the tray. The weight of these overextended areas can deform the impression, and, if they are not cut away, deformation and permanent distortion of the impression in these areas can occur.

Solution e. Finally, the alginate impression can be permanently distorted if after removal it is stored so that the impression is deformed. Two possible conditions could cause this effect: placing the impression down with the weight of the tray on it and wrapping the impression too tightly in a damp towel.

Problem 7. When an impression with polysulfide rubber material was taken, a number of voids appeared on the surface of the impressions of the teeth and abutment preparations. What is the reason for such a failure, and how can it be avoided?

Solution. Some air bubbles are always incorporated into the pastes during the manufacturing process, and these bubbles can be observed when dispensing the pastes onto the paper pad. The mixing of the base and catalyst pastes should be done carefully to avoid incorporating air into the mixture. After the two pastes are initially mixed, the material must be spatulated and spread over the widest area possible and flattened to form a thin layer over the surface of the pad. The spatula must be kept in contact with the mixture so that air bubbles are eliminated. The material is gathered with the straight edge of the blade and redeposited onto the paper pad, and then mixing is continued with a wiping, pressing motion until a homogeneous mix is obtained.

Problem 8. On critical observation of an impression obtained with a polysulfide rubber material, some areas were found that were incompletely reproduced. What is the cause of these large voids, and how can they be avoided?

Solution. The setting time of polysulfide rubber impression materials is affected by humidity. Delay in injecting the low-consistency syringe material results in a higher-viscosity material reducing the flow, and thus a large area is incompletely produced. Also, the rubber does not effectively displace saliva from the surface of the tooth.

This type of failure may be avoided by isolating the field with cotton rolls, drying it carefully with air blasts, and then using a syringe with a low-consistency material at the correct time after mixing under proper conditions to cover the teeth and gum surfaces before placing the high-consistency material with the tray.

Problem 9. When an impression with polysulfide rubber material was withdrawn from the mouth, the impression material was separated from the tray in some areas. What caused this separation, and how accurate are the dies obtained from such an impression?

Solution. The adhesion of an impression material to the custom-made tray is obtained by coating the tray with an adhesive. To get good adhesion to the tray, enough coats of the adhesive should be used. It is also necessary to wait until the volatile organic solvent evaporates and the adhesive is dry. When the tray is filled with the high-consistency material too soon after applying the adhesive, the retention fails and the impression material separates from the tray. In this instance, a distortion of the impression always occurs and results in a distorted model and dies. It is better to remake the impression than to continue with the procedure. When the failure is caused by the adhesive itself, better mechanical retention for the impression material can be obtained by making perforations with a bur in the same type of custom-made tray. These mechanical interlocks retain the impression material in position, and the uniform thickness of rubber in the custom-made tray aids in controlling the polymerization shrinkage of the material.

Problem 10. Preparation of a complete-arch fixed bridge was completed, a wash impression with a condensation silicone rubber was taken, and a single cast was obtained as a master model. The metal frame of the bridge fit perfectly on the cast but did not fit well on all abutments. Is this a problem of the impression material, and how can it be solved? What factors may have produced this problem?

Solution a. Polymerization shrinkage occurs with condensation silicone rubber material. Dimensional change in these silicone materials increases with time up to 24 hours, although about half the change takes place in the first hour. The longer the impression is left on the bench before the cast is poured, the greater the shrinkage of the material. Usually, some castings fit individual abutments, but when such a cast is used as a master model to make the fixed prosthesis, the general accuracy is unsatisfactory.

Solution b. Distortion may be produced as a result of relaxation of stresses in the impression. If the impression is removed from the mouth when polymerization has not progressed sufficiently, stresses may be induced in the mass, and a distorted impression is obtained. A distorted impression can result from excessive pressure on the material during setting, which produces residual stresses that can be relieved.

Solution c. Distortion can be produced when the impression is removed with slow movements. Like all elastic impression materials, condensation silicone rubber impressions must be removed from the mouth with a sudden motion. A slow removal induces permanent deformation in the mass, and an inaccurate cast is obtained. If a fixed appliance is made on such a cast, it will not fit on all teeth preparations. Note that less permanent deformation occurs with silicone than with polysulfide impressions.

Solution d. Distortion may result when too much space is provided between the tray and teeth. The amount of silicone rubber impression material between the tray and the abutments should be small. A thin layer is better than a thick mass because less permanent deformation occurs during the removal of the impression and more accurate dies and models will be obtained.

Problem 11. An impression of a dentulous quadrant was taken with a medium-consistency polyether impression material in a custom-made acrylic tray. The normal relief of 2 mm was provided between the tray and the oral structures. After removal of the impression, tearing was noted at several locations. What adjustments can be made so that the possibility of tearing will be minimized on retaking the impression?

Solution a. Polyether impression materials are stiff (low strain in compression) at the time of removal from the mouth; this stiffness, combined with only moderate tear strength, increases the probability of tearing of the impression. Doubling the relief space between the tray and the tissues to 4 mm increases the effective flexibility of the rubber and improves the chances for success.

Solution b. Use of an equal length of thinner paste with the base and catalyst paste increases the flexibility without a serious loss in tear strength and accuracy and thus decreases the chance of tearing the impression.

Solution c. Although polyethers are more elastic and less viscoelastic than polysulfide rubbers, the tear strength increases as the rate of removal of the impression increases. Therefore, on the retake, rather than trying to "tease" the impression out to decrease the chance of tearing, the impression should be removed as rapidly as feasible.

Problem 12. The manufacturer of an addition silicone impression specified that high-strength stone dies should not be poured until after 1 hour. An epoxy die was desired, and therefore pouring was delayed for 1 hour. On separation the die was covered with negative bubbles. What caused the problem, and how can it be avoided?

Solution. Some brands of addition silicones release hydrogen after setting. Waiting 1 hour before pouring the fast-setting, high-strength stone allows the rate of hydrogen release to decrease sufficiently so that bubble-free dies can be produced. However, many epoxy die materials set slowly compared with high-strength stone, and sufficient hydrogen is still being released at 1 hour so that it produces bubbles on the surface of the epoxy die. Even waiting 4 hours may not result in a bubble-free epoxy die. Allowing the impression to stand overnight before pouring the epoxy die solves the problem. Also note that the accuracy of addition silicone impressions is excellent at 24 hours, even with the evolution of hydrogen.

Problem 13. An impression was taken in a hydrophobic addition silicone that had been mixed by hand spatulation. The resulting high-strength stone die had enough positive and negative bubbles, especially along the line angles of the preparation, so that a retake of the impression was necessary. What could be done to reduce the number of bubbles?

Solution. Changing to an addition silicone supplied in automixing cartridges substantially reduces the number of bubbles in the mix compared with one prepared by hand spatulation and minimizes the number of positive bubbles.

In addition, changing to hydrophilic automixing addition silicone decreases the number of negative bubbles in the die because of the better wetting of the impression by the mix of high-strength stone.

■ REFERENCES

Agar and Alginate Hydrocolloids

Appleby DC, Pameijer CH, Boffa J: The combined reversible hydrocolloid/irreversible hydrocolloid impression system, *J Prosthet Dent* 44:27, 1980.

Bergman B, Bergman M, Olsson S: Alginate impression materials, dimensional stability and surface detail sharpness following treatment with disinfectant solutions, *Swed Dent J* 9:255, 1985.

Brune D, Beltesbrekke H: Levels of airborne particles resulting from handling alginate impression material, *Scand J Dent Res* 86:206, 1978.

Buchan S, Peggie RW: Role of ingredients in alginate impression compounds, *J Dent Res* 45:1120, 1966.

Carlyle LW III: Compatibility of irreversible hydrocolloid impression materials with dental stones, *J Prosthet Dent* 49:434, 1983.

Craig RG: Mechanical properties of some recent alginates and tensile bond strengths of agar/alginate combinations, *Phillip's J Rest Zahnmed* 6:242, 1989.

Craig RG: Review of dental impression materials, *Adv Dent Res* 2:51, 1988.

Durr DP, Novak EV: Dimensional stability of alginate impressions immersed in disinfection solutions, *J Dent Child* 54:45, 1987.

Ellis B, Lamb DJ: The setting characteristics of alginate impression materials, *Br Dent J* 151:343, 1981.

Farah JM, Powers JM, editors: Crown and bridge impression materials, *The Dent Advisor* 6:1, 1989.

Fish SF, Braden M: Characterization of the setting process in alginate impression materials, *J Dent Res* 43:107, 1964.

Ghani F, Hobkirk JA, Wilson M: Evaluation of a new antiseptic-containing alginate impression material, *Br Dent J* 169:83, 1990.

Herrero SP, Merchant VA: Dimensional stability of dental impressions after immersion disinfection, *J Am Dent Assoc* 113:419, 1986.

Jarvis RG, Earnshaw R: The effects of alginate impressions on the surface of cast gypsum. I. The physical and chemical structure of the cast surface, *Aust Dent J* 25:349, 1980.

Jarvis RG, Earnshaw R: The effect of alginate impressions on the surface of cast gypsum. II. The role of sodium phosphate in incompatibility, *Aust Dent J* 26:12, 1981.

Johnson GH, Craig RG: Accuracy and bond strength of combinations of agar/alginate hydrocolloid impression materials, *J Prosthet Dent* 55:1, 1986.

Lewinstein I, Craig RG: The effect of powder/water ratio of irreversible hydrocolloid on the bond strength of irreversible hydrocolloid and agar combinations, *J Prosthet Dent* 62:412, 1989.

MacPherson GW, Craig RG, Peyton FA: Mechanical properties of hydrocolloid and rubber impression materials, *J Dent Res* 46:714, 1967.

Matyas J, Dao N, Caputo AS, Lucatorto FM: Effects of disinfectants on dimensional accuracy of impression materials, *J Prosthet Dent* 64:25, 1990.

Miller MW: Syneresis in alginate impression materials, *Br Dent J* 139:425, 1975.

Peutzfeldt A, Asmussen E: Effect of disinfecting solutions on accuracy of alginate and elastomeric impressions, *Scand J Dent Res* 97:470, 1989.

Peutzfeldt A, Asmussen E: Effect of disinfecting solutions on surface texture of alginate and elastomeric impressions, *Scand J Dent Res* 98:74, 1990.

Sawyer HF, Sandrik JL, Neiman R: Accuracy of casts produced from alginate and hydrocolloid impression materials, *J Am Dent Assoc* 93:806, 1976.

Wanis TM, Combe EC, Grant AA: Measurement of the viscosity of irreversible hydrocolloids, *J Oral Rehabil* 20:379, 1993.

Woodward JD, Morris JC, Khan Z: Accuracy of stone casts produced by perforated trays and nonperforated trays, *J Prosthet Dent* 53:347, 1985.

Woody RD, Huget EF, Cutright DE: Characterization of airborne particles from irreversible hydrocolloids, *J Am Dent Assoc* 94:501, 1977.

Duplicating Materials

Craig RG, Gehring PE, Peyton FA: Aging characteristics of elastic duplicating compounds, *J Dent Res* 41:196, 1962.

Craig RG, Peyton FA: Physical properties of elastic duplicating materials, *J Dent Res* 39:391, 1960.

Finger W: Accuracy of dental duplicating materials, *Quintessence Dent Tech* 10:89, 1986.

Lyon FF, Anderson JN: Some agar duplicating materials: an evaluation of their properties, *Br Dent J* 132:15, 1972.

Peyton FA, Craig RG: Compatibility of duplicating compound and casting investments, *J Prosthet Dent* 12:1111, 1962.

Polysulfide, Silicone, and Polyether Rubbers

Bell JW, Davies EH, von Fraunhofer JA: The dimensional changes of elastomeric impression materials under various conditions of humidity, *J Dent* 4:73, 1976.

Bergman M, Olsson S, Bergman B: Elastomeric impression materials: dimensional stability and surface sharpness following treatment with disinfection solutions, *Swed Dent J* 4:161, 1980.

Braden M: Characterization of the setting process in dental polysulfide rubbers, *J Dent Res* 45:1065, 1966.

Braden M, Causton B, Clarke RL: A polyether impression rubber, *J Dent Res* 51:889, 1972.

Braden M, Inglis AT: Visco-elastic properties of dental elastomeric impression materials, *Biomaterials* 7:45, 1986.

Chong YH, Soh G: Effectiveness of intraoral delivery tips in reducing voids in elastomeric impressions, *Quintess Int* 22:897, 1991.

Cook WD: Permanent set and stress relaxation in elastomeric impression materials, *J Biomed Mater Res* 15:44, 1981.

Cook WD: Rheological studies of the polymerization of elastomeric impression materials. I. Network structure of the set state, *J Biomed Mater Res* 16:315, 1982.

Cook WD: Rheological studies of the polymerization of elastomeric impression materials. II. Viscosity measurements, *J Biomed Mater Res* 16:331, 1982.

Cook WD: Rheological studies of the polymerization of elastomeric impression materials. III. Dynamic stress relaxation modulus, *J Biomed Mater Res* 16:345, 1982.

Cook WD, Liem F, Russo P, Scheiner M, Simkiss G, Woodruff P: Tear and rupture of elastomeric dental impression materials, *Biomaterials* 5:275, 1984.

Cook WD, Thomasz F: Rubber gloves and addition silicone materials, *Aust Dent J* 31:140, 1986.

Council on Dental Materials and Devices: Status report on polyether impression materials, *J Am Dent Assoc* 95:126, 1977.

Craig RG: Composition, characteristics and clinical and tissue reactions of impression materials. In Smith DC, Williams DF, editors: *Biocompatibility of dental materials,* vol 3, *Biocompatibility of dental restorative materials,* Boca Raton, Fla, 1982, CRC Press.

Craig RG: Evaluation of an automatic mixing system for an addition silicone impression material, *J Am Dent Assoc* 110:213, 1985.

Craig RG: Properties of 12 addition silicones compared with other rubber impression materials, *Phillip's J Rest Zahnmed* 3:244, 1986.

Craig RG: Review of dental impression materials, *Adv Dent Res* 2:51, 1988.

Craig RG, Sun Z: Trends in elastomeric impression materials, *Oper Dent* 19:138, 1994.

Craig RG, Urquiola NJ, Liu CC: Comparison of commercial elastomeric impression materials, *Oper Dent* 15:94, 1990.

Drennon DG, Johnson GH : The effect of immersion disinfection of elastomeric impressions on the surface detail reproduction of improved gypsum casts, *J Prosthet Dent* 63:233, 1990.

Drennon DG, Johnson GH, Powell GL: The accuracy and efficacy of disinfection by spray atomization on elastomeric impressions, *J Prosthet Dent* 62:468, 1989.

Goldberg AJ: Viscoelastic properties of silicone, polysulfide, and polyether impression materials, *J Dent Res* 53:1033, 1974.

Gordon GE, Johnson GH, Drennon DG: The effect of tray selection on the accuracy of elastomeric impression materials, *J Prosthet Dent* 63:12, 1990.

Herfort TW, Gerberich WW, Macosko CW, Goodkind RJ: Tear strength of elastomeric impression materials, *J Prosthet Dent* 39:59, 1978.

Herfort TW, Gerberich WW, Macosko CW, Goodkind RJ: Viscosity of elastomeric impression materials, *J Prosthet Dent* 38:396, 1977.

Inoue K, Wilson HJ: Viscoelastic properties of elastomeric impression materials. II. Variation of rheological properties with time, temperature and mixing proportions, *J Oral Rehabil* 5:261, 1978.

Johansson EG, Erhardson S, Wictorin L: Influence of stone mixing agents, impression materials and lubricants on surface hardness and dimensions of a dental stone die material, *Acta Odontol Scand* 33:17, 1975.

Johnson GH, Craig RG: Accuracy of addition silicones as a function of technique, *J Prosthet Dent* 55:197, 1986.

Johnson GH, Craig RG: Accuracy of four types of rubber impression materials compared with time of pour and a repeat pour of models, *J Prosthet Dent* 53:484, 1985.

Johnson GH, Drennon DG, Powell GL: Accuracy of elastomeric impressions disinfected by immersion, *J Am Dent Assoc* 116:525, 1988.

Kim KN, Craig RG, Koran A III: Viscosity of monophase addition silicones as a function of shear rate, *J Prosthet Dent* 67:794, 1992.

Koran A, Powers JM, Craig RG: Apparent viscosity of materials used for making edentulous impressions, *J Am Dent Assoc* 95:75, 1977.

Lorren RA, Salter DJ, Fairhurst CW: The contact angles of die stone on impression materials, *J Prosthet Dent* 36:176, 1976.

Mansfield MA, Wilson HJ: Elastomeric impression materials: a comparison of methods for determining working and setting times, *Br Dent J* 132:106, 1972.

McCabe JF, Bowman AJ: The rheological properties of dental impression materials, *Br Dent J* 151:179, 1981.

McCabe JF, Storer R: Elastomeric impression materials: the measurement of some properties relevant to clinical practice, *Br Dent J* 149:73, 1980.

Neissen LC, Strassler H, Levinson PD, Wood G, Greenbaum J: Effect of latex gloves on setting time of polyvinylsiloxane putty impression material, *J Prosthet Dent* 55:128, 1986.

Norling BK, Reisbick MH: The effect of nonionic surfactants on bubble entrapment in elastomeric impression materials, *J Prosthet Dent* 42:342, 1979.

Ohsawa M, Jørgensen KD: Curing contraction of addition-type silicone impression materials, *Scand J Dent Res* 91:51, 1983.

Pratten DH, Craig RG: Wettability of a hydrophilic addition silicone impression material, *J Prosthet Dent* 61:197, 1989.

Salem NS, Combe EC, Watts DC: Mechanical properties of elastomeric impression materials, *J Oral Rehabil* 15:125, 1988.

Sandrik JL, Vacco JL: Tensile and bond strength of putty-wash elastomeric impression materials, *J Prosthet Dent* 50:358, 1983.

Schelb E, Cavazos E Jr, Troendle KB, Prihoda TJ: Surface detail reproduction of Type IV dental stones with selected polyvinyl siloxane impression materials, *Quintess Int* 22:51, 1991.

Sneed WD, Miller R, Olean J: Tear strength of ten elastomeric impression materials, *J Prosthet Dent* 49:511, 1983.

Stackhouse JA Jr: The accuracy of stone dies made from rubber impression materials, *J Prosthet Dent* 24:377, 1970.

Stackhouse JA Jr: Relationship of syringe-tip diameter to voids in elastomeric impressions, *J Prosthet Dent* 53:812, 1985.

Storer R, McCabe JF: An investigation of methods available for sterilising impressions, *Br Dent J* 151:217, 1981.

Tolley LG, Craig RG: Viscoelastic properties of elastomeric impression materials, *J Oral Rehabil* 5:121, 1978.

Vermilyea SG, Huget EF, de Simon LB: Apparent viscosities of setting elastomers, *J Dent Res* 59:1149, 1980.

Williams JR, Craig RG: Physical properties of addition silicones as a function of composition, *J Oral Rehabil* 15:639, 1988.

Zinc Oxide–Eugenol Pastes

Brauer GM, White EE, Moshonas MG: Reaction of metal oxides with o-ethoxy benzoic acid and other chelating agents, *J Dent Res* 37:547, 1958.

Copeland HI, Brauer GM, Sweeney WT, Forziati AF: Setting reaction of zinc oxide and eugenol, *J Res Nat Bur Stand* 55:133, 1955.

Harvey W, Petch NJ: Acceleration of the setting of zinc oxide cements, *Br Dent J* 80:1, 1946; 80:35, 1946.

Kelly EB: Dental impression paste, US Patent No 2,077,418, April 20, 1937.

Myers GE, Peyton FA: Physical properties of the zinc oxide–eugenol impression pastes, *J Dent Res* 40:39, 1961.

Olsson S, Bergman B, Bergman M: Zinc oxide–eugenol impression materials: dimensional stability and surface detail sharpness following treatment with disinfection solutions, *Swed Dent J* 6:177, 1982.

Smith DC: The setting of zinc oxide–eugenol mixtures, *Br Dent J* 105:313, 1958.

Tyas MJ, Wilson HJ: Properties of zinc oxide–eugenol impression pastes, *Br Dent J* 129:461, 1970.

Vieira DF: Factors affecting the setting of zinc oxide–eugenol impression pastes, *J Prosthet Dent* 9:70, 1959.

Plaster of Paris

Jørgensen KD: Study on the setting of plaster of paris, *Odont Tskr* 61:305, 1953.

Sodeau WH, Gibson CS: The use of plaster of paris as an impression material, *Br Dent J* 48:1089, 1927.

Compound

Bevan EM, Smith DC: Properties of impression compound, *Br Dent J* 114:181, 1963.

Braden M: Rheology of dental composition (impression compound), *J Dent Res* 46:620, 1967.

Combe EC, Smith DC: Further studies on impression compounds, *Dent Pract* 15:292, 1965.

Docking AR: Kneading of modelling compounds, *Aust J Dent* 59:225, 1955.

Stanford JW, Paffenbarger GC, Sweeney WT: Revision of ADA Specification No. 3 for dental impression compound, *J Am Dent Assoc* 51:56, 1955.

Die, Cast, and Model Materials

Aiach D, Malone WFP, Sandrik J: Dimensional accuracy of epoxy resins and their compatibility with impression materials, *J Prosthet Dent* 52:500, 1984.

Blum W, Hogaboom GB: *Principles of electroplating and electroforming*, ed 3, New York, 1949, McGraw-Hill.

Craig RG, Johnson KT: Accuracy of models for indirect posterior restorations, *J Oral Rehabil* 20:483, 1993.

Cummins RL: A laboratory procedure for copperplating rubber base impressions, *J Prosthet Dent* 33:342, 1975.

Eames WB, Edwards CR Jr, Buck WC Jr: Scraping resistance of dental die materials: a comparison of brands, *Oper Dent* 3:66, 1978.

Ellis RG: *Electrodeposition and its application in dentistry*, Toronto, 1943, Canadian Dental Research Foundation Bulletin No 26.

Fan PL, Powers JM, Reid BC: Surface and mechanical properties of stone, resin, and metal dies, *J Am Dent Assoc* 103:408, 1981.

Finger W, Ohsawa M: Accuracy of stone-casts produced from selected addition-type silicone impressions, *Scand J Dent Res* 91:61, 1983.

Frankel CB: A scientific approach to the solution of practical problems encountered in electro-forming copper dies, *J Am Dent Assoc* 32:1130, 1945.

Luria MA, Dennison JB: A comparison of epoxy resin, dental stone, and silver plated dies for cast gold restorations, *Mich Dent Assoc J* 63:17, 1981.

Myers GE: Electroformed die technique for rubber base impressions, *J Prosthet Dent* 8:531, 1958.

Nevers RP, Hungerford RL, Palmer EW: Effect of anode composition in acid copper plating, *Plating* 41:1301, 1954.

Novak A: Solution of difficulties encountered with copper electroformed dies, *J Am Dent Assoc* 39:554, 1949.

Östland SG: Cutting resistance tests of die materials, *J Prosthet Dent* 9:461, 1959.

Östland SG, Akesson NA: Epoxy resins as die material, *Odontol Revy* 11:225, 1960.

Peyton FA, Leibold JP, Ridgley GV: Surface hardness, compressive strength, and abrasion resistance of indirect die stone, *J Prosthet Dent* 2:381, 1952.

Schwartz HB, Leupold RJ, Thompson VP: Linear dimensional accuracy of epoxy resin and stone dies, *J Prosthet Dent* 45:621, 1981.

Stackhouse JA Jr: Impression materials and electrodeposits. I. Impression materials, *J Prosthet Dent* 45:44, 1981.

Stackhouse JA Jr: Impression materials and electrodeposits. II. Electrodeposits, *J Prosthet Dent* 45:146, 1981.

Vermilyea SG, Powers JM, Craig RG: Polyether, polysulfide and silicone rubber impression materials. I. Quality of silverplated dies, *Mich Dent Assoc J* 57:371, 1975.

Vermilyea SG, Powers JM, Craig RG: Polyether, polysulfide and silicone rubber impression materials. II. Accuracy of silverplated dies, *Mich Dent Assoc J* 57:405, 1975.

Wiktorsson G, Feder D: Quality of stone dies produced by different impression materials: a comparative study of impression techniques, *Swed Dent J* 7:77, 1983.

Williams GJ, Bates JF, Wild S: The effect of surface treatment of dental stone with resins, *Quintessence Dent Tech* 7(1):41, 1983.

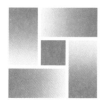

12 *Gypsum Products and Investments*

ypsum products probably serve the dental profession more adequately than any other materials used in dentistry. Dental plaster, stone, high-strength/high-expansion stone, and casting investment materials constitute this group of products, which are all closely related. With slight modification, gypsum products are used for several different purposes. For example, as impression plaster, these materials can be used to take impressions of edentulous mouths or to mount casts, as dental stone to form a die that duplicates the oral anatomy when poured into any type of impression, as a binder for silica for gold and low-melting nickel-chromium casting investments, and as soldering investment. These products are used also as a mold material for processing complete dentures. The main reason for such diversified use is that the properties of gypsum materials can be easily modified.

The dihydrate form of calcium sulfate, $CaSO_4 \cdot 2H_2O$, called gypsum, is usually white to milky yellowish in color and is found in a compact mass in nature.

The mineral gypsum has commercial importance as a source of plaster of paris. The term *plaster of paris* got its name because it was obtained by burning the gypsum from deposits near Paris, France. Deposits of gypsum, however, are found in most countries.

■ CHEMICAL AND PHYSICAL NATURE OF GYPSUM PRODUCTS

Most gypsum products are obtained from natural deposits. Because gypsum is the dihydrate form of calcium sulfate, $CaSO_4 \cdot 2H_2O$, on heating, it loses 1.5 g mol of its 2 g mol of H_2O and is converted to calcium sulfate hemihydrate, $CaSO_4 \cdot 1/2H_2O$, sometimes written $(CaSO_4)_2 \cdot H_2O$. When calcium sulfate hemihydrate is mixed with water, the reverse reaction takes place, and the calcium sulfate hemihydrate is converted back to calcium sulfate dihydrate. The reaction of calcium sulfate hemihydrate with water can be shown as:

$$CaSO_4 \cdot \tfrac{1}{2}H_2O + 1\tfrac{1}{2}H_2O \rightarrow CaSO_4 \cdot 2H_2O + 3900 \text{ cal/g mol}$$

Plaster of paris   **Water**   **Gypsum**

The reaction is exothermic, and whenever 1 g mol of calcium sulfate hemihydrate is reacted with 1.5 g mol of water, 1 g mol of calcium sulfate dihydrate is formed, and 3900 calories of heat are developed. This chemical reaction takes place regardless of whether the gypsum material is used as an impression material, a die material, or a binder in the casting investment.

Manufacture of Dental Plaster, Stone, and High-Strength Stones

The four important types of relatively pure gypsum products used in dentistry are classified as model plaster, dental stone, high-strength stone, and high-strength/high-expansion dental stone, or alternatively as Types II, III, IV, and V in revised ANSI/ADA Specification No. 25 (ISO 6873). Although these types have identical chemical formulas of calcium sulfate hemihydrate, $CaSO_4 \cdot 1/2H_2O$, they possess different physical properties, which makes each of them usable for a different purpose in dentistry. All four forms are derived from the natural gypsum deposits, with the main difference being in the manner of driving off part of the water of the calcium sulfate dihydrate. Synthetic gypsum can also be used to formulate some products, but it is less popular because of higher manufacturing costs.

Mineral gypsum $\xrightarrow[\text{or other means}]{\textbf{Heat}}$ Model plaster
Dental stone   + Water
High-strength
dental stone

Model plaster is produced when the gypsum mineral is heated in an open kettle at a temperature of about 110° to 120° C. The hemihydrate produced is called β-calcium sulfate hemihydrate. Such a powder is known to have a somewhat irregular shape and is porous in nature. Crystals of model plaster are shown in Fig. 12-1.

If gypsum is dehydrated under pressure and in the presence of water vapor at about 125° C, the product is called dental stone. The powder particles of this product are more uniform in shape and more dense than the particles of model plaster. Crystals of a dental stone are shown in Fig. 12-2. The calcium sulfate hemihydrate produced in this manner is designated as α-calcium sulfate hemihydrate.

Types IV and V are produced when the dehydration is accomplished by adding another chemical, as by boiling in a 30% calcium chloride solution, after which the chlorides are washed away with hot water (100° C) and ground to the desired fineness. The calcium sulfate hemihydrate in the presence of 100° C water does not react to form calcium sulfate dihydrate because at this temperature their solubilities are the same. The powder obtained by this process is the densest of the types. These materials are generally described as high-strength dental stone or high-strength/high-expansion dental stone.

Gypsum products may be formulated with chemicals that modify their handling characteristics and properties. Potassium sulfate, K_2SO_4, and terra alba, which is set calcium sulfate dihydrate, are effective accelerators. Sodium chloride in small amounts shortens the setting but increases the setting expansion of the gypsum mass. Borax, $Na_2B_4O_7$, is a dependable retarder. A mixture of calcium oxide (0.1%) and gum arabic (1%) reduces the amount of water necessary to mix gypsum products resulting in improved properties. Type IV gypsum differs from Type V in that Type IV contains extra salts to reduce its setting expansion.

Chemical Reaction

The chemical reaction that takes place during the setting of gypsum products determines the quantity of H_2O needed for the reaction.

The reaction of 1 g mol of plaster with 1.5 g mol of water produces 1 g mol of gypsum material. In other words, 145.15 g of plaster requires 27.02 g of water to react and form 172.17 g of gypsum. There-

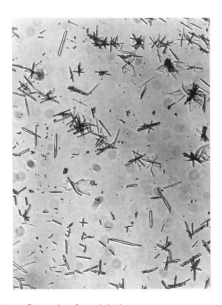

Fig. 12-1 Crystals of model plaster.

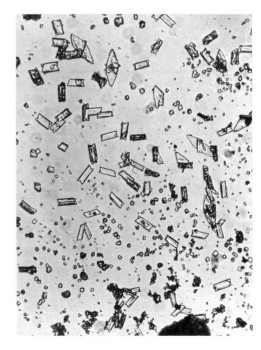

Fig. 12-2 Crystal structure typical of dental stone.

fore 100 g of plaster requires 18.61 g of water to form calcium sulfate dihydrate. As seen in practice, however, model plaster cannot be mixed with such a small amount of water and still develop a mass suitable for manipulation. To mix 100 g of model plaster to a practically usable consistency, 45 g of water should be used. Note that only 18.61 g of 45 g of water reacts with 100 g of model plaster, and the excess is distributed as free water in the set mass without taking part in the chemical reaction. The excess water is necessary to wet the powder particles during mixing. Naturally, if 100 g of model plaster is mixed with 50 g of water, which is the ratio used frequently, the resultant mass is thinner and mixes and pours easily into a mold, but the quality of the set gypsum is inferior and weaker than when more plaster is used. When model plaster is mixed with a lesser amount of water, the mixed mass is thicker, is more difficult to handle, and traps air bubbles easily when it is poured into a mold, but the set gypsum is usually stronger. Thus a careful control of the proper amount of water in the mix is necessary for proper manipulation and quality of the set mass.

Water/powder (W/P) ratio of dental stone and high-strength dental stone

The principal difference among model plaster, dental stone, and high-strength dental stones is in the shape and form of the calcium sulfate hemihydrate crystals. Some calcium sulfate hemihydrate crystals are comparatively irregular in shape and porous in nature, as are the crystals in model plaster, whereas the crystals of dental stone and the two high-strength dental stones are dense and more regular in shape, as shown in Figs. 12-1 and 12-2. This difference in the physical shape and nature of the crystals makes it possible to obtain the same consistency with less excess water with dental stone and high-strength dental stones than with model plaster.

In comparison, dental stone requires only about 30 ml of water, and high-strength dental stones require as little as 19 to 24 ml. The difference in their water/powder ratios has a pronounced effect on their compressive strength and resistance to abrasion.

When mixed with water, model plaster, dental stone, or high-strength dental stones set to a hard mass of gypsum. The gypsum products known as high-strength dental stones (Types IV and V) are the strongest, the mass produced as model plaster is the weakest, and dental stone produces an intermediate strength material. However, note that all gypsum products have the same chemical formula, that the chemical nature of the masses produced by mixing any one of them with water also is identical, and that the differences are primarily in their physical properties.

Mechanism of setting

The most important and well-recognized theory for the mechanism of the setting is the crystalline theory. It was originated in 1887 by Henry Louis Le Châtelier, a French chemist; and later, in 1907, the theory received the full support of Jacobus Hendricus van't Hoff, a famous Dutch chemist in Berlin at the turn of the century. According to the explanation of van't Hoff, the difference in the solubilities of calcium sulfate dihydrate and hemihydrate causes the setting of these materials. Dissolved calcium sulfate precipitates as calcium sulfate dihydrate because calcium sulfate dihydrate is less soluble than hemihydrate.

Also, if two types of centers are distinguished in a setting mass of plaster, one for dissolution and the other for precipitation, the dissolution centers are located around the calcium sulfate hemihydrate, and the precipitation centers are around the calcium sulfate dihydrate. The concentration of calcium sulfate also is different in these two centers and is highest around the dissolution centers and lowest close to the precipitation centers. Calcium and sulfate ions travel in solution by diffusion from the area in which the concentration is greatest to the area in which the concentration is lowest. By understanding the basic concept of the crystalline theory, the effect of different manipulative conditions can be explained.

The effect of manipulative variables and certain chemicals on setting has been studied recently by a kinetic model. An induction time and a reaction constant for crystal growth have been observed.

Volumetric contraction

Theoretically, calcium sulfate hemihydrate should contract volumetrically during the setting process. However, experiments have determined that all gypsum products expand linearly during setting. As indicated earlier, when 145.15 g of calcium sulfate hemihydrate reacts with 27.02 g of water, the result is the production of 172.17 g of calcium sulfate dihydrate.

However, if the volume rather than the weight of calcium sulfate hemihydrate is added to the volume of water, the sum of the volumes will not be equal to the volume of calcium sulfate dihydrate. The volume of the calcium sulfate dihydrate formed is about 7% less than the sum of the volumes of calcium sulfate hemihydrate and water. Instead of 7% contraction, however, about 0.2% to 0.4% linear expansion is obtained. According to the crystalline theory of Le Châtelier and van't Hoff, the expansion results from the thrusting action of gypsum crystals, $CaSO_4 \cdot 2H_2O$, during their growth from a supersaturated solution. The fact that the contraction of gypsum is not visible does not invalidate its existence, and when the volumetric contraction is measured by a dilatometer, it is determined to be approximately 7%. Because of the linear expansion of the outer dimensions, which is caused by the growth of calcium sulfate dihydrate, with a simultaneous true volumetric contraction of calcium sulfate dihydrate, these materials are porous when set.

Effect of spatulation

The mixing process, called spatulation, has a definite effect on the setting time and setting expansion of the material. Within practical limits an increase in the amount of spatulation shortens the setting time. The amount can be influenced by either the speed or time of spatulation or a combination of the two. Obviously when the powder is placed in water, the chemical reaction starts, and some calcium sulfate dihydrate is formed. During spatulation the newly formed calcium sulfate dihydrate breaks down to smaller crystals and starts new centers of nucleation, around which the calcium sulfate dihydrate can be precipitated. Because an increased amount of spatulation causes more nuclei centers to be formed, the conversion of calcium sulfate hemihydrate to dihydrate requires somewhat less time.

Effect of temperature

The temperature of the water used for mixing, as well as the temperature of the environment, has an effect on the setting reaction of gypsum products. The setting time probably is more affected by a change in temperature than any other physical property. Evidently the temperature has two main effects on the setting reaction of gypsum products.

The first effect of increasing temperature is a change in the relative solubilities of calcium sulfate hemihydrate and calcium sulfate dihydrate, which alters the rate of the reaction. The ratio of the solubilities of calcium sulfate dihydrate and calcium sulfate hemihydrate at 20° C is about 4.5. As the temperature increases, the solubility ratios decrease until 100° C when the ratio becomes one. As the ratio of the solubilities becomes lower, the reaction is slowed, and the setting time is increased. The solubilities of calcium sulfate hemihydrate and calcium sulfate dihydrate are shown in Table 12-1.

The second effect is the change in ion mobility with temperature. In general, as the temperature increases, the mobility of the calcium and sulfate ions increases, which tends to increase the rate of the reaction and shorten the setting time.

Practically, the effects of these two phenomena are superimposed, and in practice the total effect is observed. Thus, by increasing the temperature from 20° to 30° C, the solubility ratio decreases from 0.90/0.200 = 4.5 to 0.72/0.209 = 3.44, which ordinarily should retard the reaction. At the same time, however, the mobility of the ions increases, which should accelerate the setting reaction. Thus, according to the solubility values, the reaction should be retarded, and according to the mobility of the ions, the reaction should be accelerated. Experimentation has shown that increasing the temperature from room temperature of 20° C to body temperature of 37° C increases the rate of the reaction slightly and shortens the setting time. However, as the tempera-

TABLE 12-1 Solubility of Calcium Sulfate Hemihydrate and Calcium Sulfate Dihydrate at Different Temperatures

Temperature (° C)	$CaSO_4 \cdot \frac{1}{2}H_2O$ (g/100 g water)	$CaSO_4 \cdot 2H_2O$ (g/100 g water)
20	0.90	0.200
25	0.80	0.205
30	0.72	0.209
40	0.61	0.210
50	0.50	0.205
100	0.17	0.170

Adapted from Partridge EP, White AH: *J Am Chem Soc* 51:360, 1929.

ture is raised over 37° C, the rate of the reaction decreases, and the setting time is lengthened. At 100° C the solubilities of dihydrate and hemihydrate are both equal, in which case no reaction takes place, and plaster does not set.

Effect of humidity

In the manufacture of plaster it is not practical to convert all the calcium sulfate dihydrate ($CaSO_4 \cdot 2H_2O$) to calcium sulfate hemihydrate ($CaSO_4 \cdot 1/2H_2O$). During the calcination process most of the gypsum particles are changed to the hemihydrate, although a small portion may remain as the dihydrate, and possibly some particles may further dehydrate completely to form anhydrous soluble calcium sulfate ($CaSO_4$). Soluble calcium sulfate, to a greater degree, and plaster, to a lesser degree, are hygroscopic materials by nature and can easily absorb water vapor from a humid atmosphere to form calcium sulfate dihydrate, which changes the original proportion of each form of calcium sulfate. The presence of small amounts of calcium sulfate dihydrate on the surface of the hemihydrate powder provides additional nuclei for crystallization. Increased contamination by moisture produces sufficient dihydrate on the hemihydrate powder to retard the solution of the hemihydrate. Experience has shown that the common overall effect of contamination of gypsum products with moisture from the air is a lengthening of the setting time. For the best results all gypsum products should be kept in a closed container and well protected from the atmospheric humidity.

Effect of colloidal systems

Colloidal systems such as agar, alginate, and the biological fluids (blood and saliva) retard the setting of gypsum products. If these materials are in contact with $CaSO_4 \cdot 1/2H_2O$ during setting, a soft, easily abraded surface is obtained. Accelerators such as potassium sulfate are added to improve the surface quality of the set $CaSO_4 \cdot 2H_2O$ against agar or alginate.

These colloids and biological fluids do not retard the setting by altering the solubility ratio of the hemihydrate and dihydrate forms. They retard the setting by being adsorbed on the $CaSO_4 \cdot 1/2H_2O$ or on the $CaSO_4 \cdot 2H_2O$ nucleation sites and thus interfere in the hydration reaction. The adsorption of these materials on the nucleating sites retards the setting reaction more effectively than adsorption on the calcium sulfate hemihydrate.

■ PROPERTIES

The important properties of gypsum products include setting time, fineness of powder particles, compressive strength, tensile strength, hardness and abrasion resistance, reproduction of detail, and setting expansion. Some of these property requirements described by Revised ANSI/ADA Specification No. 25 (ISO 6873) are summarized in Table 12-2.

Setting Time

Definition and importance

The time required for the reaction to be completed is called the final setting time. If the rate of the reaction is too fast or the material has a short setting time, the mixed mass may harden before the operator can manipulate it properly. On the other hand, if the rate of reaction is too slow, an excessively long time is required to complete the operation. Therefore a proper setting time is one of the most important properties of gypsum materials.

The chemical reaction is initiated at the moment the powder is mixed with water, but at the early stage only a small portion of the hemihydrate is converted to gypsum. The freshly mixed mass has a semifluid consistency and can be poured into a mold of any shape. As the reaction proceeds, however, more and more calcium sulfate dihydrate crystals are produced. The viscosity of the mixed mass increases, and the mass can no longer flow easily into the fine details of the mold. This time is called the working time. The final setting time is defined as the time at which the material is completely set and can be separated from the impression without distortion or fracture. At final setting the conversion of calcium sulfate hemihydrate to calcium sulfate dihydrate is completed. However, the initial setting time is the time required for gypsum products to reach a certain arbitrary stage of firmness in their setting process. In the normal case this arbitrary stage is represented by a semihard mass that has passed the working stage but is not yet completely set.

TABLE 12-2 Property Requirements for Dental Gypsum Products

Type	Setting Time (min)	Fineness		Setting Expansion at 2 hr (%)		Compressive Strength at 1 hr (MPa)	Testing Consistency (mm)
		Passes No. 100 Sieve (minimum %)	Passes No. 200 Sieve (minimum %)	Mini-mum	Maxi-mum		
I. Impression plaster	4 + 1	98	85	0.00	0.15	4.0 ± 2.0	–
II. Model plaster	12 ± 4	98	90	0.00	0.30	8.8 minimum	30 ± 3*
III. Dental stone	12 ± 4	98	90	0.00	0.20	20.6 minimum	30 ± 3†
IV. High-strength dental stone	12 ± 4	98	90	0.00	0.10	34.3 minimum	30 ± 3†
V. High-strength high expansion dental stone	12 ± 4	98	90	0.10	0.30	48.0 minimum	30 ± 3†

Adapted from Revised ANSI/ADA Specification No. 25 for dental gypsum products, 1989.
*Cone penetration depth of modified Vicat apparatus, 0.34 N (35 g) total weight.
†Cone penetration depth of modified Vicat apparatus, 0.98 N (100 g) total weight.

Measurement

The initial setting time usually is measured arbitrarily by some form of penetration test, although occasionally other types of test methods have been designed. For example, the loss of gloss from the surface of the mixed mass of model plaster or dental stone is an indication of this stage in the chemical reaction and is sometimes used to indicate the initial set of the mass. Similarly, the setting time may be measured by the temperature rise of the mass because the chemical reaction is exothermic.

The Vicat apparatus shown in Fig. 12-3 is commonly used to measure the initial setting time of gypsum products. It consists of a rod weighing 300 g with a needle of 1-mm diameter. A ring container is filled with the mix, and the setting time will be measured. The rod is lowered until it contacts the surface of the material, and then the needle is released and allowed to penetrate the mix. When the needle fails to penetrate to the bottom of the container, the material has reached the Vicat or the initial setting time. Other types of instruments, such as Gillmore needles, can be used to obtain both the initial and final setting times of gypsum materials.

Control of setting time

The setting time of gypsum products can be altered rather easily. For example, plaster, which is able to take up water readily, can absorb moisture from the atmosphere and change to gypsum; thus this absorbance alters the setting time and the other properties of the plaster. The rate of the chemical reaction also can be changed by the addition of suitable chemicals, so that it may take from a few minutes to a few hours for the reaction to be completed. According to the crystalline theory discussed earlier, the difference between the solubilities of the calcium sulfate hemihydrate and the calcium sulfate dihydrate causes the set of the gypsum mass. At a temperature of 20° C about 4.5 times as much hemihydrate is dissolved in a given amount of water as is dihydrate. If this ratio of 4.5 is increased by the addition of certain salts, the chemical reaction progresses faster and the setting time is shortened. The salt that causes such a change is called an accelerator. On the other hand, if some salt is added and the ratio of the solubilities of hemihydrate to the dihydrate is decreased, the rate of the reaction is slowed, and the setting time is lengthened. Then the salt is considered to be a retarder.

Although not all accelerators and retarders work on this principle, the change of the solubility ratio may be considered as one way of changing the setting time. In general, the setting time can be controlled by the manufacturers when they add different chemicals to model plaster or other gypsum products and by operators when they change the manipulative conditions.

Factors controlled by the manufacturer. The easiest and most reliable way to change the setting time is to add different chemicals. Potassium sulfate, K_2SO_4, is known as an effective accelerator, and the use of a 2% aqueous solution of this salt rather than water reduces the setting time of model

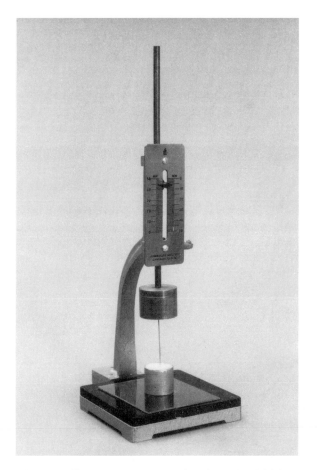

Fig. 12-3 Vicat penetrometer used to determine initial setting time of gypsum products.

plaster from approximately 10 minutes to about 4 minutes. On the other hand, borax, with the formula $Na_2B_4O_7 \cdot 10H_2O$, is a good and dependable retarder. A 2% aqueous solution of borax mixed with the powder may prolong the setting time of some gypsum products to a few hours.

If a small amount of set calcium sulfate dihydrate is ground and mixed with model plaster, it provides nuclei of crystallization and acts as an accelerator. The set gypsum used as an accelerator is called terra alba, and it has a pronounced effect at lower concentrations. The setting time changes significantly if the amount of terra alba present in the mix is changed from 0.5% to 1%. However, terra alba concentrations above 1% have less effect on the setting time. Manufacturers usually take advantage of this fact and add about 1% terra alba to plaster. Thus the setting time of model plaster is altered less in normal use because of opening and closing the container. When not in use, the model plaster container should be closed tightly to reduce the possibility of moisture contamination, which lengthens the setting time.

Water/powder ratio. The operator also can change to a certain extent the setting time of model plaster by changing the water/powder (W/P) ratio or the extent of spatulation.

The W/P ratio has a pronounced effect on the setting time. The more water in the mix of model plaster, dental stone, or high-strength dental stone, the longer the setting time, as shown in Table 12-3. The effect of spatulation on setting time of model plaster and dental stone is shown in Table 12-4. Increased spatulation shortens the setting time. Properties of a high-strength dental stone mixed by hand and by a power-driven mixer with vacuum are shown in Table 12-5. The setting time typically is shortened for power mixing compared with hand mixing.

Consistency

To compare mechanical properties of gypsum products, specimens must be prepared with a uniform consistency. The consistencies are determined according to Revised ANSI/ADA Specification No. 25 by a cone penetration test using a modified Vicat apparatus, as shown in Fig. 12-4. The test involves mixing 300 g of material in a powder form with a 1% aqueous solution of sodium citrate, pouring the mix into a mold, and allowing the conical plunger to

TABLE 12-3 Effect of Water/Powder Ratio on Setting Time

Material	W/P Ratio (ml/g)	Spatulation Turns	Initial (Vicat) Setting Time (min)
Model plaster	0.45		8
	0.50	100	11
	0.55		14
Dental stone	0.27		4
	0.30	100	7
	0.33		8
High-strength dental stone	0.22		5
	0.24	100	7
	0.26		9

TABLE 12-4 Effect of Spatulation on Setting Time

Material	W/P Ratio (ml/g)	Spatulation Turns	Setting Time (min)
Model plaster	0.50	20	14
	0.50	100	11
	0.50	200	8
Dental stone	0.30	20	10
	0.30	100	8

TABLE 12-5 Properties of a High-Strength Dental Stone Mixed by Hand and by a Power-Driven Mixer with Vacuum

	Hand Mix	Power-Driven Mix with Vacuum
Setting time	8.0	7.3
Compressive strength at 24 hr, MPa	43.1	45.5
Setting expansion at 2 hr (%)	0.045	0.037
Viscosity, centipoise, (cp)	54,000	43,000

From Garber DK, Powers JM, Brandau HE: *Mich Dent Assoc J* 67:133, 1985.

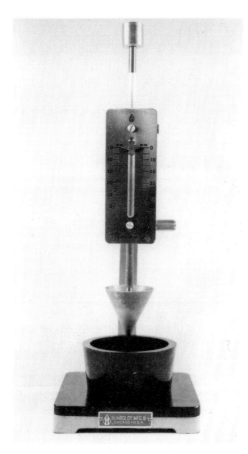

Fig. 12-4 Modified Vicat apparatus used to determine testing consistency of Types II-V gypsum products.

TABLE 12-6 Viscosity of Several High-Strength Dental Stones and Impression Plaster

Material	Viscosity (cp)
High-strength dental stone*	
A	21,000
B	29,000
C	50,000
D	54,000
E	101,000
Impression plaster	23,000

*Adapted from Garber DK, Powers JM, Brandau HE: *Mich Dent Assoc J* 67:133, 1985. Stones were mixed with 1% sodium citrate solution to retard setting. Viscosity was measured 4 min from the start of mixing.

penetrate the mix from the surface. The amount of penetration of the cone is measured at 7, 8, and 9 minutes after the start of the mix, and an average value is obtained. The W/P ratio that gives a penetration of 30 ± 3 mm (Table 12-2) is the testing consistency. The testing consistency of impression plaster results from the manufacturer's recommended W/P ratio.

Viscosity

The viscosities of several high-strength dental stones and impression plaster are listed in Table 12-6. A range of viscosities from 21,000 to 101,000 centipoises (cp) was observed for five different high-strength stones. More voids were observed in casts made from the stones with the higher viscosities. Impression plaster is used infrequently, but it has a low viscosity, which makes it possible to take impres-

sions with a minimum of force on the soft tissues (mucostatic technic).

Compressive Strength

When set, gypsum products show relatively high compressive strength values. The values are inversely related to the W/P ratio of the mix. The more water used to make the mix, the lower the compressive strength.

Model plaster has the greatest quantity of excess water, whereas high-strength dental stone contains the least excess water. The excess water is uniformly distributed in the mix and contributes to the volume but not to the strength of the material. The set model plaster is more porous than set dental stone, causing the apparent density of model plaster to be lower. Because high-strength dental stone is the densest, it shows the highest compressive strength, with model plaster being the most porous and thus the weakest.

The 1-hour compressive strength values are approximately 12.5 MPa for model plaster, 31 MPa for dental stone, and 45 MPa for high-strength dental stones. These values are representative for the normal mixes, but they vary as the W/P ratio increases or decreases. The effect of the W/P ratio on the compressive strength of these materials is given in Table 12-7. As shown in Table 12-5, the compressive strength of a high-strength dental stone is improved slightly by vacuum mixing. Evidently, when stone is mixed with the same W/P ratio as model plaster, the compressive strength of dental

TABLE 12-7   Effect of Water/Powder Ratio on the Compressive Strength of Model Plaster, Dental Stone, and High-Strength Dental Stone

Material	W/P Ratio (ml/g)	Compressive Strength, (MPa)
Model plaster	0.45	12.5
	0.50	11.0
	0.55	9.0
Dental stone	0.27	31.0
	0.30	20.5
	0.50	10.5
High-strength dental stone	0.24	38.0
	0.30	21.5
	0.50	10.5

All mixes spatulated 100 turns and tested 1 hr after the start of mixing.

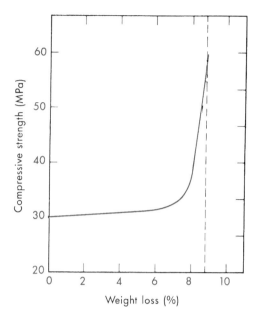

Fig. 12-5 Effect of loss of excess water on compressive strength of dental stone.

stone is almost the same as that of model plaster. Similarly, the compressive strength of high-strength dental stone with W/P ratios of 0.3 and 0.5 is similar to the normal compressive strength of dental stone and model plaster.

At 1 or 2 hours after the final setting time, the hardened gypsum material appears dry and seems to have reached its maximum strength. Actually, this is not the case. The wet strength is the strength of gypsum materials with some or all of the excess water present in the specimen. The dry strength is the strength of the gypsum material with all of its excess water driven out. The dry compressive strength usually is about twice that of the wet strength. Notice that as the hardened mass slowly loses its excess water, the compressive strength of the material does not increase uniformly. The effect of drying on the compressive strength of dental stone is shown in Fig. 12-5. Theoretically, about 8.8% of excess water is in the hardened mass of the stone. As the mass loses up to 7% of the water, no appreciable change develops in the compressive strength of the material. When the mass loses 7.5% of the excess water, however, the strength increases sharply, and when all of the excess (8.8%) is lost, the strength of the material is over 55 MPa.

The drying time for gypsum materials varies according to the size of the gypsum mass, as well as the temperature and humidity of the storage atmos-

phere. At room temperature and average humidity, approximately 7 days are necessary for an average denture flask filled with gypsum materials to lose the excess water.

Surface Hardness and Abrasion Resistance

The surface hardness of gypsum materials is related to their compressive strength. High compressive strengths of the hardened mass correspond to high surface hardnesses. After the final setting occurs, the surface hardness remains practically constant until most excess water is evaporated from the surface, after which it increases similarly to the increase of the compressive strength. The surface hardness increases at a faster rate than the compressive strength because the surface of the hardened mass reaches a dry state earlier than the inner portion of the mass.

Attempts have been made to increase the hardness of gypsum products by impregnation of the set gypsum with methyl methacrylate monomer that is allowed to polymerize. Increases in hardness were obtained for model plaster but not for dental stone or high-strength dental stone. Increases in scratch resistance of 15% to 41% were observed for a high-strength dental stone impregnated with epoxy resins or a light-cured dimethacrylate resin. Drying molds, casts, or dies in an oven to obtain a quick, dry compressive strength and dry surface hardness of a material is not practical because the gypsum would be dehydrated, which would reduce the strength instead of increasing it. Soaking the gypsum dies or casts in glycerin or different oils does not improve the surface hardness but rather makes the surface smoother, so that a wax carver or other instrument will not cut the stone as it slides over the surface. Mixing high-strength dental stone with a commercial hardening solution containing colloidal silica (about 30%) improves the surface hardness of the set gypsum. The Knoop hardnesses of two commercial high-strength dental stones were 54 and 77 kg/mm^2 when mixed with water. When the hardening solution was used, these values increased to 62 and 79 kg/mm^2, respectively. Increased surface hardness does not necessarily mean improved abrasion resistance because hardness is only one of many factors that can affect wear resistance. Two-body abrasion studies suggest that the commercial hardening solutions do not improve the abrasion resistance of high-strength dental stones. However, the clinical relevancy of the two-body abrasion test on gypsum has not been established. Further studies of abrasion resistance and methods of measurement are needed. As discussed in Chapter 11, gypsum dies abrade more readily than epoxy dies, even though the gypsum dies are harder.

Although disinfectant chemicals used on gypsum dies effectively destroy potentially dangerous organisms, some commonly used disinfectants can damage or erode the surface of a die and adversely affected the surface hardness. Other disinfectants, including sodium hypochlorite solutions, have very little effect on the surfaces of gypsum dies.

Tensile Strength

The tensile strength of model plaster and dental stone is important in structures in which bending tends to occur because of lateral force applications, such as the removal of casts from flexible impressions. Because of the brittle nature of gypsum materials, the teeth on the cast may fracture rather than bend. The diametral compression test for brittle materials normally is used to determine the tensile strength of gypsum products.

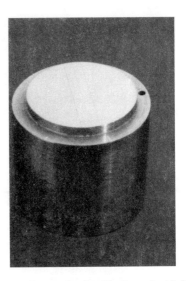

Fig. 12-6 Detail reproduction block used with Revised ANSI/ADA Specification No. 25.

Some significant observations have resulted from these studies. First, the 1-hour wet tensile strength of model plaster, 2.3 MPa, is approximately one-half the dry tensile strength, 4.1 MPa, after 40 hours at 45° C. Second, the tensile strength of model plaster in either the wet or dry condition is about one-half that of high-strength dental stone. Third, the tensile strength of model plaster in the wet or dry condition is about one-fifth the compressive strength in the same condition (dry, 4.1 MPa in tension; 20 MPa in compression). Fourth, the high-strength dental stone shows an increased difference between tensile and compressive values (for example, approximately 8 MPa in tension and 80 MPa in compression for the dry condition).

Reproduction of Detail

Revised ANSI/ADA Specification No. 25 requires that the gypsum product reproduce a groove 0.05 mm in width when tested at the consistency listed in Table 12-2. The detail reproduction block is shown in Fig. 12-6. Gypsum dies do not reproduce surface detail as well as electroformed or epoxy dies because the surface of the set gypsum is porous on a microscopic level (Fig. 12-7). Air bubbles frequently are formed at the interface of the impression and gypsum cast because freshly mixed gypsum does not wet some rubber impression materials (e.g., some silicone types) well. The incorporation of nonionic surfactants

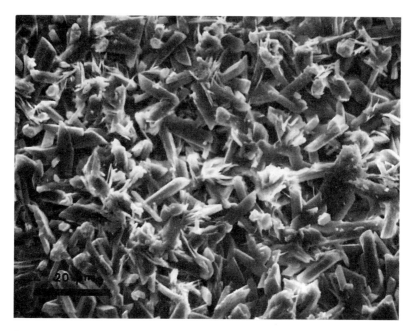

Fig. 12-7 Scanning electron photomicrograph of the surface of a set high-strength stone die. (From Craig RG, O'Brien WJ, Powers JM: *Dental materials: properties and manipulation,* ed 6, St Louis, 1996, Mosby.)

in polysulfide and silicone impression materials improves the wetting of the impression by slurry water. The use of vibration during the pouring of a cast reduces the presence of air bubbles. Contamination by saliva or blood of the impression in which the gypsum die is poured can also affect the detail reproduction. Rinsing the impression and blowing away excess water can improve the detail recorded by the gypsum die material.

Setting Expansion

When set, all gypsum products show a measurable linear expansion. The percentage of setting expansion, however, varies from one type of gypsum material to another. Under ordinary conditions model plaster has 0.2% to 0.3% setting expansion, dental stone about 0.08% to 0.1%, and high-strength dental stone only 0.05% to 0.07%. The setting expansion of high-strength/high-expansion dental stone ranges from 0.13 to 0.28%. Typically, about 70% of the expansion observed at 24 hours occurs during the first hour.

The setting expansion may be controlled by different manipulative conditions and by the addition of some chemicals. Increases in spatulation increase

the setting expansion. As shown in Table 12-5, a vacuum-mixed high-strength stone expands less at 2 hours than when mixed by hand. The power mixing appears to cause a greater initial volumetric contraction than that observed for hand mixing. The W/P ratio of the mix also has an effect, with an increase in the ratio reducing the setting expansion. The addition of different chemicals not only affects the setting expansion of gypsum products but also may change their other properties. For example, the addition of sodium chloride (NaCl) in a small concentration increases the setting expansion of the mass yet shortens the setting time. The addition of 4% potassium sulfate, on the other hand, decreases both the setting expansion and the setting time.

If during the setting process the gypsum materials are immersed in water, the setting expansion increases. This is called hygroscopic expansion and is discussed in detail in connection with dental casting investments, in which its effect is more pronounced. However, note that the hygroscopic expansion of model plaster, dental stone, and high-strength dental stone, although small, is about twice as great as their regular normal setting expansion. An average high-strength dental stone has a setting expan-

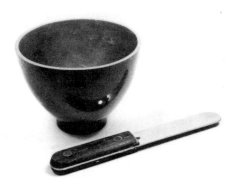

Fig. 12-8 Flexible rubber mixing bowl and metal spatula with a stiff blade. (From Craig RG, O'Brien WJ, Powers JM: *Dental materials: properties and manipulation,* ed 6, St Louis, 1996, Mosby.)

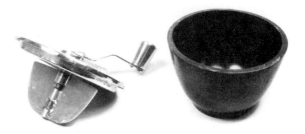

Fig. 12-9 Mechanical spatulator for use with small gypsum mixes. (From Craig RG, O'Brien WJ, Powers JM: *Dental materials: properties and manipulation,* ed 6, St Louis, 1996, Mosby.)

sion of about 0.05%. If during the setting process the mass is immersed in water, it expands about 0.1%. Such increased expansion is observed when dental stone hardens as it comes in contact with a hydrocolloid impression.

■ MANIPULATION

When any one of the gypsum products is mixed with water, it should be spatulated properly to obtain a smooth mix. Water is dispensed into a mixing bowl of an appropriate size and design (Fig. 12-8). The powder is added and allowed to settle into the water for about 30 seconds. This technic minimizes the amount of air incorporated into the mix during initial spatulation by hand. Spatulation can be continued by hand using a metal spatula with a stiff blade (Fig. 12-8), a hand-mechanical spatulator (Fig. 12-9), or a power-driven mechanical spatulator (Fig. 12-10). A summary of the effect of various manipulative variables on the properties of gypsum products is presented in Table 12-8.

Spatulation by hand involves stirring the mixture vigorously and at the same time wiping the inside surfaces of the bowl with the spatula. Spatulation to wet and mix the powder uniformly with the water requires about 1 minute at 2 revolutions per second.

Spatulation with a power-driven mechanical spatulator requires that the powder initially be wet by the water as with hand mixing. The mix is then spatulated for 20 seconds on the low-speed drive of

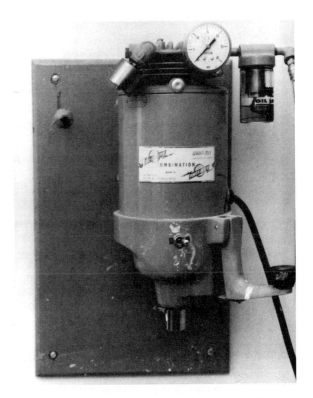

Fig. 12-10 Power-driven mechanical spatulator with a vacuum attachment. (From Craig RG, O'Brien WJ, Powers JM: *Dental materials: properties and manipulation,* ed 6, St Louis, 1996, Mosby.)

the mixer. Vacuuming during the mixing reduces the air entrapped in the mix. Vibration immediately after mixing and during pouring of the gypsum minimizes air bubbles in the set mass.

Pouring an impression with gypsum requires care to avoid entrapment of air in critical areas. The

TABLE 12-8   Summary of Effect of Manipulative Variables on Properties of Gypsum Products

Manipulative Variable	Setting Time	Consistency	Setting Expansion	Compressive Strength
Increase water/powder ratio	Increase	Increase	Decrease	Decrease
Increase rate of spatulation	Decrease	Decrease	Increase	No effect
Increase temperature of mixing water from 23° to 30° C	Decrease	Decrease	Increase	No effect

mixed gypsum should be poured slowly or added to the impression with a wax spatula. The mass should run into the rinsed impression under vibration in such a manner that it pushes air ahead of itself as it fills the impressions of the teeth. Commonly, the teeth of a cast are poured in dental stone or high-strength dental stone, whereas the base is poured in model plaster for easier trimming.

Once poured, the gypsum material should be allowed to harden for 45 to 60 minutes before the impression and cast are separated and disinfected. Models can be disinfected by immersion in 1:10 dilution of sodium hypochlorite for 30 minutes or with a spray of iodophor following manufacturer's instructions.

■ CASTING INVESTMENTS

The adoption of the casting practice in dentistry for making gold alloy inlays, crowns, bridges, and other restorations represents one of the major advances in restorative dentistry. In recent years alloys with higher melting points, the palladium and base metal alloys, have been cast into crowns, bridges, and removable partial denture restorations by using basically the same lost wax technic used for dental gold alloys. All such casting operations involve (1) a wax pattern of the object to be reproduced, (2) a suitable mold material, known as investment, which is placed around the pattern and permitted to harden, (3) suitable furnaces for burning out the wax patterns and heating the investment mold, and (4) proper facilities to melt and cast the alloy. An investment can be described as a ceramic material that is suitable for forming a mold into which a metal or alloy is cast. The operation of forming the mold is described as investing. Details of the casting technic are described in Chapter 16.

Properties Required of an Investment

1. The investment should be easily manipulated. Not only should it be possible to mix and manipulate the mass readily and to paint the wax pattern easily, but the investment also should harden within a relatively short time.

2. The investment mold must have sufficient strength at room temperature to permit ease in handling, and enough strength at higher temperatures to withstand the impact force of the molten metal. The inner surface of the mold should not break down at a high temperature.

3. On being heated to higher temperatures, the investment must not decompose to give off gases that could damage the surface of the alloy.

4. The investment should have enough expansion to compensate for shrinkage of the wax pattern and the metal that takes place during the casting procedure.

5. Casting temperatures should not be critical. Preferably the thermal expansion versus temperature curve should have a plateau of the thermal expansion over a range of casting temperatures.

6. A dental casting investment should be porous enough to permit the air or other gases in the mold cavity to escape easily during the casting procedure.

7. The investment should produce a smooth surface and fine detail and margins on the casting.

8. After the casting is completed, the investment should break away readily from the surface of the metal and should not have reacted chemically with it.

9. Because the mold is always destroyed in the casting process, the investment material must be comparatively inexpensive.

These represent the requirements for an ideal investment. No single material is known that completely fulfills all of these requirements. However, by blending different ingredients an investment can be developed that possesses most of the required qualities. These ideal qualities are the basis for considering the behavior and characteristics of casting investments.

Composition

In general, an investment is a mixture of the following three distinct types of materials:

Refractory material

This material usually is a form of silicon dioxide, such as quartz, tridymite, or cristobalite, or a mixture of these. These materials are contained in all dental investments, whether for casting gold or high-melting alloys.

Binder material

Because the refractory materials alone do not form a coherent solid mass, some kind of binder is needed. The common binder used for dental casting gold alloy is α-calcium sulfate hemihydrate. Phosphate, ethyl silicate, and other similar materials also may serve as binders for high-temperature casting investments. These latter investments are described later in conjunction with investment for high-melting alloys.

Other chemicals

Usually a mixture of refractory materials and a binder alone is not enough to produce all the desirable properties required of an investment. Other chemicals such as sodium chloride, boric acid, potassium sulfate, graphite, copper powder, or magnesium oxide often are added in small quantities to modify various physical properties. For example, small amounts of chlorides or boric acid enhance the thermal expansion of investments bonded by calcium sulfate.

Calcium Sulfate–Bonded Investments

The dental literature and patent references describe a variety of ingredients, as well as the quantity and purpose of each component in dental casting investments. In general, the investments suitable for casting gold alloys contain 60% to 65% quartz or cristobalite, or a blend of the two in varying proportions, 30% to 35% of α-calcium sulfate hemihydrate, and approximately 5% chemical modifiers. With the proper blending of these basic ingredients, the manufacturer is able to develop an investment with an established group of physical properties that is adequate for dental gold casting practices. A listing of specific compositions is of little value because the properties of the final product are influenced by both the balance of ingredients present in the investment and the manner in which the mass is manipulated and used in making the mold.

Investments with calcium sulfate hemihydrate as a binder are relatively easy to manipulate, and more information about the effect of different additives, as well as various manipulative conditions, is available for this type than for other types, such as those that use silicates or phosphates as binders. The calcium sulfate–bonded investment is usually limited to gold castings, and it is not heated above 700° C. The calcium sulfate portion of the investment decomposes into sulfur dioxide and sulfur trioxide at temperatures over 700° C, tending to embrittle the casting metal. Therefore the calcium sulfate type of binder usually is not used in investments for making castings of palladium or base metal alloys.

Properties of Calcium Sulfate–Bonded Investments

Revised ANSI/ADA Specification No. 2 (ISO 7490) for dental inlay casting investment applies to three different types of investments suitable for casting dental restorations of gold alloys. These three types are as follows:

Type I	Inlay, thermal
Type II	Inlay, hygroscopic
Type III	Partial denture, thermal

All three types have calcium sulfate as a binder material. The physical properties included in this specification are setting expansion, hygroscopic expansion, thermal expansion, compressive strength, setting time, surface defects of alloy, and fineness of powder particles. The testing consistency is the W/P ratio recommended by the manufacturer. The values allowed by the Revised ANSI/ADA Specification No. 2 for some of these tests are summarized in Tables 12-9 and 12-10. The test samples and methods

TABLE 12-9 Expansion Requirements for Gypsum-Bonded Casting Investments for Dental Gold Alloy

| Type | Setting Expansion at 2 hr (%) | | | | Thermal Expansion (%) | | Combined Setting and Thermal Expansion (%) | |
| | In Air | | In Water | | | | | |
	Minimum	Maximum	Minimum	Maximum	Minimum	Maximum	Minimum	Maximum
I. Inlay, thermal	0.0	0.6	–	–	1.0	1.6*	1.3	2.2
II. Inlay, hygroscopic	–	–	1.2	2.2	0.0	0.6†	1.3	2.7
III. Partial denture, thermal	0.0	0.4	–	–	1.0	1.5*	1.2	1.9

Modified from Revised ANSI/ADA Specification No. 2 for gypsum-bonded casting investment for dental gold alloy, *J Am Dent Assoc* 115:635, 1987.
*At 700° C.
†At 500° C.

TABLE 12-10 Property Requirements for Gypsum-Bonded Casting Investment for Dental Gold Alloy

Type	Setting Time (min)		Fineness (minimum %)			Minimum Compressive Strength at 2 hr (MPa)
	Minimum	Maximum	Passes Sieve No. 30	Passes Sieve No. 100	Passes Sieve No. 200	
I. Inlay, thermal	5	25	100	95	85	2.4
II. Inlay, hygroscopic	5	25	100	95	85	2.4
III. Partial denture, thermal	5	25	100	95	85	4.8

Modified from Revised ANSI/ADA Specification No. 2 for gypsum-bonded casting investment for dental gold alloy, *J Am Dent Assoc* 115:635, 1987.

of testing, which also apply to other types of casting investments, are described in the specification. The manipulation of investments in the inlay casting procedure is discussed in detail in Chapter 16.

Effect of Temperature on Investment

In casting with the lost wax process, the wax pattern, after being invested, is melted and removed from the investment, leaving a mold cavity into which the molten metal is cast. In this way, regardless of whether the high-heat or hygroscopic casting technic is used, the investment is heated to an elevated temperature. This temperature varies from one technic to another, but in no case is it lower than 370° C or higher than 700° C for calcium sulfate–bonded investments. During the heating process the various components of the investment respond differently to the thermal changes. For example, the refractory material is affected differently by the heat than the binder.

Effect of temperature on silicon dioxide refractories

Each of the polymorphic forms of silica, quartz, tridymite, and cristobalite expands when heated, but the percentage of expansion varies from one type to another. Pure cristobalite expands to 1.6% at 400° C, whereas quartz expands about 1.4% at 600° C, and the thermal expansion of tridymite at 600° C is less than 1%. The percentage of expansion of the three types of silica versus temperature is shown in Fig. 3-12. As seen in Fig. 3-12, none of the three forms of silica expands uniformly; instead they all show a break (nonlinearity) in their thermal expansion curves. In the case of cristobalite the expansion is somewhat uniform to about 200° C. At this temperature its expansion increases sharply from 0.5% to 1.2%, and then above 250° C it again becomes more uniform. At 573° C quartz also shows a break in the expansion curve, and tridymite shows a similar break at a much lower temperature.

The breaks on the expansion versus temperature curves indicate that cristobalite and quartz each exist in two polymorphic forms, one of which is more stable at a higher temperature and the other at a lower temperature. The form that is more stable at room temperature is called the α-form, and the more stable form at higher temperatures is designated as the β-form. Tridymite has three stable polymorphic forms. Thus the temperatures of 220° C for cristobalite, 573° C for quartz, and 105° and 160° C for tridymite are displacive transition temperatures. A displacive change involves expansion or contraction in the volume of the mass without breaking any bonds. In changing from the α-form (which is the more stable form at room temperature) to the β-form (which is stable at higher temperatures), all three forms of silica expand. The amount of expansion is highest for cristobalite and lowest for tridymite.

The quartz form of silica is found abundantly in nature, and it can be converted to cristobalite and tridymite by being heated through a reconstructive transition during which bonds are broken and a new crystal structure is formed. The α-quartz is converted to β-quartz at a temperature of 573° C. If the β-quartz is heated to 870° C and maintained at that temperature, it is converted to β-tridymite. From β-tridymite obtaining either α-tridymite or β-cristobalite is possible. If β-tridymite is cooled rapidly to 120° C and held at that temperature, it is changed to α-tridymite, which is stable at room temperature. On the other hand, if β-tridymite is heated to 1475° C and held at that temperature, it is converted to β-cristobalite. Further heating of β-cristobalite produces fused silica, but if it is cooled to 220° C and held at that temperature, α-cristobalite is formed. These transitions are shown in the diagram below.

All forms of silica are in their α-forms in the investment, and during the heating process they are converted completely or in part to their corresponding β-forms. This transition involves an expansion

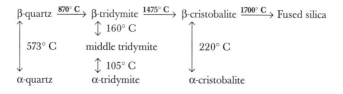

of the mass, which helps to compensate for the casting shrinkages.

Effect of temperature on calcium sulfate binders

The binder used for gold investments in dentistry usually is α-calcium sulfate hemihydrate. During the investing process some of the water mixed with the investment reacts with the hemihydrate and is converted to calcium sulfate dihydrate, whereas the remainder of the water exists uniformly distributed in the mix as excess water. During the heating process the excess water is evaporated during the early stages of heating. As the temperature rises to about 105° C, calcium sulfate dihydrate starts losing water. The investment mass then is heated further to the proper temperature for casting the metal. In this way, a mixture of anhydrous calcium sulfate, silica, and certain chemical additives remains to form the mold into which the gold alloy is cast.

It has been observed experimentally that investment expands when it is first heated from room temperature to about 105° C, then contracts slightly or remains unchanged up to about 200° C, and registers varying degrees of expansion, depending on the silica composition of the investment, between 200° and 700° C. These properties are explained as follows: up to about 105° C, ordinary thermal expansion occurs. Above 105° C, the calcium sulfate dihydrate is converted to anhydrous calcium sulfate. Dehydration of the dihydrate and a phase change of the calcium sulfate anhydrite cause a contraction. However, the α-form of tridymite (which might be present as an impurity) is expanding and sufficiently compensates for the contraction of the calcium sulfate to prevent the investment from registering a serious degree of contraction. At elevated temperatures the α-forms of silica present in the investment are converted to the β-forms, which cause some additional expansion.

The thermal expansion curves for a currently available hygroscopic type of investment containing quartz (*A*) and a thermal expansion type of investment containing cristobalite (*B*) are shown in Fig. 12-11, which illustrates the expected degree of expansion at different temperatures. The expansion of the silica content of the investment not only must be sufficiently high to overcome all the contraction

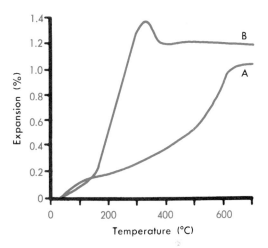

Fig. 12-11 Thermal expansion curves for calcium sulfate–bonded investments. *A,* Hygroscopic type; *B,* thermal expansion type. (Adapted from Asgar K: *Casting restorations.* In Clark JW, editor: *Clinical dentistry,* vol 4, New York, 1976, Harper & Row.)

but also should take place at temperatures close to the temperature at which contraction of the hemihydrate occurs.

Cooling of the investment

When the investment is allowed to cool, the refractory and binder contract according to a thermal contraction curve that is different from the thermal expansion curve of the investment (Fig. 12-12). On cooling to room temperature, the investment exhibits an overall contraction compared with its dimensions before heating. On reheating to the temperature previously attained, the investment does not expand thermally to the previous level; moreover, the process of cooling and reheating causes internal cracks in the investment that can affect the quality of the casting.

Setting and Hygroscopic Expansion of Calcium Sulfate–Bonded Investment

All the calcium sulfate–bonded investments currently available for casting gold alloys have thermal expansion, setting expansion, and hygroscopic expansion. The total dimensional change is a very important property of dental casting investments. The setting expansion of an investment, like that of other gypsum products discussed earlier in this chapter, is

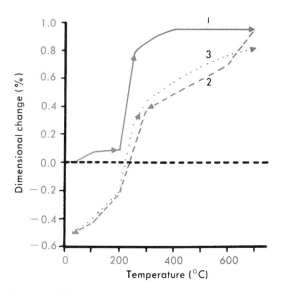

Fig. 12-12 Thermal expansion and contraction curves for calcium sulfate–bonded investment (thermal expansion type). Curve *1* is first heating, curve *2* is cooling, and curve *3* is reheating.

TABLE 12-11 Effects of Manipulative Conditions on the Expansion of Calcium Sulfate–Bonded Investments

Factor	Setting and Hygroscopic Expansion	Thermal Expansion
Water/powder ratio increased	Decreased	Decreased
Time of spatulation increased	Increased	No effect
Rate of spatulation increased	Increased	No effect
Age of investment increased	Decreased	No effect
Delay before immersion increased	Decreased	
Water bath temperature increased	Increased	
Strength of wax for some patterns	More distortion	Less effect
Location of sprue	More critical	Less critical

the linear expansion that takes place during the normal setting of the investment in air. Hygroscopic expansion, on the other hand, is the linear expansion of the investment that occurs if the investment is in contact with water from any source during the setting process after investing the wax pattern. Such contact with water can be achieved by placing the casting ring in a water bath, by putting some water on the surface of the investment in the ring, or by using a wet liner inside the casting ring.

Distinguishing between a setting expansion and hygroscopic expansion is difficult because both take place almost at the same time and end at the same time. In practice a sum of the hygroscopic and setting expansions of the investment is obtained, which is about two to four times the setting expansion alone. The mechanism of hygroscopic expansion has been studied by a number of investigators. According to some of the theories, the addition of water during the setting of an investment increases the surface-film thickness on the inert particles and gypsum crystals, thereby forcing them apart. Some believe that the added water during the setting process permits further hydration of calcium sulfate, thus causing the expansion of the investment,

whereas others believe that the added water may force gypsum gel to swell. Another theory states that hygroscopic expansion and setting expansion are the result of the same phenomenon as that occurring with dental stone, which is the outward growth of gypsum crystals. The addition of water or any other liquid provides additional volume into which the gypsum crystals can grow.

Although some question is raised about the exact mechanism of hygroscopic expansion, the effects of many of the manipulative conditions have been studied in detail. The effects of some of these conditions on the setting, hygroscopic, and thermal expansion of calcium sulfate–bonded investment are summarized in Table 12-11. These conditions also have a significant influence on the properties of the casting investment and the quality of the casting.

Water/powder ratio

As with the setting expansion of gypsum products, the more water in the mix, the thinner the mix, or the higher the water/powder ratio, the less the setting and hygroscopic expansions. Notice that less thermal expansion is also obtained with a thinner mix.

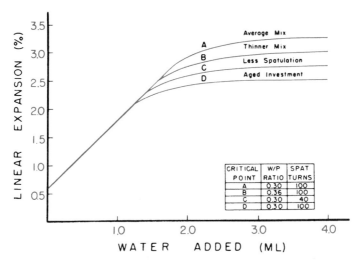

Fig. 12-13 Linear expansion of a hygroscopic investment as a function of the amount of water added and manipulative conditions.

Spatulation

The effect of spatulation on the setting and hygroscopic expansion of the investment is similar to that on the setting expansion of all gypsum products. As shown in Fig. 12-13, curve *C*, less spatulation produces lower expansion with hygroscopic investment.

Age of investment

Investments that are 2 or 3 years old do not expand as much as freshly prepared investments. Fig. 12-13, curve *D* shows the effect of aged investment on hygroscopic expansion. Occasionally the expansion may be altered in the short time of only a few months if the investment is not properly protected. Therefore the expansion changes with the age of the investment, especially if it is stored in a humid atmosphere. For this reason, the containers must be kept closed as much as possible.

Delay before immersion

After the wax pattern is invested, the investment mass may be immersed in a water bath to obtain the maximum hygroscopic expansion. The time between mixing and immersion has an effect on the total amount of expansion. Generally, the hygroscopic expansion decreases with increased time between mixing and immersion. However, some investigators claim that if the investment is

immersed at about the initial setting time, it expands more than if it is immersed earlier. However, more reproducible results are obtained from one test to another if the immersion is made before the gloss of the investment is lost.

Water bath temperature

Although the water bath temperature has little effect on the hygroscopic expansion of the investment, it has a definite effect on the wax pattern. At higher water bath temperatures, the wax pattern expands, requiring less expansion of the investment to compensate for the total casting shrinkage. In addition, higher water bath temperatures soften the wax. The softened wax then gives less resistance to the expansion of the investment, thus making the setting and hygroscopic expansions more effective. The net effect is higher expansion of the mold with higher water bath temperatures.

Choice of binder material

The investment is greatly affected if plaster or stone types of calcium sulfate hemihydrate are used with silica. Evidently when α-calcium sulfate hemihydrate (stone) is used as a binder, it produces higher setting and hygroscopic expansions than β-calcium sulfate hemihydrate (plaster). Today all dental gold investments, for thermal or hygroscopic casting technics, use α-calcium sulfate hemihydrate as their binder.

Particle size of silica

The particle size of calcium sulfate hemihydrate has little effect on the hygroscopic expansion, whereas the particle size of the silica has a significant effect. When all other conditions remain unchanged, the finer silica produce higher setting and hygroscopic expansions.

Silica/binder ratio

Investments usually contain 60% to 65% silica, 30% to 35% calcium sulfate hemihydrate, and about 4% to 7% of some additive chemicals to control the different physical properties and to color the investments. If the silica/stone ratio is increased, the hygroscopic expansion of the investment also increases, but the strength of the investment decreases.

Role of water

During the setting process, dental casting investments actually absorb water from their surroundings and expand. It also has been observed that, during setting, the more water an investment is permitted to take up from any source, the higher its hygroscopic expansion. The hygroscopic expansion of an investment during setting versus the amount of water added to its surface is shown in Fig. 12-13, curves *A* and *B*. As indicated, the more water added to the surface of the mixed investment, the higher the hygroscopic expansion, up to a point where further additions of water do not create any additional expansion. This degree of expansion or its corresponding quantity of water is called the critical point. Note that for an investment to reach its maximum hygroscopic expansion, sufficient water should be available. If hygroscopically expanding investments are in contact with less water than they are able to absorb, they will not exhibit their maximum hygroscopic expansion.

Hygroscopic-Thermal Gold Casting Investment

There is one gold casting investment on the market that was designed for use with either hygroscopic or thermal type of casting technics. Figure 12-14 shows the high thermal expansion of this investment in the range between 482° C and 649° C. This expansion is high enough to use the investment with the thermal casting technic, without water immersion. However, when immersed in a water bath, the investment expands hygroscopically

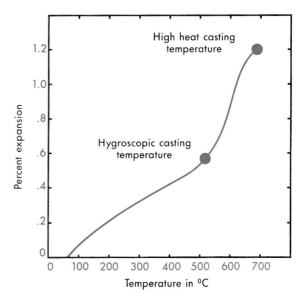

Fig. 12-14 Thermal expansion of mixed hygroscopic–thermal gold casting investment. (Courtesy Whip Mix Corp., 1992.)

(Fig. 12-15). With the hygroscopic technic the investment only needs to be heated to 482° C to provide the appropriate expansion.

Investment for Casting High-Melting Alloys

Most palladium and base metal alloys used for partial dentures and porcelain-fused-to-metal restorations have high melting temperatures. They should be cast at a mold temperature greater than 700° C. For this reason calcium sulfate–bonded investments usually are not used for casting these alloys. Only one base metal alloy for dental applications possesses a low enough melting point to be cast into a mold at 700° C with a calcium sulfate binder. This alloy is an exception because base metal alloys usually are cast into molds at 850° to 1100° C. To withstand these high temperatures, the molds require different types of binders, such as silicate and phosphate compounds. This type of investment usually has less than 20% binder, and the remainder of the investment is quartz or another form of silica.

Phosphate-bonded investment

The most common type of investment for casting high-melting alloys is the phosphate-bonded invest-

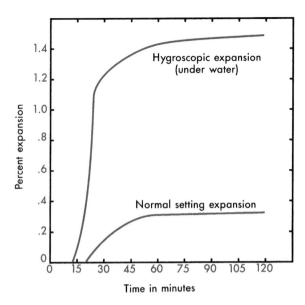

Fig. 12-15 Setting and hygroscopic expansion of mixed hygroscopic–thermal gold casting investment. (Courtesy Whip Mix Corp., 1992.)

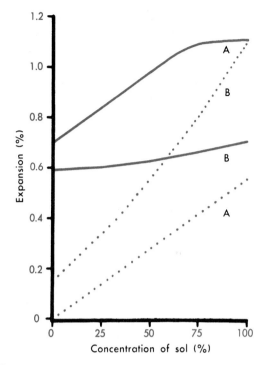

Fig. 12-16 Effect of silica sol concentration on thermal expansion (*solid lines*) (at 800° C) and setting expansion (*dotted lines*) of two phosphate-bonded investments (*A*, thermal expansion type, and *B*, hygroscopic expansion type). (Adapted from Zarb GA, Bergman G, Clayton JA, MacKay HF, editors: *Prosthodontic treatment for partially edentulous patients*, St Louis, 1978, Mosby.)

ment. This type of investment consists of three different components, each of which is responsible for certain characteristic properties. One component consists of materials that are soluble in water to yield a phosphate ion. The second component consists of materials that react with phosphate ions at room temperature. The third is a ceramic substance that hardens at a high temperature and is responsible for high-temperature strength. Different materials can be used in each group to serve as suitable components and to develop different physical properties.

Certain phosphate compounds, such as ammonium diacid phosphate ($NH_4H_2PO_4$), have been found not only to provide room-temperature strength to the investment, but also to react with silica at high temperatures to increase the strength of the investment at the casting temperature. In some investments of this type a sufficient amount of ammonium diacid phosphate is used as a component of the third group. A small amount of magnesium oxide may be used as a component of the second group, and silica may be used as a component of the first group. To produce higher expansion, a combination of different particle sizes of silica rather than a single particle size is used. At room temperature ammonium diacid phosphate reacts with mag-

nesium oxide to give the investment green strength, or room-temperature strength, according to the following chemical reaction:

$$NH_4H_2PO_4 + MgO \rightarrow NH_4MgPO_4 + H_2O$$

The ammonium diacid phosphate is used in a greater amount than necessary for this reaction so that the remainder can react with silica at an elevated temperature. The higher temperatures probably cause a superficial reaction between P_2O_5 and SiO_2 to form a silicophosphate, which increases the strength of the investment at higher temperatures. The water produced by this reaction lowers the viscosity of the mix as spatulation continues.

These investments can be mixed with water or with a special liquid supplied by the manufacturer. The special liquid is a form of silica sol in water. As shown in Fig. 12-16, phosphate-bonded investments possess higher setting expansion when they are mixed with the silica sol than when they are mixed with water. With a mix containing silica sol, the investment mass is capable of expanding hygroscopically, whereas if the mix is only water, the hygroscopic expansion of such an investment is negligible. Not all phosphate-bonded investments, however, can expand hygroscopically. Using silica sol instead of water with phosphate-bonded investment also increases its strength considerably. Fig. 12-17 shows thermal expansion curves of two commercial phosphate-bonded investments mixed according to the manufacturers' recommended liquid/powder ratio. Both the setting and thermal expansions must be considered in selecting these investments.

Proposed ANSI/ADA Specification No. 42 for dental phosphate-bonded casting investments (ISO/DIS 9694.2) specifies two types of investments for alloys having a solidus temperature above 1080° C: Type I for inlays, crowns, and other fixed restorations and Type II for partial dentures and other cast removable restoration. The following properties are specified: fluidity, initial setting time, compressive strength, and linear thermal expansion. The fluidity of Type I investment is higher than that of Type II with diameters of 90 and 70 mm, respectively, as measured by a slump test. Initial setting time must not differ by more than 30% from the time stated by the manufacturer. The compressive strengths of Types I and II at room temperature shall not be less than 2.5 and 3.0 MPa, respectively. The linear thermal expansion must not differ by more than 15% from the time stated by the manufacturer.

Silica-bonded investment

Another type of binding material for investments used with casting high-melting alloys is a silica-bonding ingredient. This type of investment may derive its silica bond from ethyl silicate, an aqueous dispersion of colloidal silica, or from sodium silicate. One such investment consists of a silica refractory, which is bonded by the hydrolysis of ethyl silicate in the presence of hydrochloric acid. The product of the hydrolysis is the formation of a colloidal solution of silicic acid and ethyl alcohol, which can be written as

$$Si(OC_2H_5)_4 + 4H_2O \xrightarrow{HCl} Si(OH)_4 + 4C_2H_5OH$$

In practice, however, the reaction is more complicated, and instead of tetrasilicic acid, which is converted into $SiO_2 \cdot 2H_2O$, a polymerized compound of silicon is formed with the following structure:

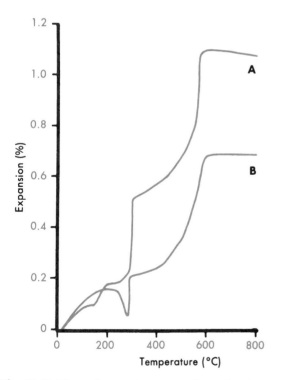

Fig. 12-17 Thermal expansion curves of two phosphate-bonded investments mixed at recommended liquid/powder ratios (*A*, thermal expansion type, and *B*, hygroscopic expansion type). (Adapted from Zarb GA, Bergman B, Clayton JA, MacKay HF, editors: *Prosthodontic treatment for partially edentulous patients,* St Louis, 1978, Mosby.)

$$
\begin{array}{c}
\quad | \qquad | \\
-Si-O-Si- \\
\quad | \qquad | \\
\quad O \qquad O \\
\quad | \qquad | \\
-Si-O-Si- \\
\quad | \qquad | \\
\quad O \qquad O \\
\quad | \qquad | \\
-Si-O-Si- \\
\quad | \qquad |
\end{array}
$$

This material has an even higher silica content and better refractory properties than the $SiO_2 \cdot 2H_2O$.

Ethyl silicate has the disadvantage of giving off flammable components during processing, and the method is expensive; thus other technics and methods have been developed to reduce the use of this material. Sodium silicate and colloidal silica currently are more common binders of the silica type.

Today this investment usually is supplied with two bottles of special liquid, instead of water, with which the investment powder should be mixed. In one of the bottles the manufacturer usually supplies a properly diluted water-soluble silicate solution. The other bottle usually contains a properly diluted acid solution such as a solution of hydrochloric acid. The contents of each bottle can be stored almost indefinitely. Before use, the equal volume of each bottle should be mixed and allowed to stand for a prescribed time according to the manufacturer's instructions, so that hydrolysis can take place and freshly prepared silicic acid formed.

Proposed ANSI/ADA Specification No. 91 for dental ethyl silicate casting investments (ISO/DIS 11246) specifies the following properties: setting time, compressive strength, and linear thermal expansion. The setting time must not differ by more than 30% from the time stated by the manufacturer. The compressive strength at room temperature shall not be less than 1.5 MPa. The linear thermal expansion must not differ by more than 15% from the time stated by the manufacturer.

Soldering Investment

When soldering the parts of a restoration, such as clasps on a removable partial denture, the parts must be surrounded with a suitable ceramic or investment material before the heating operation. The assembled parts are temporarily held together with sticky wax until they are surrounded with the appropriate investment material, after which the wax is softened and removed. The portion to be soldered is left exposed and free from investment to permit wax removal and effective heating before it is joined with solder.

The investment for soldering is similar to casting investments containing quartz and a calcium sulfate hemihydrate binder. Soldering investments are designed to have lower setting and thermal expansions than casting investments, a feature that is desirable so that the assembled parts do not shift in position during the setting and heating of the investment. Soldering investments often are made of ingredients that do not have as fine a particle size as

the casting investment because the smoothness of the mass is less important. Relatively little information is available in the dental literature on the properties of soldering investments.

Investments for All-Ceramic Restorations

Two types of investment materials have been developed recently for producing all-ceramic restorations. The first type is used for the cast glass technic (described in Chapter 16). This investment is provided by the manufacturer of the glass casting equipment and is composed of phosphate-bonded refractories. The second type of investment for making all-ceramic restorations is the refractory die materials, which are used for all-ceramic veneers, inlays, and crowns. Refractory dies are made by pouring the investment into impressions. When the investment is set, the die is removed, and it is heated to remove gases that may be detrimental to the porcelain (degassing). A refractory die spacer may be added to the surface. Next, porcelain or other ceramic powders are added to the die surface and fired. These materials must accurately reproduce the impression, remain undamaged during the porcelain firing, and have a thermal expansion compatible with that of the porcelain (otherwise the porcelain could crack during cooling). These materials are also phosphate-bonded, and they generally contain fine-grained refractory fillers to allow accurate reproduction of detail. ADA Specification No. 92 for refractory die materials is under development.

SELECTED PROBLEMS

Problem 1. High-strength dental stone dies sometimes fracture during separation from rubber impressions. How can this difficulty be minimized?

Solution a. The recommended water/powder ratio should be used. The water/powder ratio can vary from 0.19 to 0.24 for various Type IV gypsum products. The water and powder should be dispensed accurately. Optimum strength is achieved only at the correct water/powder ratio.

Solution b. Vacuum mixing of high-strength dental stone ensures maximum strength by minimizing porosity.

Solution c. The poured die should be allowed to set for at least 20 minutes or until final set before it is removed from the impression.

Solution d. Increasing the thickness of stiffer impression materials (polyether) increases the ease of removal of the die.

Problem 2. The occlusal surfaces of teeth of a Type III gypsum model poured from an alginate impression were chalky and friable. What could have happened, and how can this problem be solved?

Solution. Excess water in the depressions of an alginate impression (or any impression) from rinsing will increase the water/powder ratio of the dental stone. Blood and saliva remaining on the impression retard the setting of the dental stone. Both conditions can cause the dental stone to be chalky and friable. Carefully rinse and remove excess water from an impression before pouring it in dental stone.

Problem 3. The surface of a high-strength dental stone die was abraded during preparation of the wax pattern. Can Type IV gypsum be treated to create a more abrasion-resistant surface that is less susceptible to damage during construction of the pattern and finishing of the casting?

Solution. Apparently not, because the available hardening solutions and various impregnation technics have little effect on the abrasion resistance of Type IV gypsum. Hardening solutions do result in a slightly higher setting expansion of high-strength dental stone dies.

Problem 4. A dental stone master cast for a complete denture was placed in a bowl of water before it was mounted on an articulator. Inadvertently, the cast was left in the water overnight. After the cast was mounted and dried, an unusually rough surface appeared. What happened?

Solution. Dental stone is slightly soluble in water. Leaving the cast in water for an extended time can dissolve some of the surface, roughening the cast. This roughness is transferred to the surface of the denture. If the cast must be stored in water, use a saturated calcium sulfate dihydrate solution (slurry water).

Problem 5. The boxing edge of a dental stone master cast was trimmed on a model trimmer several days after it had been poured. Trimming was much more difficult than when done soon after the dental stone had set. Why was the cast more difficult to trim, and how can this difficulty be corrected?

Solution. As dental stone dries over a period of several days, its compressive strength increases to about twice that when wet. The wet strength may be regained by soaking the cast in slurry water, which is used to minimize dissolution of the surface during soaking.

Problem 6. A gypsum investment was mixed with water in the proportions recommended by the manufacturer, but the working time was too short to invest the wax pattern. What could have happened, and how can this problem be solved?

Solution a. The powder may have been contaminated by water during storage from high humidity or a wet dispensing spoon. Investment should be stored in an airtight and waterproof container.

Solution b. The temperature of the mixing water may have been higher than 23° C. Water at 20° to 23° C is recommended. Higher temperatures shorten the working time.

Solution c. The spatulation may have been done incorrectly with a mechanical mixer. Overmixing, too long or too rapid, shortens the working time.

Solution d. The mixing bowl or spatula may have been contaminated with particles of set investment containing calcium sulfate dihydrate that accelerated the reaction. Mixing implements should be cleaned before use.

Problem 7. A full crown casting prepared by an immersion hygroscopic technic was too loose. What conditions might have caused this problem, and how can a tighter crown be obtained?

Solution a. The water bath may have been warmer than usual. When warmer water is used, the wax pattern offers less resistance to the expansion of the investment, producing a larger mold. The temperature of the water bath should be monitored regularly.

Solution b. A thicker-than-average mix of investment may have been used, causing an increased setting and hygroscopic expansion. The water/powder ratio recommended by the manufacturer should be used, and the water and powder accurately dispensed.

■ REFERENCES

Dental Plaster and Stone

Buchanan AS, Worner HK: Changes in the composition and setting characteristics of plaster of paris on exposure to high humidity atmospheres, *J Dent Res* 24:65, 1945.

Chong JA, Chong MP, Docking AR: The surface of gypsum cast in alginate impression, *Dent Pract* 16:107, 1965.

Combe EC, Smith DC: Some properties of gypsum plasters, *Br Dent J* 117:237, 1964.

Council on Dental Materials, Instruments, and Equipment: Revised American National Standards Institute/American Dental Association Specification No. 25 for dental gypsum products, *J Am Dent Assoc* 102:351, 1981.

Docking AR: Gypsum research in Australia: the setting process, *Int Dent J* 15:372, 1965.

Docking AR: Some gypsum precipitates, *Aust Dent J* 10:428, 1965.

Earnshaw R: The consistency of gypsum products, *Aust Dent J* 18:33, 1973.

Earnshaw R, Smith DC: The tensile and compressive strength of plaster and stone, *Aust Dent J* 11:415, 1966.

Fairhurst CW: Compressive properties of dental gypsum, *J Dent Res* 39:812, 1960.

Fan PL, Powers JM, Reid BC: Surface mechanical properties of stone, resin, and metal dies, *J Am Dent Assoc* 103:408, 1981.

Garber DK, Powers JM, Brandau HE: Effect of spatulation on the properties of high-strength dental stones, *Mich Dent Assoc J* 67:133, 1985.

Hollenback GM, Smith DD: A further investigation of the physical properties of hard gypsum, *Calif Dent Assoc J* 43:221, 1967.

Jørgensen KD: Studies on the setting of plaster of paris, *Odont Tskr* 61:305, 1953.

Lindquist JT, Brennan RE, Phillips RW: Influence of mixing techniques on some physical properties of plaster, *J Prosthet Dent* 3:274, 1953.

Mahler DB: Hardness and flow properties of gypsum materials, *J Prosthet Dent* 1:188, 1951.

Mahler DB: Plasters of paris and stone materials, *Int Dent J* 5:241, 1955.

Mahler DB, Asgarzadeh K: The volumetric contraction of dental gypsum material on setting, *J Dent Res* 32:354, 1953.

Neville HA: Adsorption and reaction. I. The setting of plaster of paris, *J Phys Chem* 30:1037, 1926.

Peyton FA, Leibold JP, Ridgley GV: Surface hardness, compressive strength, and abrasion resistance of indirect die stones, *J Prosthet Dent* 2:381, 1952.

Phillips RW, Ito BY: Factors affecting the surface of stone dies poured in hydrocolloid impressions, *J Prosthet Dent* 2:390, 1952.

Sanad MEE, Combe EC, Grant AA: The use of additives to improve the mechanical properties of gypsum products, *J Dent Res* 61:808, 1982.

Sarma AC, Neiman R: A study on the effect of disinfectant chemicals on physical properties of die stone, *Quintessence Int* 21:53, 1990.

Stern MA, Johnson GH, Toolson LB: An evaluation of dental stones after repeated exposure to spray disinfectants. Part I: Abrasion and compressive strength, *J Prosthet Dent* 65:713, 1991.

Sweeney WT, Taylor DF: Dimensional changes in dental stone and plaster, *J Dent Res* 29:749, 1950.

Torrance A, Darvell BW: Effect of humidity on calcium sulphate hemihydrate, *Aust Dent J* 35:230, 1990.

von Fraunhofer JA, Spiers RR: Strength testing of dental stone: a comparison of compressive, tensile, transverse, and shear strength tests, *J Biomed Mater Res* 17:293, 1983.

Wiegman-Ho L, Ketelaar JAA: The kinetics of the hydration of calcium sulfate hemihydrate investigated by an electric conductance method, *J Dent Res* 61:36, 1982.

Williams GJ, Bates JF, Wild S: The effect of surface treatment of dental stone with resins, *Quintessence Dent Technol* 7:41, 1983.

Worner HK: Dental plasters. I. General, manufacture, and characteristics before mixing with water, *Aust J Dent* 46:1, 1942.

Worner HK: Dental plasters. II. The setting phenomenon, properties after mixing with water, methods of testing, *Aust J Dent* 46:35, 1942.

Worner HK: The effect of temperature on the rate of setting of plaster of paris, *J Dent Res* 23:305, 1944.

Casting Investments

Anderson JN: *Applied dental materials,* ed 5, Oxford, 1976, Blackwell Scientific.

Asgar K, Lawrence WN, Peyton FA: Further investigations into the nature of hygroscopic expansion of dental casting investments, *J Prosthet Dent* 8:673, 1958.

Asgarzadeh K, Mahler DB, Peyton FA: The behavior and measurement of hygroscopic expansion of dental casting investment, *J Dent Res* 33:519, 1954.

Delgado VP, Peyton FA: The hygroscopic setting expansion of a dental casting investment, *J Prosthet Dent* 3:423, 1953.

Docking AR: The hygroscopic setting expansion of dental casting investments. I. *Aust J Dent* 52:6, 1948.

Docking AR, Chong MP: The hygroscopic setting expansion of dental casting investments. IV. *Aust J Dent* 53:261, 1949.

Docking AR, Chong MP, Donnison JA: The hygroscopic setting expansion of dental casting investments. II. *Aust J Dent* 52:160, 1948.

Docking AR, Donnison JA, Chong MP: The hygroscopic setting expansion of dental casting investments. III. *Aust J Dent* 52:320, 1948.

Eames WB, Edwards CR Jr, Buck WH Jr: Scraping resistance of dental die materials: a comparison of brands, *Oper Dent* 3:66, 1978.

Earnshaw R: The effect of restrictive stress on the thermal expansion of gypsum-bonded investments. I. Inlay casting investments, "thermal expansion" type, *Aust Dent J* 11:345, 1966.

Earnshaw R: The effects of additives on the thermal behaviour of gypsum-bonded casting investments. I. *Aust Dent J* 20:27, 1975.

Higuchi T: Study of thermal decomposition of gypsum bonded investment. I. Gas analysis, differential thermal analysis, thermobalance analysis, x-ray diffraction, *Kokubyo Gakkai Zasshi* 34:217, 1967.

Jones DW: Thermal analysis and stability of refractory investments, *J Prosthet Dent* 18:234, 1967.

Jones DW, Wilson HJ: Setting and hygroscopic expansion of investments, *Br Dent J* 129:22, 1970.

Lyon HW, Dickson G, Schoonover IC: Effectiveness of vacuum investing in the elimination of surface defects in gold castings, *J Am Dent Assoc* 46:197, 1953.

Lyon HW, Dickson G, Schoonover IC: The mechanism of hygroscopic expansion in dental casting investments, *J Dent Res* 34:44, 1955.

Mahler DB, Ady AB: An explanation for the hygroscopic expansion of dental gypsum products, *J Dent Res* 39:578, 1960.

Mahler DB, Ady AB: The influence of various factors on the effective setting expansion of casting investments, *J Prosthet Dent* 13:365, 1963.

Matsuya S, Yamane M: Thermal analysis of the reaction between II-CaSO$_4$ and quartz in nitrogen flow, *Gypsum Lime* 164:3, 1980.

Miyaji T, Utsumi K, Suzuki E, Shimizu Y: Deterioration of phosphate-bonded investment on exposure to 100% relative humidity atmosphere, *Bull Tokyo Med Dent Univ* 29:53, 1982.

Moore TE: Method of making dental castings and composition employed in said method, US Patent 1,924,874, 1933.

Mori T: Thermal behavior of the gypsum binder in dental casting investments, *J Dent Res* 65:877, 1986.

Norling BK, Reisbick MH: Wetting of elastomeric impression materials modified by nonionic surfactant additions, *J Dent Res* 56B(abstr):148, 1977.

O'Brien WJ, Nielsen JP: Decomposition of gypsum investment in the presence of carbon, *J Dent Res* 38:541, 1959.

Phillips RW: Relative merits of vacuum investing of small castings as compared to conventional methods, *J Dent Res* 26:343, 1947.

Ryge G, Fairhurst CW: Hygroscopic expansion, *J Dent Res* 35:499, 1956.

Schnell RJ, Mumford G, Phillips RW: An evaluation of phosphate bonded investments used with a high fusing gold alloy, *J Prosthet Dent* 13:324, 1963.

Shell JS, Dootz ER: Permeability of investments at the casting temperature, *J Dent Res* 40:999, 1961.

Shell JS, Hollenback GM: Setting and thermal investment expansion in longitudinal and transverse directions, *J S Calif Dent Assoc* 41:511, 1965.

Weinstein LJ: Composition for dental molds, US Patent 1,708,436, 1929.

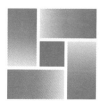

13 *Waxes*

Few procedures in restorative dentistry can be completed without the use of wax in one of its many forms. Forming an inlay pattern, boxing an impression before it is poured in dental stone, or making an impression for the registration of occlusal bite relationships each requires a specially formulated wax. Some uses for various dental waxes are shown in Fig. 13-1. These examples display how the tasks these waxes perform, and therefore their properties, vary greatly. Accuracy is a requisite for inlay or removable denture patterns, shown in the upper left of Fig. 13-1, whereas for the boxing of an impression, shown in the upper center, the ease and convenient manipulation of the wax are essential. The other applications, such as the denture forms shown in the lower left or the corrective impression wax shown in the upper right of Fig. 13-1, require equally varying qualities in the waxes, as do the applications of wax for the border and palate of the metal tray or for the attachment of a plaster splint to the model as shown in the lower right of the figure. Thus the specific use of the dental wax determines the physical properties that are most desirable for a successful application.

■ WAXES, GUMS, FATS, AND RESINS

Dental waxes may be composed of natural and synthetic waxes, gums, fats, fatty acids, oils, natural and synthetic resins, and pigments of various types. The particular working characteristics of each wax are achieved by blending the appropriate natural and synthetic waxes and resins and other additives, some of which are shown in Table 13-1.

The chemical components of both natural and synthetic waxes impart characteristic physical properties to the wax, which are of primary interest because the specific physical properties of a wax or wax blend determine its usefulness for intended applications. Natural waxes are distributed in nature, whereas synthetic waxes are produced by combination of various chemicals in the laboratory or by chemical action on natural waxes. The additives are obtained as natural materials and synthetic products.

Natural Waxes

In the past, waxes have been classified according to their origin: (1) mineral, (2) plant, (3) insect, and (4) animal; however, a better classification is based on their chemical composition. The two principal groups of organic compounds contained in waxes are hydrocarbons and esters, although some waxes contain free alcohols and acids as well.

The chief constituents of most mineral waxes are hydrocarbons ranging from 17 to over 44 carbon atoms, a fact that accounts for odd and even numbers in the chain as shown in the following formula:

$$CH_3-(CH_2)-CH_3$$
$$15 \text{ to } 42$$

The hydrocarbons in plant waxes are saturated alkanes with from 19 to 31 carbon atoms present in odd numbers. Therefore dental waxes contain molecules having a range of molecular weights that affect the melting and flow properties of the waxes.

Plant and animal waxes contain considerable concentrations of esters, and carnauba (a plant wax) contains 85% alkyl esters of various kinds. The principal ester in beeswax is myricyl palmitate,

$$C_{15}H_{31}-\overset{\displaystyle O}{\overset{\displaystyle \|}{C}}-O-C_{30}H_{61}$$

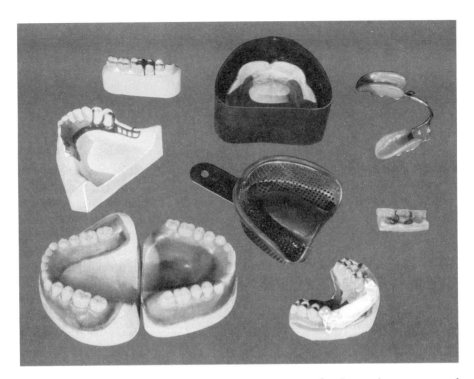

Fig. 13-1 Applications of waxes in dentistry. Inlay pattern, *upper left;* boxing of an impression, *upper center;* baseplate, *lower left;* casting wax, *left center;* utility wax, *center;* sticky wax, *lower right;* corrective impression, *upper right;* and bite, *right center.*

TABLE 13-1   Components of Dental Waxes

Natural Waxes	Synthetic Waxes	Additives
Mineral	Acrawax C	Stearic acid
Paraffin	Aerosol OT	Glyceryl
Microcrys-	Castorwax	tristearate
talline	Flexowax C	Oils
Barnsdahl	Epolene N-10	Turpentine
Ozokerite	Albacer	Colorants
Ceresin	Aldo 33	Natural resins
Montan	Durawax 1032	Rosin
Plant		Copal
Carnauba		Dammar
Ouricury		Sandarac
Candelilla		Mastic
Japan wax		Shellac
Cocoa		Kauri
butter		Synthetic resins
Insect		Elvax
Beeswax		Polyethylene
Animal		Polystyrene
Spermaceti		

which is the reaction product of myricyl alcohol and palmitic acid. Plant and animal waxes also contain acids, alcohols, hydrocarbons, and resins; whereas Montan wax (an earth wax) contains large amounts of esters, the main compound being

$$C_{28}H_{57}-\overset{\displaystyle O}{\overset{\|}{C}}-O-C_{24}H_{49}$$

However, there are other esters composed of C_{20}–C_{29} acids and C_{20}–C_{30} alcohols.

This brief description of the composition of natural waxes indicates that they are complex combinations of organic compounds of reasonably high molecular weights. Also, the composition of these waxes varies, depending on the source and the time of collection; therefore the dental manufacturers must blend the specific batches of wax to obtain the properties desired for a particular application.

Paraffin waxes are obtained principally from the high boiling point fractions of petroleum and are mixtures of chiefly straight-chain saturated hydrocarbons containing from 26 to 30 carbon atoms.

The ordinary commercial grades of paraffin melt in the range of 40° to 71° C, and the melting temperatures generally increase with increasing molecular weights. The presence of oils in the wax, however, lowers the melting temperature; paraffin waxes used in dentistry are refined waxes and have less than 0.5% oil. The paraffin waxes produced by current refining procedures crystallize in the form of plates, needles, or malcrystals but generally are of the plate type. Many hydrocarbon waxes undergo crystalline changes on cooling, and a transition from needles to plates occurs about 5° to 8° C below their melting temperature. During solidification and cooling, there is a volumetric contraction that varies from 11% to 15%. This contraction is not uniform throughout the temperature range from the melting temperature to room temperature because the wax is a mixture of hydrocarbons and the wax passes through transition points accompanied by changes in physical properties.

Microcrystalline waxes are similar to paraffin waxes, except that they are obtained from the heavier oil fractions in the petroleum industry and, as a result, have higher melting points, which range from 60° to 91° C. As their name suggests, the microcrystalline waxes crystallize in small plates and are tougher and more flexible than the paraffin waxes. In contrast to the paraffin waxes, the microcrystalline waxes largely composed of branched-chain hydrocarbons and have higher molecular weights, with the average molecule containing 41 to 50 carbon atoms. The microcrystalline waxes have an affinity for oils, and the hardness and tackiness may be altered by adding oils. Of particular interest is that microcrystalline waxes have less volumetric change during solidification than paraffin waxes.

Barnsdahl is a microcrystalline wax that has a melting point of 70° to 74° C and is an agent used for increasing the melting range and hardness and for reducing the flow of paraffin waxes.

Ozokerite is an earth wax found in central Europe and the western United States near petroleum deposits. It has a melting temperature of about 65° C and a microcrystalline structure consisting of needles or short plates. Ozokerite is similar to microcrystalline wax in that it is composed of straight- and branched-chain hydrocarbons, but it also contains some closed-chain hydrocarbons. It also has great affinity for oils and in quantities of 5% to 15% greatly improves the physical characteristics of paraffins in the melting range of 54° C.

Ceresin is a term used to describe waxes from wax-bearing distillates from natural-mineral petroleum refining or lignite refining. Like the microcrystalline waxes, they are straight- and branched-chain paraffins, but they have higher molecular weights and greater hardness than hydrocarbon waxes distilled from the crude products. These waxes also may be used to increase the melting range of paraffin waxes.

Montan waxes are obtained by extraction from various lignites, and although they are mineral waxes, their composition and properties are similar to those of the plant waxes, and they have melting temperatures from 72° to 92° C. Montan waxes are mixtures of long-chain esters of 40 to 58 carbon atoms accompanied by free high–molecular weight alcohols and acids and varying amounts of resins. As a result of their composition, the Montan waxes are hard, brittle, and lustrous; they blend well with other waxes, and therefore they are often substituted for the plant waxes to improve the hardness and melting range of paraffin waxes.

Carnauba and ouricury waxes are composed of straight-chain esters, alcohols, acids, and hydrocarbons. They are characterized by high hardness, brittleness, and high melting temperatures. Carnauba waxes have melting temperatures from 84° to 91° C, whereas ouricury waxes melt at 79° to 84° C. They both possess the outstanding quality of increasing the melting range and hardness of paraffin waxes; for example, the addition of 10% of carnauba wax to paraffin wax with a melting range of 20° C increases the melting range to 46° C. The addition of ouricury waxes produces a similar effect, but they are less effective than carnauba wax.

Candelilla waxes consist of 40% to 60% paraffin hydrocarbons containing 29 to 33 carbon atoms, accompanied by free alcohols, acids, esters, and lactones. They have melting temperatures of 68° to 75° C, and, like carnauba and ouricury wax, they harden paraffin waxes but are not so effective for increasing the melting range.

Japan wax and cocoa butter are not true waxes but are chiefly fats. Japan wax contains the glycerides of palmitic and stearic acids and higher molecular weight acids; cocoa butter is completely fat and composed of glycerides of stearic, palmitic, oleic, lauric, and lower fatty acids. Japan wax is a tough, malleable, and sticky material that melts at about 51° C, whereas cocoa butter is a brittle substance at room temperature. Japan wax may be mixed with paraffin to improve tackiness and emulsifying ability, and cocoa butter is used to protect against dehydration of soft tissues and to temporarily protect glass ionomer products from moisture during setting or from dehydrating after they are set.

Beeswax is the primary insect wax used in dentistry. It is a complex mixture of esters consisting mainly of myricyl palmitate plus saturated and unsaturated hydrocarbons and high–molecular weight organic acids. The wax has a melting temperature of 63° to 70° C. It is a brittle material at room temperature but becomes plastic at body temperature. It is used to modify the properties of paraffin waxes, and it is the main component in sticky wax.

Animal waxes such as spermaceti wax, obtained from the sperm whale, are not used extensively in dentistry but, like beeswax, are mainly ester waxes. The spermaceti wax has been used as a coating in the manufacture of dental floss.

Synthetic Waxes

In recent years both synthetic waxes and synthetic resins have become available. Although the use of synthetic waxes and resins is increasing, it is still limited in dental formulations, and the natural waxes continue to be the primary components.

Synthetic waxes are complex organic compounds of varied chemical compositions. Although they differ chemically from natural waxes, they possess certain physical properties, such as melting temperature or hardness, that are akin to those of the natural waxes. Also, synthetic waxes are highly refined, in contrast to containing contamination that is frequently present in natural waxes.

The following represent some of the synthetic waxes that are available: (1) polyethylene waxes, (2) polyoxyethylene glycol waxes, (3) halogenated hydrocarbon waxes, (4) hydrogenated waxes, and (5) wax esters from the reaction of fatty alcohols and acids. Polyethylene polymers having molecular weights from 2000 to 4000 are waxes melting at 100° to 105° C. These waxes possess properties similar to high–molecular weight paraffin waxes obtained from petroleum. The polyoxyethylene waxes are polymers of ethylene glycols and have melting temperatures from 37° to 63° C. They have limited compatibility with other waxes but do function as plasticizers and tend to toughen films of wax. The remaining synthetic waxes are prepared by reactions with natural waxes or wax products, as with chlorine in the preparation of halogenated waxes and hydrogen in the manufacture of hydrogenated waxes, and the variability of various batches of wax is similar to the original waxes.

Gums

Many waxes obtained from plants and animals resemble in appearance a group of substances described as gums. Many plants produce a variety of gums that are viscous, amorphous exudates that harden on exposure to air. Most gums are complicated substances, many of which are mixtures containing largely carbohydrates; when they are mixed with water, they either dissolve or form sticky, viscous liquids. Gum arabic and tragacanth are two natural gums that do not resemble waxes in either their properties or composition.

Fats

As a class of substances, waxes are harder and have higher melting temperatures than fats, but in some ways they resemble fat. Both are tasteless, odorless, and colorless in the pure form, and they usually feel greasy. Chemically, fats are composed of esters of various fatty acids with glycerol and are known as glycerides, which distinguishes them from waxes. Some examples of fats are glycerides of stearic acid or tristearate found in tallow and the mixed glyceride of oleic, palmitic, and butyric acids found in butter.

Glyceryl tristearate is the chief ingredient of beef tallow and is a fat with a melting temperature of about 43° C. It has a lustrous appearance and is a firm, slightly greasy solid that bears a resemblance to waxes. The fat may be used to increase the melting range and hardness of compounded wax. Oils have a pronounced effect on the properties of waxes, as mentioned earlier in connection with the discussion of paraffin waxes. Hydrocarbon oils may be used to soften mixtures of waxes, and small quantities of silicone oils may be added to improve the ease of polishing with waxes.

Resins

In some respects natural resins resemble waxes in appearance and properties, although they form a distinct classification of substances. Trees and other plants of many different species produce exudates of natural resins, such as dammar, rosin, or sandarac. The natural resins are relatively insoluble in water but vary in solubility in certain organic liquids. Resins generally are complex, amorphous mixtures of organic substances that are characterized by specific physical behavior rather than by any definite chemical composition. Most natural resins are obtained from trees and plants, except shellac, which is produced by insects. Numerous natural resins are blended with waxes to develop waxes for dental applications.

Natural resins such as dammar and kauri may be mixed with waxes. They are compatible with most natural waxes and produce harder products. Synthetic resins such as polyethylene and vinyl resins of various types may be added to paraffin waxes to improve their toughness, film-forming characteristics, and melting ranges.

Natural and synthetic resins also may be used in organic solvents to produce film-forming materials that may be used as cavity liners. Copal is a natural resin that is brittle and has a melting range well above 149° C, but when deposited as a film from an organic solvent, it serves as a liner for prepared cavities. Polystyrene is a synthetic resin that may be used in a similar manner.

■ CHARACTERISTIC PROPERTIES OF WAXES

Useful and important properties of waxes include melting range, thermal expansion, mechanical properties, flow, residual stress, and ductility.

Melting Range

Because waxes consist of similar types of molecules of different molecular weights and may contain several types of molecules, each having a range of molecular weights, they have melting ranges rather than melting points. The melting ranges of a paraffin wax, a carnauba wax, and a mixture of these two waxes are illustrated in Fig. 13-2. The curves are differential thermograms obtained in the manner described in Chapter 3 under measurement of temperature. The

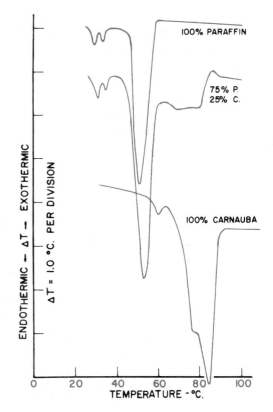

Fig. 13-2 Differential thermograms of paraffin, carnauba, and a 75% paraffin–25% carnauba wax mixture.

melting range for paraffin wax is from 44° to 62° C, and for carnauba wax, from 50° to 90° C. When a mixture of 75% paraffin and 25% carnauba wax was prepared, the paraffin component melted at essentially the same temperatures, but the melting temperature of the carnauba wax was decreased slightly. Note that adding carnauba to paraffin wax dramatically increased the melting range to 44° C, compared with 18° C for paraffin alone.

The effect of the composition of paraffin-carnauba mixtures on the melting range is shown in Fig. 13-3. The presence of 2.5% carnauba wax had little effect on the melting range, but the range increased rapidly as the concentration of carnauba wax was increased to 10%. Although concentrations of carnauba wax greater than 10% had no further effect on the melting range, higher amounts are necessary for certain applications to control the flow and mechanical properties. The melting of mixtures of paraffin and higher-melting waxes can be visualized as the melting of the

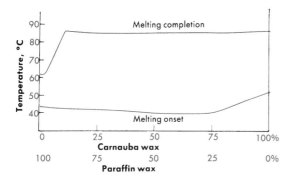

Fig. 13-3 Melting range of mixtures of paraffin and carnauba wax.

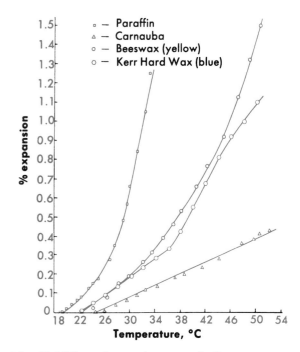

Fig. 13-4 Thermal expansion curves for four waxes.

paraffin nears its usual temperature, but the entire wax does not appear melted because the matrix of carnauba wax does not melt until a considerably higher temperature is reached.

Thermal Expansion

Like other materials, waxes expand when subjected to a rise in temperature and contract as the temperature is decreased. This fundamental property may be altered slightly when various waxes are blended (Fig. 13-4), but the response to thermal changes cannot be reduced to negligible values. The expansion and contraction of dental waxes with changes in temperature are pronounced, as is illustrated in Table 13-2. In general, dental waxes and their components have the largest coefficient of thermal expansion of any material used in restorative dentistry.

The linear thermal expansion properties of the waxes may be explained on the basis of the strength of secondary valence forces and the transition points. The mineral waxes generally have higher coefficients of linear thermal expansion than plant waxes. The mineral waxes expand more because they have weak secondary valence forces, which are overcome easily by the energy absorbed during a rise in temperature. This permits more movement of the wax components, thus allowing a greater amount of thermal expansion.

Plant waxes, on the other hand, have high secondary valence forces because of the presence of high concentrations of esters. Because the secondary valence forces restrict the movement of the wax components, small coefficients of thermal expansion

are observed until the melting range of the wax is approached. This phenomenon is illustrated by beeswax; yellow beeswax has much higher coefficients of linear thermal expansion than bleached beeswax.

Many waxes exhibit at least two rates of expansion between 22° and 52° C. These changes in rate of expansion occur at transition points. At these points the internal structural parts become freer to move. For example, during this transition hydrocarbon chains of a mineral wax become free to rotate; consequently, after a wax has been heated through a transition point, it is freer to expand. Because the ingredient waxes are undergoing transitions that do not coincide with one another, certain inlay waxes exhibit more than two changes in rate of expansion.

Different waxes may have decidedly different rates and amounts of thermal expansion, as shown in Table 13-2. As an example, carnauba and Montan wax have approximately the same melting ranges, but from 22° to 52° C they have dissimilar expansion characteristics.

Some waxes have different rates of expansion in different temperature ranges, as seen by the change of shape of the curves for paraffin, beeswax, and an

TABLE 13-2 Coefficient of Thermal Expansion of Mineral, Plant, Insect, and Inlay Waxes

Wax	Temperature Range (° C)	Coefficient $\times 10^{-6}$/° C
MINERAL		
Paraffin	20.0-27.8	307
	27.8-34.0	1631
Litene	22.0-47.5	205
	47.5-52.0	590
Barnsdahl	22.0-40.4	185
	40.4-52.0	243
Ceresin	22.0-27.4	307
	27.4-34.7	849
	34.7-42.2	471
	42.2-50.0	1434
Montan	22.0-41.5	188
	41.5-52.0	294
PLANT		
Carnauba	22.0-52.0	156
Candelilla	22.0-40.2	182
	40.2-52.0	365
Ouricury	22.0-43.0	186
	43.0-52.0	307
Japan wax	22.0-38.6	304
	38.6-45.0	755
INSECT		
Beeswax (yellow)	22.0-41.2	344
	41.2-50.0	1048
Beeswax (bleached)	22.0-38.6	271
	38.6-50.0	606
INLAY		
Kerr blue inlay	22.0-37.5	323
wax (hard)	37.5-45.0	629
	45.0-50.0	328
Kerr blue inlay	22.0-32.7	263
wax (regular)	32.7-40.9	662
	40.9-46.9	458
	46.9-50.0	1084

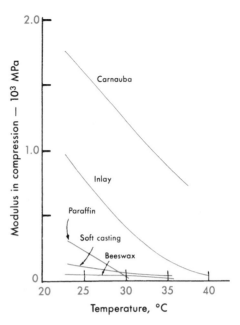

Fig. 13-5 Elastic modulus of various waxes as a function of temperature.

Mechanical Properties

The elastic modulus, proportional limit, and compressive strength of waxes are low compared with those of other materials, and these properties depend strongly on the temperature. The elastic moduli of various waxes between 23° and 40° C are shown in Fig. 13-5, with carnauba wax having the highest values and beeswax the lowest. The elastic modulus of carnauba wax decreased from 1790 to 759 MPa from 23° to 37° C. Paraffin wax showed a sharp decrease in modulus from 310 to 27.6 MPa between 23° and 30° C. The inlay wax, which simulates a mixture of 75% paraffin and 25% carnauba wax, had intermediate changes in modulus of 760 to 48.2 MPa between 23° and 40° C.

The modulus of the inlay wax is important in the hygroscopic casting procedure in which the wax pattern is subjected to stresses resulting from the expansion of the investment during setting. Nonuniform deformation of wax patterns, such as crowns, can be minimized by use of waxes having different elastic moduli for particular parts of the pattern. For example, in a crown the lateral walls can be prepared by use of inlay wax, and the occlusal surfaces can be constructed of the soft green casting wax (Fig. 13-5).

inlay wax in Fig. 13-4. Because the coefficient of thermal expansion of inlay wax is so great, temperature changes in wax patterns after the critical dimensional relationships are set may be a major contributing factor in inaccuracy of the finished restoration.

At the investing temperature the modulus ratio for the inlay and soft green casting wax is 7:1, which is the approximate ratio needed for many patterns to obtain uniform expansion in the occlusal compared with the marginal areas.

The proportional limits and the compressive strengths of the waxes shown in Fig. 13-5 exhibit the same trends as their elastic moduli. The proportional limit of carnauba wax decreased from 11 to 5.5 MPa over the range of 23° to 37° C. Inlay casting wax experienced a decrease in proportional limit of 4.82 to 0.21 MPa from 23° to 40° C. The compressive strength of inlay wax decreased from 82.7 to 0.48 MPa over the same temperature range, and the percent compression at rupture varied from 2.7% to 4.3%. Hence the inlay wax would be considered a brittle material, although it possesses flow or viscous properties at stresses below its proportional limit.

Flow

The property of flow is visualized as resulting from the slippage of molecules over each other. A measure of flow in the liquid state of wax would be synonymous with viscosity or the internal friction of the molecules during movement. Below the melting point of the wax, however, a measure of the flow actually would be a measure of the degree of plastic deformation of the material at a given temperature. Flow is decidedly dependent on the temperature of the wax, the force bringing about the deformation, and the time the force is applied, as shown in Fig. 13-6. Flow greatly increases as the melting point of the wax is approached. Although a high percentage of flow at a given temperature may be required for a specific wax, this high flow also may be extremely deleterious at a temperature a few degrees lower. This is especially true for the direct inlay wax. This material must have a relatively high flow a few degrees above mouth temperature so that when it is in a workable condition, it is not uncomfortably warm when placed in the mouth of the patient. At mouth temperature, an inlay wax to be used for a direct pattern must have essentially no flow to minimize the possibility of distortion of the pattern during removal from the tooth cavity.

The flow of wax at different temperatures is shown in Fig. 13-6. Yellow beeswax does not flow extensively until it reaches 38° C, and at 40° C it

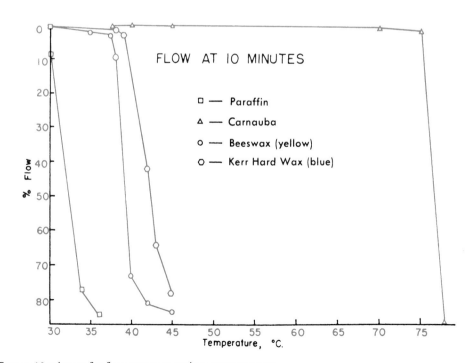

Fig. 13-6 Flow at 10 minutes for four waxes at various temperatures.

flows approximately 7%. From these data it is easy to understand why beeswax has been used as a major ingredient in dental impression wax. Many mineral waxes have about a 10° C range between 1% and 70% flow, which indicates that these waxes soften gradually over a broad temperature range. The mineral waxes, paraffin, litene, barnsdahl, and ceresin, flow 50% approximately 20° C below their melting range. This can be explained by the fact that the mineral waxes are straight- or branched-chain hydrocarbons. The secondary valence forces in these waxes are rather weak and are gradually dissipated as the temperature is increased.

Montan wax, another mineral wax, requires a temperature of 71° C, or 8° C below its melting range, to flow 50%. However, this wax is similar to the plant waxes in that it is composed mainly of esters formed in nature by the union of higher alcohols with the higher fatty acids. The plant waxes likewise require temperatures close to their melting range to produce 50% flow. As a result of the presence of ester groups in these waxes, the secondary valence forces are rather strong, and a high temperature is necessary to overcome these forces. Once the secondary valence forces are overcome, these waxes flow rapidly. Below this point they often appear to fracture in a manner similar to a brittle material.

Yellow beeswax, which is also primarily an ester wax, flows extensively 24° C below its melting range (61° to 63° C) and displays an 8° C temperature difference between 1% and 70% flow. This wax contains a large number of impurities, which interfere with the secondary valence forces. As beeswax goes through the bleaching process and some of these impurities are removed, the secondary valence forces increase. Flow data illustrate this point because bleached beeswax requires a temperature closer to its melting range to produce a large amount of flow, and the temperature difference between 1% and 70% flow is only 4° C. Note that the flow of various batches of yellow beeswax shows that significant differences may exist between batches. A similar observation is seen with paraffin and carnauba wax.

A plot of percent flow versus time for a hard inlay wax shows that at 40° C the amount of flow in relation to time is linear (Fig. 13-7). The total amount of

flow after 10 minutes at this temperature is only 2%. At 42° C the flow increases enough to cause an increase in the rate of flow. At 43° and 45° C the rate of flow is very large at the beginning of the test, and the rate decreases rapidly as a result of the increase in diameter of the sample.

The flow of dental waxes is influenced by the presence of solid-solid and melting transformations that occur in the component waxes. The transformation temperatures can be indirectly related to flow by studying the resistance of the wax to penetration as a function of temperature. Penetration thermograms are compared with a differential thermal analysis (DTA) curve for an inlay casting wax in Fig. 13-8 for annealed, A, and unannealed, U, specimens tested at two stress levels. At the lower stress level the high-melting ester component of the wax influenced the penetration. However, at a high stress level the temperature of the solid-solid transformation associated with the hydrocarbon component of the wax determined the resistance to penetration. Annealing the wax in an oven at 50° C for 24 hours before testing had the effect of increasing the resistance of the wax to penetration.

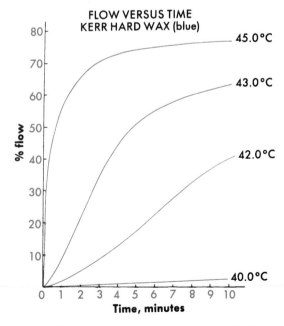

Fig. 13-7 Flow curves at various temperatures for Kerr hard (Type I) wax.

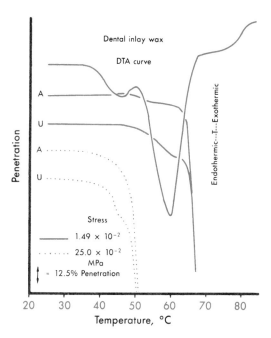

Fig. 13-8 Penetration thermograms for annealed, *A,* and unannealed, *U,* inlay wax compared with a differential thermal analysis (DTA) curve.

Residual Stress

Regardless of the method used to prepare a wax pattern, residual stress exists in the completed pattern. The presence of this residual stress can be demonstrated by comparison of the thermal expansion curves of annealed wax with wax that has been cooled under compression or tension. The thermal expansion of an annealed inlay wax is shown in Fig. 13-9, in which the same curve is obtained on heating or cooling. When the wax specimen is prepared by holding the softened wax under compression during cooling, followed by the determination of the thermal expansion, the thermal expansion is greater than for the annealed specimen. The extent of the deviation from the curve for the annealed wax is a function of the magnitude of the residual internal stress and the time and temperature of storage of the specimen before the thermal expansion curve is determined. Therefore a shaded area is shown rather than a specific curve. When the wax specimen is cooled while being subjected to tensile stress and the thermal expansion is determined, the curve for the wax specimen is lower than that for the annealed speci-

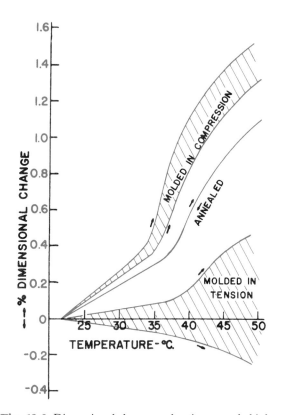

Fig. 13-9 Dimensional change on heating annealed inlay wax patterns and those formed under compression and tension.

men. If sufficient residual stress is introduced, a thermal contraction may result on heating; again a shaded area indicates the direction of the effect.

The changes in dimensions resulting from the heating of wax specimens formed under compression or tension can be explained as follows: When the specimen is held under compression during cooling, the atoms and molecules are forced closer together than when they are under no external stress. After the specimen is cooled to room temperature and the load is removed, the motion of the molecules is restricted, and this restriction results in residual stress in the specimen. When the specimen is heated, the release of the residual stress is added to the normal thermal expansion, and the total expansion is greater than normal. When the specimen is cooled while under tensile stress and the expansion is measured, the release of the residual tensile stress results in a dimensional change that is opposite to the thermal expansion. The sum of these two effects results in a lower thermal expansion curve than for annealed wax. As seen in Fig. 13-9, if a sufficiently large amount of residual stress is introduced, the overall dimensional change on heating results in a contraction of the specimen.

Ductility

Like flow, the ductility increases as the temperature of a wax sample is increased. In general, waxes with lower melting temperatures have a greater ductility at any given temperature than those with higher melting temperatures.

The ductility of a blended wax is greatly influenced by the distribution of the melting temperatures of the component waxes. A blended wax with components that have wide melting ranges generally has greater ductility than blended waxes that have a narrow range. Whenever the wide range of melting temperatures is present, the softening point of the lowest component is approached first. A further temperature rise begins to liquefy this component and approach still closer to the softening points of the higher-softening components. This tends to plasticize the entire wax mass, thereby enhancing ductility.

Generally, the highly refined waxes are quite brittle. The lower melting point, microcrystalline mineral waxes, which contain appreciable amounts of occluded oil, are moderately soft and exhibit a high degree of plasticity or ductility, even with their comparatively high melting temperatures.

■ DENTAL WAXES

A variety of natural waxes and resins have been used in dentistry for specific and well-defined applications. In some instances the most favorable qualities can be obtained from a single wax, such as beeswax, but more often a blend of several waxes is necessary to develop the most desirable qualities.

A classification of dental waxes according to their use and application is given in Table 13-3. The pattern waxes are used to form the general predetermined size and contour of an artificial dental restoration, which is to be constructed of a more durable material such as cast gold alloys, cobalt-chromium-nickel alloys, or poly(methyl methacry-

TABLE 13-3   A Classification of Dental Waxes

Pattern	Processing	Impression
Inlay	Boxing	Corrective
Casting	Utility	Bite
Sheet	Sticky	
Ready shapes		
Wax-up		
Baseplate		

late) resin. All pattern waxes have two major qualities, thermal change in dimension and tendency to warp or distort on standing, which create serious problems in their use whether an inlay pattern, a crown, or a complete denture is being constructed.

Processing waxes are used primarily as auxiliary aids in constructing a variety of restorations and appliances, either clinically or in the laboratory. The processing waxes perform numerous tasks that simplify many dental procedures in such operations as denture constructing or soldering.

One of the oldest recorded uses of waxes in dentistry is for taking impressions within the mouth. Because a wax formulated for use as an impression material exhibits high flow and ductility, it distorts readily when withdrawn from undercut areas. Therefore the use of waxes has been limited to the nonundercut edentulous portions of the mouth, and they are generally used in combination with other impression materials such as polysulfide rubber, zinc oxide–eugenol, or dental impression compound.

Inlay Pattern Wax

Such restorations as inlays, crowns, and bridge units are formed by a gold casting process that uses the lost wax pattern technic. A pattern of wax is first constructed that duplicates the shape and contour of the desired gold casting. The carved wax pattern then is embedded in a gypsum-silica investment material to form a mold with an ingate or sprue leading from the outer surface of the investment mold to the pattern, as described in Chapter 16. The wax is subsequently eliminated by heating and softening, and the mold is further conditioned to receive the molten gold by controlled heating in a furnace.

Composition

The principal waxes used to formulate inlay waxes are paraffin, microcrystalline wax, ceresin, carnauba, candelilla, and beeswax. For example, an inlay wax may contain 60% paraffin, 25% carnauba, 10% ceresin, and 5% beeswax. Therefore hydrocarbon waxes constitute the major portion of this formulation. Some inlay waxes are described as hard, regular (medium), or soft, which is a general indication of their flow. The flow can be reduced by adding more carnauba wax or by selecting a higher-melting paraffin wax. An interesting example is that a hard inlay wax may contain a lower percentage of carnauba wax than a regular inlay wax, but the flow of the hard inlay wax is less than the regular wax because of the selection of a higher-melting paraffin in the formulation of the hard wax. Resins in small amounts, such as 1%, also affect the flow of inlay waxes. Inlay waxes generally are produced in deep blue, green, or purple rods or sticks about 7.5 cm long and 0.64 cm in diameter. Some manufacturers supply the wax in the form of small pellets or cones or in small, metal ointment jars.

Properties

The accuracy and ultimate usefulness of the resulting gold casting depend largely on the accuracy and fine detail of the wax pattern. A wax that is able to function well in the gold casting technic must possess certain physical properties that are extremely critical.

Revised ANSI/ADA Specification No. 4 for dental inlay casting wax (ISO 1561) has been formulated for waxes used in both the direct and indirect waxing technics. A summary of flow requirements of this specification is given in Table 13-4. Because the wax patterns are to be melted and vaporized from the investment mold, it is essential that no excessive residue remain in the mold because of incomplete wax burnout. Excess residue may result in the incomplete casting of inlay margins. The specification therefore limits the nonvolatile residue of these waxes to a maximum of 0.10%.

Types I and II dental inlay casting waxes are recognized by Revised ANSI/ADA Specification No. 4. Type I wax is a hard wax that is prescribed for forming direct patterns in the mouth, where lower flow values at 37° C tend to minimize any tendency for distortion of the pattern on its removal from the cavity preparation. Type II wax is a softer wax that is used as an indirect technic wax. Type II wax shows greater flow than Type I wax at temperatures both below and above mouth temperature. The lower flow of Type I wax and the greater ease of carving the softer Type II waxes are desirable working characteristics for the technics associated with each.

Thermal expansion data for the Type I wax are required of the manufacturer by the specification so that compensation may be determined for the shrinkage that occurs as the wax pattern cools from mouth to room temperature (in the direct technic). The maximum linear thermal expansion allowed between 25° and 30° C is 0.20%; between 25° and 37° C, 0.60% is allowed. A proposed revision of ISO 1561 will eliminate this requirement. A similar shrinkage is found for Type II waxes and for the soft casting waxes of some manufacturers. The specification also requires the manufacturers to include instructions regarding the method of softening and the working temperature for the wax preparatory to forming a direct pattern. Both types should soften without becoming flaky, and they should not chip

TABLE 13-4   Flow Requirements for Dental Inlay Casting Wax (Flow, in %)

			Wax Temperature			
	30° C Maximum	37° C Maximum	40° C		45° C	
			Minimum	Maximum	Minimum	Maximum
Type I	–	1.0	–	20	70	90
Type II	1.0	–	50	–	70	90

Adapted from Revised ANSI/ADA Specification No. 4 for inlay wax, *J Am Dent Assoc* 108:88, 1984.

or flake when trimmed to a fine margin during the pattern-carving operation.

Flow

When forming a wax pattern directly in the mouth, the wax must be heated to a temperature at which it has sufficient flow under compression to reproduce the prepared cavity walls in great detail. The working temperature, suggested by the manufacturer, which should be satisfactory for making direct wax patterns, must not be so high as to cause damage to the vital tooth structure or be uncomfortable to the patient. Insufficient flow of the wax caused by insufficient heating not only results in the lack of cavity detail but introduces excess stress within the pattern. An overabundant amount of flow resulting from excessive heating makes compression of the wax difficult because of a lack of "body" in the material.

The values listed in Table 13-4 represent minimun or maximum values of percent flow that occur at various temperatures when Types I and II wax specimens are subjected to a 19.6 N load for 10 minutes. The temperature that the Type I wax must attain to register cavity detail is usually somewhat above 45° C. As seen from these values the flow of the hard wax is no more than 1% at body temperature. The flow of the Type II wax is about 9% at this temperature. Low flow at this temperature tends to minimize distortion of a well-carved pattern as it is withdrawn from an adequately tapered cavity in the tooth.

Thermal coefficient of expansion

The curve in Fig. 13-10 shows that the rate of expansion of the Type I inlay wax is greatest from just below mouth temperature to just above 45° C. A knowledge of the amount of wax expansion or contraction provides a basis on which to judge the compensation necessary to produce an accurate casting. Data sufficient to show the thermal contraction of the wax from its working temperature to room temperature are included in each package of inlay wax that complies with Revised ANSI/ADA Specification No. 4 for Type I wax. On completion of carving of the wax pattern, its removal from the tooth cavity and transfer to the laboratory bring about a reduction in temperature and subsequent thermal contraction. A decrease of 12° to 13° C in temperature, from mouth temperature to a room temperature

of approximately 24° C, causes a 0.4% linear contraction of the wax, or about 0.04% change for each degree change in temperature.

Warpage of wax patterns

Inlay pattern wax shows not only a high coefficient of expansion but also a tendency to warp or distort when allowed to stand unrestrained. The distortion is increased generally as the temperature and time of storage are increased. This quality of wax patterns is related to the release of residual stress developed in the pattern during the process of formation. This characteristic of stress release and warpage is present in all dental waxes but is particularly troublesome in inlay patterns because of the critical dimensional relations that must be maintained in inlay castings.

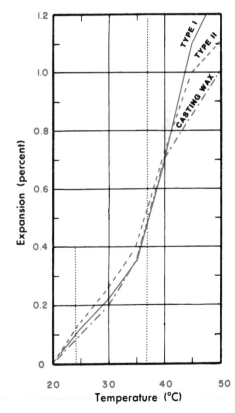

Fig. 13-10 Percent expansion of inlay and casting waxes from 20° to 50° C, showing the percent dimensional change from mouth temperature to average room temperature.

Because the warpage of the pattern is related to the temperature during pattern formation and storage, the rules related to the pattern temperature must be understood. In general, the higher the temperature of the wax at the time the pattern was adapted and shaped, the less the tendency for distortion in the prepared pattern. This is reasonable because the residual stress in the pattern causing the distortion is associated with the forces necessary to shape the wax originally. The incorporation of residual stress can be minimized by softening a wax uniformly by heating at 50° C for at least 15 minutes before use, by using warmed carving instruments and a warmed die, and by adding wax to the die in small amounts.

Because the release of internal stress and subsequent warpage are associated with the storage temperature, it follows that greater warpage results at higher storage temperatures. Lower temperature does not completely prevent distortion, but generally the amount is reduced when the storage temperature is kept to a minimum. If inlay wax patterns must be allowed to stand uninvested for a time longer than 30 minutes, they should be kept in a refrigerator. Although some distortion may take place at this temperature, it will be less than at normal room tempera-

ture. Such a practice of storage for long periods is not recommended if freedom from warpage is desired. The best way to minimize the warpage of inlay wax patterns is to invest the pattern immediately after it is completely shaped. A refrigerated wax pattern should be allowed to warm to room temperature before it is invested. During spruing, distortion can be reduced by use of a solid wax sprue or a hollow metal sprue filled with sticky wax. If the pattern was stored, the margins should be readapted. Temperature of formation, time and condition of storage, and promptness of investing the pattern are major factors related to all technics of pattern formation.

Casting Wax

The pattern for the metallic framework of removable partial dentures and other similar structures is fabricated from the casting waxes. These waxes are available in the form of sheets, usually of 28- and 30-gage (0.40 and 0.32 mm) thickness, ready-made shapes, and in bulk. As shown in Fig. 13-11, the ready-made shapes are supplied as round, half-round, and half–pear-shaped rods and wires of various gages in approximately 10-cm lengths. Although casting waxes serve the same basic purpose as inlay waxes in the formation of patterns for metallic cast-

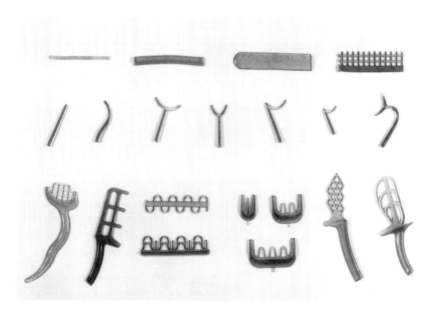

Fig. 13-11 Wax patterns for use in fabrication of metallic framework of removable partial dentures. Preformed bars and mesh, *top;* clasps, *center;* and retention forms, *bottom.*

ings, their physical properties differ slightly. Little is known of the exact composition of these sheet and shape waxes, but they include ingredients similar to those found in inlay waxes, with various combinations and proportions of paraffin, ceresin, beeswax, resins, and other waxes being used.

The casting wax sheets are used to establish minimum thickness in certain areas of the partial denture framework, such as the palatal and lingual bar, and to produce the desired contour of the lingual bar. A partial denture framework in the process of being waxed is shown in the left center of Fig. 13-1. The physical nature and form in which the sheet casting wax is supplied had resulted in its use for post damming of complete maxillary denture impressions, for checking high points of articulation, for producing wax bites of cusp tips for the articulation of stone casts, and for many other uses.

Physical characteristics

The casting sheets and ready-made shapes of certain types of casting waxes may possess a slight degree of tackiness, which helps to maintain their position on the cast and on each other during assembly of the pattern. This tackiness is not sufficient to prevent changes in position from being made with relative ease, and when the waxes are in final position, they are sealed to the investment cast with a hot spatula.

There is no ADA specification for these casting waxes, but a federal specification has been formulated that includes values for softening temperature, amount of flow at various temperatures, general working qualities, and other characteristics. A summary of the properties included in Federal Specification No. U-W-140 is given in Table 13-5. In general, the characteristics most desired include a certain degree of toughness and strength, with a true gage dimension, combined with a minimum of dimensional change with change in temperature, and the ability to be vaporized completely from the investment mold.

Because the pattern for the removable partial denture framework is constructed on and sealed to an investment cast at room temperature from which it is not separated subsequently, there is little need for the casting wax to exhibit low flow at body temperature. The flow characteristics of the casting wax, when measured similarly to the inlay wax, show a maximum of 10% flow at 35° C and a minimum of 60% flow at 38° C. These characteristics are significantly different from the flow values for inlay waxes that comply with the requirements of ANSI/ADA Specification No. 4.

The requirement for ductility of the casting waxes is high. The federal specification requires that the casting wax be bent double on itself without fracture at a temperature of 23° C and that the waxes be pliable and readily adaptable at 40° to 45° C. Heating over a flame and the compression to adapt either the ready-made shapes or the sheet casting wax easily may alter their thickness and contour because of their relatively high ductility and flow.

Because these materials are casting pattern waxes for partial denture cast restorations, as is the inlay wax, they too must vaporize at about 500° C with no residue other than carbon. The mold cavity thus produced will result in more desirable casting surfaces

TABLE 13-5 Summary of Requirements of Federal Specifications for Dental Casting Wax

Type of Wax	Flow	Breaking Point	Working Properties
Casting wax Class A–28-gage, pink Class B–30-gage, green Class C–ready-made shapes, blue	35° C–maximum, 10% 38° C–minimum, 60%	No fracture at 23° C ± 1°	Pliable and readily adaptable at 40° to 45° C Copy accurately surface against which it is pressed Shall not be brittle on cooling Vaporize at 500° C, leaving no film other than carbon

Adapted from Federal Specification No. U-W-140, March 1948, for casting wax.

because it will be free of foreign materials. Pattern waxes are being replaced to some extent by pre-formed plastic patterns.

Resin Modeling Material

Light-curing resins are available as low- and high-viscosity pastes and as a liquid for the fabrication of patterns to be used for cast metal or ceramic inlays, crowns and bridges, and precision attachments (see Fig. 13-12). The modeling pastes are based on diurethane dimethacrylate oligomers with 40% to 55% polyurethane dimethacrylate or poly(methyl methacrylate) fillers. The liquid consistency is mostly urethane dimethacrylate. These resins have a camphoroquinone activator. Self-cured acrylic plastics used as inlay patterns are described in Chapter 19.

Modeling resins are characterized by lower heat of polymerization and shrinkage than acrylics, higher strength and resistance to flow than waxes, good dimensional stability, and burnout without residue. Dimethacrylate resin patterns do not result in cracked investment from heating during burnout, which can occur with acrylic patterns. The light-cured resin pattern materials are comparable in accuracy to traditional inlay wax and self-cured acrylic as shown in Table 13-6. Gypsum and resin dies must be treated with a separator and have undercuts blocked out. The modeling resin is applied in layers 3- to 5-mm thick, with each layer cured separately in a high-intensity, light-curing

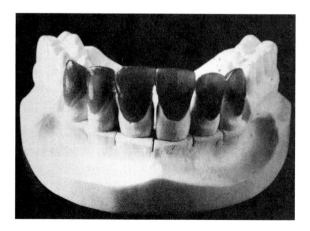

Fig. 13-12 Sculpted anterior crowns made from light-cured resin modeling material. (Courtesy Heraeus Kulzer, GmbH, Wehrheim, Germany.)

chamber for 90 seconds or by using a hand-held, light-curing unit for 20 to 40 seconds per area of irradiation. The liquid material is used first to obtain close adaptation to the die and last to provide a smooth surface. Complete elimination of modeling resins occurs between 670° to 690° C and requires about 45 minutes.

Baseplate Wax

Baseplate wax derives its name from its use on the baseplate tray to establish the vertical dimension, the plane of occlusion, and the initial arch form in the technic for the complete denture restoration. This wax also may be used to form all, or a portion, of the tray itself. The normally pink color provides some esthetic quality for the initial stage of construction of the denture before processing. Baseplate wax serves as the material to produce the desired contour of the denture after teeth are set in position. As a result, the contour wax establishes the pattern for the final plastic denture. Patterns for orthodontic appliances and prostheses other than complete dentures, which are to be constructed of plastics, also are made of baseplate wax. Although these are the primary functions of baseplate wax, it has also been widely used in many phases of dentistry to check the various articulating relations in the mouth and to transfer them to mechanical articulators.

Composition

A few formulas are found in the literature for baseplate wax. Baseplate waxes may contain 70% to 80% paraffin-base waxes or commercial ceresin,

TABLE 13-6   Average Marginal Discrepancies (μm) for Full-Crown and Inlay Patterns Measured 1 Hour and 24 Hours after Forming

Pattern Material	Full Crown	Inlay
Inlay wax (Type II)	11	15
Light-cured resin A	10	8
Light-cured resin B	12	9
Self-cured acrylic	15	7

From Iglesias A, Powers JM, Pierpont HP: Unpublished data, UT-Houston Health Science Center, Dental Branch, Houston, Texas.

with small quantities of other waxes, resins, and additives to develop the specific qualities desired in the wax. A typical composition might include 80% ceresin, 12% beeswax, 2.5% carnauba, 3% natural or synthetic resins, and 2.5% microcrystalline or synthetic waxes. Differential thermal analysis and penetration curves of a typical baseplate wax are shown in Fig. 13-13.

Physical characteristics

The baseplate waxes are normally supplied in sheets 7.60 × 15.00 × 0.13 cm in pink or red color. The manufacturer usually formulates two types of wax according to the climate in which they will be used because the flow of the wax is influenced greatly by the temperature.

The requirements for dental baseplate wax are listed in Table 13-7, which summarizes Revised ANSI/ADA Specification No. 24. Three types of wax are included: Type I is a soft wax for building contours and veneers, Type II is a medium wax to be used for patterns to be tried in the mouth in temperate climates, and Type III is a hard wax for patterns to be tried in the mouth in tropical weather. The flow values are listed for 23°, 37°, and 45° C when they are applicable. The maximum flow allowed at any given temperature decreases rapidly from Type I to Type III. The flow requirements of Type III baseplate wax are comparable to those of the Type I direct inlay wax, with less flow allowed for the baseplate wax at 45° C.

Because baseplate wax is used both to set denture teeth and to adapt around these teeth to develop proper contour, the dimensional changes that may take place because of variations in temperature are important. Although the need for dimensional stability is not as critical as with the inlay wax, the maintenance of good tooth relationship is important. Although no shrinkage value from a molten state to room temperature is stated, the linear thermal expansion from 26° to 40° C should be less than 0.8%.

A summary of practical requirements is also given in Table 13-7. Baseplate waxes should be easily trimmed with a sharp instrument at 23° C and should yield a smooth surface after gentle flaming. These waxes should not leave any residue on porcelain or

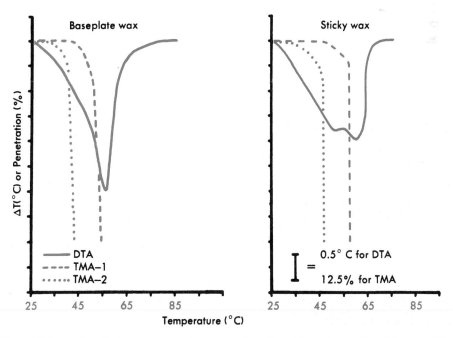

Fig. 13-13 Differential thermal analysis and penetration curves for a dental baseplate and a sticky wax. The stresses for TMA-1 and TMA-2 are 14.9×10^{-3} and 25.0×10^{-2} MPa. (Adapted from Powers JM, Craig RG: Thermomechanical analysis of dental waxes in the penetration mode. In Porter RS, Johnson JF, editors: *Analytical calorimetry,* vol 3, New York, 1974, Plenum.)

TABLE 13-7   Requirements for Dental Baseplate Wax

		Flow (%)		
	Temperature (° C)	Minimum	Maximum	Practical Requirements
Type I–Soft, building	23	–	1.0	Linear thermal expansion from 25°
contours and veneers	37	5.0	90.0	to 40° C < 0.8%
	45	–	–	Softened sheets shall cohere readily
Type II–Medium, patterns	23	–	0.6	without becoming flaky or
in mouth, temperate	37	–	10.0	adhering to fingers
weather	45	50.0	90.0	No irritation of oral tissues
Type III–Hard, patterns	23	–	0.2	Trim easily with a sharp instrument
in mouth, hot weather	37	–	1.2	at 23° C
	45	5.0	50.0	Smooth surface after gentle flaming
				No residue on porcelain or plastic
				teeth
				Coloring shall not separate or
				impregnate plaster during processing
				No adhesion to other sheets of wax
				or separating paper on storage

Adapted from Revised ANSI/ADA Specification No. 24, 1991.

plastic teeth, and the coloring agents in the wax should not separate or impregnate the plastic mold during processing.

There is residual stress within the baseplate wax that holds and surrounds the teeth of a wax denture pattern. This stress results from differential cooling, "pooling" the wax with a hot spatula, and physically manipulating the wax below its most desirable working temperature. Remember that both time and temperature affect the relief of these residual stresses; the waxed and properly articulated denture should not be allowed to stand for long periods of time, especially when subjected to elevated temperatures. Such treatment often results in distortion of the wax and movement of the teeth. The waxed denture should be flasked soon after completion to maintain the greatest accuracy of tooth relations.

Boxing Wax

To form a plaster or stone cast from an impression of the edentulous arch, first a wax box must be formed around the impression, into which the freshly mixed plaster or stone is poured and vibrated. This boxing procedure is necessary also for some other types of impressions. The boxing operation usually consists of first adapting a long, narrow stick or strip of wax around the impression below its peripheral height, followed by a wide strip of wax, producing a form around the entire impression, as seen in the upper center of Fig. 13-1.

The dental literature occasionally refers to carding wax for use in the boxing operation. Carding wax was the original material on which porcelain teeth were fixed when received from the manufacturer. The terms *carding wax* and *boxing wax* have been used interchangeably, although *boxing wax* is more acceptable.

The requirements of Federal Specification No. U-W-138 for boxing wax, which are summarized in Table 13-8, stipulate that this wax should be pliable at 21° C and should retain its shape at 35° C. This broadly defines its lower temperature limit of ductility and flow. Because the impression may be made from a viscoelastic material that is easily distorted, a boxing wax that is readily adaptable to the impression at room temperature is desirable. This property reduces the chance of distortion of the impression, from the standpoint of both temperature and stress involved in the boxing procedures. In general, boxing wax should be slightly tacky and have sufficient strength and toughness for convenient manipulation.

TABLE 13-8   Summary of Requirements of Federal Specifications for Dental Boxing, Utility, and Sticky Waxes

Type of Wax	Flow	Color	Working Properties
Boxing	–	Green or black	Smooth, glossy surface on flaming Pliable at 21° C; retains shape at 35° C Seals easily to plaster with hot spatula
Utility	37.5° C–minimum, 65% –maximum, 80%	Orange or dark red	Pliable at 21° to 24° C Tacky at 21° to 24° C; sufficient adhesion to build up
Sticky	30° C–maximum, 5% 43° C–minimum, 90%	Dark or vivid	Sticky when melted Adheres closely Not more than 0.2% residue on burnout Not more than 0.5% shrinkage from 43° to 28° C

Adapted from Federal Specification No. U-W-138, May 1947, for boxing wax; Federal Specification U-W-156, August 1948, for utility wax; Federal Specification U-W-00149a (DSA-DM), September 1966, for sticky wax.

Utility Wax

An easily workable, adhesive wax is desired in numerous instances. For example, a standard perforated tray for use with the hydrocolloids may easily be brought to a more desirable contour by such a wax, as shown in the center view of Fig. 13-1. This is done to prevent a sag and distortion of the impression material. A soft, pliable, adhesive wax may be used on the lingual portion of a bridge pontic to stabilize it while a labial plaster splint is poured. These and many other tasks are performed by the utility wax, justifying its name.

The utility wax is usually supplied in both stick and sheet form in a dark red or orange color. The ductility and flow of utility waxes, as indicated by the summarized requirements of Federal Specification No. U-W-156 in Table 13-8, are the highest of any of the dental waxes. The utility wax should be pliable at a temperature of 21° to 24° C, which makes it workable and easily adaptable at normal room temperature. The flow of this wax should not be less than 65% or more than 80% at 37.5° C. Because building one layer on top of another is often desirable, the specification requires a sufficient adhesiveness at 21° to 24° C. Utility wax most likely consists of beeswax, petrolatum, and other soft waxes in varying proportions.

Sticky Wax

A suitable sticky wax for prosthetic dentistry is formulated from a mixture of waxes and resins or other additive ingredients. Such a material is sticky when melted and adheres closely to the surfaces on which it is applied. However, at room temperature the wax is firm, free from tackiness, and brittle. Sticky wax should fracture rather than flow if it is deformed during soldering or repair procedures. Although this wax is used to assemble metallic or resin pieces in a fixed temporary position, it is primarily used on dental stones and plasters. The lower right portion of Fig. 13-1 shows an application of sticky wax to seal a plaster splint to a stone model in the process of forming porcelain facings.

According to Federal Specification No. U-W-00149a (DSA-DM), the sticky wax should have a dark or vivid color so that it is readily distinguishable from the light-colored gypsum materials. The specification, summarized in Table 13-8, also limits the shrinkage of sticky wax to 0.5% at temperatures between 43° and 28° C.

The literature contains several formulas for sticky wax, representing both a high and a low resin content. In addition to the rosin and yellow beeswax, which are the usual major constituents, coloring matter and other natural resins such as gum dammar may be present. Differential thermal analysis and penetration curves for a typical dental sticky wax are shown in Fig. 13-13.

Corrective Impression Wax

Corrective impression wax is used as a wax veneer over an original impression to contact and register the detail of the soft tissues. It is claimed that this type of impression material records the

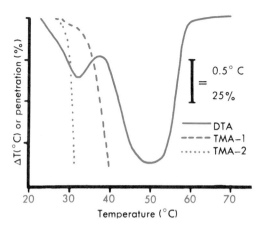

Fig. 13-14 Differential thermal analysis and penetration curves for a dental corrective impression wax. The stresses for TMA-1 and TMA-2 are 14.9×10^{-3} and 25.0×10^{-2} MPa. Observe that the solid-solid transition temperature occurs below 37° C.

mucous membrane and underlying tissues in a functional state in which movable tissue is displaced to such a degree that functional contact with the base of the denture is obtained. Corrective waxes are formulated from hydrocarbon waxes such as paraffin, ceresin, and beeswax and may contain metal particles. There are no ADA or federal specifications for corrective impression waxes. The flow of several corrective waxes measured by penetration at 37° C is 100%. Differential thermal analysis and penetration curves for a typical corrective impression wax are shown in Fig. 13-14. These waxes are subject to distortion during removal from the mouth.

Bite Registration Wax

Bite registration wax is used to accurately articulate certain models of opposing quadrants. The wax bite registration for the copper-formed die must provide proximal and occlusal relations. Bite registrations are frequently made from 28-gage casting wax sheets or from hard baseplate wax, but waxes identified as bite waxes seem to be formulated from beeswax or hydrocarbon waxes such as paraffin or ceresin. Certain bite waxes contain aluminum or copper particles. There are no ADA or federal specifications for bite waxes. The flow of several bite waxes as measured by penetration at 37° C ranges

from 2.5% to 22%, indicating that these waxes are susceptible to distortion on removal from the mouth.

SELECTED PROBLEMS

Problem 1. The investing of a wax pattern was delayed for a day, and the gold alloy casting that was produced did not fit. What probably caused this problem and can it be corrected?

Solution a. Residual stresses are always present in wax patterns from manipulation, and they may be released during storage. To minimize distortion, invest the wax pattern promptly.

Solution b. Distortion of the wax pattern may have occurred during spruing or during removal of the pattern from the die. A sprued pattern may be replaced on the die to evaluate and readapt the margins.

Problem 2. A wax pattern that had been refrigerated was invested, and the gold alloy casting that was produced did not fit. What probably caused this problem, and how can it be corrected?

Solution. Inlay waxes have high coefficients of thermal expansion. Cooling and heating of a pattern can result in a nonuniform dimensional change. A refrigerated wax pattern should be allowed to warm to room temperature, and its margins should be readapted before proceeding with investing.

Problem 3. The internal surface of a wax pattern prepared on a silver-plated die showed a wrinkled appearance. What caused this problem, and how can it be corrected?

Solution. When molten wax is flowed incrementally onto a cool metal die, the wax next to the die solidifies rapidly. Solidification of adjacent wax occurs more slowly and pulls the previously congealed wax away from the die, resulting in poor surface adaptation. A metal die should be warmed to about 32° C under an electric light or on a heating pad during waxing. An alternative solution is to use a soft wax at the cervical margins.

Problem 4. A wax-up of a complete denture was completed and stored overnight on an articulator. The next day the posterior teeth were no longer in contact. What happened during the storage period, and how can the problem be corrected?

Solution. The art portion of the wax-up is done after the teeth have been articulated. A hot spatula and an alcohol torch are used for shaping the wax, causing it to expand. Subsequent contraction of the wax can occur overnight, thereby moving the teeth out of articulation. This contraction can be minimized by not working in any one area for too long and by not applying too much heat. The waxed denture should be flasked soon after completion of the wax-up to minimize distortion caused by the release of residual stresses in the wax.

Problem 5. The impression wax forming a posterior palatal seal to a maxillary denture impression pulled away from the polysulfide rubber impression material in several areas when the impression was removed from the mouth. What caused this problem, and how can it be corrected?

Solution. Impression wax adheres poorly to polysulfide and silicone impression materials. The separation can be prevented by applying a very thin layer of sticky wax to the area of the impression material where the impression wax is to be applied. The impression wax will adhere to the sticky wax.

Problem 6. The broken pieces of a denture were joined with baseplate wax, flasked, and processed with heat-cured acrylic. However, the repaired denture did not fit. What may have caused this problem, and how can it be corrected?

Solution. Baseplate wax will flow somewhat if subjected to stress. The denture pieces held together by wax may move relative to each other during the repair process. Pieces to be repaired should be joined with sticky wax. It is brittle and will break rather than distort, thus readily indicating that the pieces have moved.

■ REFERENCES

Anderson JN: *Applied dental materials,* ed 5, Oxford, 1976, Blackwell Scientific.

Bennett H: *Industrial waxes,* vols 1 and 2, Brooklyn, 1963, Chemical Publishing.

Coleman RL: Physical properties of dental materials, US Bureau of Standards, Research Paper No. 32, *J Res Nat Bur Stand* 1:867, 1928.

Council on Dental Materials, Instruments, and Equipment: Revised ANSI/ADA Specification No. 4 for inlay wax, *J Am Dent Assoc* 108:88, 1984.

Craig RG, Eick JD, Peyton FA: Flow of binary and tertiary mixtures of waxes, *J Dent Res* 45:397, 1966.

Craig RG, Eick JD, Peyton FA: Properties of natural waxes used in dentistry, *J Dent Res* 44:1308, 1965.

Craig RG, Eick JD, Peyton FA: Strength properties of waxes at various temperatures and their practical application, *J Dent Res* 46:300, 1967.

Craig RG, Powers JM, Peyton FA: Differential thermal analysis of commercial and dental waxes, *J Dent Res* 46:1090, 1967.

Craig RG, Powers JM, Peyton FA: Thermogravimetric analysis of waxes, *J Dent Res* 50:450, 1971.

Dirksen LC: Composition and properties of a wax for lower impressions, *J Am Dent Assoc* 26:270, 1939.

Grajower R: A new method for determining the thermal expansion of dental waxes, *J Dent Res* 57:659, 1978.

Grossman LI: *Dental formulas and aids to dental practice,* Philadelphia, 1952, Lea & Febiger.

Hollenback GM, Rhodes JE: A study of the behavior of pattern wax, *J South Calif State Dent Assoc* 27:419, 1959.

Kotsiomiti E, McCabe JF: Stability of dental waxes following repeated heatings, *J Oral Rehabil* 22:135, 1995.

Lasater RL: Control of wax distortion by manipulation, *J Am Dent Assoc* 27:518, 1940.

Ludwig FJ, Jr: Modern instrumental wax analysis, *Soap & Chem Spec* 42(3):70, 1966.

Markley MR: *The wax pattern,* Dental Clinics of North America, Symposium on Dental Materials, Philadelphia, Nov 1958, Saunders.

Maves TW: Recent experiments demonstrating wax distortion on all wax patterns when heat is applied, *J Am Dent Assoc* 19:606, 1932.

McCrorie JW: Corrective impression waxes, *Br Dent J* 152:95, 1982.

McCrorie JW: Dental modelling waxes: A new approach to formulation, *Br Dent J* 132:189, 1972.

Morrison JT, Duncanson MG, Jr, Shillingburg HT, Jr: Wetting effects of surface treatments on inlay wax-investment combinations, *J Dent Res* 60:1858, 1981.

Nelson EA: Practical applications of crowns and inlay casting technics, *J Am Dent Assoc* 27:588, 1940.

Ohashi M, Paffenbarger GC: Melting, flow, and thermal expansion characteristics of some dental and commercial waxes, *J Am Dent Assoc* 72:1141, 1966.

Ohashi M, Paffenbarger GC: Some flow characteristics at 37° C of ternary wax mixtures that may have possible dental uses, *J Nihon Univ Sch Dent* 11:109, 1969.

Phillips RW: *Skinner's science of dental materials,* ed 8, Philadelphia, 1982, Saunders.

Phillips RW, Biggs DH: Distortion of wax patterns as influenced by storage time, storage temperature, and temperature of wax manipulation, *J Am Dent Assoc* 41:28, 1950.

Powers JM, Craig RG: Penetration of commerical and dental waxes, *J Dent Res* 53:402, 1974.

Powers JM, Craig RG: Thermal analysis of dental impression waxes, *J Dent Res* 57:37, 1978.

Powers JM, Craig RG, Peyton FA: Calorimetric analysis of commercial and dental waxes, *J Dent Res* 48:1165, 1969.

Smith DC, Earnshaw R, McCrorie JW: Some properties of modelling and baseplate waxes, *Br Dent J* 118:437, 1965.

Taylor NO: Progress report. Research on dental materials: the research program; cooperative work on inlay casting technic, *J Am Dent Assoc* 18:294, 1931.

Taylor NO, Paffenbarger GC: A survey of current inlay casting technics, *J Am Dent Assoc* 17:2058, 1930.

Taylor PB: Inlay casting procedure—its evolution and the effect of manipulatory variables. In Anderson GM, editor: *Proceedings of the Dental Centenary Celebration,* Baltimore, 1940, Maryland State Dental Association.

U.S. General Services Administration, Federal Supply Service, Federal Specification No. U-W-135, July 31, 1947, Wax, baseplate, dental; No. U-W-138, May 12, 1947, Wax, boxing, dental; No. U-W-140, March 16, 1953, Wax, casting, dental; No. U-W-141a, Dec 6, 1956, Wax, dental (casting inlay); No. U-W-00149a (DSA-DM), Sept 9, 1966, Wax, sticky, dental; No. U-W-156, Aug 17, 1948, Wax, utility, dental.

Warth AH: *The chemistry and technology of waxes,* ed 2, New York, 1956, Reinhold.

Washburn KC: Inlay wax and its manipulation, *Ill Dent J* 16:409, 1947.

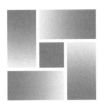

14 *Noble Dental Alloys and Solders*

Noble dental alloys have undergone a tremendous evolution since the U.S. government lifted its support on the price of gold in 1969. Before then, over 95% of fixed dental protheses in the United States were made of alloys containing a minimum of 75% by weight gold and other noble metals. However, when the price of gold increased from $35 per ounce to over $400 per ounce in the early 1980s, the development of alternative alloys increased dramatically to reduce the cost of cast dental restorations. These alternative alloys included alloys with reduced gold content, but also included alloys that contained no gold and alloys that contained no noble metal. Today, alternative alloys compose the majority of alloys used in the United States and a significant portion of alloys used in other countries.

This chapter will focus on dental casting alloys that have a noble metal content of at least 25% by weight. In addition, wrought noble alloys and solders will be discussed. The limit of 25 wt% is somewhat arbitrary, but represents the limit established by the American Dental Association for alloys that can be classified as noble alloys. Alloys with less than 25% noble metal will be discussed in Chapter 15. The first section of the chapter will survey the metallic elements that compose the noble dental alloys. In subsequent sections, the physical and chemical properties of the noble dental alloys, both cast and wrought, will be presented. Finally, soldering and soldering techniques using noble solders will be discussed.

■ METALLIC ELEMENTS USED IN DENTAL ALLOYS

For dental restorations, it is necessary to combine various elements to produce alloys with adequate properties for dental applications because none of the elements themselves have properties that are suitable. These alloys may be used for dental restorations as cast alloys, or may be manipulated into wire or other wrought forms. The metallic elements that make up dental alloys can be divided into two major groups, the noble metals and the base metals.

Noble Metals

Noble metals are elements with a good metallic surface that retain their surface in dry air. They react easily with sulfur to form sulfides, but their resistance to oxidation, tarnish, and corrosion during heating, casting, soldering, or use in the mouth is very good. The noble metals are gold, platinum, palladium, iridium, rhodium, osmium, and ruthenium (Fig. 14-1). These metals can be subdivided into two groups. The metals of the first group, consisting of ruthenium, rhodium, and palladium, have atomic weights of approximately 100 and densities of 11-12 g/cc. The metals of the second group, consisting of osmium, iridium, platinum, and gold, have atomic weights of about 190 and densities of 19-22 g/cc. The melting points of members of each group decrease with increasing atomic weight. Thus, ruthenium melts at 2310° C, rhodium at 1966° C, and palladium at 1554° C. In the second group the melting points range from 3045° C for osmium to 1064° C for gold. The noble metals, together with silver, are sometimes called precious metals. However, the terms *noble* and *precious* are not synonymous because silver is not a noble metal.

Gold (Au)

Pure gold is a soft, malleable, ductile metal that has a rich yellow color with a strong metallic luster. Although pure gold is the most ductile and malleable

Periodic table of the elements

1																	18
1 H 1.0079	2																2 He 4.00260
3 Li 6.941	4 Be 9.01218											5 B 10.81	6 C 12.011	7 N 14.0067	8 O 15.9994	9 F 18.9984	10 Ne 20.179
11 Na 22.9898	12 Mg 24.305	3	4	5	6	7	8	9	10	11	12	13 Al 26.9815	14 Si 28.0855	15 P 30.9738	16 S 32.06	17 Cl 35.453	18 Ar 39.948
19 K 39.0983	20 Ca 40.08	21 Sc 44.9559	22 Ti 47.88	23 V 50.9415	24 Cr 51.996	25 Mn 54.9380	26 Fe 55.847	27 Co 58.9332	28 Ni 58.69	29 Cu 63.546	30 Zn 65.39	31 Ga 69.72	32 Ge 72.59	33 As 74.9216	34 Se 78.96	35 Br 79.904	36 Kr 83.80
37 Rb 85.4678	38 Sr 87.62	39 Y 88.9059	40 Zr 91.224	41 Nb 92.9064	42 Mo 95.94	43 Tc (98)	44 Ru 101.07	45 Rh 102.906	46 Pd 106.42	47 Ag 107.868	48 Cd 112.41	49 In 114.82	50 Sn 118.71	51 Sb 121.75	52 Te 127.60	53 I 126.905	54 Xe 131.29
55 Cs 132.905	56 Ba 137.33	57 La ★ 138.906	72 Hf 178.49	73 Ta 180.948	74 W 183.85	75 Re 186.207	76 Os 190.2	77 Ir 192.22	78 Pt 195.08	79 Au 196.967	80 Hg 200.59	81 Tl 204.383	82 Pb 207.2	83 Bi 208.980	84 Po (209)	85 At (210)	86 Rn (222)
87 Fr (223)	88 Ra 226.025	89 Ac ▲ 227.028	104 Unq (261)	105 Unp (262)	106 Unh (263)	107 Uns (262)											

★ Lanthanide series	58 Ce 140.12	59 Pr 140.908	60 Nd 144.24	61 Pm (145)	62 Sm 150.36	63 Eu 151.96	64 Gd 157.25	65 Tb 158.925	66 Dy 162.50	67 Ho 164.930	68 Er 167.26	69 Tm 168.934	70 Yb 173.04	71 Lu 174.967
▲ Actinide series	90 Th 232.038	91 Pa 231.036	92 U 238.029	93 Np 237.048	94 Pu (244)	95 Am (243)	96 Cm (247)	97 Bk (247)	98 Cf (251)	99 Es (252)	100 Fm (257)	101 Md (258)	102 No (259)	103 Lr (260)

Fig. 14-1 Periodic table of the elements; note the location of the noble metals 44-46 and 76-79. Elements 104 and higher are not shown here. (Adapted from *Chemical and Engineering News,* Feb 4, 1985, p. 27.)

of all metals, it ranks much lower in strength. Gold melts at 1064° C and has a density of 19.32 g/cc. The density depends somewhat on the condition of the metal, whether it is cast, rolled, or drawn into wire. Small amounts of impurities have a pronounced effect on the mechanical properties of gold and its alloys. The presence of less than 0.2% lead causes gold to be extremely brittle. Mercury in small quantities also has a harmful effect on its properties. Therefore scrap of other dental alloys such as technic alloy or other base metal alloys including amalgam should not be mixed with gold used for dental restorations. The addition of calcium to pure gold improves the mechanical properties of gold used for gold foil restorations.

Air or water at any temperature does not affect or tarnish gold. Gold is not soluble in sulfuric, nitric, or hydrochloric acids. However, it readily dissolves in combinations of nitric and hydrochloric acids (aqua regia) to form the trichloride of gold ($AuCl_3$). It is also dissolved by a few other chemicals such as potassium cyanide and solutions of bromine or chlorine.

Because gold is nearly as soft as lead, it must be alloyed with copper, silver, platinum, and other metals to develop the hardness, durability, and elasticity necessary in dental alloys, coins, and jewelry. Through appropriate refining and purification, gold with an extremely high degree of purity may be produced. Such highly refined ingots of pure gold (99.99% by weight) serve as the starting material for gold foil.

Gold foil is formed by a process known as gold beating. High-purity gold is first passed through a series of rollers and then annealed until the gold is in a ribbon form about 0.0025 mm thick, which is comparable to the thickness of tissue paper. The ribbon of gold is cut into small pieces, and each piece is placed between two sheets of paper, which are then

TABLE 14-1   Physical and Mechanical Properties of Cast Pure Gold, Gold Alloys, and Condensed Gold Foil

Material	Density (g/cc)	Hardness (VHN/BHN) (kg/mm^2)	Tensile Strength (MPa)	Elongation (%)
Cast 24 k gold	19.3	28 (VHN)	105	30
Cast 22 k gold	–	60 (VHN)	240	22
Coin gold	–	85 (BHN)	395	30
Typical Au-based casting alloy (70 wt% Au)*	15.6	135/195 (VHN)	425/525	30/12
Condensed gold foil†	19.1	60 (VHN)	250	12.8

*Values are for softened/hardened condition.
†Adapted from Rule RW: *J Am Dent Assoc* 24:583, 1937.

placed one over the other to form a packet. The packet, which may contain 200 to 250 pieces of the small gold ribbons, is then beaten by a hammer until the desired thickness of gold is obtained, usually 0.00064 mm. Once the desired thickness is obtained, the foil is carefully weighed and annealed. Purity in the process of manufacturing the gold foil is critical to maintaining its cohesive properties.

If uncontaminated, gold foil is cohesive, that is it can be welded together at room temperature. This cohesive property has been exploited in the use of gold foil as a dental restorative material. If manipulated properly, small pieces of foil can be inserted and condensed into cavity preparations in teeth, providing a restoration with considerable longevity. As Table 14-1 shows, condensed gold foil has a tensile strength and hardness over twice that of pure cast gold. The reduced elongation of foil compared to cast gold is evidence of the considerable work-hardening, which the condensation process has accomplished. It is this improvement of physical properties by work hardening that makes the gold acceptable as a restorative material in some areas of the mouth. Without the improvement in properties, cast gold would lack sufficient strength and hardness to serve as a restorative material. The use of gold foil restorations is less in recent years because of the time and skill required to properly place these materials and the development of more esthetic (tooth-colored) restorative materials for areas where foil restorations were placed.

Platinum (Pt)

Platinum is a bluish-white metal with a melting point of 1772° C and a density of 21.45 g/cc. It is tough, ductile, and malleable and can be produced as foil or fine-drawn wire. Platinum has a hardness similar to copper. Pure platinum has numerous applications in dentistry because of its high fusing point and resistance to oral conditions and elevated temperatures. Platinum foil serves as a matrix for the construction of fused porcelain restorations because it does not oxidize at high temperatures. Platinum foil also has a higher melting point than porcelain and has a coefficient of expansion sufficiently close to that of porcelain to prevent buckling of the metal or fracture of the porcelain during changes in temperature. Platinum has been used as pins and posts in crown and bridge restorations, and alloys may be cast or soldered to the posts without damage.

Platinum adds greatly to the hardness and elastic qualities of gold, and some dental casting alloys and wires contain quantities of platinum up to 8% combined with other metals. Platinum is a major component of alloys used for precision attachments in complex crown and bridge restorations because these alloys have excellent wear characteristics and high melting ranges. The high melting range is necessary because other gold alloys must be cast to these attachments without distortion of the attachment. Platinum tends to lighten the color of yellow gold-based alloys.

Palladium (Pd)

Palladium is a white metal somewhat darker than platinum. It is malleable and ductile with a melting point of 1554° C and a density of 12.02 g/cc. Its density is a little more than half that of platinum and gold. Palladium has the quality of absorbing or occluding large quantities of hydrogen gas when heated. This can be an undesirable quality when alloys containing palladium are heated with an improperly adjusted gas-air torch.

Palladium is not used in the pure state in dentistry, but it is used extensively in dental alloys. Palladium can be combined with gold, silver, copper, cobalt, tin, indium, or gallium for dental alloys. Because it imparts many of the properties of platinum to dental alloys but is cheaper, it is often used as a replacement for platinum. Alloys are readily formed between gold and palladium, and palladium quantities of as low as 5% by weight have a pronounced effect on whitening the color of yellow gold-based alloys. Palladium-gold alloys with a palladium content of ≥10% by weight are white. Alloys of palladium and the other elements previously mentioned are available as substitutes for yellow gold alloys, and the mechanical properties of the palladium-based alloys may be as good or better than many traditional gold-based alloys. Although many of the palladium-based alloys are white in color, some, such as palladium-indium-silver alloys, are yellow.

Iridium (Ir), ruthenium (Ru), and rhodium (Rh)

Iridium and ruthenium are used in small amounts in dental alloys as grain-refiners to keep the grain size in the alloy small. A small grain size is desirable because it improves the mechanical properties of the alloys and improves the uniformity of properties within an alloy. As little as 0.005% (50 ppm) of iridium is effective in reducing the grain size. Ruthenium has a similar effect. The grain refining properties of these elements occur largely because of their extremely high melting points. Iridium melts at 2410° C and ruthenium at 2310° C. Thus, these elements do not melt during the casting of the alloy and serve as nucleating centers for the melt as it cools, resulting in a fine-grained alloy.

Rhodium also has a high melting point (1966° C) and has been used in alloys with platinum to form wire for thermocouples. These thermocouples help measure the temperature in porcelain furnaces used to make dental restorations.

Base Metals

Several base metals are combined with noble metals to develop alloys with properties that are suitable for dental restorations. Base metals used in dental alloys include silver, copper, zinc, indium, tin, gallium, and nickel (see Fig. 14-1).

Silver (Ag)

Silver is a white metal that is malleable and ductile. It is the best-known conductor of heat and electricity, is stronger and harder than gold, but is softer than copper. Silver has a density of 10.49 g/cc and melts at 961.9° C, which is below the melting points of both copper and gold. It is unaltered in clean, dry air at any temperature but combines with sulfur, chlorine, and phosphorus, or vapors containing these elements or their compounds. Foods containing sulfur compounds cause severe tarnish on silver. Pure silver occludes appreciable quantities of oxygen in the molten state, which makes it difficult to cast because the gas is evolved during solidification. As a result, small pits, porosity, and a rough casting surface develop. This tendency is reduced when 5-10% by weight of copper is added to the silver, for which reasons castings are made of the alloy rather than the pure metal.

Pure silver is not used in dental restorations because of the black sulfide that forms on the metal in the mouth. Adding small amounts of palladium to silver-containing alloys prevents the rapid corrosion of such alloys in the oral environment. The electroforming of silver of high purity is readily accomplished and represents a popular method of forming metal dies, as described in Chapter 11.

Silver forms a series of solid solutions with both gold and palladium and is therefore common in gold- and palladium-based dental alloys. In gold-based alloys, silver is effective in neutralizing the reddish color of alloys containing appreciable quantities of copper. Silver also hardens the gold-based alloys. In palladium-based alloys, silver is important in developing the white color. Although silver is soluble in palladium, the addition of other elements to these alloys such as copper or indium may cause the formation of multiple phases and increased corrosion.

Copper (Cu)

Copper is a malleable and ductile metal with high thermal and electrical conductivity and a characteristic red color. Pure copper melts at 1083.4° C and has a density of 8.92 g/cc. Copper forms a series of solid solutions with both gold and palladium and is therefore an important component of noble dental alloys. When added to gold-based alloys, copper imparts a reddish color to the gold and hardens the alloy. The presence of copper in gold-based alloys in quantities between approximately 40% and 88% by weight causes the ability to further improve the hardness and strength by heat treatment by formation of an ordered phase. Copper is also commonly used in palladium-based alloys where it can be used to reduce the melting point of the alloy and strengthen the alloy through solid solution hardening and formation of ordered phases. The ratio of silver and copper must be carefully balanced in both gold- and palladium-based alloys because silver and copper are not miscible. Copper is also a common component of most hard dental solders.

Zinc (Zn)

Zinc is a blue-white metal with a tendency to tarnish in moist air. Zinc melts at 419.6° C and has a density of 7.14 g/cc. In its pure form, it is a soft, brittle metal with low strength. When heated in air, zinc oxidizes readily to form a white oxide of relatively low density. It is this oxidizing property that is exploited in dental alloys. Although zinc may only be present in quantities of 1-2% by weight, it acts as a scavenger of oxygen when the alloy is melted. Thus zinc is referred to as a deoxidizing agent. Because of its low density, the resulting zinc oxide lags behind the denser molten mass during casting, and is therefore excluded from the casting. If present in too high of quantities, zinc will markedly increase the brittleness of the alloy.

Indium (In)

Indium is a soft, gray-white metal with a low melting point of 156.6° C and a density of 7.31 g/cc. Indium is not tarnished by air or water. It is used in some gold-based alloys as a replacement for zinc, and is a common minor component of some noble ceramic dental alloys. Recently, indium has been used in greater amounts (up to 30% by weight) in palladium-silver alloys to impart a yellow color to the alloy.

Tin (Sn)

Tin is a lustrous, soft, white metal that is not subject to tarnish in normal air. Tin has a melting point of 232.0° C and a density of 7.29 g/cc. Some gold-based alloys contain limited quantities of tin, usually less than 5% by weight. Tin is also an ingredient in gold-based dental solders. It combines with platinum and palladium to produce a hardening effect, but it also increases the brittleness.

Gallium (Ga)

Gallium is a grayish metal that is stable in dry air but tarnishes in moist air. It has a very low melting point of 29.8° C and a density of 5.91 g/cc. Gallium is not used in its pure form in dentistry, but is used as a component of some gold- and palladium-based dental alloys, especially ceramic alloys. The oxides of gallium are important to the bonding of the ceramic to the metal.

Nickel (Ni)

Nickel has limited application in gold- and palladium-based dental alloys, but is a common component in non-noble dental alloys. Nickel has a melting point of 1453° C and a density of 8.91 g/cc. When used in small quantities in gold-based alloys, nickel whitens the alloy and increases its strength and hardness. Ni-based alloys have increased in usage over the past 15 years. A more extensive discussion of these alloys can be found in Chapter 15.

Binary Combinations of Metals

Although most noble casting alloys have three or more elements, the properties of certain binary alloys are important because these binary combinations compose the majority of the mass of many noble alloys. An understanding of the physical and manipulative properties of these binary alloys is therefore useful in understanding the behavior of the more complex alloys. Among the noble alloys, six binary combinations of elements are important: Au-Cu, Pd-Cu, Au-Ag, Pd-Ag, Au-Pd, and Au-Pt. Phase diagrams are powerful tools for understanding the physical and manipulative properties of binary alloys. Phase diagrams for the most important binary alloys are shown in Fig. 14-2. A review of the theory of phase diagrams can be found in Chapter 5.

Alloy composition and temperature

In each phase diagram in Fig. 14-2, the horizontal axis represents the composition of the binary alloy.

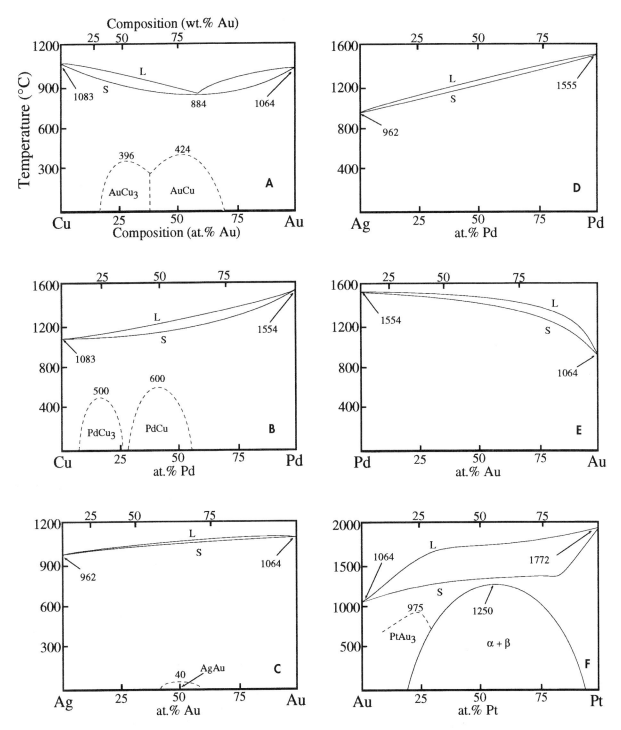

Fig. 14-2 Phase diagrams for binary combinations of **A,** copper and gold, **B,** copper and palladium, **C,** silver and gold, **D,** silver and palladium, **E,** palladium and gold, and **F,** gold and platinum. Atomic percentages are shown along the bottom of each graph; weight percentages are shown along the top. L = liquidus, S = solidus. (Adapted from Hansen M: *Constitution of Binary Alloys,* New York, 1958, McGraw Hill, p. 5 (Ag- Au), p. 41 (Ag-Pd), p. 224 (Au-Pd), p. 226 (Au-Pt), p. 612 (Cu-Pd).)

For example, in Fig. 14-2, *A*, the horizontal axis represents a series of binary alloys of gold and copper ranging in composition from 0% gold (or 100% copper) to 100% gold. The composition can be given in atomic percent (at%) or weight percent (wt%). Note that for the binary alloys shown in Fig. 14-2, the atomic percent composition is shown along the bottom of the phase diagram whereas the weight percent composition is shown along the top. The atomic and weight percent compositions of the binary alloys can differ considerably. For example, for the Au-Cu system shown in Fig. 14-2, *A*, an alloy that is 50% gold by weight is only 25% gold by atoms. For other systems, such as the Au-Pt system in Fig. 14-2, *F*, there is little difference between atomic and weight percentages. The difference between atomic and weight percentage depends on the differences in the atomic masses of the elements involved. The bigger the difference in atomic mass, the bigger the difference between the atomic and weight percentages in the binary phase diagram. From a marketing and sales standpoint, most alloy compositions are given in weight percentages because the weight percentages of gold are higher for this massive element. However, the physical and biological properties of these alloys relate best to atomic percentages. Therefore it is important to keep the difference between atomic and weight percent in mind when selecting and using noble dental casting alloys. Alloys that appear high in gold by weight percentage may in reality contain far fewer gold atoms than might be thought.

A second aspect of the phase diagrams that deserves attention is the liquidus and solidus lines. The *y* axes in Fig. 14-2 show temperature. If the temperature is above the liquidus line (marked *L*), then alloy will be completely molten. If the temperature is below the solidus line (marked *S*), then the alloy will be solid. If the temperature lies between the liquidus and solidus lines, the alloy will be partially molten. Note that the distance between the liquidus and solidus lines varies among systems in Fig. 14-2. For example, the temperature difference between these lines is small for the Ag-Au system (Fig. 14-2, *C*), much larger for the Au-Pt system (Fig. 14-2, *F*) and varies considerably with composition for the Au-Cu system (Fig. 14-2, *A*). From a manipulative standpoint, it is desirable to have a narrow liquidus-solidus

range because the alloy should be in the liquid state as little time as possible before casting. While in the liquid state, the alloy is susceptible to significant oxidation and contamination. If the liquidus-solidus line is broad, then the alloy will remain at least partially molten longer before it can be cast. The temperature of the liquidus line is also important and varies considerably among alloys and with composition. For example the liquidus line of the Au-Ag system ranges from 962-1064° C (Fig. 14-2, *C*) but the liquidus line of the Au-Pd system ranges from 1064-1554° C (Fig. 14-2, *E*). It is often desirable to have an alloy with a liquidus line at lower temperatures because the method of heating is easier, fewer side reactions occur, and shrinkage of the alloy is generally less of a problem (see Chapter 16 on Casting Procedures).

Hardening of alloys

The area below the solidus lines in Fig. 14-2 is also important to the behavior of the alloy. If this area contains no boundaries, then the binary system is a series of *solid solutions*. This means that the two elements are completely soluble in one another at all temperatures and compositions. The Ag-Pd system (Fig. 14-2, *D*) and Pd-Au system (Fig. 14-2, *E*) are examples of solid-solution systems. If the area below the solidus line contains dashed lines, then an *ordered solution* is present. An ordered solution occurs when the relationship among the two elements in the alloy assume specific and regular positions in the crystal lattice of the alloy. This situation differs from the solid solution where the positions of the elements in the crystal lattice are random. Examples of systems containing ordered solutions are the Au-Cu system (Fig. 14-2, *A*) the Pd-Cu system (Fig. 14-2, *B*) and the Au-Ag system (Fig. 14-2, *C*). Note that the ordered solutions occur over a limited range of compositions because the ratios between the elements must be correct to support the regular positions in the crystal lattices. If the area below the solidus line contains a solid line, it indicates the existence of a *second phase*. A second phase is an area with a composition distinctly different from the first phase. In the Au-Pt system (Fig. 14-2, *F*) a second phase forms between 20 and 90 at% platinum. For these compositions, if the temperature is below the phase boundary line, two phases, α and β, exist in the alloy. The presence of a second phase is important because it significantly changes the corrosion properties of an alloy.

The use of pure cast gold is not practical for dental restorations because cast gold lacks sufficient strength and hardness. Solid-solution and ordered-solution hardening are two common ways of strengthening noble dental alloys sufficiently for use in the mouth. By mixing two elements in the crystal lattice randomly (forming a solid solution), the force needed to distort the lattice may be significantly increased. For example, adding just 10% by weight of copper to gold, the tensile strength increases from 105 to 395 MPa and the Brinell hardness increases from 28 to 85 (Table 14-1). The 90-10 Au-Cu mixture is the composition used in U.S. gold coins. If the positions of the two elements become ordered (forming an ordered solution), the properties of the alloy are improved further (Table 14-1). For a typical gold-based casting alloy, the formation of an ordered solution may increase the yield strength by 50%, the tensile strength by 25%, and the hardness by at least 10%. It is important to note that the elongation of an alloy is reduced by the formation of the ordered solution. For the typical gold-based alloy the percentage elongation will decrease from 30% to about 12%.

The formation of ordered solutions has been commonly used to strengthen cast dental restorations, particularly in gold-based alloys. As shown in Fig. 14-2, *A*, the Au-Cu system supports ordered solutions between 20 and 70 at% gold. However, the manipulation of the alloy during casting will determine if the ordered solution will form. If a Au-Cu alloy containing about 50 at% gold is heated to the molten state and then cooled slowly, the mass will solidify at about 880° C as a solid solution. As the mass cools slowly to 424° C, the ordered solution will then form and will remain present at room temperature. However, if the mass is cooled rapidly to room temperature after the initial solidification, the ordered solution will not form because there is insufficient time for the mass to reorganize. Thus the alloy is trapped in a nonequilibrium state of a solid solution and will be softer, weaker, and have greater elongation. The conversion between the ordered solution and solid solution is reversible in the solid state. By heating an alloy in either condition above 424° C (but below the solidus), the state of the alloy can be selected by picking the cooling rate. Rapid cooling will preserve the solid solution and the soft condition whereas slow cooling will allow the formation of the ordered solution and the hardened condition. In alloys of gold and copper with other elements, Au-Cu ordered solutions are still possible as long as the ratio of copper to gold is greater than 30:70 (at%). As shown in Fig. 14-2, the formation of ordered solutions is possible in other noble alloy systems such as Pd-Cu and Au-Pt. The ordered solution of the Ag-Au system exists but cannot be used in practice because the transition temperature is too low (almost body temperature).

The formation of a second phase has also been used to harden dental alloys, but this method is not commonly used for noble dental alloys. The dispersion of the second phase is very important to the effectiveness of the hardening. Furthermore, the advantages of the hardening must be balanced against the liabilities of the increased corrosion often seen with multiple-phase systems. It should be noted that unlike the ordered solutions, the formation of second phases is not easily controlled by heat treatments and may not be reversible in the solid state. In fact, heat treatment commonly causes a deterioration of properties with these systems. Further discussion can be found in Chapter 15 on Cast and Wrought Base Metal Alloys.

Formulation of noble alloys

The desired qualities of noble dental casting alloys determine the selection of elements that will be used to formulate the alloys. The ideal noble casting alloy should have (1) a low melting range and narrow solidus-liquidus temperature range, (2) adequate strength, hardness and elongation, (3) a low tendency to corrode in the oral environment, and (4) low cost, among other properties. The noble elements gold and palladium are generally the foundation to which other elements are added to formulate dental casting alloys. Gold and palladium are used over other noble elements because they have relatively low melting points, have low corrosion, and form solid solutions with other alloys elements such as copper or silver (Fig. 14-2). Solid-solution systems are desirable for the formulation of alloys because they are generally easier to manufacture and manipulate, have a lower tendency to corrode than multiple phase systems, and provide increased strength through solid-solution or ordered-solution hardening. Furthermore, the systems shown in Fig. 14-2 generally have narrow liquidus-solidus ranges. Thus it is not surprising that combinations of these elements have been extensively used in the formulation of noble dental casting alloys.

The Au-Pt alloys have been developed out of fear that palladium poses a biological hazard despite no evidence that any hazard exists. These "palladium-free" alloys have the disadvantages of high cost and limited compositional flexibility. As Fig. 14-2, *F*, shows, addition of more than 20 at% platinum to gold forms a multiple phase alloy. Thus these alloy systems generally have platinum concentration below 20 at%. Furthermore, the cost of platinum is significantly higher than that of gold.

Carat and fineness of gold-based alloys

For many years the gold content of gold alloys has been described on the basis of the carat, or in terms of fineness, rather than by weight percentage. The term *carat* refers only to the gold content of the alloy and represents a 1/24 part of the whole. Thus 24 carat indicates pure gold. The carat of an alloy is designated by a small letter *k* (for example, 18k or 22k gold).

The use of the term *carat* to designate the gold content of dental alloy is less common now. It is not unusual to find the weight percentage of gold listed or to have the alloy described in terms of fineness. The fineness also refers only to the gold content and represents the number of parts of gold in each 1000 parts of alloy. Thus 24k gold is the same as 100% gold or 1000 fineness (i.e., 1000 fine). The fineness represents a precise measure of the gold content of

the alloy and often is the preferred measurement when an exact value is to be listed. An 18k gold would be designated as 750 fine, or when the decimal system is used, it would be 0.750 fine, to indicate that 750/1000 of the total is gold. A comparison of the carat, fineness, and weight percentage of gold is given in Table 14-2. Both the whole number and the decimal system are in common use, especially for noble dental solders. The fineness system is somewhat less relevant today because of the introduction of alloys that are not gold-based. It is important to emphasize that the terms *carat* and *fineness* refer only to gold content, not noble-metal content.

■ CASTING ALLOYS

Types and Composition

The number of dental casting alloys has increased dramatically in recent years. Formerly, the American Dental Association Specification No. 5 classified these alloys as types I-IV, with the content of gold and platinum group metals ranging from 83-75 wt%, respectively. Thus alloys approved by the ADA all contained high amounts of noble metal. The new ADA specification classifies alloys in a much more inclusive manner, dividing alloys into three groups: (1) *high-noble,* with a noble metal content of ≥60 wt% and a gold content of ≥40%; (2) *noble,* with a noble metal content ≥25 wt% (no stipulation for gold); and (3) *predominately base metal,* with a noble metal content <25 wt%. The newer specification therefore includes non-noble alloys as well as those with no gold but high palladium. Under the current classification, all of the older

TABLE 14-2   Comparison of Carat, Fineness, and Weight Percentage of Gold in Gold Alloys

Carat	Amount of Gold by Carats	Weight (%) of Gold	Fineness Parts/1000	Decimal
24	$^{24}/_{24}$	100.0	1000.00	1.000
22	$^{22}/_{24}$	91.7	916.66	0.916
20	$^{20}/_{24}$	83.3	833.33	0.833
18	$^{18}/_{24}$	75.0	750.00	0.750
16	$^{16}/_{24}$	66.7	666.66	0.666
14	$^{14}/_{24}$	58.3	583.33	0.583
9	$^{9}/_{24}$	37.5	374.99	0.375

TABLE 14-3 Typical Compositions (wt%) of Noble Dental Casting Alloys

Alloy Type	Ag	Au	Cu	Pd	Pt	Zn	Other
HIGH-NOBLE							
Au-Ag-Pt	11.5	78.1	–	–	9.9	–	Ir (trace)
Au-Cu-Ag-Pd-*I*	10.0	76.0	10.5	2.4	0.1	1.0	Ru (trace)
Au-Cu-Ag-Pd-*II*	25.0	56.0	11.8	5.0	0.4	1.7	Ir (trace)
NOBLE							
Au-Cu-Ag-Pd-*III*	47.0	40.0	7.5	4.0	–	1.5	Ir (trace)
Au-Ag-Pd-In	38.7	20.0	–	21.0	–	3.8	In 16.5
Pd-Cu-Ga	–	2.0	10.0	77.0	–	–	Ga 7
Ag-Pd	70	–	–	25.0	–	2.0	In 3

alloy "types" are considered high-noble alloys. The percentages used as boundaries in the new specification are somewhat arbitrary.

Although the number of casting alloys is immense, it is possible to subdivide each ADA group into several classes (Table 14-3). The predominately base metal alloys are not shown, but will be discussed in Chapter 15. These classes are simply a convenient way of organizing the diverse strategies that have been used to formulate casting alloys. For each class of alloy shown in Table 14-3, there are many variations, and the compositions shown are meant only to be representative. All of the alloys contain some zinc as a deoxidizer and either Ir or Ru as grain refiners. Some of these compositions are used for both full metal castings and porcelain-metal restorations.

There are three classes of *high-noble alloys:* the Au-Ag-Pt alloys, the Au-Cu-Ag-Pd alloys with a gold content of >70 wt% (Au-Cu-Ag-Pd-*I* in Table 14-3), and the Au-Cu-Ag-Pd alloys with a gold content of about 50-65% (Au-Cu-Ag-Pd-*II*). The Au-Ag-Pt alloys typically consist of 78 wt% gold with roughly equal amounts of silver and platinum. These alloys have been used as either casting alloys or as porcelain-metal alloys. The Au-Cu-Ag-Pd-*I* alloys are typically 75 wt% gold with approximately 10 wt% each of silver and copper and 2-3 wt% palladium. These alloys are identical to the Type III alloys under the old ADA classification. The Au-Cu-Ag-Pd-*II* alloys typically have <60 wt% gold, with the silver content increased to accommodate the reduced gold content. Occasionally, these alloys will have slightly higher palladium and lower silver percentages.

There are four classes of *noble* alloys: the Au-Cu-Ag-Pd alloys (Au-Cu-Ag-Pd-*III* in Table 14-3), Au-Ag-Pd-In alloys, Pd-Cu-Ga alloys, and Ag-Pd alloys. The Au-Cu-Ag-Pd-*III* alloys typically have a gold content of ≤40 wt%. The reduced gold is compensated primarily with silver, thus the copper and palladium contents are not changed much from the Au-Cu-Ag-Pd-*II* alloys. The Au-Ag-Pd-In alloys have a gold content of only 20 wt%, and have about 40 wt% silver, 20 wt% palladium, and 15 wt% indium. The Pd-Cu-Ga alloys have little or no gold, with about 75 wt% palladium and about equal copper and gallium. Finally, the Ag-Pd alloys have no gold, but have 70 wt% silver and 25 wt% palladium. By the ADA specification, these alloys are considered noble because of their palladium content.

As Tables 14-3 and 14-4 show, the wt% and at% of dental casting alloys can differ considerably. For example, by weight, the Au-Cu-Ag-Pd-*I* alloys have 76% gold. However, only 57% of the atoms in these alloys are gold. Other elements that have less mass than gold increase in atomic percentage. For these same alloys, the copper content by weight is 10%, but by atoms is 24%. For other alloys whose elements have similar mass, the differences between wt% and at% are less pronounced. For example, in the Ag-Pd alloys the weight and atomic percentages are similar. Weight percentages of the alloys are most commonly used by manufacturers in the production and sales of the alloys. However, the physical, chemical, and biological properties are best understood in terms of atomic percentages.

TABLE 14-4   Typical Compositions (at%) of Noble Dental Casting Alloys

Alloy Type	Ag	Au	Cu	Pd	Pt	Zn	Other
HIGH-NOBLE							
Au-Ag-Pt	19.3	71.4	–	–	9.2	–	Ir (trace)
Au-Cu-Ag-Pd-*I*	13.6	56.5	24.2	3.4	0.1	2.2	Ru (trace)
Au-Cu-Ag-Pd-*II*	30	36.6	23.9	6.1	0.3	3.4	Ir (trace)
NOBLE							
Au-Cu-Ag-Pd-*III*	53.3	24.8	14.4	4.7	–	2.8	Ir (trace)
Au-Ag-Pd-In	36.1	10.3	–	33.3	–	5.8	In 16.6
Pd-Cu-Ga	–	1.0	15.8	73.1	–	–	Ga 10.1
Ag-Pd	69.0	–	–	25.0	–	3.3	In 2.3

Note: Percentages may not add to exactly 100.0 because of rounding error in calculation of the atomic percentages.

TABLE 14-5   Physical and Mechanical Properties of Several Types of Noble Dental Casting Alloys

Alloy	Solidus (° C)	Liquidus (° C)	Color	Density (g/cc)	0.2% Yield Strength (Soft/Hard) (MPa)	Elongation (Soft/Hard) (%)	Vickers Hardness (Soft/Hard) (kg/mm^2)
HIGH-NOBLE							
Au-Ag-Pt	1045	1140	Yellow	18.4	420/470	15/9	175/195
Au-Cu-Ag-Pd-*I*	910	965	Yellow	15.6	270/400	30/12	135/195
Au-Cu-Ag-Pd-*II*	870	920	Yellow	13.8	350/600	30/10	175/260
NOBLE							
Au-Cu-Ag-Pd-*III*	865	925	Yellow	12.4	325/520	27.5/10	125/215
Au-Ag-Pd-In	875	1035	Light yellow	11.4	300/370	12/8	135/190
Pd-Cu-Ga	1100	1190	White	10.6	1145	8	425
Ag-Pd	1020	1100	White	10.6	260/320	10/8	140/155

The compositions of casting alloys determine their color. In general, if the palladium content is >10 wt%, the color of the alloy will be white. Thus the Pd-Cu-Ga and Ag-Pd alloys in Table 14-5 are white, whereas the other alloys are yellow. The Au-Ag-Pd-In alloys are an exception because they have a palladium content of >20% and retain a light-yellow color. The color of this alloy results from interactions of the indium with the palladium in the alloy. Among the alloys with yellow color, the composition will modify the shade of yellow. Generally, copper adds a reddish color and silver lightens either the red or yellow color of the alloys.

Grain Size

Recent studies have described the influence of minute quantities of various elements on the grain size of dental casting alloys. In the past, many alloys had relatively coarse grain structures. Now, by the addition of small amounts (0.005% or 50 ppm) of elements such as iridium and ruthenium, fine grain castings are produced. Adding one of these elements to the alloy is believed to develop centers for nucleating grains throughout the alloy. Most alloy manufacturers use grain refinement in present-day products. The mechanical properties of tensile strength and elongation are improved significantly (30%) by the fine grain structure in castings, which contributes to uniformity of properties from one casting to another. Other properties, however, such as hardness and yield strength, show less effect from the grain refinement.

Properties

Melting range

Dental casting alloys do not have melting points, but they do have melting ranges because they are mixtures of elements rather than pure elements. The width of the solidus-liquidus melting range is important to the manipulation of the alloys (Table 14-5). The solidus-liquidus range should be narrow to avoid having the alloy in a molten state for extended times during casting. If the alloy spends a long time in the partially molten state during casting, there is increased opportunity for the formation of oxides and contamination. Most of the alloys in Table 14-5 have solidus-liquidus ranges of 70° C or less. The Au-Ag-Pt alloys, Pd-Cu-Ga alloys, and Ag-Pd alloys have wider ranges, which makes them more difficult to cast without problems.

The liquidus temperature of the alloys determines their burnout temperature, the type of investment, and the type of heat-source that must be used during casting. In general, the burnout temperature must be about 500° C below the liquidus temperature. Thus, for the Au-Cu-Ag-Pd-*I* alloys, a burnout temperature of about 450-475° C should be used. If the burnout temperature approaches 700° C, a gypsum-bonded investment cannot be used because the calcium sulfate will decompose and embrittle the alloys. At temperatures near 700° C or greater, a phosphate-bonded investment is used. From Table 14-5, a gypsum-bonded investment may be used with the Au-Cu-Ag-Pd-*I, II,* and *III* and the Au-Ag-Pd-In alloys, but a phosphate-bonded investment is advisable for the other alloys. The gas-air torch will adequately heat alloys with liquidus temperatures below 1100° C. Above this temperature, a gas-oxygen torch or electrical induction method must be used. Again from Table 14-5, a gas-air torch would only be acceptable for the Au-Cu-Ag-Pd-*I, II,* and *III* and the Au-Ag-Pd-In alloys.

The composition of the alloys determines the liquidus temperatures. If the alloy contains a significant amount of an element that has a high melting point, then the alloy is likely to have a high liquidus. Thus alloys that contain significant amounts of palladium or platinum, which both have high melting points, will have high liquidus temperatures. In Table 14-5, these include the Pd-Cu-Ga, Ag-Pd, and Au-Ag-Pt alloys.

The solidus temperature is important to both soldering and formation of ordered phases, because during both of these operations, the shape of the alloys is to be retained. Therefore during soldering or hardening-softening, the alloy may only be heated to the solidus before melting occurs. In practice, it is desirable to limit heating to 50° C below the solidus to avoid local melting or distortion of the casting.

Density

Density is important during the acceleration of the molten alloy into the mold during casting. Alloys with high densities will generally accelerate faster and tend to form complete castings more easily. Among the alloys shown in Table 14-5, all have densities sufficient for convenient casting. Lower densities (7-8 g/cc) seen in the predominately base metal alloys sometimes present problems in this regard. Alloys in Table 14-5 with high densities generally contain higher amounts of denser elements such as gold or platinum. Thus the Au-Ag-Pt alloys and Au-Cu-Ag-Pd-*I* alloys are among the most dense of the casting alloys.

Strength

Strength of alloys can be measured by either the yield strength or tensile strength. Although tensile strength represents the maximum strength of the alloy, the yield strength is more useful in dental applications because it is the stress at which permanent deformation of the alloys occurs. Because permanent deformation of dental castings is generally undesirable, the yield strength is a reasonable practical maximum strength for dental applications. The yield strengths for the different classes of alloys are shown in Table 14-5. Where applicable, the hard and soft conditions, resulting from the formation of ordered solutions, are shown. For several alloys, such as Au-Cu-Ag-Pd-*I, II,* and *III,* the formation of the ordered phase increases the yield strength significantly. For example, the yield strength of the Au-Cu-Ag-Pd-*II* alloys increases from 350 to 600 MPa with the formation of an ordered phase. For other alloys, such as the Au-Ag-Pt and Ag-Pd alloys, the increase in yield strength is more modest in the hardened condition. The Pd-Cu-Ga alloys do not support the formation of ordered phase because the ratio of palladium and copper are not in the correct range for ordered phase formation (Table 14-3 and Fig. 14-2, *B*).

The yield strengths of these alloys range from 320-1145 MPa (hard condition). The strongest alloy is the Pd-Cu-Ga alloy with a yield strength of 1145 MPa. The other alloys range in strength from 320-600 MPa. These latter yield strengths are adequate for dental applications and are generally in the same range as those for the base metal alloys, which range from 495-600. The effect of solid-solution hardening by the addition of copper and silver to the gold or palladium base is significant for these alloys. Pure cast gold has a *tensile* strength of 105 MPa (see Table 14-1). With the addition of 10 wt% copper (coin gold), solid-solution hardening increases the tensile strength to 395 MPa. With the further addition of 10 wt% silver and 3 wt% palladium (Au-Cu-Ag-Pd-*I*), the tensile strength increases to about 450 MPa and 550 MPa in the hard condition.

Hardness

Hardness is a good indicator of the ability of an alloy to resist local permanent deformation under occlusal load. Although the relationships are complex, hardness is related to yield strength and gives some indication of the difficulty in polishing the alloy. Alloys with high hardness generally will have high yield strengths and are more difficult to polish. As Table 14-5 shows, the values for hardness generally parallel those for yield strength. In the hard condition, the hardness of these alloys ranges from 155 kg/mm^2 for the Ag-Pd alloys to 425 kg/mm^2 for the Pd-Cu-Ga alloys. More typically the hardness of the noble casting alloys is around 200 kg/mm^2. The Ag-Pd alloys are particularly soft because of the high concentration of silver, which is a soft metal. The Pd-Cu-Ga alloys are particularly hard because of the high concentration of Pd, which is a hard metal. The hardness of most noble casting alloys is less than that of enamel (343 kg/mm^2), and typically less

than that of the base metal alloys. If the hardness of an alloy is greater than enamel, it will tend to wear the enamel of the teeth opposing the restoration.

Elongation

The elongation is a measure of the ductility of the alloy. For crown and bridge applications, the value of elongation for an alloy is generally not a big concern because permanent deformation of the alloys is generally not desirable. However, the elongation will indicate if the alloy can be burnished. Alloys with high elongation can be burnished without fracture. Elongation is sensitive to the presence or absence of an ordered phase, as shown in Table 14-5. In the hardened condition, the elongation will drop significantly. For example, for the Au-Cu-Ag-Pd-*II* alloys, the elongation is 30% in the soft condition versus only 10% in the hard condition. In the soft condition, the elongation of noble dental casting alloys ranges from 8 to 30%. These alloys are substantially more ductile than the base metal alloys which have elongation on the order of 1-2%.

Gold-Based Alloys for Porcelain-Metal Restorations

Alloys used for porcelain-to-metal restorations are discussed in detail in Chapter 18.

■ WROUGHT ALLOYS

Alloys that are worked and adapted into prefabricated forms for use in dental restorations are described as wrought alloys. The work done to the alloy is usually at a temperature far below the solidus of the alloys, and is therefore referred to as cold work. Wrought forms may include precision attachments, backings for artificial teeth, and wire in various cross-sectional shapes. Wrought alloys are used in two ways in dental prostheses. First, they can be soldered to an existing appliance, as a wrought wire clasp is soldered to a previously cast partial denture framework. Second, they can be embedded into a cast framework by "casting to" the alloy, as a precision attachment is "cast-to" the retainer of a crown, bridge, or partial denture. The physical properties that are required of the wrought alloy will depend on the technique used and the composition of the alloy in the existing appliance.

Microstructure

As indicated in Chapter 5, the microstructure of wrought alloys is fibrous. This fibrous structure results from the cold work applied during the operations that shape the alloy into its final form. Wires or other wrought forms normally have a measurable increase in tensile strength and hardness when compared with corresponding cast structures. The increase in properties results from the entangled, fibrous internal structure created by the cold work.

Wrought forms will recrystallize during heating operations unless caution is exercised. During recrystallization, the fibrous microstructure is converted to a grained structure similar to the structure of a cast form. In general, the amount of recrystallization increases as both the heating time and temperature become excessive. For example, in most noble dental wires, a short heating cycle during the soldering operation is not sufficient to appreciably recrystallize the wire, even though the temperature approaches the fusion temperature. However, a prolonged heating period of 30-60 seconds or longer may cause recrystallization, depending on the time, temperature, alloy composition, and manner in which the wire was fabricated. Recrystallization results in a reduction in mechanical properties in proportion to the amount of recrystallization. Severe recrystallization can cause the wrought forms to become brittle in the area of recrystallization. Therefore, heating operations must be minimized when working with wrought forms.

Composition

By the current ADA definitions, all alloys used for wrought forms are high-noble alloys, except one, which is a noble alloy (Table 14-6). As with the casting alloys, several strategies have been used to formulate alloys with appropriate properties. The compositions in Table 14-6 are not inclusive of all available wrought alloys but are intended to demonstrate typical alloys. These compositions are designed to provide a range of melting ranges and mechanical properties that are appropriate for wrought alloy applications. The Pt-Au-Pd alloys contain primarily platinum with equal amounts (27 wt%) of palladium and gold. These "PGP" alloys have been commonly used as clasping wires on removable partial dentures. The Au-Pt-Pd alloys are primarily gold with platinum and palladium. The Au-Pt-Cu-Ag, Au-Pt-Ag-Cu, and Au-Ag-Cu-Pd alloys all contain approximately 60 wt% gold, but have adopted different strategies for the remaining 40% of the mass. The first two of these alloys contain about 15 wt% platinum with the balance in silver, copper, and palladium, whereas the third of these alloys contains no platinum and higher amounts of silver. The last alloy shown in Table 14-6 contains no appreciable gold or platinum, but consists of palladium and silver in approximately equal amounts with about 16 wt% copper. The Au-Ag-Cu-Pd wrought alloy (Table 14-6) is similar to the Au-Cu-Ag-Pd-*II* casting alloy (see Table 14-3). These alloys differ only slightly in the gold to silver ratio. Other wrought alloys differ from the casting alloys primarily in their higher platinum contents and absence of iridium or ruthenium grain refiners. Platinum is added to increase the melting temperature of the alloys. The grain refinement is not necessary because these alloys will be cold-worked into their final forms.

Properties

The properties of alloys used for wrought applications are shown in Table 14-7. The solidus of

TABLE 14-6 Composition of Typical Wrought Dental Alloys (wt%)

Alloy	Ag	Au	Cu	Pd	Pt	Other
Pt-Au-Pd*	–	27	–	27	45	
Au-Pt-Pd	–	60	–	15	24	Ir 1.0
Au-Pt-Cu-Ag	8.5	60	10	5.5	16	
Au-Pt-Ag-Cu	14	63	9	–	14	
Au-Ag-Cu-Pd	18.5	63	12	5	–	Zn 1.5
Pd-Ag-Cu*	39	–	16	43	1	

*Adapted from Lyman T: *Metals Handbook,* vol 1, *Properties and selection of metals,* ed 8, Metals Park, Ohio, 1961, American Society for Metals.

these alloys ranges from 875° C for the Au-Ag-Cu-Pd alloy to 1500° C for the Pt-Au-Pd alloy. If the wrought form is to be cast-to or soldered-to, the solidus must be sufficiently high so that the form does not melt or lose its fibrous structure. The solidus that is required will depend on the metals to be joined, the solder, and the burnout and casting temperatures to be used. In general, alloys with high solidus temperatures also have higher recrystallization temperatures. The color of these alloys are mostly white because of the high platinum and palladium contents. Exceptions are the Au-Pt-Ag-Cu and Au-Ag-Cu-Pd alloys, which are light yellow and yellow, respectively. Yield strength, elongation, and hardness are all properties that are relevant to wrought alloys (Table 14-7). The wrought form must generally have a yield strength low enough to allow for adjustment (of a clasp or attachment), but be high enough that permanent distortion does not occur in service. Furthermore, the elongation must be sufficient to allow for adjustment without fracture. Three of the wrought alloys shown in Table 14-7 can be hardened by formation of ordered phases. The Au-Pt-Ag-Cu and Au-Ag-Cu-Pd alloys are hardened by a Au-Cu ordered phase, whereas the Pd-Ag-Cu alloys are hardened by a Pd-Cu ordered phase. As with the casting alloys, the ordered phase imparts significantly more strength and hardness to the alloy and lower elongation.

■ SOLDERS AND SOLDERING OPERATIONS

It is often necessary to construct a dental appliance in two or more parts and then join them together by either a soldering or welding process. The terms *soldering, welding,* and *brazing* have specific meanings in industry. The term *welding* is used if two pieces of metal are joined together without adding another metal; that is, the metal pieces are heated to a high enough temperature so they attach to each other. The words *soldering* and *brazing* are used if two pieces of metal are joined by adding a third metal. If the temperature used in the process is below 425° C, the operation is called soldering; however, if the temperature is above 425° C, the operation is called brazing. In dentistry the parts are joined at temperature above 425° C, so the operation should be called brazing. However, it is most commonly called soldering. Therefore in this chapter such an operation is called soldering.

Types of Solders

In general, solders may be divided into two major groups: soft and hard. The soft solders include the lead-tin alloys of eutectic type with a low melting point, sometimes known as "plumber's" solder. The soft solders have several interesting properties, including a low fusion range of about 260° C or less, which permits them to be applied by simple means, such as by a hot soldering iron. Many also possess good

TABLE 14-7   Properties of Typical Wrought Dental Alloys

Alloy	Solidus (° C)	Color	Property 0.2% Yield Strength (Soft/Hard) (MPa)	Elongation (Soft/Hard) (%)	Vickers Hardness (Soft/Hard) (kg/mm^2)
Pt-Au-Pd*	1500	White	750	14	270
Au-Pt-Pd	1400	White	450	20	180
Au-Pt-Cu-Ag	1045	White	400	35	190
Au-Pt-Ag-Cu	935	Light yellow	450/700	30/10	190/285
Au-Ag-Cu-Pd	875	Yellow	400/750	35/8	170/260
Pd-Ag-Cu*	1060	White	515/810	20/12	210/300

*Adapted from Lyman T: *Metals Handbook,* vol 1, *Properties and selection of metals,* ed 8, Metals Park, Ohio, 1961, American Society for Metals.

working or mechanical properties, making them favorable for use in industry. However, the soft solders lack corrosion resistance, which makes them impractical for dental applications.

Hard solders have a much higher melting temperature than soft solders and also possess greater hardness and strength. The high melting range of these solders precludes the use of soldering irons for melting. In industry, special melting methods are used, such as heating with a gas torch, in a furnace, or with other special heating devices.

Two types of hard solders are used in dentistry. Gold solders that have good tarnish and corrosion resistance are extensively used in crown and bridge applications. Silver solders are commonly used in orthodontic appliances. For dental applications, the gold or silver solders are normally melted with a specifically designed dental type of gas blowtorch. Occasionally a method involving an electric furnace or other heating equipment is used, but this is the exception rather than common practice.

Two techniques of dental soldering are used to assemble dental appliances. One is known as "freehand" soldering, commonly used in assembling orthodontic and other appliances, and the other is "investment" soldering, customarily used in assembling bridges and similar restorations. In freehand soldering the parts to be assembled are manually held in contact while the heat and solder are applied. As soon as the solder has flowed to position, the heating is discontinued, and the appliance is cooled. In investment soldering the parts to be assembled are mounted in a soldering investment and held in intimate contact by the hardened investment while the heat and solder are applied. These two techniques are described in detail in appropriate textbooks or manuals on orthodontics, crown and bridge protheses, or operative dentistry.

Basis of selecting solders

Certain principles must be observed in selecting solders, regardless of the type of application. The ideal solder includes qualities such as (1) ease of flow at relatively low temperature, (2) sufficient fluidity to freely flow when melted, (3) strength compatible with that of the structure being soldered, (4) acceptable color to give an inconspicuous joint, (5) resistance to tarnish and corrosion, and (6) resistance to pitting during heating and application. No single dental gold solder has all of these qualities; therefore manufacturers provide solders that cover a range of fineness as well as a number of solders that have special qualities. The properties of solders are significantly influenced by the method used during the soldering operation. Thus a recommended procedure must be faithfully followed to obtain the maximum quality from a product.

Composition

Gold solders for dental use are primarily alloys of gold, silver, and copper, with small quantities of tin, zinc, and sometimes phosphorus included to modify the fusion temperature and flow qualities. The typical composition and resulting fusion temperature values of a variety of gold solders are given in Table 14-8. The compositions of different solders vary

TABLE 14-8 Typical Compositions and Fusion Temperatures of Dental Gold Solders

| Solder | Fineness | Composition (% of weight) | | | | | Fusion Temperature (° C) |
		Au	Ag	Cu	Sn	Zn	
1*	0.809	80.9	8.1	6.8	2.0	2.1	868
2†	0.800	80.0	3–8	8–12	2–3	2–4	746–871
3*	0.729	72.9	12.1	10.0	2.0	2.3	835
4*	0.650	65.0	16.3	13.1	1.7	3.9	799
5†	0.600	60.0	12–32	12–22	2–3	2–4	724–835
6†	0.450	45.0	30–35	15–20	2–3	2–4	691–816

*Adapted from Coleman RL: Res Paper No 32, *J Res, Nat Bur Stand* 1:894, 1928.
†Adapted from Lyman T: *Metals handbook,* vol 1, *Properties and selection of metals,* ed 8, Metals Park, Ohio, 1961, American Society for Metals.

considerably from one another. For example, the gold content may vary from 45-81 wt%, silver from 8-30%, and copper from 7-20%, with little variation in the tin or zinc content. Most solders have a copper-to-gold ratio to support the formation of a Au-Cu ordered phase. The fusion temperature is lower for alloys that have reduced gold content, but the reduction is not as great as sometimes believed. For example, the difference in fusion temperature between solders 1 and 4 is only 69° C when the gold content is reduced by approximately 16%.

In the past, solders were commonly referred to by a carat number. The number did not describe the actual carat of the solder but rather the carat of the gold alloy on which the solder was to be used. This permitted a wide range of compositions, or actual carat values, to be used for solders described as a specific carat because the solder was intended for use with an alloy of a definite carat. For example, solders that varied in gold content from 58.5-65 wt% might be described as 18k because they were to be used on a casting made of an 18k alloy. The gold content of an 18k alloy should be 75 wt% gold, but the solders contained only 58.5-65 wt% gold. This system led to much confusion. In recent years the degree of fineness has been used to describe the various solders, such as those values designated in Table 14-8 and 14-9. This designation is appropriate because it is specific, and when the fineness is changed, the actual carat change is indicated.

Easy-flowing and free-flowing qualities

Dental gold solders are frequently described by terms such as *easy-flowing* or *free-flowing*. Although these terms are sometimes interchanged, they refer to two different qualities in the solder alloys. The easy-flowing solder is one that has a relatively low fusion temperature, and the lower the temperature of fusion, the easier to melt and form the joint. However, the difference in fusion temperatures of high- and low-fineness gold solder is approximately 56° C, so differences in flow caused by a lower fusion temperature are small among these solders (Table 14-8).

The fusion temperature of the solder must be below that of the alloys being soldered, or the joined pieces will melt during the operation. Previous discussion of casting alloys indicated that the lowest solidus values for the casting alloys are for the Au-Cu-Ag-Pd-*II* and -*III* alloys and the Au-Ag-Pd-In alloys from 865-875° C (Table 14-5). For wrought alloys, the lowest solidus values ranged from 875-935° C, although most of the wrought alloys have substantially higher solidus temperatures (Table 14-7). As Table 14-8 indicates, most of the solders have fusion temperatures below the solidus temperatures for the casting or wrought alloys. Thus solders are available for even the lowest fusing alloys. In general, the fusion temperature of the solder should be at least 56° C below that of the parts being joined to prevent distortion.

The free-flowing quality refers specifically to the ability of the solder to spread and flow freely over the surfaces of the parts being joined. This quality is closely related to the surface tension of the melted solder. The surface tension (and free-flowing qualities) also control the capillary action, which causes the melted solder to penetrate into fine openings between the parts being assembled. In general, the

TABLE 14-9   Typical Mechanical Properties of Dental Gold Solders

Solder	Fineness	Tensile Strength (Soft/Hard) (MPa)	Proportional Limit (Soft/Hard) (MPa)	Elongation (Soft/Hard) (%)	BHN (Soft/Hard) (kg/mm^2)
1*	0.809	259	142	18	78
3*	0.729	248/483	166/424	7/<1	103/180
4*	0.650	303/634	207/532	9/<1	111/199
	0.730†	221/483	166/405	3/1	112/154
	0.650†	219/436	176/376	3/1	143/192

*Adapted from Coleman RL: Res Paper No 32, *J Res, Nat Bur Stand* 1:902, 1928.
†Adapted from Gabel AB, editor; *American textbook of operative dentistry,* ed 9, Philadelphia, 1954, Lea & Febiger, p. 546.

lower-fineness solders are more fluid in the molten state than the higher-fineness solders because of the lower gold content and presence of small quantities of alloying metals such as zinc and tin. For this reason, the lower-fineness solders are preferred when joining parts because the solder flows promptly and freely into the available spaces. Solders that spread slowly are often described as being sticky, and they resist spreading even though properly heated. As a result, they tend to penetrate or "burn through" the part being soldered if the solder is forced to spread by overheating. Obviously the easy- and free-flowing qualities work together because the lower-fineness gold solders have the lowest melting range and greatest freedom of flow.

Mechanical properties

The values in Table 14-9 illustrate typical mechanical properties for dental solders. There are a wide range of strengths and hardness available. As stated previously, it is most desirable to use a solder with a strength similar to that of the parts being joined. All solders in Table 14-9 are subject to hardening by ordered-phase formation except solder 1, which does not form an ordered phase because the gold-to-copper ratio is not appropriate (Table 14-8). A considerable increase in strength and hardness can be obtained by slow-cooling the solder and allowing the ordered phase to form.

The percentage of elongation in noble solders are notably less than those of many noble casting alloys (Table 14-9 and 14-5). Even in the soft condition, the elongation ranges only from 3-9% for all of the solders except solder 1. In the hard condition the elongation is most often ≤1%, which is quite brittle. In general, it is more desirable in most appliances to obtain an improved hardness and proportional limit that accompany the ordered-phase formation than to sacrifice these properties for a small increase in elongation.

Color and tarnish resistance

The color of dental noble solders varies from deep yellow to light yellow and white in much the same manner as casting alloys. Although the ability to match the color of the appliances is an important quality of a solder, producing an inconspicuous solder joint is not difficult in practice. Obviously the location of the solder junction on the restoration and the total amount of solder applied are factors that influence color matching.

On the basis of gold content, the solders of high fineness are assumed to be more resistant to tarnish, discoloration, and corrosion in the mouth than the lower-fineness solders. However, there is little evidence or data to support such claims because no good tests are available for tarnish and discoloration of such structures. High-fineness solders are often recommended to prevent tarnish in service. However, the qualities of increased fluidity and mechanical properties associated with the lower fineness (0.650 or less) may outweigh any increased tendency of those solders to tarnish in service. Actually, the lower-fineness solders are used extensively for the assembly of dental appliances without serious tendencies to discolor.

Pitted solder joints

Hard solders have a tendency to be pitted after the soldering operation. In general, pitting results from improper heating of the solder, although some compositions of solder may be more susceptible to pitting than others. When solders of typical fineness are used, a pitted solder can often be associated with either excessive heating during the fusion of the solder or with improper fluxing during heating.

If the solder is heated to too high a temperature or for prolonged periods, the lower-melting tin and zinc in the solder can boil or oxidize and form pits or porosities as the solder solidifies. These pits often become apparent only during finishing and polishing operations. If the solder is underheated and the flux is applied in excess or improperly melted, it may be trapped in the melted solder and form pits, which are uncovered during polishing. To avoid pitting from these causes, the solder should be heated promptly to the fusion temperature, and heating should be stopped as soon as the solder has flowed into position.

Microstructure of Soldered Joints

Microscopic examination of well-formed soldered joints has shown that the solder does not combine excessively with the parts being soldered. When the solder has fused properly and has not been overheated, a well-defined boundary forms between the solder and the soldered parts. When the joint is heated too high or for too long, diffusion of elements between the solder and the parts occurs in proportion to the time and temperature excess. Studies indicate that diffusion in the soldered joint reduces the strength and quality of the joint.

Fig. 14-3 shows a microscopic view of a soldered joint between a high-noble casting alloy and a section of a Pt-Au-Pd wire used as a clasp on a removable partial denture. The sample has been etched with acid to reveal its microstructure. The wire has a typical fibrous appearance of a wrought form, and the alloy has a typical granular appearance of a cast form. The solder also has a normal granular appearance, and a sharp boundary exists between the solder and wire and the solder and the cast alloy, indicating that time or temperature of the soldering procedure was not excessive.

A less favorable soldered joint is shown in Fig. 14-4. The boundary between the wire and the solder is less sharp and is wider. This poorer adaptation may have resulted from either improper fluxing or improper heating when the solder was applied. The solder is also not ideally adapted to the cast alloy. However, there is no evidence of recrystallization of

the wire and the grain size in the alloy is unchanged, indicating that the time and temperature of heating was not excessive. Overheating would also cause diffusion between the alloys. Recrystallization of the wire, grain growth of the casting alloy, and diffusion are all undesirable because they result in a loss of physical properties, which are necessary for the successful function of the dental appliance.

The microstructure of an overheated wire is shown in Fig. 14-5. Some evidence of the original fibrous wire remains, but recrystallization has taken place throughout most of the wire. The section of wire shown in Fig. 14-5 was 2 mm from the soldered joint. More severe recrystallization occurred close to the solder, and the wire broke in service within the area adjacent to the solder. When cast structures are overheated in the presence of solder, the solder will diffuse into the alloy resulting in a new alloy that lacks strength and ductility. Overheating can also cause warpage and distortion of the appliance from large dimensional changes.

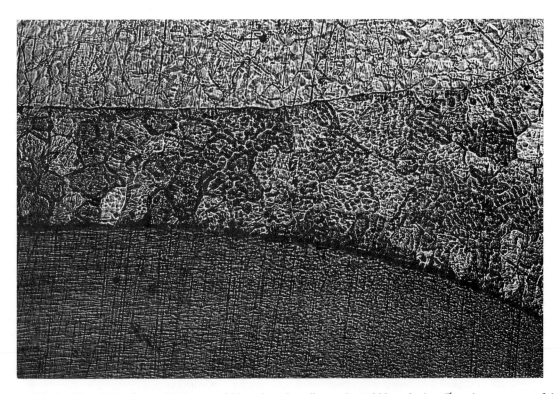

Fig. 14-3 Ideal soldered joint formed between gold-based casting alloy and a gold-based wire. *Top,* microstructure of the cast alloy; *bottom,* microstructure of the wire.

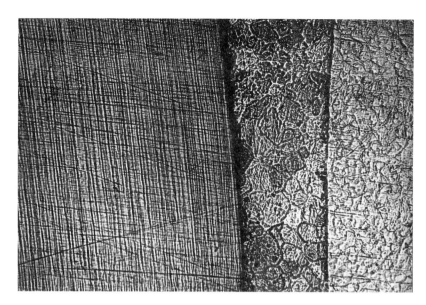

Fig. 14-4 Solder well attached to cast alloy but with less satisfactory attachment to the wire. *Left,* microstructure of wire; *right,* microstructure of the cast alloy.

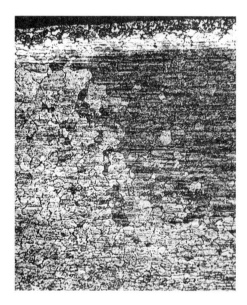

Fig. 14-5 Evidence of recrystallization resulting from excessive heating of gold wire. *Right,* original fibrous microstructure of the wire; *bottom and left,* granular structure resulting from recrystallization.

Silver Solder

Hard solders composed of silver alloys are used extensively in some industries, but their application in dentistry has been limited. These solders are also commonly known as silver solders and are used when a low-fusing solder is needed for soldering onto stainless steel or other base metal alloys. Orthodontic appliances are commonly soldered using silver solders. In general, the resistance of silver solders to tarnish is not as good as gold-based solders, but the strengths of the two types of solders are comparable.

The silver solders are composed of silver (10-80 wt%), copper (15-30%), and zinc (4-35%) with some products containing small percentages of cadmium, tin, or phosphorus to further modify the fusion temperature. The formation of the silver-copper eutectic is responsible for the low melting range found in the silver solders. The liquidus temperatures for these solders range from 620-700° C, which is slightly below those of gold solders. This difference is important in the soldering of stainless steel.

General Suggestions for Soldering

The details for dental soldering are adequately described in textbooks related to other fields of dentistry. Certain principles of both the freehand and investment techniques are emphasized. For successful soldering, both the technique and the selection of solder are important.

Dental solders are supplied in a variety of shapes, such as strips, rods, wires, or cubes, all of which are convenient for certain operations. Thin strips are the conventional form for general applications, and small cubes, approximately 1-mm square, are convenient for soldering a contact area on an inlay or crown. The rods are often notched along two sides, which permits them to hold flux better than a smooth form. Also, when melted, the notched forms do not roll back into a ball as easily as smooth forms. The choice of the shape of the solder depends on the operation to be performed; each shape is available in a range of fineness.

Proper application of fluxes during the soldering operation is important to provide a protective coating that prevents oxidation of the solder and parts being soldered. The flux dissolves surface oxides and allows the melted solder to wet and flow onto the adjoining alloy surfaces. The fluxes used for soldering gold alloys are combinations of borax and boric acid, with potassium fluoride added to some. As discussed previously, too much flux is as undesirable as not enough flux. Fluxes are discussed further in Chapter 16.

The careful and skillful use of the soldering torch flame is important to a high-quality soldered joint. A well-defined and pointed flame of not too large dimensions is advisable for the final heating of the solder in a localized area, but a larger, less well-defined flame of the "brush" type may be used for the initial heating. The flame should not be applied directly to the parts to be joined until the flux has melted and formed a uniform layer over the surface. Applying a hot flame to the flux too quickly causes the flux to form droplets rather than a film. Once the flame has been applied to the spot to be soldered, it should not be withdrawn until soldering is completed. A protective envelope should be created around the spot to be soldered with the reducing portion of the flame. The operation should be completed in the shortest time possible to avoid oxidation of the base metal ingredients of the alloys involved and to prevent damage to the microstructures of the alloys.

Overheating during the soldering operation will cause (1) pits in the solder as described previously, (2) penetration or burning through thin sections, and (3) a loss of strength because of diffusion of the solder into the other metals or loss of fibrous microstructure. Underheating will cause pitting from the retention of unmelted flux and failure of the solder to flow and

adhere to all surfaces. Good wetting of the soldered surfaces by the solder is imperative for satisfactory joining of the parts. Solder that is not well heated tends to "ball" and fails to spread properly. Both over- and underheating will result in a weaker solder joint. For this reason, the proper and careful heating and fluxing of the solder are essential.

Sometimes the flow of the solder should be restricted from parts of the restoration such as the margins or the occlusal grooves. Flow into these areas can be prevented with an antiflux material, which should be applied to the surface before the flux or solder is applied. Solder does not flow into an area contaminated with graphite; therefore a soft lead pencil serves as an effective antiflux. Other materials such as rouge (iron oxide) or whiting (calcium carbonate) in an alcohol and water suspension serve as an effective antiflux for prolonged heating or high-temperature heating, which can burn off the graphite.

The distance between the parts to be joined can influence the accuracy of the final appliance. If the parts are in intimate contact, they tend to expand and push apart on heating, whereas if the distance is too great, the parts tend to draw together as the solder solidifies. A clearance of a few hundredths of a millimeter (0.13 mm) between the parts to be joined is optimum when using the investment-soldering technique. When attempting free-hand soldering of wires for orthodontic or other appliances, a closer adaptation of the parts is possible. The shape of the joint and the purpose of the appliance will ultimately determine the appropriate distance between the soldered parts.

Despite certain well-established principles, soldering is an art. The timing and type of heating, selection of the type and shape of the solder, contour of parts to be joined, and application of flux are all factors that cannot always be dictated by specific rules. Ultimately, the experience of the operator plays a significant role in any successful soldering operation.

Infrared Soldering

Instead of using a torch to provide heat, an infrared heating unit is available specifically for dental soldering. The unit uses the light from a 1000-watt tungsten filament quartz-iodine bulb, which is mounted at the primary focal point of a gold-plated, elliptical reflector. The material to be soldered is

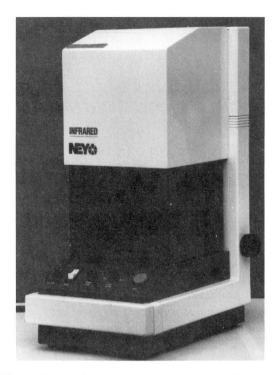

Fig. 14-6 An infrared soldering unit that uses a focused light beam for melting the solder.

placed at the reflector's secondary focal point, at which the reflected infrared energy of the tungsten light source is focused. This equipment, shown in Fig. 14-6, can be used for the high-temperature soldering of alloys for porcelain-fused-to-metal bridges at 1150° C. The main problem in the use of this unit is locating the focal center of the light on the spot to be soldered. The infrared energy must be focused on the crowns and not on the solder itself. Failure to focus on the right spot on the crown can result in cold joints that are porous.

Casting to Embedded Metals or Alloys

Certain types of dental appliances require that a wrought or cast form be embedded into the appliance. To accomplish this, the prefabricated form, such as a clasp wire or precision attachment, is attached to the wax pattern in the same position that it will be in the finished appliance. The wax pattern and metal form are then invested as usual. The wax is eliminated from the mold during burnout and the metal form remains in the investment. A casting alloy is then cast into the mold where it surrounds and becomes attached to the metal insert upon cooling.

Casting to embedded forms may be more practical than trying to solder the form to a casting because of the design of the appliance or the precision required for the appliance. If done correctly, the strength of the union between an embedded form and casting is equally satisfactory to a form that is soldered. In addition, the time and effort of the soldering procedure are eliminated. To successfully cast to an embedded metal, the following conditions are necessary: (1) the fusion temperature of the embedded alloy must be above that of the casting alloy, (2) the investment mold must not be overheated to avoid damage to the embedded structure (which is often wrought), and (3) the recommended technique for the casting procedure must be followed carefully.

SELECTED PROBLEMS

Problem 1. Table 14-1 shows that cast 24k gold has a hardness and strength that are not sufficient for dental restorations, yet gold foil, which is also 24k gold, has three times the hardness and over twice the tensile strength. Why?

Solution. The manufacturing of gold foil starts with the cast form of the element, then imparts severe cold work until it is very thin. Thus gold foil has a wrought microstructure and exhibits superior mechanical properties because of its fibrous form. Condensation of the foil into the restoration imparts further work hardening to the metal.

Problem 2. Inspection of Table 14-3 shows that most casting alloys are based either on gold, palladium, or silver with smaller amounts of copper, platinum, and zinc added. Why do dental manufacturers pick these elements for noble dental casting alloys?

Solution. Gold and palladium are selected as major elements for noble casting alloys because they impart corrosion resistance to the alloys and are miscible (freely soluble) with the other elements (see Fig. 14-2). Palladium is often used because it is considerably cheaper than gold. Silver is used as a less expensive alternative to palladium, but cannot provide corrosion resistance because it is not a noble metal. Furthermore, silver is not miscible with copper. The other elements in Table 14-3 (copper, zinc, gallium, iridium ruthenium, and indium) are inappropriate as major elements. Copper, zinc, gallium, and indium lack corrosion resistance, and iridium and ruthenium have extremely high melting points and are very expensive. These minor elements are used because they enhance the properties of the major elements. For example, copper provides solid-solution hardening, zinc is a deoxidizer during casting, and iridium is a grain refiner.

Problem 3. An alloy was listed by a manufacturer as an 11k alloy containing 4.2% Pd, 25% Cu, and 25% Ag (all wt%). What is the atomic percentage of Au in this alloy? Is the carat based on the atomic or weight percent?

Solution. The alloy contains 25.9 atomic percentage of gold. The answer is arrived at in the following manner: an 11-carat alloy contains $11/24 \times 100 = 45.8$ wt% gold. Thus the carat is based on weight percentage. The weight percentage of each element is divided by the respective atomic weight, giving the following results: Au $45.8/197 = 0.232$; Cu $25/63.5 = 0.394$; Ag $25/208 = 0.231$; Pd $4.2/106.5 = 0.039$. The atomic percentage of Au is $0.232 \times 100/(0.232 + 0.394 + 0.231 + 0.039) = 25.9$ atomic percent.

Problem 4. In Table 14-4, the atomic percentages of elements in the alloys are sometimes different than their corresponding weight percentages in Table 14-3 and sometimes quite similar. Why?

Solution. If an alloy contains elements with vastly different atomic weights, then the atomic percentages and weight percentages will be significantly different. The heaviest elements will be lower in atomic percentage than weight percentage and the lightest elements will be higher in atomic percentages than weight percentages. If an alloy contains elements that are comparable in atomic weights, then the atomic and weight percentages of the elements will not differ as much. Thus in Tables 14-3 and 14-4, the atomic and weight percentages of the Ag-Pd alloys are similar because the majority of the alloy is composed of silver, palladium, and indium, which are very close to the same atomic weight (Ag = 107.9, Pd = 106.4, and In = 114.8). The other element in this alloy, zinc, does not change much because it is a minor component. If zinc were more prevalent in this alloy, its atomic and weight percentages would be significantly different because its atomic weight (Zn = 65.4) is quite different than the other components.

Problem 5. A gold crown made of Au-Cu-Ag-Pd-*I* alloy was inadvertently allowed to slowly cool to room temperature after casting. Because the crown was then in the hardened condition, it was placed into an oven at 400° C for 20 minutes and then quenched in water. However, the casting was still as difficult to finish. Why?

Solution. To convert the hardened alloy to the softened condition, it must be heated above 424° C to affect the conversion (see phase diagram in Fig. 14-2, *A*). Frequently, alloys of this composition are heated to 700° C, which is above the transition temperature of the ordered phase but well below the solidus, to affect the conversion. At this temperature, the alloy converts to the softened condition, then quenching maintains it in the softened condition by cooling it so fast that it does not have enough time to form the ordered phase.

Problem 6. A casting composed of Ag-Pd alloy produced incomplete margins. Why might this have happened?

Solution. Centrifugal casting depends on the density of the molten alloy to create hydrostatic pressure. Low-carat alloys have a lower density, which requires that the casting machine be wound tighter (more turns) for compensation. Alternatively, the fluidity of low-carat alloys is difficult to judge when casting because of a heavier oxide, which forms on the surface of the molten mass. If the alloy was not heated sufficiently, then the molten metal cooled before it could reach the fine margin areas of the mold.

Problem 7. A bridge broke at the soldered joint after 2 years in the mouth. What factors might cause such a failure, and how can this problem be avoided in the future?

Solution a. An excessively large gap between the parts might cause a failure. When the distance between the units is too large, the solder fills the space. As a result, a low-strength joint is obtained because the physical properties of the solders are generally inferior to the alloys. The distance between the parts to be soldered should be carefully gauged to have a small, but sufficient amount of solder alloy occupying the space.

Solution b. A very small gap or a close contact between the parts might be a factor. When the invested bridge is heated, thermal expansion of the metallic units tends to close the gap and produce a close contact between the parts. When the solder is melted, it flows around that contact point but leaves a void in the center of the solder mass. That space is the weakest part of the bridge and may break when a sudden high stress is applied. With a minimal distance of 0.1 mm between the units to be soldered, the solder alloy flows in by capillary action without any problem.

Solution c. The soldered connector might be to narrow. For esthetic reasons, the soldered connectors are sometimes made narrower than the retainer and pontics that they join. [As a result, a weaker joint is obtained.] A wider and more solid-soldered connector should be made despite esthetic considerations.

Problem 8. A soldered joint showed a large number of porosities. What might be the cause of those porosities, and how can they be avoided?

Solution a. Porosities in the soldered joint are usually associated with excessive heat applied during the melting of the solder or with improper fluxing at the time of heating. When the area to be soldered is not absolutely clean or has been contaminated or improperly fluxed, the solder forms globules that make it difficult for the solder to flow over the surfaces. Then excessive heat is usually applied to the solder to make it flow between the parts. Consequently, porosities are formed.

Solution b. Cleaned and properly fluxed surfaces combined with careful application of heat eliminate the possibility of porosity formation. Before the retainers and pontics are assembled, they should be finished and scrupulously cleaned. Dirt, pencil marks, and a heavy layer of oxide cannot be removed with flux.

Solution c. Before the assembled and invested bridge is put into the furnace, a coating of flux should be placed on the parts to be soldered to prevent oxidation. During the soldering procedure the solder should also be covered with a thin coating of flux, and the reducing part of the flame should be used. If the gold solder does not immediately flow smoothly over the area to soldered, the surface is not clean or is oxidized and certainly further heating will not decrease oxide formation. If a further application of flux does not reduce the oxide layer, then the soldering operation should be discontinued, and the operator should again clean the area to be soldered.

Problem 9. During soldering, the fine margins of the retainers were fused. What might have caused this problem, and how can it be avoided when soldering is repeated?

Solution a. Improper investing technique might be a cause. When the assembled bridge is invested, care should be taken to protect the fine margins of the retainers with a thick layer of investment. If this layer is too thin, the refractory material will not act as a thermal barrier, and the fine margins will melt when the flame is applied.

In addition, when air bubbles exist close to the margins, voids in the investment will leave the metal without protection, and it will be easily melted when heat is applied. To avoid trapping air bubbles, the investment should be painted carefully into the occlusal areas and along the proximal walls.

Solution b. A causative factor might be an investment prepared with a high water/powder ratio. When a thin mixture of investment is prepared, the strength of the set investment is low, and when heat is applied, it may be easily broken, leaving the fine margins of the retainers exposed during soldering.

Solution c. Overheating the investment assembly may cause brittleness. When the retainers are well protected by the investment and the assembled units are overheated for a long time, the temperature of the investment may be increased sufficiently to melt the fine margins.

Solution d. Improper use of antiflux may also cause brittleness and a friable surface. Antifluxing is the most effective method for protecting fine margins during soldering. An antiflux is any substance that, when applied on a metallic surface, precludes the attachment of the solder and at the same time prevents the metal from being easily melted. In general, antifluxes are oxides mixed in a volatile solvent; zinc oxide in alcohol or rouge (iron oxide) in chloroform. Graphite may also act as an antiflux. The area to protect is marked off with a lead pencil. A graphite layer may also be obtained by painting the margins with a mixture of graphite powder in a volatile solvent. This antiflux is often used at lower temperatures. A very effective antiflux made of rouge and chloroform can be used to protect the fine margins at higher temperatures produced during soldering. A small amount of chloroform is placed in a dappen dish. A camel's hair brush is wet with chloroform and then placed on a stick of rouge to make a rouge paint. A small amount of this paint mixture is painted on margins inside the retainers adjacent to the areas for soldering. The fine margins of the retainers are protected by the thin layer of iron oxide that is left after the evaporation of the chloroform.

■ REFERENCES

Gold Foil

Cartwright CB: Gold foil restorations, *Mich Dent Assoc J* 43:231, 1961.

Hodson JT: Compaction properties of various gold restorative materials, *J Am Acad Gold Foil Op* 12:52, 1969.

Hollenback GM, Collard AW: An evaluation of the physical properties of cohesive gold, *J South Calif Dent Assoc* 29:280, 1961.

Mahan J, Charbeneau GT: A study of certain mechanical properties and the density of condensed specimens made from various forms of pure gold, *J Am Acad Gold Foil Op* 8:6, 1965.

Richter WA, Cantwell KR: A study of cohesive gold, *J Prosthet Dent* 15:772, 1965.

Richter WA, Mahler DB: Physical properties vs clinical performance of pure gold restorations, *J Prosthet Dent* 29:434, 1973.

Shell JS, Hollenback GM: Tensile strength and elongation of pure gold, *J South Calif Dent Assoc* 34:219, 1966.

Casting Alloys and Wrought Forms

Asgar K, Peyton FA: Casting dental alloys to embedded wires, *J Prosthet Dent* 15:312, 1965.

Böning K, Walter M: Palladium alloys in prosthodontics: selected aspects, *Int Dent J* 40:289, 1990.

Corso PP, German RM, Simmons HD: Corrosion evaluation of gold-based dental alloys, *J Dent Res* 64:854, 1985.

Council on Dental Materials, Instruments, and Equipment: Revised ANSI/ADA Specification No. 5 for dental casting alloys, *J Am Dent Assoc* 118:379, 1989.

Council on Dental Materials, Instruments, and Equipment: Status report on low-gold-content alloys for fixed prostheses, *J Am Dent Assoc* 100:237, 1980.

Farah JW, Dennison JB, Powers JM: Effects of design on stress distribution of intracoronal gold restorations, *J Am Dent Assoc* 94:1151, 1977.

Federation Dentaire Internationale: Alternative casting alloys for fixed prothosthodontics, *Int Dent J* 40:54, 1990.

German RM, Wright DC, Gallant RF: *In vitro* tarnish measurement on fixed prosthodontic alloys, *J Prosthet Dent* 47:399, 1982.

Gettleman L: Noble alloys in dentistry, *Curr Opin Dent* 2:218, 1991.

Glantz PO: Intraoral behaviour and biocompatibility of gold versus non precious alloys, *J Biol Buccale* 12:3, 1984.

Johansson BI, Lemons JE, Hao SQ: Corrosion of dental copper, nickel, and gold alloys in artificial saliva and saline solutions, *Dent Mater* 5:324, 1989.

Keller JC, Lautenschlager EP: Metals and alloys. In von Recum AF: *Handbook of biomaterials evaluation*, New York, 1986, Macmillan.

Leinfelder KF, Price WG, Gurley WH: Low-gold alloys: a laboratory and clinical evaluation. *Quintessence Dent Technol* 5:483, 1981.

Malhotra ML: Dental gold casting alloys—a review, *Trends and Techniques in the Contemporary Dental Laboratory* 8:73, 1991.

Malhotra ML: New generation of palladium-indium-silver dental cast alloys: a review, *Trends and Techniques in the Contemporary Dental Laboratory* 9:65, 1992.

Mezger PR, Stols ALH, Vrijhoef MMA, Greener EH: Metallurgical aspects and corrosion behavior of yellow low-gold alloys, *Dent Mater* 5:350, 1989.

Moffa JP: Alternative dental casting alloys, *Dent Clin North Am* 27:733, 1983.

Nielsen JP, Tuccillo JJ: Grain size in cast gold alloys, *J Dent Res* 45:964, 1966.

Sarkar NK, Fuys RA Jr, Stanford JW: The chloride corrosion of low-gold casting alloys, *J Dent Res* 58:568, 1979.

Stub JR, Eyer CS, Sarkar NK: Heat treatment, microstructure and corrosion of a low-gold casting alloy, *J Oral Rehabil* 13:521, 1986.

Taylor DF, Peyton FA: A comparison of the tensile and bending properties of dental gold wires, *J Dent Res* 30:290,1951.

Wise EM: Cast gold dental alloys. In *ASM metals handbook*, Cleveland, 1948, American Society of Metals.

Wise EM, Eash JT: The role of the platinum metals in dental alloys. III. The influence of platinum and palladium and heat treatment upon the microstructure and constitution of basic alloys, Tr AIME, *Inst Metal Div* 104:276, 1933.

Dental Solders and Soldering

Anderson JN: *Applied dental materials,* ed 5, Oxford, 1976, Blackwell Scientific.

Brumfield RC: Load capacities of posterior dental bridges, *J Prosthet Dent* 4:530, 1954.

Coleman RL: Physical properties of dental materials, Research Paper No. 32, *J Res Nat Bur Stand* 1:867, 1928.

Coleman RL: Some effects of soldering and other heat treatments on orthodontic alloys, *In J Orthod* 19:1238, 1933.

Crowell WS: Dental gold solders. In *ASM metals handbook*, Cleveland, 1948, American Society for Metals.

Federal Specification: Solder; gold, dental, No. QQ-S-554, Mar 29, 1946, Washington, CD, US Government Printing Office.

Mebs RW, Roeser WF: Solders and soldering, National Bureau of Standards Circular No. 492, Washington, DC, 1940, US Government Printing Office.

Meyer FS: The elimination of distortion during soldering, *J Prosthet Dent* 9:441, 1959.

Moyers RE: *Handbook of orthodontics,* ed 4, St Louis, 1988, Mosby.

O'Brien WJ, Hirthe WM, Tyge G: Wetting characteristics of dental gold solders, *J Dent Res* 42:675, 1963.

Rasmussen EJ, Goodkind RJ, Gerberich WW: An investigation of tensile strength of dental solder joints, *J Prosthet Dent* 41:418, 1979.

Ryge G: *Dental soldering procedures,* Dental Clinics of North America, Symposium on Dental Materials, Nov 1958, Philadelphia, WB Saunders.

Steinman RR: Warpage produced by soldering with dental solders and gold alloys, *J Prosthet Dent* 4:384, 1954.

Taylor NO, Teamer CK: Gold solders for dental use, *J Dent Res* 28:219, 1949.

15 Cast and Wrought Base Metal Alloys

ase metal alloys are used extensively in dentistry for appliances and instruments, as shown in the outline below. Cast cobalt-chromium and nickel-chromium alloys have been used for many years for fabricating partial denture frameworks and have replaced Type IV gold alloys almost completely for this application. Cast nickel-chromium alloys are used in fabricating crowns and bridges. These alloys were developed as substitutes for Type III gold alloys. Nickel-chromium and cobalt-chromium alloys are used in porcelain-fused-to-metal restorations, and these alloys are discussed in greater detail in Chapter 18. Titanium and titanium alloys are used in both cast and wrought forms for crowns, bridges, implants, orthodontic wires, and endodontic files. Stainless steel alloys are used principally for orthodontic wires, in fabricating endodontic instruments, and for preformed crowns.

Dental applications of cast and wrought base metal alloys are summarized as follows:
1. Cast cobalt-chromium alloys
   a. Partial denture framework
   b. Porcelain-metal restorations (see Chapter 18)
2. Cast nickel-chromium alloys
   a. Partial denture framework
   b. Crowns and bridges
   c. Porcelain-metal restorations (see Chapter 18)
3. Cast titanium and titanium alloys
   a. Crowns
   b. Bridges
   c. Partial dentures
   d. Implants
4. Wrought titanium and titanium alloys
   a. Implants
   b. Crowns
   c. Bridges

5. Wrought stainless steel alloys
   a. Endodontic instruments
   b. Orthodontic wires and brackets
   c. Preformed crowns
6. Wrought cobalt-chromium-nickel alloys—orthodontic wires and endodontic files
7. Wrought nickel-titanium alloys—orthodontic wires and endodontic files
8. Wrought beta-titanium alloys—orthodontic wires

■ GENERAL REQUIREMENTS OF A DENTAL ALLOY

The metals and alloys used as substitutes for gold alloys in dental appliances must possess certain minimal fundamental characteristics:
1. The alloy's chemical nature should not produce harmful toxologic or allergic effects in the patient or the operator.
2. The chemical properties of the appliance should provide resistance to corrosion and physical changes when in the oral fluids.
3. The physical and mechanical properties, such as conductivity, melting temperature, coefficient of thermal expansion, and strength, should all be satisfactory, meeting certain minimum values and being variable for various appliances.
4. The technical expertise needed for fabrication and use should be feasible for the average dentist and skilled technician.
5. The metals, alloys, and companion materials for fabrication should be plentiful, relatively inexpensive, and readily available, even in periods of emergency.

A list of requirements, such as the above for the ideal substitute for dental gold alloys, calls attention to the fact that a combination of chemical, physical, mechanical, and biological qualities is involved in the evaluation of each alloy. Properties depend on material-, compositional-, and processing-related factors.

Cast and wrought base metal alloys, including cobalt-chromium-nickel, nickel-chromium-iron, commercially pure titanium, titanium-aluminum-vanadium, stainless steel, nickel-titanium, and titanium-molybdenum (beta-titanium) alloys, are discussed in this chapter. The discussion is based on the synergistic relationship between processing, composition, structure, and properties of the materials.

■ COBALT-CHROMIUM AND NICKEL-CHROMIUM CASTING ALLOYS

During the years since the cobalt-chromium casting alloys became available for cast removable partial denture restorations, they have continued to increase in popularity. It was estimated as early as 1949 that more than 80% of all partial denture appliances were cast from the cobalt-chromium alloys. By 1969, over 87% of all partial denture appliances made in this country were cast from some type of base metal alloy. Currently, almost all the metal frameworks of partial denture appliances are made from cobalt-chromium or nickel-chromium alloys.

ANSI/ADA Specification No. 14

According to this specification, the total weight of chromium, cobalt, and nickel should be no less than 85%, or no less than 20% chromium. Alloys having other compositions may also be accepted by the ADA provided that the alloys comply satisfactorily with requirements on toxicity, hypersensitivity, and corrosion. Composition to the nearest 0.5% must be marked on the package, along with the presence and percentage of hazardous elements and recommendations for processing the materials. The specification also requires minimum values for elongation (1.5%), yield strength (500 MPa), and elastic modulus (170 GPa).

An important feature of this specification is that it has made a standardized method of testing available, which has, in turn, made possible comparisons of results from one investigation with those of another.

Composition

The principal elements present in cast base metals for partial dentures are chromium, cobalt, and nickel, which together account for approximately 90 weight percent of most alloys used for dental restorations. Representative compositions of the two major commercially available dental casting alloys are listed in Table 15-1. Chromium, cobalt, and nickel compose about 85% of the total weight of these alloys, yet their effect on the physical properties is rather limited. As is discussed in this chapter, the physical properties of these alloys are controlled by the presence of minor alloying elements such as carbon, molybdenum, beryllium, tungsten, and aluminum.

Function of various alloying elements

Chromium is responsible for the tarnish resistance and stainless properties of these alloys. When the chromium content of an alloy is over 30%, the alloy is more difficult to cast. With this percentage of chromium, the alloy also forms a brittle phase, known as the sigma (σ) phase. Therefore cast base metal dental alloys should not contain more than 28% or 29% chromium. In general, cobalt and nickel, up to a certain percentage, are interchangeable elements. Cobalt

TABLE 15-1   Composition of Major Cast Base Metal Alloys Used in Dentistry

Elements	Alloys (% of Weight)	
	Vitallium	**Ticonium**
Chromium	30.0	17.0
Cobalt	Balance	—
Nickel	—	Balance
Molybdenum	5.0	5.0
Aluminum	—	5.0
Iron	1.0	0.5
Carbon	0.5	0.1
Beryllium	—	1.0
Silicon	0.6	0.5
Manganese	0.5	5.0
Gallium	—	—

Data from Asgar K: *An overall study of partial dentures,* USPHS Research Grant DE-02017, National Institutes of Health, Bethesda, Md, September 1, 1968.

increases the elastic modulus, strength, and hardness of the alloy more than does nickel.

The effect of other alloying elements on the properties of these alloys is much more pronounced. One of the most effective ways of increasing the hardness of cobalt-base alloys is by increasing their carbon content. A change in the carbon content of approximately 0.2% changes the properties to such an extent that the alloy would no longer be usable in dentistry. For example, if the carbon content is increased by 0.2% over the desired amount, the alloy becomes too hard and brittle and should not be used for making any dental appliances. Conversely, a reduction of 0.2% in the carbon content would reduce its yield and ultimate tensile strengths to such low values that, once again, the alloy would not be usable in dentistry. Furthermore, almost all elements in these alloys, such as chromium, silicon, molybdenum, cobalt, and nickel, react with carbon to form carbides, which change the properties of the alloys. The presence of 3% to 6% molybdenum contributes to the strength of the alloys.

Aluminum in nickel-containing alloys forms a compound of nickel and aluminum (Ni_3Al). This compound increases the ultimate tensile and yield strengths of the alloy considerably. The addition of as little as 1% to 2% beryllium to nickel-base alloys lowers the fusion range by about 100° C. However, recent studies suggest that this concentration of beryllium may adversely affect ductility. Corrosion resistance is also compromised, as corrosion occurs preferentially in the Ni-Be eutectic phase, presumably releasing quantities of beryllium greater than the nominal alloy composition of 1 to 2%. Silicon and manganese are added to increase the fluidity and castability of these alloys. Nitrogen, which cannot be controlled unless the castings are made in a controlled atmosphere, such as in a vacuum or under argon, also contributes to the brittle qualities of these cast alloys. When the nitrogen content of the final alloy is more than 0.1%, the castings lose some of their ductility. Numerous other modifications in composition are being proposed to develop more ductile and stronger alloys. There is a remarkable similarity in properties of different alloys having a relatively wide variation in composition. However, as is discussed below, it is the minor alloying elements of carbon, nitrogen, and oxygen are what mainly influence casting and the properties of a final casting.

Microstructure of Cast Base Metal Alloys

The microstructure of any substance is the basic parameter that controls the properties. In other words, a change in the physical properties of a material is a strong indication that there must have been some alteration in its microstructure. Sometimes this variation in microstructure cannot be distinguished by ordinary means. Neither cobalt-chromium nor nickel-chromium alloys have simple microstructures, and their microstructures change with slight alterations of manipulative conditions.

The microstructure of cobalt-chromium alloys in the cast condition is inhomogeneous, consisting of an austenitic matrix composed of a solid solution of cobalt and chromium in a cored dendritic structure. The dendritic regions are cobalt-rich, whereas the interdendritic regions can be a quaternary mixture consisting of a cobalt-rich γ-phase; a chromium-rich $M_{23}C_6$ phase, where M is Co, Cr, or Mo; an M_7C_3 phase; and a chromium and molybdenum-rich σ-phase. Interdendritic casting porosity is also associated with this structure.

Many elements present in cast base metal alloys, such as chromium, cobalt, and molybdenum, are carbide-forming elements. Depending on the composition of a cast base metal alloy and its manipulative condition, it may form many types of carbide. Furthermore, the arrangement of these carbides may also vary depending on the manipulative condition.

The microstructure of a commercial cobalt-chromium alloy is illustrated in Fig. 15-1. In Fig. 15-1, *A*, the carbides are continuous along the grain boundaries. Such a structure is obtained when the metal is cast as soon as it is completely melted. In this condition, the cast alloy possesses low elongation values with a good and clean surface. Carbides that are spherical and discontinuous like islands are shown in Fig. 15-1, *B*. Such a structure can be obtained if the alloy is heated about 100° C above its normal melting temperature, and this results in a casting with good elongation values but with a very poor surface. The surface is so poor that the casting cannot be used in dentistry. Dark eutectoid areas, which are lamellar in nature, are shown in Fig. 15-1, *C*. Such a structure is responsible for very low elongation values but a good and clean casting. From these three examples, it is clear that microstructure can strongly effect physical and mechanical properties.

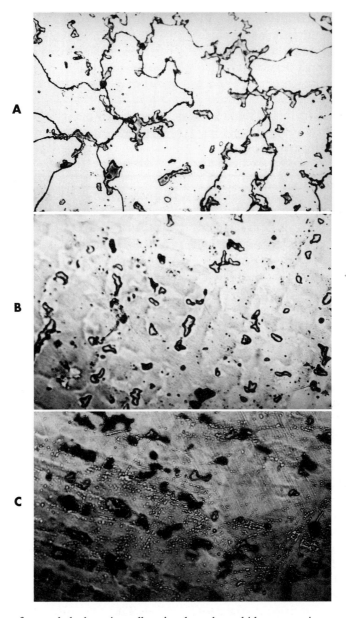

Fig. 15-1 Microstructure of cast cobalt-chromium alloy, **A,** where the carbides are continuous around the grain boundaries. **B,** The islandlike structures are carbides, which are dispersed throughout the entire area. **C,** The dark areas are eutectoid, which are lamellar in nature. (×500). (From Asgar K, Peyton FA: *J Dent Res* 40:68, 1961.)

The Co-Cr-Mo alloy exhibits an eutectic point at approximately 1235° C. At temperatures above the eutectic point, localized melting of the solute-rich zones occurs. Cooling to below the eutectic point yields a microstructure consisting of grain boundary σ, γ, and $M_{23}C_6$, which embrittle the alloy.

Heat Treatment of Base Metal Alloys

The early base metal alloys used in partial denture prostheses were primarily cobalt-chromium and were relatively simple. Heat treating these alloys up to 1 hour at 1000° C did not change their mechanical properties appreciably. Base metal alloys available today for partial denture prostheses, however, are more complex alloys. Presently, complex cobalt-chromium alloys, as well as nickel-chromium and iron-chromium alloys, are used for this purpose.

Studies have shown that many heat treatments of cobalt-base alloys reduce both the yield strength and elongation. If for any reason some soldering or welding must be performed on these partial dentures, the lowest possible temperature should be used with the shortest possible time of heating to the elevated temperature.

On heating, the Co-Cr-Mo alloy undergoes an allotropic phase transformation from a hexagonal close-packed (HCP) structure to a face-centered cubic (FCC) structure, at approximately 890° C. This phase transformation is slow, and the FCC structure is retained on cooling to room temperature. Subsequent aging below 890° C can lead to the formation of HCP bands, rich in carbides, $M_{23}C_6$.

The coarse grain size and interdendritic carbide and σ-phases present in cast Co-Cr-Mo limit the strength and ductility of the as-cast alloy. Because the interdendritic phases are associated with reduced ductility and reduced corrosion resistance, cast Co-Cr-Mo is typically solution-annealed at approximately 1225° C. Such a thermal treatment results in the transformation of σ to $M_{23}C_6$ and the partial dissolution of the $M_{23}C_6$ phase, leading to increased yield strength and ductility, if the treatment and chemical composition are well controlled. In general, yield and fatigue strengths of this alloy are believed to be controlled by the ability of the solute atoms C, Cr, and Mo to inhibit dislocation motion.

Slow cooling to temperatures below those at which incipient melting occurs enhances ductility. A reduction in the carbon content also enhances ductility. However, these increases in ductility are at the expense of yield strength. In general, excess grain boundary carbide decreases ductility, whereas structures with carbide-free grain boundaries are characterized by markedly reduced yield and tensile strengths.

Physical Properties

Melting temperature

The melting temperature of the base metal alloys differs significantly from that of the dental gold casting alloys. Most base metal alloys melt at temperatures of 1400° to 1500° C, as compared to cast gold alloy Types I to IV, which have a melting range of 800° to 1050° C. Only one commonly used nickel-chromium alloy (Ticonium) melts below 1300° C, at a temperature of 1275° C. The addition of 1% to 2% beryllium lowers the melting temperature of Ni-Cr alloys about 100° C. The melting temperature is important in the selection of casting equipment and control of the casting technic.

Density

The average density of the cast base metal alloys is between 7 and 8 g/cm^3, which is approximately half the density of most dental gold alloys. The property of density is of some importance in bulky maxillary appliances, in which the force of gravity causes the relative weight of the casting to place additional forces on the supporting teeth. With certain appliances, therefore, the reduction of weight resulting from the lower density of the cast base metal alloys can be considered an advantage.

Mechanical Properties

Typical mechanical properties of the alloys listed in Table 15-1 have been assembled in Table 15-2, together with a representative range of values for Type IV casting gold alloys subjected to a hardening heat treatment.

Yield strength

The yield strength gives an indication when a permanent deformation of a device or part of a device, such as a clasp, will occur. As such, it is one of the important properties of alloys intended for removable partial denture restorations. It is believed that dental alloys should have yield strengths of at least 415 MPa to withstand permanent deformation when used as partial denture clasps. It may be seen from Table 15-2 that the base metal dental alloys have yield strengths of greater than 600 MPa.

Tensile strength

The ultimate tensile strength of the cast base metal alloys is less influenced by variations in specimen preparation and test conditions than are some other properties, such as elongation. Table 15-2 shows that the ultimate tensile strength of cast base metal dental alloys is greater than 800 MPa. Table 15-2 also demonstrates that the hardened partial denture gold

TABLE 15-2   Mechanical Properties of Alloys Used in Partial Dentures

	Yield Strength, 0.2% Offset (MPa)	Tensile Strength (MPa)	Elongation (%)	Elastic Modulus (GPa)	Vickers Hardness (kg/mm^2)
Cast base metal alloys*					
Vitallium	644	870	1.5	218	380
Ticonium	710	807	2.4	186	340
Hardened partial denture gold alloys†	480-510	700-760	5-7	90-100	220-250

*Data from Asgar K, Techow BO, Jacobson JM: *J Prosthet Dent* 23:36, 1970; Morris HF, Asgar K: *J Prosthet Dent* 33:36, 1975; Moffa JP, Lugassy AA, Guckes AD, Gettleman L: *J Prosthet Dent* 30:424, 1973.
†Data from Oilo G, Gjerdet NR: *Acta Odontal Scand* 41:111, 1983.

alloys can have ultimate tensile strengths almost equal to those of the cast base metal alloys.

Elongation

The percent elongation of an alloy is important as an indication of the relative brittleness or ductility that a restoration will exhibit. There are many occasions, therefore, when elongation is an important property for comparison of alloys for removable partial denture appliances. For example, as described in Chapter 4, the combined effect of elongation and ultimate tensile strength is an indication of toughness of a material. Partial denture clasps cast of alloys with a high elongation and tensile strength do not fracture in service as often as do those with low elongation because of their toughness.

The percent elongation is one of the properties that is critical to accurately test and to properly control during test preparation. For example, a small amount of microporosity that may exist in the test specimen will alter the elongation considerably, whereas its effect on yield strength, elastic modulus, and tensile strength is rather limited. One can therefore assume that practical castings may exhibit similar variations in elongation from one casting to another. To some degree this is borne out in practice, with some castings from the same product showing a greater tendency toward brittleness than do others. This observation indicates that control of the melting and casting variables is of extreme importance if reproducible results are to be obtained.

Although nickel and cobalt are interchangeable in cobalt-nickel-chromium alloys, increasing the nickel content with a corresponding reduction in cobalt generally increases the ductility and elongation. High values of elongation are obtained by casting at the normal melting temperature and by not heating the alloy 100° C above its normal casting temperature. High elongation is achieved without sacrificing strength and is the result of the precise and proper combination of the carbon and molybdenum contents of the alloy.

Elastic modulus

The higher the elastic modulus, the more rigid a structure can be expected, provided the dimensions of the casting are the same in both instances. Some within the profession recommend the use of a well-designed, rigid appliance on the basis that it gives the proper distribution of forces on the supporting tissues when in service. With a greater elastic modulus, one can design the restoration with slightly reduced dimensions. The elastic modulus of the cast base metal alloys is at least twice that of the dental gold alloys. From Table 15-2, it can be seen that the elastic modulus of base metal alloys is approximately double the modulus of Type IV cast dental gold alloys.

Hardness

Differences in composition of the cast base metal alloys have some effect on their hardness, as indicated by the values given in Table 15-2. In general, the cast base metal alloys have a hardness about one-third greater than gold alloys used for the same purpose.

Hardness is an indication of the ease of finishing the structure and the resistance to scratching in service. The higher hardness of the cast base metal alloys as compared with gold alloys requires the use of special polishing equipment, which may be considered a disadvantage, but the finishing operation can be completed without difficulty by experienced operators. It is a common practice to use electrolytic polishing for a portion of the finishing operation, which reduces the time and effort necessary for mechanical finishing operations. With an electrolytic polishing procedure, cast base metal restorations are deplated, and only a very small amount of alloy (a few angstroms) is removed from the surface. Electrolytic polishing works on the reverse principle of electroplating, with the restoration serving as the anode. The deplating exposes a new surface, which is smoother than the cast surface because the rough areas are deplated more readily than the smooth ones. The cast base metal appliances retain their polish well in service. Deplating such a small amount of alloy from the tissue-bearing side of the prosthesis produces a clean shiny surface, but does not alter the fit. The nontissue-bearing side of the partial denture can be further polished on a high-speed lathe.

Corrosion

Recent research on dental casting alloys has been dominated by studies on corrosion and potential biological effects of metal ion release. In general, *in vitro* corrosion tests have evaluated a number of important variables, including effects of electrolytic media and artificial saliva, alloy composition, alloy microstructure, and surface state of the metal. These variables account for 2 to 4 orders of magnitude variation in the amount of species released. The surface state of the metal is an extremely important factor influencing corrosion because the surface composition is almost always different from that of the bulk alloy. Another important consideration is corrosion coupled with wear. Up to three times the mass of metal ions, such as Ni and Be, is released during occlusal rubbing in combination with corrosion than during corrosion alone for Ni-Cr alloys.

Crown and Bridge Casting Alloys

The nickel-chromium alloys can be divided into those containing or not containing beryllium. Most of the alloys contain 60% to 80% nickel, 10% to 27% chromium, and 2% to 14% molybdenum. As a comparison, cobalt-chromium alloys contain 53% to 67%

cobalt, 25% to 32% chromium, and 2% to 6% molybdenum. Those alloys that contain beryllium contain 1.6% to 2.0% of the element. They may also contain small amounts of aluminum, carbon, cobalt, copper, cerium, gallium, iron, manganese, niobium, silicon, tin, titanium, and zirconium. The low atomic weight of about 9 for beryllium compared with about 59 for nickel and 52 for chromium results in atomic percentages of beryllium in these alloys of about 11%.

The properties of these alloys are similar to those reported in Table 15-2 for the cobalt-chromium alloys. The crown and bridge casting alloys exhibit a higher hardness and elastic modulus than do noble alloys, but they prove more difficult in casting and soldering. They are also more technic sensitive, and because of their higher solidification shrinkage, the production of a restoration with a satisfactory fit is more difficult.

Precautions should be taken to avoid exposure to metallic vapor, dust, or grindings containing beryllium and nickel. The safety standard for beryllium dust is 2 $\mu g/m^3$ of air for a time-weighted, 8-hour day. A higher limit of 25 $\mu g/m^3$ is allowed for a minimum exposure time of less than 30 minutes. Physiologic responses may range from contact dermatitis to severe chemical pneumonitis. Therefore efficient local exhaust and filtration systems should be used when casting, finishing, and polishing these beryllium-containing alloys.

The presence of nickel is of greater importance because it is a known allergen. The incidence of allergic sensitivity to nickel has been reported to be from 5 to 10 times higher for females than for males, with 5% to 8% of females showing sensitivity. However, no correlation has been found between the presence of intraoral nickel base restorations and sensitivity. A cobalt-chromium alloy without nickel or other nonnickel-containing alloy should be used on patients with a medical history indicating an allergic response to nickel. The safety standard for nickel is 15 $\mu g/m^3$ of air for a 40-hour week. To minimize exposure of patients to metallic dust containing nickel or beryllium, intraoral finishing should be done with a high-speed evacuation system.

Other Applications of Cast Base Metal Alloys

Cast cobalt-chromium alloys serve a useful purpose in appliances other than removable partial denture restorations. In the surgical repair of bone fractures, alloys of this type have been used for bone plates, screws, various fracture appliances, and splints. Metallic obturators and implants for various purposes are formed from cast base metal alloys. The use of cobalt-chromium alloys for surgical purposes is well established, and these alloys have numerous oral surgical uses. They can be implanted directly into the bone structure for long periods without harmful reactions. This favorable response of the tissue is probably attributable to the low solubility and electrogalvanic action of the alloy used, with the result that the metal is inert and produces no inflammatory response. The product known as surgical Vitallium® is used extensively for this purpose. The primary metal used today in oral implantology is titanium.

■ TITANIUM AND TITANIUM ALLOYS

Titanium's resistance to electrochemical degradation; the benign biological response that it elicits; its relatively low weight; and its low density, low modulus, and high strength make titanium-based materials attractive for use in dentistry. Titanium forms a very stable oxide layer with a thickness on the order of angstroms, and it repassivates in a time on the order of nanoseconds (10^{-9} seconds). This oxide formation is the basis for the corrosion resistance and biocompatibility of titanium. Titanium has therefore been called the "material of choice" in dentistry.

Commercially pure titanium (c.p. Ti) is used for dental implants, surface coatings, and, more recently, as crowns, partial and complete dentures, and orthodontic wires. Several titanium alloys are also used. Of these alloys, Ti-6Al-4V is the most widely used. Wrought alloys of titanium and nickel and of titanium and molybdenum are used for orthodontic wires. The term *titanium* is frequently used to include all types of pure and alloyed titanium. However, it should be noted that the processing, composition, structure, and properties are quite different, and also that for a given type of titanium, differences exist between the wrought and cast forms.

Commercially Pure Titanium

Commercially pure Ti is available in four grades, which vary according to the oxygen (0.18 to 0.40 wt%)

and iron (0.20 to 0.50 wt%) contents. These apparently slight concentration differences have a substantial effect on the physical and mechanical properties.

At room temperature, c.p. Ti has a HCP crystal lattice, which is denoted as the alpha (α) phase. On heating, an allotropic phase transformation occurs. At 883° C, a body centered cubic (BCC) phase, which is denoted as the beta (β) phase, forms. A component with a predominantly β phase is stronger but more brittle than a component with an α-phase microstructure. As with other metals, the temperature and time of processing and heat treatment dictate the amount, ratio, and distribution of phases, overall composition and microstructure, and resultant properties. As a result, casting temperature and cooling procedure are critical factors in ensuring a successful casting.

The density of c.p. Ti (4.5 g/cm³) is about half the value of many of the other base metals. The modulus (100 GPa) is also about half the value of the other base metals. The yield and ultimate strengths vary, respectively, from 170 to 480 MPa and 240 to 550 MPa, depending on the grade of titanium.

Titanium Alloys: General

Alloying elements are added to stabilize either the α or the β phase by changing the β to α transformation temperature. For example, in Ti-6Al-4V, aluminum is an α stabilizer, which expands the α phase field by increasing the (α + β) to β transformation temperature, whereas vanadium, as well as copper and palladium, are β stabilizers, which expand the β phase field by decreasing the (α + β) to β transformation temperature.

In general, α-titanium is weldable but difficult to form or work with at room temperature. Beta-titanium, however, is malleable at room temperature and is thus used in orthodontics. The (α + β) alloys are strong and formable but difficult to weld. Thermal and thermochemical treatments can refine the postcast microstructures and improve properties.

Ti-6Al-4V

At room temperature, Ti-6Al-4V is a two-phase α + β alloy. At approximately 975° C, an allotropic phase transformation takes place, transforming the microstructure to a single-phase BCC β alloy. Thermal treatments dictate the relative amounts of the α and β phases and the phase morphologies and yield a variety of microstructures and a range of mechanical properties. Microstructural variations depend on whether working and heat treatments were performed above or below the β-transition temperature and on the cooling rate.

Following forging at temperatures in the range of 700° to 950° C, thermal treatments below the β-transition temperature (typically performed at approximately 700° C) produce recrystallized microstructures having fine equiaxed α grains (Fig. 15-2, *A*). Equiaxed microstructures are characterized by small (3 to 10 μm), rounded grains that have aspect ratios near unity. This class of microstructure is recommended for Ti-6Al-4V surgical implants.

Thermal treatments above the β-transition temperature lead to various microstructures, which depend primarily on the cooling rate in the (α + β) field. Slow cooling from the β phase into the (α + β) phase (β-annealing) produces an (α + β) lamellar microstructure (Fig. 15-2, *B*). Cast Ti-6Al-4V and high-temperature sintering of Ti-6Al-4V produce lamellar microstructures. On cooling into the (α + β) field, coarse (approximately 5 to 20 μm thick), plate-like α grains, which have a parallel orientation, nucleate. The amount of nucleation and growth and the colony size depend on the thermal cycling and quenching rate.

A frequent thermal treatment used to refine lamellar microstructures is a solution treatment at a temperature slightly above the β transition (e.g., 1000° to 1050° C) and subsequent aging at a temperature high in the (α + β) phase field (e.g., 800° to 950° C). Such treatments refine the platelet thickness, but do not truly break up the microstructural lamellarity.

The mechanical properties of (α + β) titanium alloys are dictated by the amount, size, shape, and morphology of the α phase and the density of α/β interfaces. The tensile and fatigue properties of Ti-6Al-4V have been studied extensively. Microstructures with a small (<20 μm) α grain size, a well-dispersed β phase and a small α/β interface area, such as equiaxed microstructures, resist fatigue crack initiation best and have the best high-cycle fatigue strength (approximately 500 to 700 MPa). Lamellar microstructures, which have a greater α/β surface area and more oriented colonies, have lower fatigue strengths (approximately 300 to 500 MPa) than do equiaxed microstructures.

Cast Titanium

Based on the attributes, extensive knowledge, and clinical success of wrought titanium implants, interest has developed in cast titanium for dental applications. Although titanium has been cast for over 50 years, it has only been recently that nearly precision castings have been attainable. For aerospace and medical components, hot isostatic pressing (HIPing) and specific finishing technics are routinely practiced. However, these technics are beyond the capabilities and affordability of most dental laboratories.

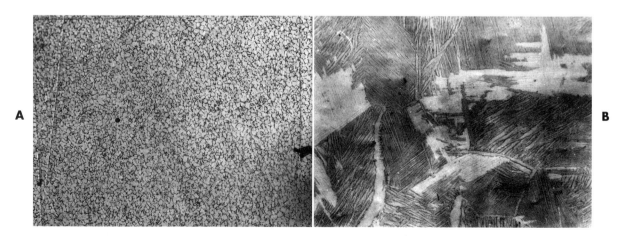

Fig. 15-2 Microstructures of **A,** equiaxed and **B,** lamellar (β annealed at 1300° C for 4 hrs.) Ti-6Al-4V (×200). Equiaxed microstructures are characterized by small, rounded α-grains, with aspect ratios near unity. Lamellar microstructures are characterized by α-platelets in a β matrix, with grain boundary α.

The two most important factors in casting titanium-based materials are the high melting point (≈ 1700° C for c.p. Ti) and chemical reactivity. Because of the high melting point, special melting procedures, cooling cycles, mold material, and casting equipment to prevent metal contamination are required. Titanium is a getter material, which readily reacts with gaseous elements such as hydrogen, oxygen, and nitrogen, particularly at high temperatures (>600° C). As a result, any manipulation of titanium at elevated temperatures must be performed in a well-controlled vacuum. Without a well-controlled vacuum, titanium surfaces will be contaminated with α case, an oxygen enriched and hardened surface layer, which can be as thick as 100 μm. Surface layers of this thickness reduce strength and ductility and promote cracking because of the embrittling effect of the oxygen. The technology required to overcome these factors is what makes casting titanium so expensive.

Because of the high affinity titanium has for hydrogen, oxygen, and nitrogen, standard crucibles and investment materials cannot be used. Investment materials must have oxides that are more stable than the very stable titanium oxide and must also be able to withstand a temperature sufficient to melt titanium. If this is not the case, then diffusion of oxygen into the molten metal is likely to occur. Investment materials such as phosphate-bonded silica and phosphate investment materials with added trace elements achieve this goal. It has been shown that with magnesium oxide–based investments, internal porosity results.

Because of the low density of titanium, it is difficult to cast in conventional, centrifugal-force casting machines. In the last 10 to 15 years, advanced casting technics, which combine centrifugal, vacuum, pressure, and gravity casting, new investment materials, and advanced melting technics (e.g., electric arc melting) have been developed. These advances have improved the feasibility of casting titanium-based materials in the dental laboratory.

Pure titanium has been cast into crowns, partial dentures, and complete denture bases. Titanium alloys have a lower melting point than pure titanium. By alloying titanium, the melting temperature can be lowered to the same temperature as that of nickel-chromium and cobalt-chromium alloys. For example,

the Ti-Pd and Ti-Cu alloys have melting points of 1350° C. Lower casting temperatures may also reduce the reactivity of titanium with oxygen and other gases. Binary and ternary titanium-based alloys have been cast. Ti-13Cu-4.5Ni has been cast into crowns and partial dentures using vacuum investment casting technology. Other titanium alloys, such as Ti-6Al-4V, Ti-15V, Ti-20Cu, Ti-30Pd, Ti-Co, and Ti-Cu are still in the experimental stages and have not yet been implemented in any large clinical studies.

Microstructures of cast titanium materials are similar to those described previously, namely coarse lamellar grains, a result of the slow cooling through the β to α or β to (α + β) transformation temperature (Fig. 15-3).

The mechanical properties of cast c.p. Ti are similar to those of Types III and IV gold alloy, whereas cast Ti-6Al-4V and Ti-15V exhibit properties, except for modulus, similar to those of nickel-chromium and cobalt-chromium alloys. Because of the coarse and heterogeneous microstructure, the properties of cast titanium can be nonuniform.

Recently, cast Ti-6Al-4V microstructures have been refined by temporary alloying with hydrogen. The resulting microstructures (Fig. 15-4) can have α grain sizes less than 1 μm, aspect ratios near unity, and discontinuous grain boundary α, microstructural attributes that increase tensile and fatigue strength. These changes in microstructural form and structure result in significant increases of the yield strength (974 to 1119 MPa), ultimate strength (1025 to 1152 MPa), and fatigue strength (643 to 669 MPa) as

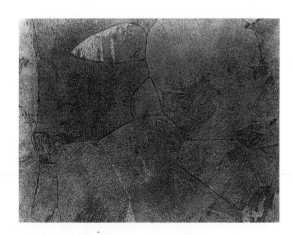

Fig. 15-3 Microstructure of as-cast Ti-6Al-4V.

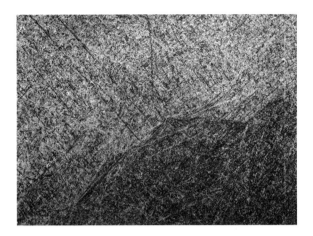

Fig. 15-4 Microstructure of hydrogen-alloy–treated Ti-6Al-4V (×200).

compared with respective values for lamellar (902, 994, and 497 MPa) and equiaxed microstructures (914, 1000, and 590 MPa).

Pure titanium has been cast with a pressure-vacuum casting machine. Other researchers have developed a casting machine that uses an electric arc that melts the titanium in an argon atmosphere. Melting is followed by pressurized casting in a copper crucible and investment in phosphate-bonded silica investment. Such a machine provides a relatively oxygen-free environment and, with the use of a tungsten arc, can reach temperatures of 2000° C. This latter casting regime has been used to cast c.p. Ti crowns and full denture bases. Crowns cast in this manner have been evaluated clinically, and results revealed that, although fitness was inferior to that of silver-palladium alloy, it was superior to that of nickel-chromium. Occlusal adjustment was no more difficult than with conventional crowns, and discoloration, occlusal wear, and plaque retention were similar to other metals. The clinical results of full denture bases cast such as this have not been as good.

Observations of randomly chosen cast crowns have revealed gross surface porosities, to a depth of 75 μm, on both the inside and outside of the surfaces. Mechanical polishing is insufficient to remove this porosity. Internal porosities, sometimes measuring up to 30% of the cross-sectional area, are also readily observed. Surfaces of castings can also be contaminated with α case. The cause of the α case is proba-

bly poor vacuum control or mold contamination. For optimum functionality of the final casting, the surface layer must be removed during finishing. However, even after the α case is removed, internal oxidation can remain and compromise the mechanical properties of the final appliance. Further examination of such castings has also revealed multiple microcracks at the edges of the margins. Some cracks are as long as 100 μm. Cracks of this length are catastrophic to a notch-sensitive material such as titanium.

As outlined, the difficulties with cast titanium for dental purposes include high melting point and high reactivity, low casting efficiency, inadequate expansion of investment, casting porosity, and difficulty in finishing this metal. From a technical standpoint, titanium is difficult to weld, solder, machine, finish, and adjust. Casting titanium requires expensive equipment. As with any new material or technology, specific casting technics must be developed, which take time, effort, and money.

Dental Implants

The objectives and intended function of dental implants are to restore function to the oral cavity. To fulfill this requirement over an extended period, several other objectives must be met. The implant must be capable of carrying occlusal stresses. Additionally, stresses must be transferred to the adjacent bone. Not only must stresses be transferred, but these stresses must be of a "correct" orientation and magnitude so that tissue viability is maintained in as near a physiological state as possible. The ability to transmit stress largely depends on attaining interfacial fixation. Thus two additional requirements are that (1) the interface stabilize in as short a time as possible post-operatively and that once stable, (2) the interface remain stable for as long a time as possible. Designing an "optimal" implant that meets all of the above objectives requires the integration of material, physical, chemical, mechanical, biological, and economic factors.

In analyzing an implant/tissue system, three aspects are important: (1) the individual constituents, namely the implant material(s) and tissue(s); (2) the effect of the implant and its breakdown products on the local and systemic tissues; and (3) the interfacial zone between the implant and tissue. Regarding the ultrastructure of the implant/tissue interface, it is important to understand that, although this zone is relatively thin (on the order of angstroms), the constituents of the zone–heterogeneous metallic oxide, proteinacious layer, and connective tissue–have a substantial effect on the maintenance of interfacial integrity. Furthermore, interfacial integrity depends on material, mechanical, chemical, surface, biological, and local environmental factors, all of which change as functions of time *in vivo*. Thus implant "success" is a function of biomaterial and biomechanical factors, as well as of surgical technics, tissue healing, and a patient's overall medical and dental status.

The physical and material factors affecting implants may be summarized as follows: (1) materials and material processing; (2) mechanisms of implant/tissue attachment; (3) mechanical properties; (4) implant design; (5) loading type; (6) tissue properties; (7) stress distribution; (8) initial stability and mechanisms of enhancing osseointegration; (9) biocompatibility of the implant materials; and (10) surface chemistry, mechanics, and bone-bonding ability of the implant.

Implant materials and processing

In general, two basic classes of materials are used in implantology–metals and ceramics–either alone or in hybrid fashion. Metallic implant materials are largely titanium based–either c.p. Ti or Ti-6Al-4V. However, it is essential to note that the synergistic relationships between processing, composition, structure, and properties of both the bulk metals and their surface oxides effectively leaves more than two metals. Casting, forging, and machining to form near net shape end-products can all alter the bulk microstructure, surface chemistry, and properties. Similarly, densification of ceramics and deposition of ceramic and metal coatings by hot isostatic pressing and/or sintering can change bulk and surface composition, structure, and properties. Thus the many material processing sequences necessary to yield the end-stage dental implant have a strong influence on the properties and functionability of the implant, primarily through temperature and pressure effects.

Although cobalt-based alloys have been used experimentally in dentistry, clinically used metallic dental implants are almost exclusively titanium based. The attributes of titanium (namely, corrosion resistance and high strength) have been discussed previously.

The initial rationale for using ceramics in dentistry was based on the relative biological inertness of ceramics as compared with that of metals. Ceramics are fully oxidized materials and therefore chemically stable. Thus ceramics are less likely to elicit an adverse biological response than metals, which oxidize only at their surface. Recently, a greater emphasis has been placed on bioactive and bioresorbable ceramics, materials that not only elicit normal tissue formation, but that may also form an intimate bond with bone tissue and even be replaced by tissue over time.

Mechanisms of implant/tissue attachment

Various surface configurations have been proposed as means of improving the cohesiveness of the implant/tissue interface, maximizing load transfer, minimizing relative motion between the implant and tissue, minimizing fibrous integration and loosening, and lengthening the service-life of the construct. The concept of osseointegration around screw-threaded implants represents a situation of bone ongrowth. An alternative method of implant fixation is based on bone tissue ingrowth into roughened or three-dimensional porous surface layers. Such a composite system has been shown to have a higher bone/metal shear strength than have other types of fixation. Increased interfacial shear strength results in a better stress transfer from the implant to the surrounding bone, a more uniform stress distribution between the implant and bone, and lower stresses in the implant. In principle, the result of a stronger interfacial bond is a decreased propensity for implant loosening. A progression of surfaces from the lowest implant/tissue shear strength to the highest is as follows: smooth, textured, screw threaded, plasma sprayed, and porous coated.

Enhancing osseointegration

Because of the necessity of developing a stable interface before loading, effort has been placed on developing materials and methods of accelerating tissue apposition to dental implant surfaces. Materials developments that have been implemented into clinical practice include using surface-roughened implants and ceramic coatings. Other, more experimental, technics include electrical stimulation, bone grafting, and the use of growth factors.

Important examples of bioactive materials are bioactive glasses and glass ceramics and calcium-phosphate ceramics. Bioactive glasses and glass ceramics include Bioglass®, which is a synthesis of several glasses containing mixtures of silica, phosphate, calcia, and soda; Ceravital®, which has a different alkali oxide concentration from that of Bioglass®; and a glass-ceramic–containing crystalline oxyapatite and fluorapatite ($Ca_{10}[PO_4])6[O,F_2]$) and β-wollastonite (SiO_2-CaO) in a MgO-CaO-SiO_2 glassy matrix (denoted glass-ceramic A-W). The calcium-phosphate ceramics are ceramic materials with varying calcium:phosphate ratios, depending on processing-induced physical and chemical changes. Among them, the apatite ceramics, one of which is hydroxyapatite (HA), have been studied most.

The impetus for using synthetic HA as a biomaterial stems from the perceived advantage of using a material similar to the mineral phase in bone and teeth for replacing these materials. As such, better tissue bonding is expected. Additional perceived advantages of bioactive ceramics include low thermal and electrical conductivity, elastic properties similar to those of bone, control of *in vivo* degradation rates through control of material properties, and the possibility of the ceramic functioning as a barrier to metallic corrosion products when it is coated onto a metal substrate.

However, processing-induced phase transformations provoke a considerable change in the *in vitro* dissolution behavior, and the different structures and compositions alter the biologic reactions. Given the range of chemical compositions available in bioactive ceramics and the resultant fact that pure HA is rarely used, the broader term *calcium-phosphate ceramics* (CPC) has been proposed in lieu of the more specific term *hydroxyapatite*. Each individual CPC is then defined by its own unique set of chemical and physical properties.

Mixtures of HA, tricalcium phosphate (TCP), and tetracalcium phosphate may evolve as a result of plasma-spraying deposition processes. Physical properties of importance to the functionality of calcium phosphate ceramics include powder particle size, particle shape, pore size, pore shape, pore size distribution, specific surface area, phases present, crystal structure, crystal size, grain size, density, coating thickness, hardness, and surface roughness.

Results of *ex-vivo* push-out tests indicate that the ceramic/metal bond fails before the ceramic/tissue bond and is the "weak link" in the system. Thus the weak ceramic/metal bond and integrity of that interface over a lengthy service-life of functional loading causes reason for concern.

Surface state and biocompatibility

Implant materials may corrode and/or wear, leading to the generation of particulate debris, which may in turn elicit both local and systemic biological responses. Metals are more susceptible to electrochemical degradation than are ceramics. Therefore a fundamental criterion for choosing a metallic implant material is that it elicit a minimal biological response. Titanium-based materials are well tolerated by the body because of their passive oxide layers. The main elemental constituents, as well as the minor alloying constituents, can be tolerated by the body in trace amounts. However, larger amounts of metals usually cannot be tolerated. Therefore minimizing mechanical and chemical breakdown of implant materials is a primary objective.

Titanium and other implant metals are in their passive state under typical physiological conditions, and breakdown of passivity should not occur. Both c.p. Ti and Ti-6Al-4V possess excellent corrosion resistance for a full range of oxide states and pH levels. It is the extremely coherent oxide layer and the fact that titanium repassivates almost instantaneously through surface-controlled oxidation kinetics that renders titanium so corrosion resistant. The low dissolution rate and near chemical inertness of titanium dissolution products allow bone to thrive and therefore osseointegrate with titanium. However, even in its passive condition, titanium is not inert. Any titanium ion release that does occur is a result of the chemical dissolution of titanium oxide.

Analyses of implant surfaces are necessary to ensure a two-fold requirement. First, implant materials cannot adversely affect local tissues, organ systems, or organ functions. Second, the *in vivo* environment cannot degrade the implant and compromise its long-term function. The interface zone between an implant and the surrounding tissue is therefore the most important entity in defining the biological response to the implant and the response of the implant to the body.

The success of any implant depends on its bulk and surface properties, the site of implantation, tissue trauma during surgery, and motion at the implant/tissue interface. Surface analysis in implantology therefore aids in characterizing material, determining structural and composition changes occurring during processing, identifying biologically induced surface reactions, and analyzing environmental effects on the interfaces.

The surface of a material is most always different in chemical composition, form, and structure than is the bulk material. These differences arise from the molecular arrangement, surface reactions, and contamination. In this regard, the interface chemistry is primarily determined by the properties of the metal oxide and not as much by the metal itself. Little or no similarity is found between the properties of the metal and the properties of the oxide, but the adsorption and desorption phenomena can still be influenced by the properties of the underlying metal. Therefore characterization of surface composition, binding state, and form and function are all important in the analysis of implant surfaces and implant/tissue interfaces.

Metallic oxides dictate the type of cellular and protein binding at the implant surface. Surface oxides are continually altered by the inward diffusion of oxygen, by hydroxide formation, and by the outward diffusion of metallic ions. Thus a single oxide stoichiometry does not exist.

Summary

Although there is no consensus regarding methods of evaluating dental implants and what parameters are most important, clinical evaluations have generally shown that dental implants are successful in about 75% of the cases, 5 years postimplantation. Despite advances in materials' synthesis and processing, surgical technic, and clinical protocols, clinical failures do occur, at rates of approximately 2% to 5% per year. Causes of failure and current problems with dental implants include: (1) early loosening, stemming from a lack of initial osseointegration; (2) late loosening, or loss of osseointegration; (3) bone resorption; (4) infection; (5) fracture of the implant and/or abutment; and (6) delamination of

the coating from the bulk implant. The most common failure mechanism is alveolar crest resorption, leading to progressive periodontal lesions, decreased areas of supporting tissues, and ultimately implant loosening. Aseptic failures are most often the cumulative result of more than one of the above-mentioned factors.

Other Applications of Wrought Titanium

Based on the clinical experience with wrought titanium dental implants, wrought titanium crown and bridge applications have been pursued. With the advent of reproducible, high-tolerance machining and processing technics, such as spark erosion, laser welding, and micromachining, and computer-aided design/computer-aided manufacturing (CAD/CAM), wrought titanium crowns are now possible. Future applications are likely to include partial denture work, other precision work, implant-supported restorations, and orthodontic components.

◾ WROUGHT STAINLESS STEEL ALLOYS

Steel is an iron-carbon alloy. The term *stainless steel* is applied to alloys of iron and carbon that contain chromium, nickel, manganese, and perhaps other metals to improve properties and give the stainless quality to the steel. These alloys differ in composition from the cobalt-chromium, nickel-chromium, and titanium casting alloys. Usually, stainless steel alloys are not cast, but instead are used in the wrought form in dentistry, which represents the second way that stainless steel differs from the cast base metal alloys. As a result, the types of appliances formed from these two materials differ. Currently, the most common applications of stainless steel for dental purposes are in the preparation of orthodontic appliances and in the fabrication of endodontic instruments, such as files and reamers. Some specialized applications of stainless steel exist for temporary space maintainers, prefabricated crowns, or other appliances placed in the mouth, and for various clinical and laboratory instruments.

Composition

Several broad classifications of stainless steel are generally recognized. The various groups are referred to as ferritic, martensitic, and austenitic, and they have different compositions, properties, and applications. The ferritic stainless steels are chromium steels employed in the manufacture of instruments or equipment parts in which some degree of tarnish resistance is desirable. A wide range of compositions is available in this group, in which amounts of chromium, the principal element contributing to stainless qualities, may vary from 15% to 25%. Elements such as carbon, silicon, and molybdenum are included but are all held within narrow limits.

The martensitic steels also are primarily chromium steels with a lower chromium content (about 12% to 18%). These steels can be hardened to some degree by heat treatment, and they have a moderate resistance to tarnish. They are used chiefly in the manufacture of instruments and, to a limited degree, for orthodontic appliances.

The austenitic steels represent the alloys used most extensively for dental appliances. The most common austenitic steel used in dentistry is 18-8 stainless steel, so named because it contains approximately 18% chromium and 8% nickel. The carbon content is between 0.08% and 0.20%, and titanium, manganese, silicon, molybdenum, niobium, and tantalium are present in minor amounts to give important modifications to the properties. The balance ($\approx72\%$) is, of course, iron.

Function of Alloying Elements and Chemical Resistance

The corrosion resistance of stainless steel is attributed largely to the presence of chromium in the alloy, and no other element added to iron is as effective in producing resistance to corrosion. Iron cannot be used without chromium additions because iron oxide (Fe_2O_3), or rust, is not adherent to the bulk metal. Approximately 11% chromium is needed to produce corrosion resistance in pure iron, and the necessary proportion is increased with the addition of carbon to form steel. Chromium resists corrosion well because of the formation of a strongly adherent coating of oxide on the surface, which prevents further reaction with the metal below the surface. The formation of such an oxide layer is called passivation. The surface coating is not visible, even at high magnification, but the film adds to the metallic luster of the metal. The degree of

passivity is influenced by a number of factors, such as alloy composition, heat treatment, surface condition, stress in the appliance, and the environment in which the appliance is placed. In dental applications, the stainless characteristics of the alloys can therefore be altered or lost by excessive heating during assembly or adaptation; using abrasives or reactive cleaning agents, which can alter the surface conditions of the appliance; and even by poor oral hygiene practices over prolonged periods.

Of the stainless steel alloys in general use, the austenitic type of 18-8 stainless steel shows the greatest resistance to corrosion and tarnish. In these alloys, the chromium and nickel form solid solutions with the iron, which gives corrosion protection. The chromium composition in these alloys must be between 13% and 28% for optimal corrosion resistance. If the chromium content is less than 13%, the adherent chromium oxide layer does not form. If there is more than 28% chromium, chromium carbides form at the grain boundaries, embrittling the steel. The amount of carbon must also be tightly controlled. If not, carbon will react with chromium, forming these grain boundary chromium-carbides, which lead to depletion of grain boundary chromium and decrease corrosion resistance in a process known as sensitization. Molybdenum increases the resistance to pitting corrosion.

The elements present in small amounts tend to prevent the formation of carbides between the carbon present in the alloy and the iron or chromium and, as a result, often are described as stabilizing elements. Some steels, termed *stabilized stainless steels,* contain titanium, niobium, or tantalum, so that the carbides that do form are titanium carbides rather than chromium carbides.

The chemical resistance of stainless steel alloys is improved if the surface is clean, smooth, and polished. Irregularities promote electrochemical action on the surface of the alloy. Soldering operations on stainless steel with gold and silver solder may contribute to a reduction in stainless qualities because of electrogalvanic action between dissimilar metals or because of localized, improper composition of the stainless steel wire.

Stress-Relieving Treatments

The 18-8 alloys are not subject to an increase in properties by heat treatment, but they do respond to strain hardening as a result of cold work during adjustment or adaptation of the alloy to form the appliance. Heat treatment above 650° C results in recrystallization of the microstructure, compositional changes, and formation of chromium-carbides, three factors that can reduce mechanical properties and/or corrosion resistance.

Appliances formed from these alloys may, however, be subjected to a stress-relieving operation to remove the effects of cold working during fabrication, to increase the ductility, or to produce some degree of hardening with some alloys. If heat treatment is to be performed, it should be held to temperatures between 400° and 500° C for 5 to 120 seconds, depending on the temperature, type of appliance, and alloy being heated. A time of 1 minute at 450° C would represent an average treatment to be used on an orthodontic appliance. Keep in mind that temperatures above 650° C will soften or anneal the alloy, and the properties cannot be restored by further treatment. The main advantage of a low-temperature heat-treating operation is that it establishes a uniformity of properties throughout the appliance after adaptation and fabrication, which may reduce the tendency toward breakage in service. Factors affecting an alloy's ability to be heat treated and stress relieved include alloy composition, working history (i.e., fabrication procedure), and the time, temperature, and atmosphere of the heat treatment.

Stainless Steel Orthodontic Wires

Manipulation

Stainless steel wires are processed in the wrought form, through rolling or drawing. The word *wrought* means that the near net shape is formed from the material in a solid state. Stainless steel wires can be formed easily into appliances with special orthodontic pliers and instruments. Once an appliance is fabricated, it should be heat-treated for 1 minute at 450° C to relieve stresses induced in the wire during fabrication.

The soldering of stainless steel appliances requires skill, and the use of suitable materials is essential. As pointed out in Chapter 14, borax fluxes are not satisfactory, and the use of fluoride-containing flux is required for a successful solder joint. Gold and silver solders may be employed to form the union. Silver solders are considered easier

to use than most gold solders, and they also provide a stronger solder joint than gold solder. Silver solders also have the advantage of having slightly lower melting temperatures, 600° to 650° C, than most gold solders, which reduces the hazard of overheating the steel during the soldering operation and thus reducing properties.

The strength of a wire in the vicinity of the soldered joint formed with gold solder is lower than the one formed with silver solder. Many operators therefore use silver solder with stainless steel or rely entirely on spot welding to assemble the appliance. In one study, which used a standard orthodontic blowtorch as a source of heat with a low-fineness gold solder and a fluoride type of flux, the temperature recorded in the center of a joint was 700° C when the least possible amount of heat was used and 800° C when the maximum amount was applied. At 1 mm from the joint the temperature was 650° C and at 3 mm it was 635° C, whereas at 5 mm the temperature in the wire was only 440° C. These observations indicate that higher temperatures are being developed during soldering than were believed to exist, and no doubt these are responsible for some of the reduction in strength of stainless steel adjacent to the solder joint.

Cleaning and polishing of stainless steel appliances are troublesome operations that become necessary after soldering, heat treating, or periods of service in the mouth. The appliance may be pickled in warmed nitric acid, but a gray satin finish will result that requires buffing or mechanical brushing with a fine abrasive to restore the luster of the original material. An electrolytic polishing bath, also known as an anodic polisher, is useful for restoring the surface appearance to stainless steel appliances, the same as for the cast cobalt-chromium structures mentioned previously.

Properties

ANSI/ADA Specification No. 32 for orthodontic wires not containing precious metals describes Type I (low-resilience) and Type II (high-resilience) wires. The requirements for flexure yield strength and number of bend cycles are listed in Table 15-3.

Some properties of stainless steel wires when tension, bending, and torsion are applied are listed in Table 15-4 and are compared with the properties of

TABLE 15-3   Requirements of ANSI/ADA Specification No. 32 for Orthodontic Wires Not Containing Precious Metals

	Type I–Low Resilience		Type II–High Resilience
Flexure yield strength at 2.9-degree offset, MPa	1700 minimum 2400 maximum		2500 minimum
Number of 90-degree bend cycles(minimum)	0.30-mm diameter 15	0.30-mm to 0.64-mm diameter 10	0.64-mm diameter 5

TABLE 15-4   Properties of Orthodontic Wires in Tension, Bending, and Torsion

Property	18-8 Stainless Steel	Nickel-Titanium	Beta-Titanium
TENSION			
0.1% yield strength, MPa	1200	343	960
Elastic modulus, GPa	134	28.4	68.6
Springback (YS/E), 10^{-2}	0.89	1.40	1.22
BENDING			
2.9-degree offset yield strength, MPa	1590	490	1080
Elastic modulus, GPa	122	32.3	59.8
Spring rate, mm-N/degree	0.80	0.17	0.37
TORSION			
Spring rate, mm-N/degree	0.078	0.020	0.035

Adapted from Drake SR, Wayne DM, Powers JM, Asgar K: *Am J Orhtod* 82:206, 1982. Values are for a 0.43 × 0.64-mm rectangular wire.

nickel-titanium and beta-titanium wires. Of the three types of wires, the stainless steel wire has the highest values of yield strength, elastic modulus, and spring rate and the lowest springback (yield strength/elastic modulus).

Mechanical properties of stainless steel orthodontic wires are listed in Table 15-5 for two sizes of wires in as-received and stress-relieved conditions. The higher values of proportional limit and yield strength of the 0.36-mm diameter wire reflect the increased amount of cold-working used to fabricate this size of wire as compared with that for the 0.56-mm diameter wire. The properties of these wires (except tensile strength) are improved by the stress-relieving heat treatment.

Curves of bending moment versus angular deflection are strongly affected by three factors: (1) the geometry of the wire; (2) the direction of loading, with respect to the wire orientation; and (3) the thermal history of the wire. Curves of bending moment

versus angular deflection are shown in Fig. 15-5 for stainless steel wires having square and rectangular cross sections. The direction of bending of the rectangular wire has an important effect on the bending moment because the wire is much stiffer in bending in the larger dimension (upper curve versus the middle curve). The curves for the square wire are nearly the same for bending in the direction of the square or the diagonal (bottom curve). The effect of heating on the bending moment–angular deflection curves for round stainless steel wires is shown in Fig. 15-6. Heating the wire even for a short time (15 seconds) causes a decrease in the stiffness in bending and in the angle at which permanent deformation starts as compared with that of the as-received wire. Similarly, increased temperature also leads to recrystallization and reduced properties.

Both soldering and spot welding can cause a deterioration in properties if the wire is overheated or underheated. Cross sections of a spot-welded

TABLE 15-5   Mechanical Properties of 18-8 Stainless Steel Wires

Property	0.36-mm Diameter		0.56-mm Diameter	
	As Received	Stress Relieved*	As Received	Stress Relieved*
Proportional limit,[†] MPa	1200	1380	1060	912
Yield strength, 0.1% offset,[†] MPa	1680	1950	1490	1640
Tensile strength, MPa	2240	2180	2040	2160
Hardness (Knoop), kg/mm^2	525	572	536	553
Cold-bending, number of 90-degree bends	37	45	13	21

Adapted from Craig RG, editor: *Dental materials: a problem oriented approach,* St Louis, 1978, Mosby.
*Heated at 482° C for 3 min.
[†]Properties are measured in tension.

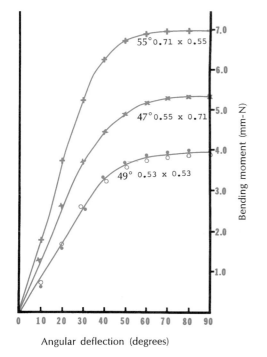

Fig. 15-5 Bending moment–angular deflection curves for square and rectangular 18-8 stainless steel wires. The dimensions of the wires are in mm. (From Craig RG, editor: *Dental materials: a problem-oriented approach,* St Louis, 1978, Mosby.)

wire are shown in Fig. 15-7. The low setting of the spot welder (underheating) produced an inadequate joint, whereas the high setting (overheating) caused excessive melting and recrystallization of the wrought structure of the wire.

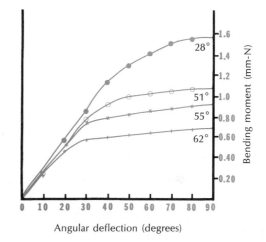

Fig. 15-6 Bending moment–angular deflection curves for 0.46-mm diameter 18-8 stainless steel wire in the as-received condition (•••) and after 15 seconds (ooo), 60 seconds (×××), and 120 seconds (+++) at 816° C. (From Craig RG, editor: *Dental materials: a problem-oriented approach,* St Louis, 1978, Mosby.)

Stainless Steel Endodontic Instruments

Numerous endodontic instruments are classified for hand use or as motor-driven instruments. The most common instruments are the K type of root canal files and reamers. These are manufactured by machining a stainless steel wire into a pyramidal blank, either square or triangular in cross section, and then twisting the blank to form a spiral cutting edge. A file with a rhombohedral cross section has also been introduced. Examples of a K file, a K reamer, and a rhombohedral file are shown in Fig. 15-8.

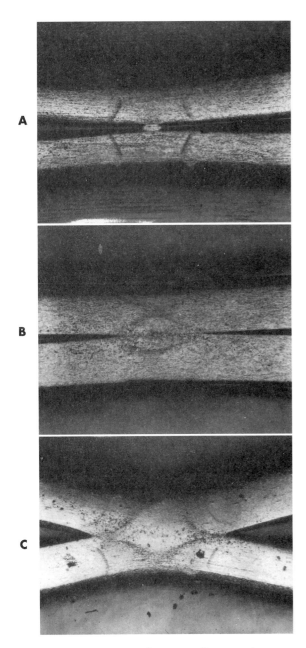

Fig. 15-7 Cross sections of 0.56-mm diameter wires welded at low **A**, medium **B**, and high **C** setting of the spot welder. (From Craig RG, editor: *Dental materials: a problem-oriented approach,* St Louis, 1978, Mosby.)

Properties

Root canals are rarely straight. Therefore, endodontic files need to be able to follow a curved path. As such, bending and torsional properties of

files are important. Similar to orthodontic wires, mechanical properties of endodontic files are dependent upon file geometry, direction of loading, and material composition. An example of this is illustrated by the bending moment–angular deflection curves of K and rhombohedral endodontic files (sizes 10 to 35) shown in Fig. 15-9. In bending, the rhombohedral files are less stiff than the K files, and the increase in stiffness for increasing sizes is smaller and more uniform for the rhombohedral files.

Torsional moment–angular rotation curves of K and rhombohedral endodontic files (sizes 20 and 25) are shown for clockwise and counterclockwise rotation in Fig. 15-10. The rhombohedral files are also less stiff than the K files in torsion, in both directions of rotation. Both types of files fail at lower angular rotation when tested in the counterclockwise direction because counterclockwise rotation increases the tightness of the twist, resulting in brittle fracture, as shown in Fig. 15-11, *A*. Clockwise rotation causes untwisting of the instrument, thereby allowing more rotation before failing in a ductile manner (Fig. 15-11, *B*). Operators are therefore cautioned against twisting a file more than a fourth turn in the counterclockwise direction when a file binds in a canal.

ANSI/ADA Specification No. 28 for endodontic files and reamers defines geometry, minimum values of torque and angular deflection, and maximum values of stiffness in bending for various sizes of files and reamers. Mechanical tests are made in the clockwise direction. No requirements exist for the counterclockwise direction. Stainless steel instruments are required to be resistant to corrosion when tested according to the specification.

A property not covered in the ANSI/ADA specification, but of importance clinically, is cutting ability. Measurement of cutting ability requires construction of machines that simulate the cutting motion of the instrument. Dentin substrates have been used but produced variation in the data as a result of biological differences in hardness of teeth. To overcome this problem, some investigators use acrylic specimens. Cutting ability of individual files varies considerably but is reproducible for the same file with various numbers of strokes. Wear of a file does not appear to affect its cutting ability. Sterilization by dry heat or salt has no effect on the cutting ability of stainless steel files, but autoclave

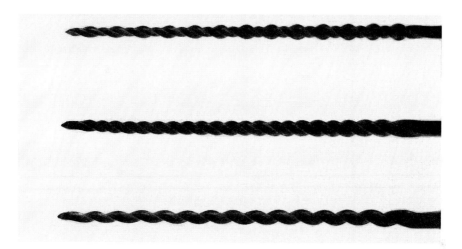

Fig. 15-8 *Top* to *bottom,* examples of rhombohedral file, K file, and K reamer. (Courtesy Corcoran JF, Ann Arbor, 1983, University of Michigan School of Dentistry.)

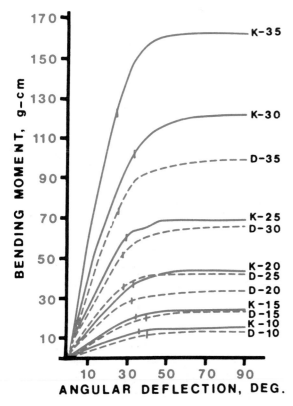

Fig. 15-9 Bending moment–angular deflection curves of endodontic files, sizes 10 to 35. *Vertical marks on curves,* permanent deformation after 90-degree bending. (From Dolan DW, Craig RG: *J Endodont* 8:260, 1982.)

sterilization causes a reduction. Irrigants such as sodium hypochlorite, hydrogen peroxide, and EDTA-urea cause a reduction in cutting ability, whereas a saline irrigant does not cause a reduction. These solutions, excluding saline, also corrode stainless steel at room temperature. Therefore irrigants should be rinsed from the instruments as soon as possible after use.

Base Metal Prefabricated Crowns

Stainless steel crowns were introduced in 1950 and are recommended for the permanent restoration of primary teeth, particularly in children suffering from rampant caries or in situations where the crowns of the teeth are destroyed. The approximate composition of stainless steel used for crowns and its mechanical properties are listed in Table 15-6. Additionally, a titanium-stabilized stainless steel may be used. For purposes of comparison, the properties of a nickel-base alloy used for permanent prefabricated crowns and a tin-base and an aluminum-base alloy used for temporary prefabricated crowns are also shown.

The mechanical properties of the stainless steel and the nickel-base materials are similar, and the high ductility is important in the clinical adaptation of the crowns. In addition, they have reasonable hardness and strength and, as a result, are classified as permanent restorations. The tin-base and

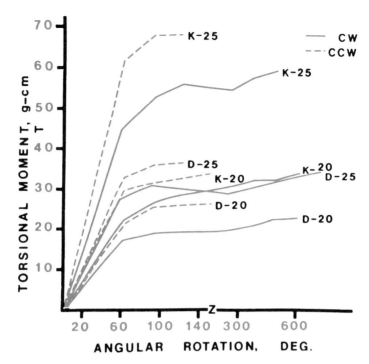

Fig. 15-10 Torsional moment–angular rotation curves of endodontic files, sizes 20 and 25. Clockwise, CW, and counterclockwise, CCW, rotation. (From Dolan DW, Craig RG: *J Endodont* 8:260, 1982.)

aluminum-base temporary types also have high ductility but are soft and have lower yield and tensile strengths and thus do not resist clinical wear as do the stainless steel and nickel-base types.

■ WROUGHT COBALT-CHROMIUM-NICKEL ALLOY

Composition

A cobalt-chromium-nickel alloy known as Elgiloy® is available in wire and band form for various dental appliances. Elgiloy® is composed of 40% cobalt, 20% chromium, 15% nickel, 7% molybdenum, 2% manganese, 0.4% beryllium, 0.15% carbon, and 15.4% iron. Of particular interest is the fact that beryllium decreases the alloy's melting point, facilitating manufacturing. In composition, this alloy resembles the cast base metal alloys more than it does stainless steel.

Processing and Manipulation

The orthodontic wire is supplied in various tempers (amounts of cold work): soft, ductile, semispring

temper, and spring temper. The wires are typically formed in a ductile condition, allowing them to be easily deformed and shaped into appliances and then heat treated to maximize strength. The standard heat treatment, similar to the treatment used to relieve stress in a stainless steel wire, is 482° C for 7 minutes. Low-temperature heat treatment causes a phase change and stress relief. Excessive heat treatment can cause embrittlement.

The fabrication and soldering technics used with Elgiloy® are similar to those used with stainless steel wires. Elgiloy® wires should be soldered with a silver solder in the presence of a fluoride flux or should be joined by spot welding.

Properties

The properties of Elgiloy® as received are similar to those of stainless steel wires; however, its properties can be modified slightly by the heat treatment (7 minutes at 482° C) that is used to stress relieve a stainless steel wire. The mechanical properties of spring-temper Elgiloy® wire are proportional limit, 1610 MPa; 0.2% yield strength, 1930 MPa; tensile

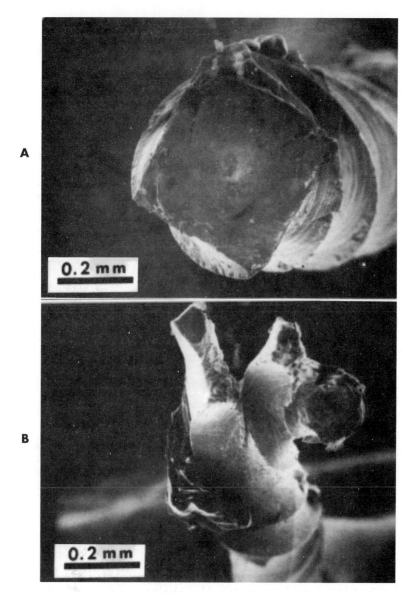

Fig. 15-11 Fracture of K file by counterclockwise torque, **A,** and clockwise torque, **B.** (From Chernick LB, Jacobs JJ, Lautenschlager EP, Heuer MA: *J Endo* vol. 2, #4, 1976.)

strength, 2540 MPa; and Vickers hardness number, 700 kg/mm^2. The number of 90-degree bends until failure for 0.36-mm and 0.46-mm wires is listed in Table 15-7 for as-received and heat-treated conditions. Note that temper, heat treatment, and wire size all affect this property. Bending moment–angular deflection curves for several Elgiloy® wires are shown in Fig. 15-12. The stiffness in bending of the wires is similar; however, the angle at which permanent deformation occurs increases from soft-temper to spring-temper types. The permanent set after a 90-degree bend decreases from soft-temper to spring-temper types. Heat treatment for 7 minutes at 482° C causes an increase in the angle at which permanent deformation occurs but decreases the permanent set.

TABLE 15-6 Mechanical Properties of Prefabricated Base Metal Crowns

Types	0.2% Yield Strength (MPa)	Tensile Strength (MPa)	Elongation (%)	Brinell Hardness (kg/mm^2)
PERMANENT TYPES				
Stainless steel 17%-19% Cr, 9%-13% Ni, 0.08%-0.12% C, 0.4%-0.6% Ti	248	593	55	154
Nickel base 76% Ni, 15.5% Cr, 8% Fe, 0.04% C, 0.35% Mn, 0.2% Si	207	519	42	210
TEMPORARY TYPES				
Tin base 96% Sn, 4% Ag	24.8	31.7	49	19
Aluminum base 87% Al, 1.2% Mn, 10% Mg, 0.7% Fe, 0.3% Si, 0.25% Cu	41.4	110	40	28

TABLE 15-7 Cold Bending of Cobalt-Chromium-Nickel (Elgiloy®) Wires

	Number of 90-Degree Bends until Fracture		
	0.46 mm Diameter		0.36 mm Diameter
Wire Type	**As Received**	**Heat Treated***	**As Received**
Soft	15	12	—
Ductile	13	9	—
Semispring temper	12	9	—
Spring temper	5	<1	11

From Craig RG, editor: *Dental materials: a problem oriented approach,* St Louis, 1978, Mosby.
*Heated at 482° C for 7 min.

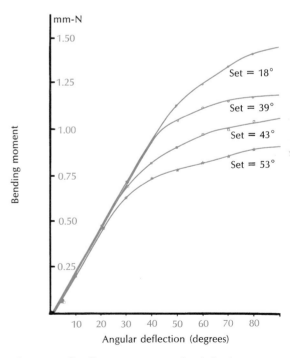

Fig. 15-12 Bending moment–angular deflection curves for 0.46-mm diameter cobalt-chromium-nickel (Elgiloy®) wires from bottom to top of the soft (***), ductile (□□□), ductile heat-treated for 7 minutes at 482° C (ooo), and spring temper (•••) types. (From Craig RG, editor: *Dental materials: a problem-oriented approach,* St Louis, 1978, Mosby.)

■ WROUGHT NICKEL-TITANIUM ALLOY

A wrought nickel-titanium alloy known as Nitinol® was introduced as a wire for orthodontic appliances in 1972. Nitinol® is characterized by its high resiliency, limited formability, and thermal memory.

Composition and Shape-Memory Effect

The industrial alloy is 55% nickel and 45% titanium and possesses a temperature transition range (TTR). At temperatures below the TTR, the alloy can be deformed plastically. When the alloy is then heated from below to above the TTR, a temperature-induced crystallographic transformation from a martensitic to an austenitic microstructure occurs and the alloy will return to its original shape. Hence, nickel-titanium is called a shape-memory alloy. The orthodontic alloy contains several percent cobalt to lower the TTR. A number of variations of the Ni-Ti alloy have been developed in dentistry. Compositional variations lead to changes in the martensitic and austenitic start and finish temperatures and mechanical properties. Only those wires with austenitic finish temperatures less than 37° C exhibit superelasticity.

Properties and Manipulation

Mechanical properties of an orthodontic nickel-titanium alloy are compared with those of stainless steel and a beta-titanium alloy in tension, bending, and torsion in Table 15-4. The nickel-titanium alloy has the lowest elastic modulus and yield strength but the highest springback (maximum elastic deflection). As shown in Figs. 15-13 and 15-14, nickel-titanium has the lowest spring rate but the highest resiliency in bending and torsion of the three alloys used for orthodontic wires. Clinically, the low elastic modulus and high resiliency mean that lower and more constant forces can be applied with activations and an increased working range. The high springback is important if large deflections are needed, such as with poorly aligned teeth.

Nitinol® wire requires special bending technics and cannot be bent over a sharp edge or into a complete loop; thus the wire is more suited for use with pretorqued, preangulated brackets. The alloy is brittle and therefore cannot be soldered or welded, and so wires must be joined mechanically.

■ WROUGHT BETA-TITANIUM ALLOY

Composition and Microstructure

A titanium-molybdenum alloy known as beta-titanium was introduced in 1979 as a wrought orthodontic wire. As discussed previously, c.p. Ti exists in a

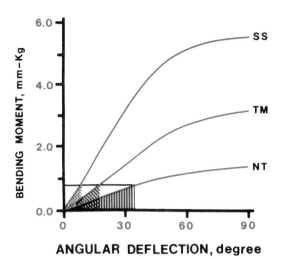

Fig. 15-13 Stored energy at a fixed bending moment below the proportional limit for 0.48-mm by 0.64-mm wires of alloys stainless steel (SS), beta titanium (*TM*), and nickel-titanium (*NT*). The stored energy is equal to the shaded areas under the curve for each wire. The spring rate is equal to the slope of each curve. (From Drake SR, Wayne DM, Powers JM, Asgar K: *Am J Orthod* 82:206, 1982.)

hexagonal close-packed crystal lattice at temperatures below 883° C and in a body-centered cubic crystal lattice at higher temperatures. These structures are referred to as alpha-titanium and beta-titanium, respectively. The beta form of Ti can be stabilized at room temperature by alloying with certain elements. Beta-titanium alloy for dental use has the composition 78% titanium, 11.5% molybdenum, 6% zirconium, and 4.5% tin and is supplied as wrought wire.

Manipulation

Beta-titanium wires can be shaped easily, and the wires can be soldered and welded. Joints can be made by electrical resistance welding. Under proper welding conditions, minimum distortion of the cold-worked microstructure occurs.

Properties

Compared with stainless steel and Elgiloy® wires, the beta-titanium wire has lower force magnitudes, a lower elastic modulus, higher springback (maximum elastic deflection), a lower yield strength, and good ductility, weldability, and corrosion resistance. The mechanical properties of beta-titanium alloy in

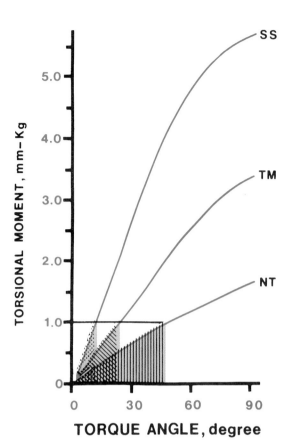

Fig. 15-14 Stored energy at a fixed torsional moment below the proportional limit for 0.48-mm by 0.64-mm wires of alloys stainless steel (*SS*), beta titanium (*TM*), and nickel-titanium (*NT*). The stored energy is equal to the shaded area under the curve for each wire. The spring rate is equal to the slope of each curve. (From Drake SR, Wayne DM, Powers JM, Asgar K: *Am J Orthod* 82:206, 1982.)

tension, bending, and torsion are compared with stainless steel and nickel-titanium alloys in Table 15-4 and Figs. 15-13 and 15-14. The beta-titanium alloy has values of yield strength, modulus of elasticity, and springback intermediate to those of stainless steel and Nitinol®. Its formability and weldability are advantages over Nitinol®, and it has a larger working range than have stainless steel or Elgiloy® wires.

■ NEW/EXPERIMENTAL ORTHODONTIC WIRES

Recent developments in orthodontic wires include a titanium-based alloy (Ti-15V-3Cr-3Al-3Sn), which is reported to offer a yield strength to modulus ratio slightly greater than that of beta-titanium. Fiber-reinforced thermoplastic wires have also been studied. Candidate fibers include fiberglass and aramid. Candidate resins include polycarbonate and polyethylene terephthalate glycol. For each resin/fiber system, there is a heating or working range where the material can be formed without property degradation. This temperature range is primarily related to the glass transition temperature (T_g) of the resin matrix. A temperature above the T_g is necessary to allow sufficient softening. However higher temperatures will lead to structural changes and reduction in flexural modulus.

Summary of Orthodontic Wires

Properties of stainless steel, nickel-titanium, and beta-titanium wires in tension, bending, and torsion are compared in Table 15-4. Of the three types of wires, the stainless steel wire has the highest values of yield strength, elastic modulus, and spring rate and the lowest springback (elastic deflection or yield strength/elastic modulus). Elgiloy® is easily deformed and shaped. The nickel-titanium alloy has the lowest elastic modulus and yield strength but the highest springback. Nickel-titanium has the lowest spring rate but highest resiliency in bending and torsion of the three alloys used for orthodontic wires. The disadvantages are that it is hard to bend and cannot be soldered, welded, or heat treated. Beta-titanium offers an intermediate force delivery system and greater formability and weldability.

■ SOME OTHER ALLOYS

Certain alloys find considerable use for dental instruments and equipment because of their special properties. For example, Monel® Metal is an alloy of copper and nickel used for equipment parts because of its good physical properties and resistance to tarnish or corrosion. It has not been popular for constructing appliances placed in the mouth because of difficulties in manipulation. Such an alloy has a composition of approximately 28% copper, 68% nickel, 2% iron, 1.5% manganese, and 0.2% silicon.

Other stainless steels are also used, to lesser extents. A steel with 3% Al offers the ability to be heat treated and can be used in wrought condition.

Following forming, heat treatment at 900° C for 1 hour leads to an increase in properties. The heat treatment forms coherent precipitate Ni_3Al, which strain hardens the lattice.

Another recently developed alloy is Zr-Pd-Ru with an intermetallic compound structure. This alloy undergoes transformation toughening and has good fracture toughness. The stress-induced microstructural changes are also hypothesized to provide good wear resistance. The 30Ni-30Cu-40Mn alloy is an experimental base metal casting alloy. The hypothesized advantage of this alloy include a melting point of less than 1000° C and a resultant reduced tendency to absorb oxygen. The secondary alloying elements, Al, In, and Sn, further reduce the melting point, refine and reduce the dendritic microstructure, and increase hardness and casting accuracy. The secondary alloying elements also segregrate to the intermetallic regions, leading to an increase in corrosion resistance.

The possibility of developing satisfactory substitutes for gold in dental appliances is far from being exhausted. Numerous new alloys are being developed for use by the engineering profession, some of which eventually may be found to be satisfactory for dental purposes. Many metals such as tantalum, molybdenum, columbium, vanadium, and gallium are becoming available in increasing quantities. These metals and their alloys, along with chromium, nickel, cobalt, titanium, stainless steel, and various copper, aluminum, or magnesium alloys, may be developed to possess physical and chemical qualities that satisfy the requirements of various dental applications.

SELECTED PROBLEMS

Problem 1. The elastic modulus values of nickel-chromium and cobalt-chromium alloys are about twice those of gold alloys, thus the thickness of a restoration in the direction of a bending force can be about halved and still have the same deflection. Is this a justifiable conclusion? (Defend your answer.)

Solution. No. Although a stress-strain curve in tension might lead you to respond affirmatively, it should be remembered that, although the deflection of a beam is directly proportional to the modulus, it is inversely proportional to the cube of the thickness. As a result, halving the thickness of the nickel-chromium beam will dramatically increase the deflection as compared with that of the gold beam, even though it has twice the elastic modulus. It can be shown that only small decreases in thickness of the nickel-chromium beam can be done and yet maintain the same stiffness as the gold alloy beam.

Problem 2. During the soldering of a cobalt-chromium partial denture, the temperature of the torch became very high. What might be the expected effect on the properties of the cast framework?

Solution. Excessive heating of the framework will result in a decrease in the yield strength as well as the percent elongation. This can result from migration of atoms and formation of carbides, resulting in chromium depletion in the grains, which can cause increased corrosion.

Problem 3. Nickel-chromium alloys that can be cast into gypsum-bonded investments contain up to 2% beryllium to reduce the melting temperature. An alloy labeled as containing 77% nickel, 21% chromium, and 2% beryllium will contain 2 atomic % of Be. Is that statement correct? Defend your response.

Solution. No. The values listed are weight percentages. To obtain the atomic percent, you must first divide the weight percent of each element by the respective atomic number. Next these quotients are added, and the percentage calculated by division of each quotient by the sum times 100. For example, 77 wt% Ni ÷ 59 = 1.305, 21 wt% Cr ÷ 52 = 0.404, and 2 wt% Be ÷ 9 = 0.222. The sum is 1.931 and 0.222 ÷ 1.931 = 11.5 atomic % Be.

Problem 4. An austenitic 18-8 stainless steel orthodontic wire was bent and then was heat-treated for 3 minutes, but it was inadvertently heated to 816° C rather than the recommended 482° C. What effect would this have on the wire?

Solution. Substantial recrystallization and precipitation of trapped carbon atoms in the iron lattice of the wrought wire would occur, which would result in reduced stiffness and reduced resistance to permanent bending. The recommended heating to 482° C is to relieve stresses introduced during bending of the wire and is sufficiently low so that changes in stiffness and resistance to bending do not occur.

Problem 5. If you wished to select an orthodontic wire with the most constant force without reactivation as the tooth moved, would you select a 18-8 stainless steel, beta-titanium, or nickel-titanium wire? Why?

Solution. Based on the bending and torsional moment versus deflection curves, a nickel-titanium wire should be chosen. This wire has the lowest spring rate for a given size but has the highest resiliency and the smallest decrease in force with movement of the tooth. Therefore longer times between activations and a more constant force result.

Problem 6. Endodontic stainless steel K files are used with a 90-degree clockwise rotation and withdrawal. If the tip of a file becomes bound in a root canal, why should care be taken not to rotate it much in the counterclockwise direction?

Solution. The files are twisted during construction so that if the tip is bound in a root canal, continued clockwise rotation will untwist the file, but counterclockwise rotation will twist the file tighter and possibly result in brittle rather than ductile fracture. As a result, these instruments fracture more readily in counterclockwise rotation, frequently in as little as a one-quarter turn.

■ REFERENCES

Cast Base Metal Alloys

Asgar K, Allan FC: Microstructure and physical properties of alloy for partial denture castings, *J Dent Res* 47:189, 1968.

Asgar K, Peyton FA: Effect of casting conditions on some mechanical properties of cobalt-base alloys, *J Dent Res* 40:73, 1961.

Asgar K, Peyton FA: Effect of microstructure on the physical properties of cobalt-based alloys, *J Dent Res* 40:63, 1961.

Asgar K, Peyton FA: Flow and fracture of dental alloys determined by a microbend tester, *J Dent Res* 41:142, 1962.

Asgar K, Techow BO, Jacobson JM: A new alloy for partial dentures, *J Prosthet Dent* 23:36, 1970.

Bates JF: Studies related to the fracture of partial dentures, *Br Dent J* 118:532, 1965.

Ben-Ur Z, Pataei H, Cardash HS, Baharov H: The fracture of cobalt-chromium alloy removable partial dentures, *Quintessence Internat* 17:797, 1986.

Bergman M, Bergman B, Soremark R: Tissue accumulation of nickel released due to electrochemical corrosion of non-precious dental casting alloys, *J Oral Rehabil* 7:325, 1980.

Brune D, Beltesbrekke H: Dust in dental laboratories: types and levels in specific operations, *J Prosthet Dent* 43:687, 1980.

Bumgardner JD, Lucas LC: Surface analysis of nickel-chromium dental alloys, *Dent Mater* 9:252, 1993.

Cecconi BT: Removable partial denture research and its clinical significance, *J Prosthet Dent* 39:203, 1978.

Cecconi BT, Asgar K, Dootz ER: Fit of the removable partial denture base and its effect on abutment tooth movement, *J Prosthet Dent* 25:515, 1971.

Cheng TP, Tsai WT, Chern Lin JH: The effect of beryllium on the corrosion resistance of nickel-chromium dental alloys, *J Mater Sci: Mater Med,* 1:211, 1990.

Council on Dental Materials, Instruments, and Equipment: Report on base metal alloys for crown and bridge applications: benefits and risks, *J Am Dent Assoc* 111:479, 1985.

Cunningham DM: Comparison of base metal alloys and Type IV gold alloys for removable partial denture frameworks, *Dent Clin North Am* 17:719, 1973.

Frank RP, Brudvik JS, Nicholls JI: A comparison of the flexibility of wrought wire and cast circumferential clasps, *J Prosthet Dent* 49:471, 1983.

Geis-Gerstorfer J, Passler K: Studies of the influence of Be content on corrosion behaviour and mechanical properties of Ni25Cr10Mo alloys, *Dent Mater* 9:177, 1993.

Hinman RW, Lynde TA, Pelleu GB, Jr, Gaugler RW: Factors affecting airborne beryllium concentrations in dental space, *J Prosthet Dent* 33:210, 1975.

Lucas LC, Lemons JE: Biodegradation of restorative metal systems, *Adv Dent Res* 65:32, 1992.

Mohammed H, Asgar K: A new dental super alloy system, I, II, III. *J Dent Res* 52:136, 145, 151, 1973.

Morris HF, Asgar K: Physical properties and microstructure of four new commercial partial denture alloys, *J Prosthet Dent* 33:36, 1975.

Morris HF, Asgar K, Rowe AP, Nasjleti CE: The influence of heat treatments on several types of base-metal removable partial denture alloys, *J Prosthet Dent* 41:388, 1979.

Rowe AP, Bigelow WC, Asgar K: Effect of tantalum addition to a cobalt-chromium-nickel base alloy, *J Dent Res* 53:325, 1974.

Smith DC: Tissue reaction to noble and base metal alloys. In Smith DC, William DF, editors: *Biocompatibility of dental materials,* vol 4, Boca Raton, FL, 1982, CRC Press.

Strandman E: Influence of different types of acetylene-oxygen flames on the carbon content of dental Co-Cr alloy, *Odontol Revy* 27:223, 1976.

Wakasa K, Yamaki M: Corrosive properties in experimental Ni-Cu-Mn based alloy systems for dental purposes, *J Mater Sci: Mater Med* 1:171, 1990.

Wakasa K, Yamaki M: Dental application of the 30Ni-30Cu-40Mn ternary alloy system, *J Mater Sci: Mater Med* 1:44, 1990.

Wakasa K, Yamaki M: Tensile behaviour in 30Ni-30Cu-30Mn based alloys for a dental application, *J Mater Sci: Mater Med* 2:71, 1991.

Wataha JC, Craig RG, Hanks CT: The effects of cleaning on the kinetics of *in vitro* metal release from dental casting alloys, *J Dent Res* 71:1417, 1992.

Wataha JC, Craig RG, Hanks CT: The release of elements of dental casting alloys into cell-culture medium, *J Dent Res* 70:1014, 1991.

Waterstrat RM: New alloys, *J Am Dent Assoc* 123:33, 1992.

Yong T, De Long B, Goodkind RJ, Douglas WH: Leaching of Ni, Cr and Be ions from base metal alloys in an artificial oral environment, *J Prosthet Dent* 68:692, 1992.

Wrought Base Metal Alloys

Andreasen GF, Barrett RD: An evaluation of cobalt-substituted Nitinol wire in orthodontics, *Am J Orthod* 63:462, 1973.

Andreasen GF, Bigelow H, Andrews JG: 55 Nitinol wire: force developed as a function of 'elastic memory,' *Aust Dent J* 24:146, 1979.

Andreasen GF, Brady PR: A use hypothesis for 55 Nitinol wire for orthodontics, *Angle Orthod* 42:172, 1972.

Andreasen GF, Morrow RE: Laboratory and clinical analyses of Nitinol wire, *Am J Orthod* 73:142, 1978.

Braff MH: A comparison between stainless steel crowns and multisurface amalgams in primary molars, *J Dent Child* 46:474, Nov-Dec 1975.

Brantley WA, Augat WS, Myers CL, Winders RV: Bending deformation studies of orthodontic wires, *J Dent Res* 57:609, 1978.

Burstone CJ, Goldberg AJ: Beta titanium: a new orthodontic alloy, *Am J Orthod* 77:121, 1980.

Chen R, Zhi YF, Arvy Stas MG: Advanced Chinese NiTi alloy wire and clinical observations, *Angle Orthod* 62:15, 1992.

Council on Dental Materials, Instruments, and Equipment: New American Dental Association Specification No. 32 for orthodontic wires not containing precious metals, *J Am Dent Assoc* 95:1169, 1977.

Council on Dental Materials, Instruments, and Equipment: Status report on beta titanium orthodontic wires, *J Am Dent Assoc* 105:684, 1982.

Dolan DW, Craig RG: Bending and torsion of endodontic files with rhombus cross sections, *J Endodont* 8:260, 1982.

Drake SR, Wayne DM, Powers JM, Asgar K: Mechanical properties of orthodontic wires in tension, bending, and torsion, *Am J Orthod* 82:206, 1982.

Goldberg AJ, Burstone CJ: An evaluation of beta titanium alloys for use in orthodontic appliances, *J Dent Res* 58:593, 1979.

Goldberg AJ, Burstone CJ, Hadjinikolaoa I, Jancar J: Screening of matrices and fibers for reinforced thermoplastics intended for dental applications, *J Biomed Mater Res* 28:167, 1994.

Kapila S, Sachdeva R: Mechanical properties and clinical applications of orthodontic wires, *Am J Orthod Dentofac Orthop* 96:100, 1989.

Kusy RP: Comparison of nickel-titanium and beta-titanium wire sizes to conventional orthodontic arch wire materials, *Am J Orthod* 79:625, 1981.

Neal RG, Craig RG, Powers JM: Cutting ability of K-type endodontic files, *J Endodont* 9:52, 1983.

Neal RG, Craig RG, Powers JM: Effect of sterilization and irrigants on the cutting ability of stainless steel files, *J Endodont* 9:93, 1983.

Newman JG, Brantley WA, Gorstein H: A study of the cutting efficiency of seven brands of endodontic files in linear motion, *J Endodont* 9:316, 1983.

Parmiter OK: Wrought stainless steels. In *ASM metals handbook,* Cleveland, 1948, American Society for Metals.

Patel AP, Goldberg AJ, Burstone CJ: The effect of thermoforming on the properties of fiber-reinforced composite wires, *J Appl Biomat* 3:177, 1992.

Peterson DS, Jubach TS, Katora M: Scanning electron microscope study of stainless steel crown margins, *ASDC J Dent Child* 45:376, Sept-Oct 1978.

Schwaninger B, Sarkar NK, Foster BE: Effect of long-term immersion corrosion on the flexural properties of Nitinol, *Am J Orthod* 82:45, 1982.

Shastry CV, Goldberg AJ: The influence of drawing parameters on the mechanical properties of two beta-titanium alloys, *J Dent Res* 62:1092, 1983.

Waters NE: Superelastic nickel-titanium wires, *Br J Orthod* 19:319, 1992.

Wilkinson JV: Some metallurgical aspects of orthodontic stainless steel, *Am J Orthod* 48:192, 1962.

Wilson DF, Goldberg AJ: Alternative beta-titanium alloys for orthodontic wires, *Dent Mater* 3:337, 1987.

Yoneyama T, Doi H: Superelasticity and thermal behaviour of NiTi orthodontic archwires, *Dent Mater* 11:1, 1992.

Titanium

Ducheyne P, Kohn D, Smith TS: Fatigue properties of cast and heat treated Ti-6Al-4V alloy for anatomic hip prostheses, *Biomat* 8:223, 1987.

Ida K, Tani Y, Tsutsumi S, Togaya T, Toshiyuki N, Kazuhiro S, Takayoshi K, Nakamura M, Wada H: Clinical applications of pure titanium crowns, *Dent Mater J* 4:191, 1985.

Ida K, Togaya T, Tsutsumi S, Takeuchi M: Effect of magnesia investments on the dental casting of pure titanium or titanium alloys, *Dent Mater J* 1:8, 1982.

Kimura H, Izumi O, editors: *Titanium '80 science and technology,* Warrendale, Penn, 1980, The Metallurgical Society of AIME.

Kohn DH, Ducheyne P: A parametric study of the factors affecting the fatigue strength of porous coated Ti-6Al-4V implant alloy, *J Biomed Mater Res* 24:1483, 1990.

Kohn DH, Ducheyne P: Microstructural refinement of beta-sintered and porous coated Ti-6Al-4V by temporary alloying with hydrogen, *J Mater Sci* 26:534, 1991.

Kohn DH, Ducheyne P: Tensile and fatigue strength of hydrogen treated Ti-6Al-4V alloy, *J Mater Sci* 26:328, 1991.

Lutjering G, Gysler A: Critical review-fatigue. In Lutjering G, Zwicker U, Bunk W, editors: *Titanium, science and technology,* Oferursel, West Germany, 1985, Deutsche Gesellschaft Fur Metallkunde.

Margolin H, Williams JC, Chesnutt JC, Lutjering G: A review of the fracture and fatigue behavior of Ti alloys. In Moser JB, Lin JHC, Taira M, Greener EH: Development of dental Pd-Ti alloys, *Dent Mater* 1:37, 1985.

Okabe T, Hero H: The use of titanium in dentistry, *Cells and Mater* 5:211, 1995.

Peters M, Gysler A, Lutjering G: Influence of microstructure on the fatigue behavior of Ti-6Al-4V. In Kimura H, Izumi O, editors: *Titanium '80 science and technology,* Warrendale, Penn, 1980, The Metallurgical Society of AIME.

Szurgot KC, Marker BC, Moser JB, Greener EH: The casting of titanium for removable partial dentures, *Dent Mater Sci QDT Yearbook*, 1988.

Taira M, Moser JB, Greener EH: Studies of Ti alloys for dental castings, *Dent Mater* 5:45, 1989.

Voitik AJ: Titanium dental castings, cold worked titanium restorations—yes or no? *Trends and Techniques* 8(10):23, Dec 1991.

Waterstrat RM: Comments on casting of Ti-13Cu-4.5Ni alloy, Pub No (NIH) 77-1227, DHEW, 1977.

Yamauchi M, Sakai M, Kawano J: Clinical application of pure titanium for cast plate dentures, *Dent Mater J* 7:39, 1988.

Implants

Adell R, Lekholm U, Rockler B, Brånemark PI: A 15-year study of osseointegrated implants in the treatment of the edentulous jaw, *Int J Oral Surg* 10:387, 1981.

Albrektsson T, Brånemark PI, Hansson HA, Kasemo B, Larsson K, Lundstrom I, McQueen DH, Skalak R: The interface zone of inorganic implants in vivo: titanium implants in bone, *Ann Biomed Engr* 11:1, 1983.

Brånemark PI, Hansson BO, Adell R, Breine U, Lindstrom J, Hallen O, Ohman A: Osseointegrated implants in the treatment of the edentulous jaw: experience from a 10-year period, *Scand J Plast Reconstr Surg* 11(suppl 16):1-132, 1977.

Brånemark PI, Zarb GA, Albrektsson T: *Tissue-integrated prostheses—osseointegration in clinical dentistry,* Chicago, 1987, Quintessence.

Brunski JB, Hipp JA: *In vivo* forces on endosteal implants: a measurement system and biomechanical considerations, *J Prosthet Dent* 51:82, 1984.

Brunski JB, Moccia AF, Pollack SR, Korostoff E, Trachtenberg DI: The influence of functional use of endosseous dental implants on the tissue-implant interface. I. Histological aspects, *J Dent Res* 58:1953, 1979.

Cook SD, Thomas KA, Kay JF, Jarcho M: Hydroxyapatite-coated porous titanium for use as an orthopedic biologic attachment system, *Clin Orthop* 230:303, 1988.

Deporter DA, Friedland B, Watson PA, Pilliar RM, Howley TP, Abdulla D, Melcher AH, Smith DC: A clinical and radiographic assessment of a porous-surfaced, titanium alloy dental implant system in dogs, *J Dent Res* 65:1071, 1986.

Ducheyne P: Bioceramics: material characteristics versus in vivo behavior, *J Biomed Mater Res; Appl Biomat* 21(suppl A2):219, Aug 1987.

Ducheyne P, Hench LL, Kagan A II, Martens M, Bursens A, Mulier JC: The effect of hydroxyapatite impregnation on skeletal bonding of porous coated implants, *J Biomed Mater Res* 14:225, 1980.

Healy KE, Ducheyne P: The mechanisms of passive dissolution of titanium in a model physiological environment, *J Biomed Mater Res* 26:319, 1992.

Hench LL, Ethridge EC: *Biomaterials: an interfacial approach,* New York, 1982, Academic Press.

Hench LL, Splinter RJ, Allen WC, Greenlee TK, Jr: Bonding mechanisms at the interface of ceramic prosthetic materials, *J Biomed Mater Res Symp* 2:117, 1972.

Kasemo B: Biocompatibility of titanium implants: surface science aspects, *J Prosthet Dent* 49:832, 1983.

Koeneman J, Lemons J, Ducheyne P, Lacefield W, Magee F, Calahan T, Kay J: Workshop on characterization of calcium phosphate materials, *J Appl Biomat* 1:79, 1990.

Kohn DH: Overview of factors important in implant design, *J Oral Implantol* 18:204, 1992.

Kohn DH: Structure-property relations of biomaterials for hard tissue replacement. In Wise DL, editor, *Encyclopedia of Biomaterials and Bioengineering,* Matawan, NJ, 1995, Marcel Dekker.

Lemons JE: Dental implant retrieval analyses, *J Dent Ed* 52:748, 1988.

Luthy H, Strub JR, Scharer P: Analysis of plasma flame-sprayed coatings on endosseous oral titanium implants exfoliated in man: preliminary results, *Int J Oral Maxillofac Imp* 2:197, 1987.

Maniatopoulos C, Pilliar RM, Smith DC: Threaded versus porous-surfaced designs for implant stabilization in bone-endodontic implant model, *J Biomed Mater Res* 20:1309, 1986.

National Institutes of Health Consensus Development Conference Statement on Dental Implants, June 13-15, 1988, *J Dent Ed* 52:824, 1988.

Schnitman PA, Schulman LB: Dental implants: benefit and risk. In US Department Health and Human Services, publication no 81-1531, 1980.

16 *Casting Procedures*

In dentistry the lost-wax casting technic was not popular until 1907 when W.H. Taggart introduced his technic and casting machine. Today the lost-wax technic is common practice and is used for a variety of casting operations; these range from the simplest inlay to all forms of cast crowns, bridge structures, and removable partial dentures, each of which involves the same fundamental practices in forming the cast restoration.

■ CASTING PRACTICES FOR LOW-FUSING GOLD ALLOYS

The casting method consists of forming a wax pattern, surrounding it with investment material, and later heating the investment mold to remove the wax before casting the molten metal into the mold. Glass can be cast in a manner similar to that used with metals; thus esthetic dental crowns can be produced. The procedure for casting glass is described briefly at the end of this chapter. Regardless of the technic used or the type of restoration to be cast, an exact duplicate pattern of the finished restoration must first be prepared in wax or plastic. After an acceptable pattern is formed, it is surrounded with dental investment, and the investment hardens to form the mold into which the alloy is cast.

All investment materials display some setting expansion and hygroscopic expansion on hardening, and they display thermal expansion when they are heated to eliminate the wax from the mold or when they are heated to more elevated temperatures. The amount of each type of expansion varies with the technic selected and the method used to manipulate the investment. However, with any acceptable technic, the combined setting, hygroscopic, and thermal expansion should be consistent

and should produce a total of 1.5% to 2% mold expansion before the casting is made. The choice of the technic is optional, depending on the facilities available and the operator's preference. Each technic is influenced by variables of manipulation; therefore, to obtain reproducible and accurate results, attention must be given to all details of the procedure.

When the investment mold has been formed and the wax eliminated by heating, the mold is then ready to receive the molten metal to form the casting. Proper and careful heating of the investment mold is necessary for at least three reasons: (1) complete wax elimination occurs only with adequate time and temperature of heating, (2) proper heating permits the correct thermal expansion to occur before making the casting, and (3) overheating of calcium sulfate–bonded investment produces a chemical decomposition of the calcium sulfate.

This decomposition of the investment mold is damaging to the surface quality and physical properties of the alloys if the decomposition is excessive. Excessive heating of the investment is especially undesirable when embedded alloy backings, wire clasps, and other forms are included in the mold as part of the restoration. The decomposition gases within the mold embrittle the embedded alloy and prevent the formation of a good union with the cast alloy. To prevent the damaging effects of decomposition gases from calcium sulfate–bonded investment, avoid heating the investment mold to temperatures above 700° C and keep the heating time to the required minimum. Some calcium sulfate–bonded investments contain special ingredients, such as oxalic acid and oxalate salts; on heating, such ingredients decompose and form carbon dioxide. The presence of carbon dioxide in the mold cavity depresses the decomposition of calcium sulfate.

437

■ DIMENSIONAL CHANGES

The purpose of the dental casting is to provide a metallic replacement for missing tooth structure. Some castings serve as a framework to support artificial replacements of missing teeth, such as bridges or removable partial denture restorations. A casting should be as accurate as possible, although a tolerance of ±0.05% for an inlay casting is acceptable. If the linear dimension of an average dental inlay casting is assumed to be 4 mm, ±0.05% of this value is equal to only ±2 μm, which indicates that if two castings made for the same tooth have a variation of 4 μm, the difference may not be noticeable. To visualize this dimension, recall that the thickness of an average human hair is about 40 μm. Therefore the tolerance limits of a dental casting are approximately one-tenth of the thickness of a human hair. To obtain castings with such small tolerance limits, rigid requirements must be placed not only on the investment material but also on the impression materials, waxes, and die materials. Naturally, technical procedures and the proper handling of these materials are equally important. The absolute values for the setting, hygroscopic, and thermal expansions of investment materials may vary from one product to another, and slightly different technics may be used with different investments. In each case the values that are obtained for any one property should be reproducible from one batch to another and from one casting to another.

In general, three distinct contractions that require compensation may take place during the casting process.

1. Shrinkage of the wax pattern results from the change in the temperature at which the wax pattern is prepared and subsequently invested. The wax pattern may be prepared in the patient's mouth. This factor of wax shrinkage is discussed in greater detail in Chapter 13.

2. Contraction can also result from phase changes. Recall that most materials contract during solidification. However, when casting alloys solidify, this contraction is minimized, and it is negligible if the wax pattern is sprued properly and an adequate casting pressure is delivered by the casting machine during the casting operation.

3. Shrinkage of cast alloys results from the thermal coefficient of expansion. Remember that dental castings cool after solidification from the solidus temperature of the alloy to room temperature. This cooling involves contraction, the amount of which depends on both the alloy composition and the casting shape. For dental gold alloys, this shrinkage may vary from 1.25% to 1.7% for different alloys and castings of different shapes.

These three contractions take place in all castings, and adequate compensation is required to properly fit the restoration.

Means of Compensation

A portion of the compensation for shrinkage might be accomplished by thermal expansion of the wax before investment of a wax pattern. However, this method is impractical because it tends to distort the wax pattern. The wax expansion and distortion are discussed in Chapter 13. The more practical way to compensate for the shrinkages during casting is by expansion of the investment mold. As described in Chapter 12, the investments currently available exhibit three types of expansion–setting, hygroscopic, and thermal. Theoretically, the type of investment expansion that compensates for the shrinkages is not important as long as the sum of the effective setting, hygroscopic, and thermal expansions is sufficient to compensate for all the shrinkages. The dimensional changes that occur in the casting operation are summarized at the end of this section.

Because wax expansion is not a practical method, the compensation is accomplished by expansion of the investment. In general, the various technics used in casting operations can be classified into two main groups: (1) the high-heat or thermal expansion technic and (2) the low-heat or hygroscopic technic. If the majority of the compensation for shrinkages is produced by the thermal expansion of the investment, the investment is called a thermal type of investment, and the technic is described as a high-heat, or thermal expansion, technic. Conversely, if the majority of the compensation for the shrinkage is accomplished by the hygroscopic expansion of the investment, the investment is known as a hygroscopic type of investment, and the technic is described as a low-heat, or hygroscopic, technic.

$$\underset{\text{shrinkage}}{\text{Wax}} + \underset{\text{shrinkage}}{\text{Gold}} =$$

$$\underset{\text{expansion}}{\text{Wax}} + \underset{\text{expansion}}{\text{Setting}} + \underset{\text{expansion}}{\text{Hygroscopic}} + \underset{\text{expansion}}{\text{Thermal}}$$

■ FORMATION OF INLAY PATTERNS

The factors of flow, expansion, warpage, and others are all important in preparing an inlay wax pattern that will produce an accurate gold casting. Regardless of the procedure followed, the physical principles that govern the basic nature of the wax also control the behavior of the pattern during and following formation. The method of preparing a wax pattern is called direct if the wax pattern is prepared in the patient's mouth. Conversely, if an impression of the cavity preparation is taken and a die is formed from the impression on which the pattern is prepared, the method is called indirect.

Direct Wax Patterns

As mentioned in Chapter 13, the Type I wax for a direct wax pattern must be heated sufficiently to have adequate flow and plasticity under compression to reproduce all details of the cavity walls. Adequate compression of the wax is required in forming direct wax patterns. Also, overheating of the wax should be avoided because of possible tissue damage and discomfort to the patient, as well as the difficulty encountered in compression of the very fluid overheated wax.

When the wax is heated to the proper working temperature of approximately 50° to 52° C for a short period, the previously induced stress from manufacturing and handling tends to be dissipated. A stress-free piece of wax at the proper consistency should be obtained so that the pattern, when formed under pressure, remains relatively stress-free. Thus minimal distortion results when the pattern is subsequently removed from the tooth. This heating and annealing of the wax before insertion into the cavity preparation is accomplished most easily and effectively in a small dry-heat oven. A nonuniform consistency and possible volatilization of some of the wax mass tends to result from excessively heating the wax over a Bunsen burner flame. Prolonged heating of the wax in water, especially at high temperatures, may result in a crumbly mass. Although wax may be annealed in water that is at a proper temperature, it should not be stored for long periods under these conditions.

Because wax has a rather low thermal conductivity, cooling from the working temperature to mouth temperature occurs slowly, and ample time for cooling should be allowed. The decrease in temperature of the wax to mouth temperature results in a contraction. This contraction is offset to some degree when the pattern is held under pressure until mouth temperature is reached because the compression stresses tend to be released, to some degree, when the wax is removed from the prepared tooth. However, the degree and distribution of these stresses vary from one pattern to another. Although these induced stresses are undesirable, their presence is unavoidable.

Because carving a wax pattern directly in the mouth is a task demanding a high degree of dexterity, any property that eases manipulation is desirable. Therefore ANSI/ADA Specification No. 4 for wax states that the wax should be of a color that contrasts with the hard and soft tissues of the mouth; the wax should soften without becoming flaky; and the wax should not show appreciable chipping or flaking when trimmed to a fine margin. Carving instruments that have been sufficiently warmed are desirable to soften, but not melt, the wax as the marginal adaptation and contour are developed. The warm instrument brings the portion of the wax that is being manipulated to its proper working temperature, so that less stress is induced in these areas. A cool carving instrument burnishing over or cutting through the wax introduces both tension and compression stresses into the pattern, which are detrimental to the ultimate fit of the casting.

Indirect Wax Patterns

When a wax pattern is formed by the indirect method, a metal or stone die is used, which is the positive replica of at least a portion of the surrounding tooth structure and the cavity preparation. This tooth replica permits the pattern to be formed outside of the mouth. Forming the wax pattern on a die permits a change in the type of wax (Type II) and certain manipulative procedures that are necessary for the direct inlay technic. The convenience provided by the indirect method makes the property of flow less critical, because the pattern may be removed from the die at a lower temperature and with greater ease.

When adapting wax to stone or some metal dies, some form of lubricant must be used to release the wax pattern from the die. In the mouth no such lubricant is required because a thin film of saliva or dentinal fluid serves as a lubricant. A variety of fluids are currently available to prevent the attachment of the wax to the die. These fluids produce a separator film of minimum thickness. An excess of separator is to be avoided because it leads to inaccuracies in the wax pattern and poor surface of the cast alloy.

The wax may be adapted to the die either by the flowing of small melted increments from a spatula to build up the desired contour or by the compression method, as is suggested in the direct technic methods. By either method the temperature of a stone die is of little concern in wax adaptation, because the stone is a poor thermal conductor. Likewise, the temperature of a metal die is not critical when compression of the wax is used to form the pattern. However, this temperature is critical when molten increments are used to build up the pattern because the manner of solidification of the wax depends on the temperature of the metal die.

When molten wax flows onto a cool metal die, the wax immediately adjacent to the die solidifies rapidly because the heat from the molten wax is rapidly dissipated. The wax adjacent to the air stays molten for a longer period, and as it solidifies and contracts, it pulls the previously congealed wax away from the metal, resulting in poor surface adaptation, as shown in Fig. 16-1, *A*. Conversely, if the metal die is warmed throughout to near body temperature, the wax solidifies more evenly throughout its mass, resulting in better adaptation, as shown in Fig. 16-1, *B*. The die can be warmed by placing it under an electric lamp or placing it with the carving instruments on an electric heating pad that is at a suitable temperature. The indirect wax pattern is carved with a warm instrument, as is the direct pattern, again to minimize the formation of stresses in the wax.

Because of the basic physical nature of the wax, distortion of the pattern is a continual hazard. Not only does wax have one of the highest coefficients

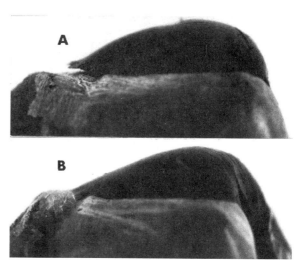

Fig. 16-1 Evidence of wax pulling away when applied on a cold metal die, **A**, and lying flat with good adaptation on warmed metal die, **B**.

of thermal expansion of any dental material, but it also possesses a relatively low softening temperature that may cause stress release or flow to occur. Stresses are easily induced in forming any pattern; in fact, the formation of a completely stress-free wax pattern would appear improbable. With knowledge of the physical characteristics of the inlay wax, the operator must minimize the stress within the pattern by applying manipulative procedures that permit proper temperature and stress control of the wax.

Spruing the Pattern

The removal of any wax pattern from a cavity preparation within the mouth or from a die should be accomplished with the forces applied symmetrically. If the wax pattern is for a small inlay, removal from an indirect die can be accomplished without difficulty after attaching a single or double sprue pin of appropriate diameter. However, if the wax pattern is for a large crown, it should be carefully released to ensure ease of removal from the die. The die is then cleaned with a cloth or tissue paper and lubricated again. The pattern is reseated, marginal adjustments are completed, and the sprue is attached. In any case the type, size, location, and direction of the sprue are factors that contribute to the quality of the casting. A hollow sprue pin provides a stronger attachment to the pattern and is recommended over the solid pin. The core of the pin should be filled with sticky wax before its use so that wax from the pattern is not sucked into it during attachment, which would result in a void. Where the solid sprue pin is necessary, as in some types of double sprues having a Y shape, a minute amount of sticky wax should be used to enhance the union of the pin and the wax.

The diameter of the sprue, in conjunction with the pressure of the casting machine and density of the molten metal, controls the rate of flow of the molten metal into the mold cavity. The larger the diameter of the sprue or the higher the pressure of the casting machine and density of the molten metal, the faster the molten metal should enter the mold cavity. However, the mold cavity is filled with various gases before the entry of the molten metal, and the mold cavity cannot be filled completely unless all gases are driven out through the pores of the investment. As mentioned in Chapter 12, a requirement of dental investments is that they be sufficiently porous to allow gases to escape. Thus not only do the sprue diameter and the pressure of the casting machine have an effect on the rate of filling the mold cavity, but the rate of the elimination of gases from the mold cavity also has an effect. With dense investments and large castings, the addition of vents might be necessary to allow gases to escape. These vents are made of small-diameter wax wire and run from the casting to the sprue base. Incomplete castings may result also from using a sprue with a diameter that is too small. In this case the molten metal may solidify before completely filling the mold cavity. The proper sprue diameter for dental casting, depending on the size of the wax pattern, may vary between 6 and 12 gage (4.1 and 2.0 mm, respectively). Theoretically the diameter of the sprue should be larger than the thickest part of the wax pattern; however, practically it could be slightly smaller.

The sprue should be attached to the bulkiest portion of the wax pattern, as shown in Fig. 16-2. Placing the sprue away from the fine margins minimizes distortion of the wax pattern. When attaching the sprue, remember to flare the point of contact, as shown in insert *x* of Fig. 16-2, *B*. This allows more even flow of the metal into the mold and less porosity in the casting at the point of contact. In addition, not flaring the sprue connections, as shown in insert *y*, results in the formation of sharp projections of investment that can break off and incorporate into

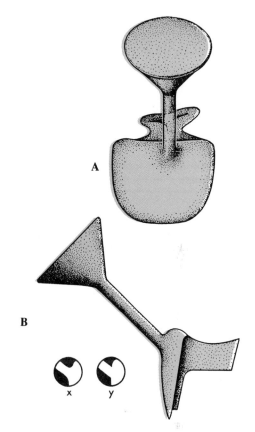

Fig. 16-2 Position and angle of attachment of the sprue to the wax pattern.

the metal during casting. The direction of the sprue is another factor to consider. In general, the sprue should be directed toward the margins so that it minimizes the turbulence of the flow of the molten metal and favors the fine margins of the wax pattern.

The wax pattern should be positioned approximately 6 mm from the end of the casting ring. This position provides sufficient thickness of investment to contain the casting and reduces the amount of investment through which gases must escape. Positioning the pattern close to the surface also ensures that the casting cools more rapidly than the more centrally located sprue. When this is done the metal in the sprue remains liquid and provides flow of metal to the casting until it is completely solidified.

Wettability

Wax surfaces generally are not easily wetted by water. The surface of a wax pattern that is not completely covered with investment develops surface irregularities in the casting alloy restoration that destroy the accuracy of the casting. These irregularities can be minimized by applying a surface-active wetting agent on the wax, using the hand-investing technic.

The function of the wetting agents is to reduce the contact angle of a liquid with the wax surface. Also, they remove any oily film that is left on the wax pattern from the separating medium used on the die. This spreading is illustrated by comparisons in Fig. 16-3, which show silhouettes of advancing water droplets on a polished inlay wax surface, *A,* and on the same surface treated with the surface-active agent before the water droplet was applied, *B.* In *B,* the agent was applied and blotted dry with lens paper. The contact angles are 98 degrees for the plain wax surface and 61 degrees for the treated wax surface. The lower contact angle indicates that the treated wax surface has an affinity for water, which results in the investment being able to spread easier over the wax. Because the surface-active agents are quite soluble, rinsing the wax pattern with water after the application defeats the purpose of their use, as shown in Fig. 16-3, *C.* The same wax as that used in Fig. 16-3, *B,* was rinsed with tap water and blotted dry. The contact angle in this case is 91 degrees, closely approaching that of the original plain wax surface.

Inlay patterns are usually coated with a surface-active solution or wetting agent made specifically for

the purpose, and the excess is removed with a damp-dry inlay brush. After the traces of solution remaining on the pattern are removed, the investment mix is brought into contact with the wax.

Distortion

The distortion of the wax pattern after its removal from the cavity is a function of the temperature and time interval before investing. The nearer the softening point of the wax is approached, the more readily the stress is released. Also, the longer a pattern is allowed to remain before investing, the greater the deformation that may occur, even at room temperature. Therefore a pattern should be invested as soon as possible after its removal from the tooth cavity or die, and it should not be subjected to a warm environment during this interval. In any case, a pattern should not stand for more than 20 to 30 minutes before being invested. Once it is properly invested and the investment has set, there is no danger of further pattern distortion, even though it remains for some hours before the final stages of wax elimination and casting.

During the investing procedures, a further distortion of the wax pattern may occur due to improper handling of the pattern or a specific compensating technic. This problem is discussed in Chapter 12 under casting investments, in which the effect of a warm water bath on hygroscopic investment is described.

■ INVESTING PROCEDURE FOR WAX PATTERNS

After the wax pattern for an inlay or other small restoration, such as a crown or bridge abutment, has been prepared and sprued, and a surface tension–reducing agent has been applied, it then should be invested promptly. The correct water/powder ratio of the investment mix, a required number of spatulation turns, and a proper investing technic are essential to obtain acceptable casting results. There are two different methods of investing the wax pattern: hand investing and vacuum investing.

Hand-Investing Procedure

The recommended water/powder ratio always should be followed for best results. Usually 50 g of

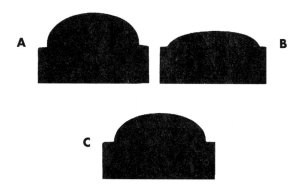

Fig. 16-3 Spreading of water droplet on polished wax surface, **A;** on polished wax that is coated with wetting agent, **B;** and on wax from which wetting agent was rinsed with water before application of droplet, **C.**

calcium sulfate–bonded investment powder or 60 g of phosphate–bonded investment powder is sufficient to fill an inlay ring. A correct amount of water or special liquid is measured and placed in a rubber mixing bowl, and then the investment powder is added. The powder and liquid are mixed briefly with a plaster spatula until all the powder is wetted. The cover of the bowl, which carries the mechanical mixer, is placed over the bowl, and the mix is spatulated. The mixing bowl and a hand mechanical spatula are shown in Fig. 16-4. While spatulating, the manufacturer's recommendations should be followed carefully; usually 100 turns of the spatulator are adequate. As discussed with the hygroscopic investment, the setting of an investment depends critically on the number of spatulation turns, which affects the hygroscopic expansion.

The investment, after being spatulated, is placed on the vibrator to eliminate some of the air bubbles from the mix and to collect all of the mix from the sides of the rubber bowl into the center. A sprue base with sprue, wax pattern, and ring are shown in Fig. 16-5. The sprue base, which holds the sprue and wax pattern, is held with one hand, and the investment is painted over the wax pattern with a camel-hair brush. In painting the pattern, the investment should be teased ahead of the brush to prevent incorporation of air adjacent to the pattern. After the painting is completed, the pattern is vibrated very gently with the sprue base held firmly with the fingers and the under-

side of the hand resting on the vibrator. This method relieves any minor air bubbles that might have been trapped around the wax pattern. Then the inlay ring is placed over the sprue base and filled.

For the setting and hygroscopic expansion of an investment to take place more uniformly, some allowance must be made for the lateral expansion of the investment. Solid rings do not permit the investment to expand laterally during the setting, hygroscopic, and thermal expansions of the mold. To overcome this lateral restriction, a ceramic paper liner is placed inside the ring. A drawing of a sprue base, wax pattern, inlay ring, and liner in position is shown in Fig. 16-6. The ceramic paper liner is cut to fit the inside of the metal ring and is held in place with the fingers. The ring containing the liner is then dipped into water until the liner is completely wet and water is dripping from it. The ring is shaken gently to remove the excess water. Variable amounts of water in the liner produce different amounts of hygroscopic expansion in the investment, regardless of the type of investment used. After the liner has been soaked, it should not be touched or adapted further with the fingers because this reduces its cushioning effect, which is needed for the lateral expansion of the investment. A liner that is about 3 mm short at each end of the ring is preferred. When the liner is equally short at each end of the ring, the investment is locked into the ring, and uniform expansion of the cavity form occurs.

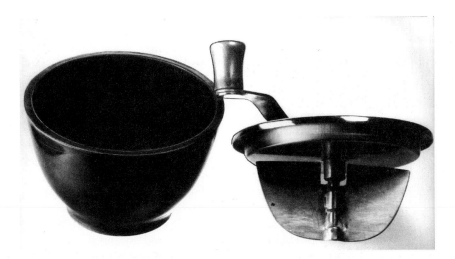

Fig. 16-4 Mixing bowl and hand mechanical spatula.

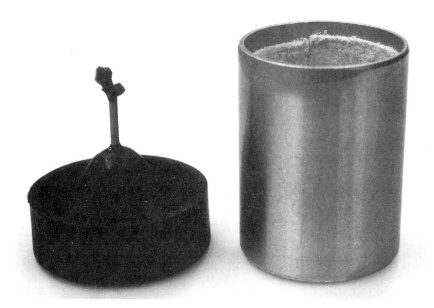

Fig. 16-5 Sprue base, sprue pin with wax pattern, and ceramic paper-lined casting ring.

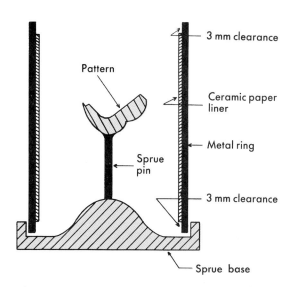

Fig. 16-6 Assembled sprue base and metal casting ring.

After the pattern has been painted with investment, the liner is properly adapted, and the ring is properly assembled on the sprue base, the mixed investment is poured into the ring, which is held at a slight angle so that the investment flows slowly down its side to fill from the bottom to the top. In this manner the possibility of trapping quantities of air in the ring, or around the pattern, is reduced to a minimum.

It is often helpful to hold the assembled ring and sprue base in one hand, which rests gently on a vibrator while the investment is being poured into the ring. When the ring is completely filled, it is leveled with the top by the edge of a plaster spatula. The filled ring is then set aside for the investment to set completely, which usually requires 45 to 60 minutes.

When a phosphate investment is used the ring is slightly overfilled, the top of the ring is not leveled off, and the investment is allowed to set. After the investment has set, the excess investment is ground off using a model trimmer. This procedure is necessary because a nonporous, glassy surface results, which must be ground off in order to improve the permeability of the investment and allow for gases to readily escape from the mold during the casting step.

Vacuum-Investing Procedure

Vacuum-investing equipment is available to facilitate the investing operation. A popular vacuum machine that is used in dentistry is shown in Fig. 16-7. With this equipment the powder and water, or special liquid, are mixed under vacuum, and the mixed investment is permitted to flow into the ring and around the wax pattern with the vacuum present. Although vacuum investing does not remove all the air from the investment and the inlay

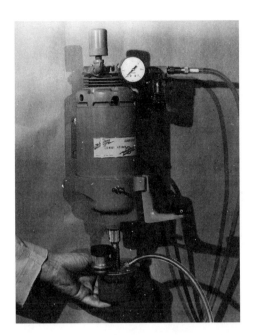

Fig. 16-7 One type of vacuum unit for investing small wax patterns.

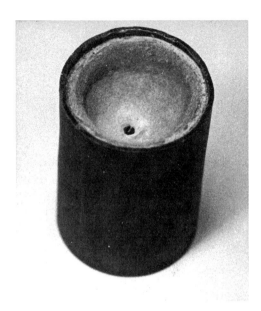

Fig. 16-8 Investment mold ready for burnout. (From Craig RG, O'Brien WJ, Powers JM: *Dental materials: properties and manipulation,* ed 6, St Louis, 1996, Mosby.)

ring, the amount of air usually is reduced enough to obtain a smooth adaptation of the investment to the pattern. Vacuum investing often yields castings with improved surfaces when compared with castings produced from hand-invested patterns. The degree of difference between the two procedures depends largely on the care used in hand investing.

Whether hand- or vacuum-investing procedures are used in filling the casting ring, the investment should be allowed to harden in air if the thermal expansion technic is used. Conversely, if the hygroscopic water-immersion technic is used, the casting ring containing the investment should be placed immediately in a water bath at 37° C, and the investment should be allowed to harden under water. As described in Chapter 12 under casting investments, some water from the bath penetrates the investment, causing it to expand hygroscopically. An inlay casting ring containing a ceramic paper liner and investment after setting using the water bath immersion technic is ready for burnout of the wax (Fig. 16-8).

Investing Patterns for Water-Added Technic

The hand- and vacuum-investing procedures apply to any technic and can be practiced regardless of whether a high-heat or hygroscopic casting technic is used. However, certain technics may require some minor changes to accommodate the particular method. For example, with the water-added hygroscopic technic, in which a controlled amount of water is added to the investment in the ring to provide the desired hygroscopic expansion of the investment, a regular metal ring with ceramic paper liner cannot be used.

In the water-added technic a flexible rubber ring capable of expanding laterally without any liner is used. A set of commercially available equipment for the water-added technic is shown in Fig. 16-9 and it consists of a flexible sprue base, a flexible ring that fits the sprue base, a metallic sleeve to facilitate the handling of the flexible ring, a reservoir to provide extra room for water to be added after the wax pattern is invested and the metallic sleeve removed, and a hypodermic syringe to accurately deliver a prescribed amount of water. With this equipment the wax pattern can be invested by either a hand-investing or a vacuum-investing technic, as described previously.

Heating the Mold

After the wax pattern has been invested, it should be set aside until the investment mass is hardened.

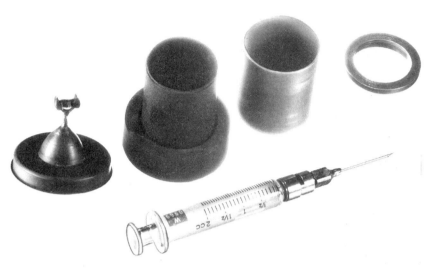

Fig. 16-9 Equipment needed for water-added hygroscopic expansion technic.

A requirement in all investments is to wait until the final set of the investment before placing it in an oven for elimination of the wax pattern. Usually 45 to 60 minutes are required after the start of the mix for the investment to reach its final set and to possess a sufficiently high wet strength to be transferred to the oven.

As discussed previously, the strength of the investment is an important property of an investment in any technic, especially with the water-added technic, in which a flexible rubber ring is used instead of a metallic ring with a ceramic liner. With regular technics the metallic ring containing the investment and the wax pattern is placed in the oven for wax elimination. After the wax has been eliminated and the mold has reached the casting temperature, the molten metal is cast into the mold cavity while the mold is supported by the metallic ring. In this way the mold can better withstand the impact force exerted by the molten metal entering the hot mold.

With water-added technics, the water reservoir, flexible ring, sprue, and sprue base are removed, and a cylinder of the investment without a supporting ring is placed in the oven. Such a mold ready to be heated after removal of the sprue is shown in Fig. 16-10. After the wax is eliminated, the molten metal is forced into the investment without support of a metal ring. Therefore, the investment used with

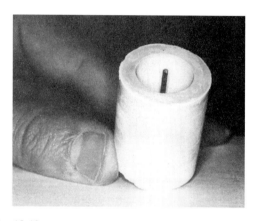

Fig. 16-10 Mold with invested wax pattern ready for removal of the sprue and heating for wax elimination.

this technic should not only have a high strength, but also should have adequate time (at least 45 minutes) to reach its maximum wet strength before being placed into the oven.

Wax Elimination

The mold is placed in an oven to completely eliminate the wax, thereby forming a cavity into which the molten metal is cast. During wax elimination the investment expands thermally, which is necessary to compensate for the casting shrinkages. Although wax melts at a comparatively low temperature, its complete elimination requires much higher

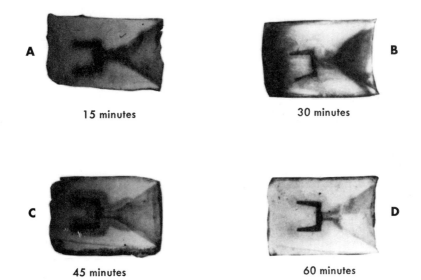

A   15 minutes

B   30 minutes

C   45 minutes

D   60 minutes

Fig. 16-11 Effect of burnout time of wax in investment molds on the presence of carbon residue. Each mold was placed in a room-temperature furnace that was then set at 500° C, heated for the times indicated, and sectioned to examine the internal appearance. Notice the dark gray area of carbon residue around the mold cavity in **C** even after 45 minutes of heating.

temperatures. Usually, if elimination is not complete, small bits of the wax residue are retained in the fine margins of the mold and prevent the formation of a complete casting. When the molten metal enters the sprue hole, the resulting force causes the air in the mold cavity to be driven out through the pores of the investment, and thus the mold cavity is filled completely. The presence of any foreign material in the mold cavity slows down or possibly prevents the air or other gases from being driven out of the mold before the molten metal solidifies. As a result, the castings are incomplete or the margins are irregular, in which case the casting should be repeated, starting with a new wax pattern.

Because the ingredients of inlay waxes are organic materials, they are composed of carbon, hydrogen, and nitrogen. When heated to higher temperatures, any organic material decomposes and forms carbon dioxide (CO_2), water (H_2O), or nitrogen oxide (NO), all of which are gaseous and can be easily eliminated. However, formation of these gases depends on the presence of a sufficient supply of oxygen, the relatively high temperature of the oven, and adequate heating time of the ring. If the amount of oxygen available to the wax in the mold cavity is

not sufficient, the temperature of the oven is not high enough, or the wax pattern is heated only for a short time, incomplete reaction between the wax and oxygen may result. The internal walls of mold cavities placed in a room-temperature oven set at 500° C and left for different times are shown in Fig. 16-11. The longer the ring remained in the oven, the better the elimination of carbon residue from the mold cavity. Castings made under these four conditions showed that for conditions seen in Fig. 16-11, *A,* and Fig. 16-11, *B,* the castings were not complete and part of the pattern did not cast. For the condition seen in Fig. 16-11, *C,* depending on the total amount of wax used, the number of investment rings in the oven, and other such variables, the castings either were incomplete (as under conditions shown in Fig. 16-11, *A,* and Fig. 16-11, *B,*) or appeared to be complete but had short and round margins. These results indicated that elimination of gases from mold cavities was rather slow because of the presence of carbon deposits, and the molten alloy solidified before all the gases around the marginal area could escape. For all three conditions, the surfaces of the castings were black and could not be cleaned by normal pickling action. This black color indicated that the surfaces were covered with fine particles of carbon residue, because the acid in pickling solutions is not effective in dissolving or removing carbon particles. Castings made under the condition shown in Fig. 16-11, *D,* were complete, with sharp margins, and on pickling the casting surfaces had a typical yellow color.

A satisfactory way of eliminating the wax pattern is to set the mold in the furnace with the sprue hole placed downward at first, so that most of the wax drains out and is eliminated as a liquid. The ring is then inverted with the sprue hole placed upward. In this position the oxygen in the oven atmosphere can circulate more readily into the cavity, react with the wax, and form gases rather than the fine carbon that interferes with the venting of the mold cavity. The lower the mold temperature and the larger the wax pattern, the longer the mold should be left in the oven. For a 500° C mold temperature and larger wax patterns, the mold should remain in the oven for approximately 1 hour, with the sprue hole placed downward during half of this time and upward during the other half. If more than one ring is placed in an oven, a longer period is required for wax elimination. The general rule is to add 5 minutes to the wax elimination time for every extra ring placed in the oven at 500° C. With an oven temperature of 600° to 700° C, a shorter time may be sufficient to completely eliminate the wax.

Oven Temperature

Investment materials are poor heat conductors, which results in some temperature difference between the inner core and the outside portion of the mold. Although this difference is relatively great at the beginning of the heating cycle, it diminishes as the time progresses and may cease to exist at the time of casting. The difference in temperature between the inner and outer portions of the mold becomes greater if the mold is placed in a preheated oven or if the heating rate of the oven is too rapid. The outside of the mold, being exposed to a higher temperature, expands somewhat more than does the inner part. This expansion may cause the mold to crack during the heating period. Because of the high thermal expansion of investments containing cristobalite, the difference in the temperatures of different portions of the mold may create uneven expansion.

For best results this type of investment should always be placed in a room-temperature oven, with the oven temperature increased slowly. The difference in the temperature of different portions of the mold does not affect quartz-containing investments as much as it affects cristobalite investments, probably because the rate of thermal expansion of the quartz investment is slower than that of the cristobalite investment. With hygroscopic investments, in which the thermal expansion of the investment is only about 0.5%, the mold can be placed in a preheated oven of 500° C and not crack during the heating.

When the wax pattern is completely eliminated and the mold has reached the casting temperature, the gold alloy is melted by an appropriate method and cast into the mold cavity.

■ PRACTICAL DIFFERENCES BETWEEN HYGROSCOPIC AND HIGH-HEAT TECHNICS

In the hygroscopic technic the setting and hygroscopic expansions of the investment are major factors in compensating for the shrinkage of the cast alloy and wax pattern. The thermal expansion of such investments is rather low. In the high-heat technic the thermal expansion of the investment compensates mainly for the shrinkage, and the setting and hygroscopic expansions of such investments are rather low. The net expansion should be the same with either type of investment. When heating the investment to eliminate the wax pattern and to obtain thermal expansion of the investment, the wax pattern melts and the mold cavity can expand without any interference from the wax pattern. However, during setting and hygroscopic expansions of the investment, the wax pattern is present and offers some resistance to the expansion forces. For example, the setting and hygroscopic expansions of the investment inside the core of the full crown type of pattern are restricted by the strength of the wax pattern. A bulkier pattern offers more resistance than the normal-sized wax pattern. Similarly, full crowns made of hard inlay wax offer more resistance than those made of regular or soft wax. However, note that the type of wax used for making one-surface inlays has very little effect. In this instance the investment expands away from the wax pattern, and the strength of the wax cannot alter the expansion. In all other cases, the type of the wax used with the hygroscopic technic is important in the fit of the resulting castings. In general, regular or soft waxes should be used with the hygroscopic technic. The use of hard inlay wax or a plastic pattern in the hygroscopic technic should be avoided. The effect of the type of wax used with the water-added hygroscopic technic is even greater than with the water bath immersion hygroscopic technic. In the water bath immersion technic the temperature of the water bath is about 37° to 38° C, which tends to soften the wax pattern, reducing any restrictions of the pattern because of its thermal expansion. In the water-added technic the invested wax pattern remains near room temperature, and neither its rigidity nor its dimensions are altered.

■ CASTING FACILITIES

To cast a metal restoration, a suitable torch or other heating equipment to melt the alloy and a suitable means of forcing the molten metal into the mold are necessary. Various devices are available for each of these operations.

Methods of Melting Alloys

The most common method of heating gold alloys for full cast metal restorations is by using a gas-air torch. A properly adjusted torch develops an adequate temperature for melting dental gold alloys, whose melting range is between 870° and 1000° C. Completing the melting operation promptly also depends on the proper adjustment of the torch flame. Poorly adjusted flames can lead to wasted time during melting and can considerably damage the alloy through excessive oxidation or gas inclusion. Small and irregularly shaped flames should not be used to melt moderate or large quantities of alloys for casting purposes. A well-defined torch flame is the hottest and most effective for such melting operations.

The literature contains many descriptions of the proper flame for heating metals and alloys. One practical method of checking and interpreting the flame condition is to apply the flame to a small piece of copper, approximately the size of a coin, placed on a soldering block. The torch is adjusted as it would be for making a casting and is then directed on the copper. If the copper turns bright and clean as it is heated, the flame and the torch manipulation are correct. If the copper turns to a dark, dull red color, oxidation is occurring and the heating is ineffective. The operator should make the necessary adjustments to eliminate these conditions.

The properly adjusted flame contains well-defined component parts described as inner and outer cones or portions having differing color intensities. For example, the inner, well-defined light blue central cone is usually accepted as the most effective for heating because it is the least oxidizing portion of the flame. Although an improper flame is the frequent cause of oxidation of the base metals in the alloys, a properly adjusted flame also causes oxidation if it is held too closely to the metal being heated, too far from it, or to one side or another, or if it is moved over the surface or away from the alloy. The dramatic oxidation and ineffective heating that can be seen on the copper are not as evident with gold alloys, yet may be observed by the operator who is aware of such conditions.

Modified torches may be used that combine natural gas and oxygen or certain "tank" gases, such as acetylene and oxygen. The natural gas and oxygen combination is mainly used for melting alloys designed for constructing porcelain-metal restorations. The combination of acetylene and oxygen has been used mostly to melt cobalt-chromium base alloys, which have higher fusion temperatures and are used in fabricating removable partial denture prostheses.

Electric melting units of various designs are used in some laboratories to melt the alloys to make the castings. The advantage of using these units is that slightly less skill is required than that necessary for controlling the torch; however, many of these electric heating units have no limiting controls, and as a result, the operator must exercise judgment regarding the proper condition of the alloy to be cast. The electric units are heated either by induction or by resistance heating systems. Those units heated by induction melt alloys much faster than do those heated by torch; therefore, if the procedure is not watched closely, the alloy can easily be overheated. An electronic monitor is useful for indicating the proper temperature. Melting units with resistance heating require a longer time to complete the heating and casting operation as compared with torch-melting. The slightly longer heating time does not appreciably increase the temperature of the molten alloy, nor does it cause any significant problems.

Casting Machines

Several types and designs of casting machines are used to make dental castings. All casting machines can be divided into two general types. One is described as a centrifugal force type, and the other depends on air pressure to force the metal into the mold. Numerous modifications and variations of these principles are used in different instruments.

A variety of centrifugal machines are available, with some designed to spin the mold in a plane parallel to the table top on which the machine is mounted and others designed to rotate in a plane vertical to the table top. Some are spring-driven, and others are operated by electric power. An electric heating unit is attached to some machines to melt the alloy before spinning the mold to throw in the metal. Others have a simple refractory crucible mounted on the machine in which the alloy is placed to be melted by a torch before the casting operation is completed. Each of these machines depends on the centrifugal force applied to the molten metal to cause it to completely fill the mold with properly melted metal. Concerning the quality of the casting, a preference for either machine is not known. The main advantage of the centrifugal machines is the simplicity of design and operation, with the opportunity to cast both large and small castings on the same machine.

With the air pressure type of machine, either compressed air or some other gas, such as carbon dioxide or nitrogen, can be used to force the molten metal into the mold. The gas pressure is applied to the molten metal through a suitable valve mechanism. This type of machine is satisfactory for making small castings, and little preference is noted between the gas pressure and centrifugal type of machine for this kind of casting.

Casting machines, both the centrifugal and gas pressure, are available with an attached vacuum system designed to assist the molten metal in filling the mold. In some castings the added vacuum may be advantageous, but in general, this addition shows little evidence of a superior quality of castings.

Regardless of the method of melting the alloy or the manner of casting it into the mold, keep in mind certain objectives when making the casting: (1) heat the alloy as quickly as possible to a completely molten condition, (2) prevent oxidation by heating the metal quickly with a well-adjusted torch or other method and a small amount of flux on the metal surface, and (3) produce a casting with sharp details by having adequate pressure applied to the well-melted metal to force it into the mold. Although each of these operations demands care and attention, they are not difficult to master.

After the molten metal is forced into the mold cavity, the casting machine should be allowed to provide necessary pressure on the metal while the metal is solidifying. This pressure leads to complete casting of the margins. After the centrifugal casting machine stops and the color of the sprue button has changed from red to black, which indicates that the temperature of the metal is lower than 700° C, the ring should be placed in a bowl of water (quenched). Such an operation not only simplifies the separation of the casting from the investment but also cools the metal quickly. Quenching the ring leaves the casting metal in a softened condition, as discussed in Chapter 14 under heat treating of gold alloys.

Gold alloys in the softened condition can be more easily burnished and finished than those in the hardened condition. Whether the burnishing of margins of cast gold alloy restorations permits them to be burnished (pulled) to the extent that a casting with a short or poor marginal fit can be properly adjusted is questionable. Depending on the type of gold alloy, the shape of the cavity, and the type of finishing line on the cavity preparation, cast gold alloys may or may not be able to be burnished to offset a poor marginal fit. In general, it is more practical to burnish Types I and II gold alloys, used for casting gold inlays, than Type III gold alloys, used for casting full crowns. Regardless of the type of alloy and the shape of the cavity preparation, castings should be finished to have smooth surfaces with no observable catches when an explorer is drawn over the casting and the tooth surface.

■ SOME COMMON CASTING PROBLEMS

Unless every step in the casting operation is handled properly, the cast gold restoration may not fit the prepared tooth with the desired accuracy. Naturally, a proper cavity design, an accurate impression of the prepared cavity, a good and accurate die, and proper waxing and casting all are important steps in achieving an acceptable gold restoration. Some of the problems related to the casting operation are described in the following paragraphs.

Improper solidification of metal causes many casting problems. As discussed earlier in this chapter, the shrinkage of wax and alloy is compensated for by various types of expansion of the investment. However, the shrinkage of alloys takes place in two stages as a result of (1) the transformation of the alloy from liquid to solid and (2) the coefficient of expansion of the solid alloy. While the molten alloy is cooling, the temperature eventually reaches the solidification range, causing the alloy to change from a liquid to a solid. This change of state is accompanied by a large shrinkage, which is compensated for only by adhering to a proper casting technic because the expansion of the investment cannot offset such a large shrinkage. In a correct technic, molten alloy located farthest from the sprue button should freeze first and alloy in the sprue and the sprue button should feed the rest of the pattern, thus compensating for the shrinkage as a result of the change of state. As shown in Fig. 16-12, *A,* the part farthest from the sprue button freezes first and changes from the liquid to the solid state, and this change involves some shrinkage that is compensated for by the metal feeding from the sprue and the sprue button.

As long as the remaining alloy is in the liquid state and the casting machine is rotating, molten alloy will feed the solidified portion of the casting, thereby compensating for the shrinkage. The next layer then solidifies, and this process continues until all the shrinkage resulting from the change of state is compensated for by the available molten alloy in the casting, the sprue, and the sprue button. If the solidification did not occur in this systematic manner and a portion of the alloy in the sprue froze before the alloy in the casting, then what is known as suckback

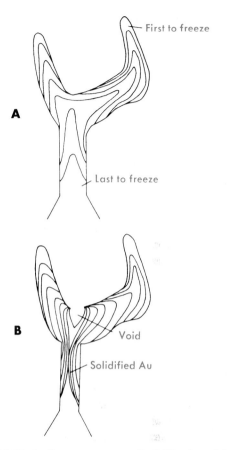

Fig. 16-12 A, Correct sequence of solidification of the gold alloy. **B,** Incorrect sequence of solidification resulting in suckback porosity.

porosity would occur, as shown in Fig. 16-12, *B.* Expansion of the investment material cannot compensate for this type of porosity.

As seen in Fig. 16-12, molten alloy enters the mold cavity through a single sprue. Investment at the pulpal floor of a full crown pattern therefore heats up because of the higher temperature of the molten alloy, and it keeps the alloy in this area molten somewhat longer than other areas. Thus if alloy in the sprue solidifies before the alloy in the pulpal floor area, the molten alloy in this area would feed the solidifying alloy in the sprue area. When molten alloy in the pulpal-floor area solidifies and shrinks because of the change of state, it cannot be fed. As a result, a large porosity under the sprue is observed. Because the cause of suckback porosity is the improper sequence of solidification of the alloy, the following precautions would help to eliminate it:

1. A Y-shaped sprue should be used instead of a single sprue. In this instance only half of the molten alloy enters the mold cavity through each leg of the Y-shaped sprue, so that the temperature of the investment under the sprue does not rise as high. However, the arms of the Y must be widely separated to prevent the investment between the arms from overheating, which could also cause suckback porosity.

2. The mold temperature could be increased from 500° C, which is used with many investments and technics, to 650° to 700° C. With a higher mold temperature, the difference in temperature of the investment located around the sprue and the investment in the area of the pulpal floor of the full crown is decreased. This decrease helps the molten alloy at the pulpal floor to solidify before the alloy at the sprue. Studies have shown that when a gold alloy with a solidification temperature of 940° C was heated to 1040° C and cast into a mold with a temperature of 500° C, the temperature of the mold varied from one location to another. The temperature of the investment 1 mm away from the sprue reached only 585° C, whereas the temperature of the investment 1 mm away from the area of the pulpal floor was as high as 900° C. Thus the difference between the solidification temperature of the alloy and the temperature of the investment at the pulpal floor was only 40° C, whereas the difference near the sprue was 355° C. Therefore molten alloy decreases in temperature faster around the sprue than at the pulpal floor, and the sprue solidifies sooner. When the temperature of the mold was increased from 500° to 700° C, the temperature of the investment 1 mm away from the pulpal floor increased from 900° C to 905°–910° C, whereas the temperature of the investment around the sprue area increased from 585° to 800° C. Thus the difference between the solidification temperature of the alloy and the temperature of the investment in the area of the pulpal floor was 30° to 35° C, whereas around the sprue it was 140° C. In other words, by increasing the mold temperature before casting, the variation of the mold temperature in different areas after casting is reduced.

   Note that with hygroscopic technics, a mold temperature of 700° C would produce an over-expanded mold and an oversized cast restoration and thus should not be used. With the hygroscopic water immersion technic, if a mold temperature of 700° C must be used, the ring should not be placed in a water bath after investing the wax pattern. Bench-hardening of hygroscopic investments with a mold temperature of 700° C produces a sufficient amount of expansion of the mold cavity. Routine use of a mold temperature of 700° C with hygroscopic investments should be avoided because the high mold temperature produces somewhat rougher surfaces on the casting.

3. The diameter of each leg of the Y-shaped sprue could be increased, or an extra 1 or 2 g of gold alloy could be used, which would keep the alloy in the sprue and the sprue button in the molten phase somewhat longer and would feed the solidifying alloy better.

Increasing the temperature of the molten alloy or using an extra turn on a centrifugal casting machine does not help eliminate the suckback porosity and may increase the chances of creating the porosity.

A miscast is also obtained by incomplete wax elimination, overheating of gold alloys, insufficient casting pressure, or incorrect spruing.

With today's calcium sulfate–bonded investments, when the color of the cast alloy is black, the cause is probably one of the following: (1) the wax was not completely eliminated, (2) the mold remained in the oven too long, (3) the oxidizing flame was used in melting the gold alloy, or (4) the investment did not contain any deoxidizing agent. As mentioned earlier, when wax is not completely eliminated, very fine particles of carbon cover the pores of the investment through which the gas in the mold cavity is supposed to escape. Depending on the amount of carbon remaining on the walls of the mold cavity when the molten metal enters, the casting may be complete but be black in color, or it may be incomplete. The black color in this instance cannot be cleaned by the routine pickling action, which is described later in this chapter, because most pickling solutions are acid solutions and most acids are not effective in removing carbon from the surface of gold castings.

However, if the black color of the gold casting is removed by the normal pickling procedure, the black color was caused mainly by copper oxides formed during casting. As mentioned in Chapter 14, most casting investments contain some deoxidizers. Manufacturers add deoxidizers to dental gold casting investments to provide a reducing atmosphere when the molten gold alloys are entering the mold cavity. If the investment mold is left too long in an oven, all the deoxidizers will be decomposed and eliminated. Thus when the molten alloy enters the mold cavity, the oxidation of the copper is not prevented, and the casting will be black. Some investments routinely produce blackened gold castings because the manufacturers do not add any deoxidizing agents. Also, if an oxidizing flame is used in melting the gold alloy, the castings will be black. Castings that are black because of oxidation of some of the elements in the alloy can easily be cleaned, and the gold color can be restored by normal pickling procedures.

Insufficient casting pressure or underheating of gold alloys usually results in castings with rounded margins, which are caused by freezing of molten alloy before the gases are forced from the mold cavity. Therefore gases in the mold cavity should be forced out before the alloy solidifies so that the alloy completely occupies the cavity. Too few turns on the casting machine or a weak spring in the casting machine produces insufficient casting pressure, and all the gases are not forced out of the mold cavity. Similarly, underheating of the alloy does not keep the molten metal in the liquid state long enough. Both of these conditions result in castings with rounded margins.

As mentioned earlier, the location, size, and direction of the sprue are important. The sprue and sprue button should be the last portions to freeze because they feed the alloy to the pattern. The pattern should be located about 6 mm from the end of the ring to ensure that it solidifies first. Attaching the sprue to a thin area, using a sprue with a diameter that is too small, or not directing the sprue toward the fine margins usually results in a miscast or a casting with short margins.

■ CASTING AND SOLDERING FLUXES

A flux is a substance applied to the surface of molten metal primarily to prevent oxygen from contacting the hot metal and thereby causing oxidation. In addition, the flux dissolves oxides that may form while the metal is heated, and the resulting solution of oxides or other extraneous matter in the flux constitutes a slag. A flux also assists in the free flow of solder and permits the solder to wet and spread over the metal surface. For a flux to be effective, it must have a fusion temperature below that of the alloy that is being heated; at the same time, it should not burn or volatilize readily.

Borax, or sodium tetraborate ($Na_2B_4O_7 \cdot 10\ H_2O$), can dissolve the metal oxides that are in gold alloys, mainly copper oxides, and therefore is frequently used as a flux in dentistry. Dehydrated sodium tetraborate is known as borax glass and can be used in the dry powder form. When melted, the borax glass is a clear, viscous liquid that does not volatilize readily when heated. It can be made more fluid by the addition of boric acid or other salts, which aid in spreading the flux on the hot metal surface. Boric acid is not used alone for fluxing purposes, as is sometimes done with borax. Dehydrated borax glass is preferred to the ordinary hydrated borax, which liberates water vapor on being heated and, as a result, effervesces and bubbles up over the surface of the hot metal without forming an effective surface covering.

Fluxes are available in a variety of forms. Generally, the forms are designated for specific applications for soldering or casting operations. The liquid form is principally a solution of borax and boric acid in water, and it is applied in soldering operations of orthodontic appliances and bridge structures in which a minimum of flux is desired. A saturated solution, or lower concentration, of the ingredients may be used, and smaller quantities of other salts, such as potassium carbonate or ammonium chloride, may be added to some liquid fluxes. Also available are paste forms of flux that are formed from mixtures of about one-third borax added to a mineral grease, such as petroleum jelly, with other chemicals added as desired. Pastes are a convenient form for soldering operations in which a large quantity of flux is desired and its application is directed to a specific area. A flux in powder form is normally used for metals during the melting for a casting operation. When this form is used, it is sprinkled lightly on the metal. The powder fluxes may contain finely divided charcoal or other ingredients mixed with borax and boric acid; this combination gives added protection by producing what is described as a reducing flux. The charcoal not only helps prevent the formation of oxides on the metal surface but also reduces oxides that have already formed to free metal. Fluxes in the powder form also may contain a very small percentage (1% to 2%) of finely divided silica flour, which holds the molten flux in position on the surface of the hot metal.

When soldering stainless-steel or cast cobalt-base alloys that contain chromium, a special flux is required because borax and boric acid alone do not dissolve the chromium oxides. Normally the fluxes for these soldering operations should contain about 50% to 60% potassium fluoride, or another fluoride, mixed with 25% to 35% boric acid (H_3BO_4), 6% to 8% borax glass, and 8% to 10% potassium or sodium carbonate. An equal mixture of boric acid and the fluoride salt may be formed into a paste for soldering when they are ground together with a few drops of water, which is considered effective in such soldering operations. Other similar compositions have been recommended. Pastes should not be formulated with petroleum grease for these applications because the carbon formed in heating alters the properties of the alloy being soldered.

Choosing the proper flux, borax or fluoride, for the soldering operation is important. The choice of flux is dictated by the type of alloy to be soldered and not by the type of solder used. If the alloy contains chromium, such as stainless steel wires for orthodontics or cobalt-chromium alloys for partial dentures, the proper choice is fluoride flux, regardless of whether gold or silver solder is used. Similarly, if gold alloys are to be soldered, the proper choice is borax flux, regardless of the solder employed.

As indicated earlier, a principle governing the use of fluxes for any purpose is that neither too much nor too little should be applied to the metal during the heating operation. When too little flux is applied, it tends to burn off and be ineffective; when too much flux is applied, it may become entangled in the molten metal to produce a defect by inclusion.

■ CASTING PORCELAIN VENEER METAL STRUCTURES

Because of the characteristically high melting temperature of the noble or base alloys used in the porcelain-fused-to-metal restorations, special investments and casting facilities are necessary. The calcium sulfate–bonded investment materials and conventional melting facilities are inadequate for most of the alloys available. Generally, the phosphate-bonded investments are used in casting this type of alloy. The phosphate investments are stronger and denser than are the gypsum-bonded investments normally used for gold alloy casting. Although the technic for using these special alloys and investments is not complicated or elaborate, the technic recommended by the manufacturers should be followed faithfully to achieve satisfactory surface conditions and fit of the casting.

The dental literature describes steps in the construction of porcelain veneer restorations and the metal casting operation; all details of the procedure are not discussed here. Because the investment is dense, special attention should be given to the manner of spruing of the wax pattern. Proper spruing should facilitate the escape of gases from the mold cavity before complete solidification of the molten metal. The bar type of spruing used for casting these alloys is shown in Fig. 16-13. With this type of spruing, the sprue bar is placed inside the mold as a reservoir to help keep the alloy in the molten stage for a longer time so that a more complete casting can be attained. Note that with a normal spruing method, the pattern is sprued in such a manner as to reduce turbulence in the flow of molten alloy. However, with the bar spruing method, an attempt is made to increase the turbulence so that the investment close to the sprue maintains a higher temperature, which keeps the alloy in the molten state for a longer time. The main disadvantage of the bar type of sprue is the increased amount of alloy required to make castings; for this reason, the bar type is not used to make castings of ordinary gold alloys.

If a bar type of sprue is used with a centrifugal casting machine, the casting ring should be placed in the casting machine so that the bar sprue is vertical. The leaders from the sprue button to the bar should be attached 1 to 2 mm below the height of the bar.

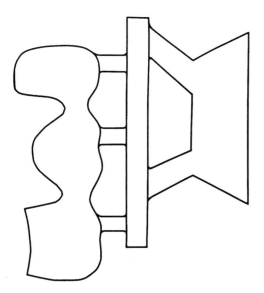

Fig. 16-13 Bar type of spruing of three copings.

In this manner when the alloy at the tip of the bar sprue freezes, the alloy 1 to 2 mm below the tip remains molten, and feeding from the sprue button to the bar is still possible. The leaders from the bar to the wax pattern should be attached to the highest part of the wax pattern. Centrifugal casting machines tend to feed molten alloy straight (as a result of centrifugal force) and down (from gravity). If the leaders from the sprue button to the bar or from the bar to a one-piece cast bridge are placed in the middle of the bar or in the middle of the bridge, there is a high probability for a miscast. In such a sprue arrangement, the molten alloy must fill the lower portion of the bar and the mold cavity before being forced upward against gravity to fill the upper portion of the bar and the bridge. Proper attachment of the leaders to the bar and to three copings is shown in Fig. 16-13.

Other steps in the investing and casting procedure normally include vacuum-investing practice, careful wax elimination, a gas-oxygen torch or other high-temperature melting facilities, and centrifugal casting with adequate casting pressure. Special solders may be required with these alloys for certain technics, and with some alloys and solders the operation requires skillful management for a successful bridge assembly.

■ CLEANING AND "PICKLING" GOLD ALLOYS

The surface oxidation or other contamination of dental gold alloys is a troublesome occurrence. The oxidation of the base metals in the alloy approved by ANSI/ADA Specification No. 5 can be kept to a minimum or avoided completely by combining a properly adjusted method of heating the alloy and a suitable amount of flux when melting the alloy. Despite these precautions, as the hot metal enters the mold, certain alloys tend to become contaminated on the surface because of combination with the hot mold gases, reaction with investment ingredients, or physical inclusion of mold particles in the metal surface. The surface of cast, soldered, or otherwise heated metal dental appliances is cleaned by warming the structure in suitable solutions, by mechanical polishing, or by other treatment of the alloy to restore the normal surface condition.

Surface tarnish or oxidation can be removed by the process of pickling. Gold alloy castings may be cleaned in this manner by warming them in a 50% sulfuric acid and water solution. Today, most commercially available pickling solutions are not made of the ordinary inorganic acid solutions and do not release poisonous gases on boiling. In either case, the casting to be cleaned is placed in a suitable porcelain casserole, or glass beaker, to which the pickling solution is added. It is then warmed gently, but not to the boiling point, until the surface becomes bright, which normally requires only a few moments of heating to a temperature slightly below boiling. When the heating is completed, the acid may be poured from the casserole into the original storage container before the casting is rinsed thoroughly with water.

Although castings or other appliances may have their surface appearance restored by being heated to redness and then dropped into room-temperature acid, this practice is discouraged. The uncontrolled heating to redness softens gold alloys that are subject to heat treatment and tends to relieve any internal stress that may exist in the structure, with resulting warpage or distortion. Thin, delicate castings may have the margins of the restoration damaged by excessive heating or by striking the container when they are dropped into the pickling solution.

Removal of gold restorations from the pickling solution with steel or stainless steel tweezers should be avoided. The pickling solution attacks and dissolves the tweezers, causing the plating of some of the base metals from the tweezers over the gold restorations. This plating may lead to pitting and corroding of gold restorations. Rubber-coated tweezers are recommended for this purpose. If rubberized tweezers are not available, gold restorations may be rinsed with water two or three times before they are removed from the porcelain casserole or glass beaker.

Any contamination of the acid cleaning solutions must be avoided. The solution should be periodically replaced with a fresh quantity of acid, before it becomes severely contaminated and before the bath appears discolored.

Other solutions of an acid salt in water have been suggested for cleaning or pickling operations. In general, the practices followed for their use are the same as those followed for the acid baths. Although they work effectively, their advantages are not pronounced. With proper care and control of the cleaning procedure, acid solutions are acceptable.

The sprue buttons cut from castings may be recast without further treatment if the contamination during the original casting operation was not excessive and the surface of the metal is completely free from the investment. Evidence indicates that the dental gold casting alloys may be recast without loss of properties if the casting procedure is properly conducted. Gold alloys used for metal-ceramic restorations may be recast if 50% new alloy is used to ensure that minor ingredients required for bonding of the ceramic and hardening of the alloy have not been burned out and are in adequate concentration. If the investment material has adhered to the surface of the alloy, it should be removed by sandblasting or brushing with soap and water before it is remelted. Melting the sprue button to clean investment from the surface should be avoided because the investment materials decompose, forming gases that react with noble metal alloys and damage their physical properties.

■ CASTING OF COBALT-CHROMIUM AND NICKLE-CHROMIUM ALLOYS

Posterior crowns may be cast in base metal alloys but because of their high melting temperatures phosphate investments are frequently used. Also, as a result of their high freezing temperatures more shrink-

age of the alloy must be compensated for than in crown and bridge gold alloys in order to obtain accurately fitting castings. The extra compensation can be obtained by (1) painting a die spacer (varnish) on the die but short of the margins before preparing the wax pattern and/or (2) using two layers of ceramic paper liner in the invensing ring in order to make the setting expansion of the investment more effective.

The methods of casting relatively large partial denture frameworks in base metals (Fig. 16-14) differs from the casting of simple restorations such as single inlays or crowns, although the two operations are similar in principle. In cast partial denture construction, a suitable cast of refractory material, or investment, serves as the structure on which the wax pattern is formed. The investment cast is prepared by duplicating the master stone model, usually by using an agar duplicating material described in Chapter 11. A duplicating flask containing the master model is shown in Fig. 16-15 prior to pouring the duplicating material. Fig. 16-15 also shows the duplicate impression in agar and the separated refractory investment cast that was prepared in the agar mold. A gypsum-bonded investment is used when a low-fusing nickel-chromium alloy (Ticonium) is to be cast and a phosphate- or silica-bonded investment is used when high-fusing alloys are to be cast (Nobilium or Vitallium). When a gypsum- or phosphate-bonded investment is used, part of the casting shrinkage of the metal is compensated for by expansion of the investment during setting. Thus the investment cast is intentionally slightly larger than the master model.

The wax pattern is prepared on the investment cast because the large wax pattern is too fragile and easily distorted to be handled as a free-standing wax pattern such as those for a crown or inlay. Fig. 16-16 shows a wax pattern on an investment cast. Note that the pattern is sprued through the base of the cast. After the wax pattern is formed the investment cast with the wax pattern is invested in a casting ring as shown in Fig. 16-16, where the sprue button former has been removed. The invested pattern is burned out and the investment is heated to the casting temperature causing thermal expansion. As for smaller gold castings the sum of the setting and thermal expansions compensates for the casting shrinkage of the base metals.

When casting any of the base metals into molds designed to accommodate the higher melting

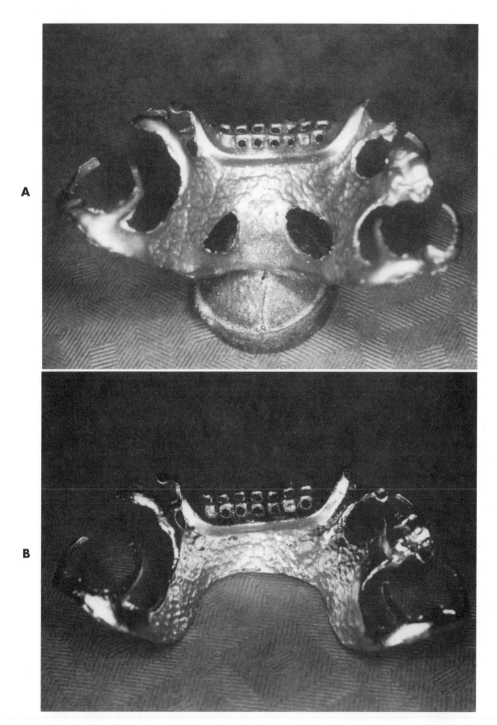

Fig. 16-14 Base metal partial denture framework after casting with sprues and sprue button attached, **A,** and after removing the sprues and finishing, **B**. (Courtesy Dootz ER, Ann Arbor, 1995, University of Michigan School of Dentistry.)

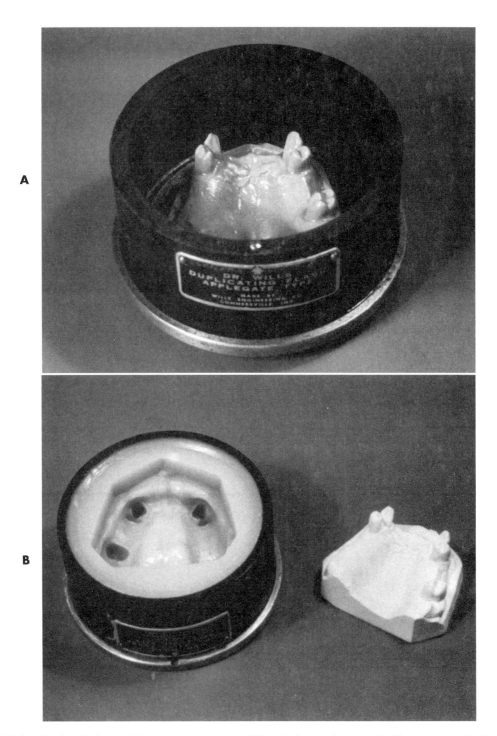

Fig. 16-15 Duplicating flask containing a master stone model ready for pouring agar duplicating material, **A,** and the agar mold and gypsum-bonded investment cast after separation, **B**. (Courtesy Dootz ER, Ann Arbor, 1995, University of Michigan School of Dentistry.)

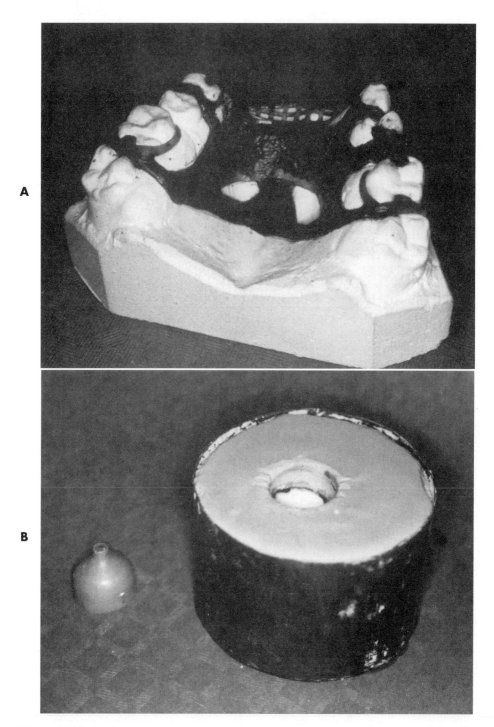

Fig. 16-16 Wax pattern on an investment cast sprued through the base, **A,** and invested wax pattern and investment cast with the sprue button former removed, **B**. (Courtesy Dootz ER, Ann Arbor, 1995, University of Michigan School of Dentistry.)

temperatures of these alloys, certain problems may be encountered that are less common when casting alloys of lower melting temperatures. One problem is that of trapping gases in the mold during the casting process. To have sufficient strength and resistance to thermal shock, some investments for the cast base metal alloys lack sufficient porosity for the rapid escape of gases from the mold cavity when the hot metal enters. As a result, the gases may be trapped in the mold cavity and produce voids and casting defects. The effect of such trapped gases on one casting of a cobalt-chromium alloy is clearly shown in Fig. 16-17. This general view of the casting shows the location of the defect in a critical area of the appliance. The magnified view of the defective area (Fig. 16-17) reveals that a large gas bubble became trapped in the molten metal at the time the mold was filled. Before it could be dissipated, the metal solidified. Because similar observations have been made when certain dense investments are used to make gold castings, this problem is not unique to base metal alloys and molds. A higher temperature of the casting alloy would have assisted in overcoming this difficulty. Numerous other methods have been proposed to overcome such defects, such as venting to the surface of the mold to permit rapid elimination of gases. Such a method is used in the preparation of cast test bars for specification testing purposes. The skillful spruing and venting of the mold, combined with complete elimination of the wax residue and adequate heating of the metal, tend to reduce this type of defective casting.

The melting of base metal alloys must be carefully controlled to avoid severe damage to the alloy during the melting and casting process. Oxidation of the ingredient metals and carbide or nitride formation at the high temperatures required to melt these alloys demand precise control of the melting and casting operation. Regardless of the method employed to melt the alloy, it is possible to cause severe damage to the properties of the casting if proper melting practices are not observed. Two sprue buttons from base metal alloy castings, one sound and free from defects and the other with some porosity and surface irregularities, are shown in Fig. 16-18. More severe damage is not uncommon and results from excessive overheating and resulting porosities and surface reactions with the mold materials. Such castings with poor surface

appearance usually possess inferior physical properties. It is probable that the proper control of the factors related to the casting operation is more important in controlling the properties of the finished structure than are the variations in composition or the choice of different products.

When properly designed and cast, the cast base metal alloys give acceptable removable partial denture restorations. A typical appliance of this type, with an acrylic plastic denture base material and artificial teeth attached in the proper relationship, is shown in Fig. 16-19. Much clinical study has been given to the choice of clasp materials and the proper design of the appliance to give stability and support both to the appliance and to the remaining teeth. The mechanics of the design of such restorations represent an important aspect of clinical procedures.

Because the minor alloying elements of carbon, nitrogen, and oxygen influence the properties of a base metal casting, it is generally recognized that a pronounced variation in properties can result from the use of variable casting conditions. Variables such as mold temperature, temperature of the molten alloy, and the sprue size and arrangement affect the properties of the finished casting as much as does the composition. Therefore these alloys are generally considered to be technic-sensitive. One reason for this sensitivity is that almost all elements in these alloys, such as chromium, silicon, molybdenum, cobalt, and nickel, react with carbon to form carbides, even though only a relatively small amount of carbon is present in the alloys. Depending on the mold and alloy-casting temperature, cooling rate, and other technical variables, carbides of any one of these elements may form, which changes the properties of the alloys. As a result, careful control of manipulative variables in the casting operations is essential.

The melting temperature is an important factor in the selection and control of the melting and casting equipment and in the choice of technic and mold equipment used for the casting operation. Gold alloys for complete metal restorations are cast into calcium sulfate–bonded investment molds after the alloys have been melted with gas-air blowtorches. Only a base metal alloy that melts below 1300° C (e.g., Ticonium) can be cast into a calcium sulfate–bonded investment. It is also possible to cast a low melting nickel–chromium alloy

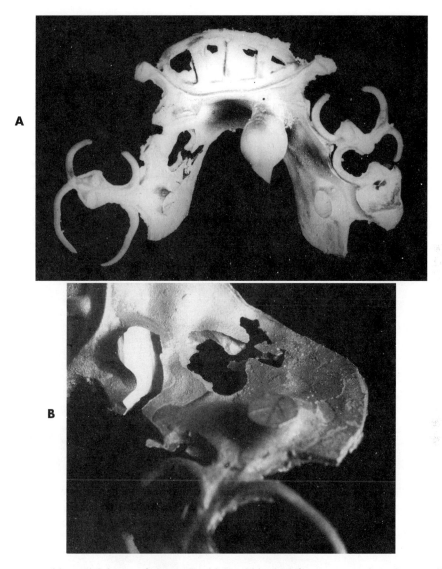

Fig. 16-17 Cast removable partial denture framework with a void in the left center area, **A,** and a magnified view of a defect caused by metal that was too cold and gas inclusion in the mold, **B**.

(e.g., Ticonium) against wrought platinum-gold-palladium wire when a more flexible partial denture clasp than a cast clasp is required. Because of their higher melting point, other cast base metal alloys cannot be melted with the conventional blowtorch used for gold alloys. It has therefore been necessary to develop special electric melting facilities or, less commonly, to melt the alloys with an oxyacetylene torch. Either method is acceptable in the hands of a skillful operator. However, if prolonged heating or excessive temperatures are developed during the melting and casting process, either method of heating will damage the alloy.

Even when base metal alloys are cast properly and normal heating is used, some metal always remains in the crucible. Tensile specimens cast from overheated, underheated, and normally heated alloy are shown in Fig. 16-20. As can be seen, some investment material remains adhered to the base metal alloys, and it should be removed by sandblasting.

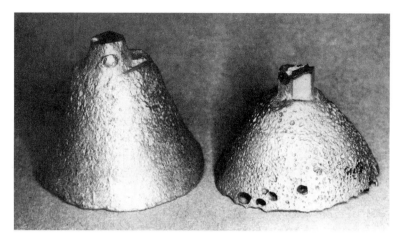

Fig. 16-18 Sprue buttons, showing an alloy that was properly heated, *left,* and one that slightly overheated, *right.*

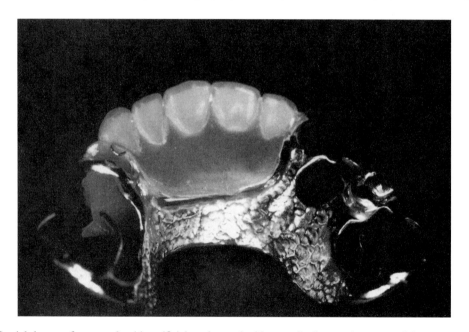

Fig. 16-19 Partial denture framework with artificial teeth attached by acrylic denture base material. (Courtesy Dootz ER, Ann Arbor, 1995, University of Michigan School of Dentistry.)

Casting shrinkage compensation

The cast base metal alloys have a casting shrinkage of 2.3%, which requires that the mold be expanded more than is necessary when dental gold alloys are cast. Thermal expansion represents the principal method of mold expansion for compensation of the alloy shrinkage. The use of special gypsum- , phosphate- , or silicate-bonded investments permits adequate setting and thermal expansion of the molds when they are properly heated, and one can produce castings that display the proper fit and adequate compensation.

Porosity in castings

Castings with porosity present in a portion of the structure that is subject to severe stress concentration are likely to fail in the area of the defect because the effective cross-sectional area of the casting is reduced

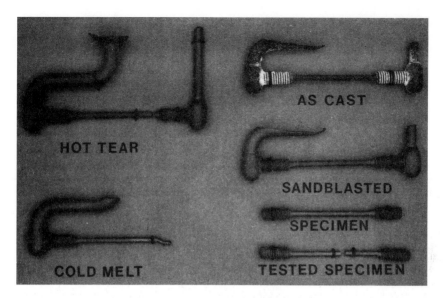

Fig. 16-20 Specimens cast from over-heated (*top left*), under-heated (*bottom left*), and normally heated (*right*) alloy.

by the amount equal to the area of the defect and stresses concentrate at the defect. Subsurface porosity and other defects may occur in castings of gold alloys as well as in base metal alloys, and the tendency toward these defects is closely related to the size and shape of the casting, the manner of spruing, and the metal and mold temperatures when the casting is made. For these reasons, care and attention to details of the casting technic are of extreme importance in all types of dental castings.

Finishing of base metal partial denture castings

Because there is always some metal-investment interaction, the castings are sandblasted to remove any scale and particles of investment. Any areas of flash where the inner and outer investment separated are ground off. The casting is then electropolished, which is the reverse of electroplating with the casting being made the anode. Atoms in the area of rough projections go into solution in preference to those in smooth areas resulting in a satinlike smooth surface. No further polishing is done to tissue-bearing surfaces. However, other surfaces are polished using rubber wheels impregnated with abrasives. These alloys are difficult to polish compared with gold alloys, and the electropolishing procedure saves a great deal of laboratory time.

■ CASTING OF TITANIUM

Titanium has many desirable properties for use in dentistry, but it is difficult to cast in comparison with the common dental casting alloys because it requires relatively complex and expensive equipment. For this reason few laboratories presently cast titanium dental restorations. Two problems in casting titanium are its high melting point and the tendency for the molten metal to become contaminated. The melting point of commercially pure titanium is about 1671° C, whereas the base metal alloys have liquidus temperatures of 1300 to 1500° C, and the gold alloys melt at even lower temperatures. Titanium readily absorbs several gases when in the molten state. If hydrogen, oxygen, and nitrogen are absorbed, the mechanical properties are adversely effected. To prevent absorption of gases, titanium is cast under the protective atmosphere of argon or in a vacuum. To achieve the high melting temperatures, arc melting in either graphite or water-cooled copper crucibles is used. The casting systems force the metal into the mold using either pressure or centrifugal casting technics.

The casting design is similar to that of other more common dental alloys. A wax pattern is prepared and sprued, as before, but here only the more temperature resistant investments can be used. Both phosphate-bonded silica and magnesia investments produce good castings and give casting dimensions that are within the accepted range for base metal partial denture castings.

■ CASTING OF GLASS

A castable glass (ceramic) inlay or crown is prepared in a manner similar to that of a metal casting. A wax pattern is made on a high-strength stone die, and all sections of the pattern should be more than 1 mm thick, with the occlusal surfaces and marginal edges being 1.5 mm thick. The wax pattern is sprued with 8- or 10-gage sprues. One or two sprues are used, depending on the size and whether it is an anterior or posterior pattern. The pattern is positioned 6 to 7 mm from the top end of the casting ring. The ring is lined with ceramic paper, and the pattern is invested in a phosphate-bonded investment and allowed to set for 1 hour. The invested pattern is placed in a room-temperature oven, heated to 250° C, and held at that temperature for 30 minutes, after which the temperature is raised to 955° C for an additional 30 minutes.

A special centrifugal casting machine is used that has an electric furnace and is motor-driven. The glass is heated to 1360° C and then cast and spun for a sufficient time to allow the casting to cool. The casting is allowed to set at room temperature for 45 minutes before divesting. At this point, the casting is transparent (see Chapter 17). After the sprue is cut off and the area is finished, it must be "cerammed" (devitrified or crystallized from the glassy state) to produce a translucent crown. The restoration is embedded in phosphate-bonded investment before ceramming for 6 hours at 1075° C. The cerammed restoration is one color and must be shaded with ceramic stains to yield an esthetic restoration.

SELECTED PROBLEMS

Problem 1. An invested casting ring was removed from the oven in preparation for melting and casting the gold alloy; however, a delay of several minutes occurred before the alloy was cast. The 3-unit fixed bridge did not fit. What probably caused this problem, and how can it be corrected?

Solution. When the casting ring is removed from the oven and placed in the casting machine, the investment begins to cool and contract. A delay of more than a minute generally results in sufficient shrinkage to produce an undersized casting. The recommended procedure is to premelt the gold alloy in the crucible of the casting machine before removing the casting ring from the oven and to cast promptly.

Problem 2. A casting that did not seat well had external and internal surface irregularities. How were these surface irregularities produced, and how might they be avoided?

Solution a. Air bubbles become attached to the wax pattern during investing, thereby producing nodules on the casting. Their removal can alter the fit of the casting. To avoid air bubbles, a wetting agent should be applied to the wax pattern, and the investment should be mixed and the pattern should be invested under vacuum.

Solution b. When too much water is used in mixing the investment, a rougher surface on the casting can result. The powder and liquid of the investment should be dispensed accurately.

Solution c. The position and direction of the sprue affects the turbulence of the molten alloy as it is introduced into the mold cavity. Localized roughness can result from abrasion of the mold. Attach the sprue to the bulkiest portion of the wax pattern. The point of contact should be flared, and the sprue should be directed toward the margins.

Solution d. Prolonged heating of a gypsum-bonded investment at a temperature above 650° C causes a breakdown of the investment, resulting in a rough surface on the casting. Casting should be prompt when wax burnout has been achieved.

Problem 3. A full crown casting was made by reheating an invested casting ring that had been heated to the burnout temperature and then cooled the day before when the procedure could not be completed. The resulting crown did not fit. What caused this problem, and how can it be corrected?

Solution. Chemical and physical changes in the binder and refractory of the investment occur when the investment is heated and then cooled. On reheating, the dimensional changes of the mold will be less than normal. If a casting procedure cannot be completed promptly with a heated investment, a new wax pattern should be invested and cast.

Problem 4. A soldered joint showed a large amount of porosity. What caused the porosity, and how can it be avoided?

Solution. Porosity in the soldered joint is usually associated with excessive heat applied during the fusion of the solder or with improper fluxing. Scrupulously clean and properly flux the surfaces to be soldered. The reducing part of the flame should be used.

Problem 5. During a soldering operation, the fine margins of a casting were fused. What factor produced this problem, and how can it be avoided when the operation is repeated?

Solution a. If the layer of investment protecting the margins of a casting is too thin or is porous, the refractory material will not be able to act as a thermal barrier. The margins of a casting should be protected with a thick layer of investment carefully painted onto the occlusal areas and along the proximal walls.

Solution b. If the investment is mixed with a high water/powder ratio, the strength of the investment will be low. Portions of the investment may fracture during heating, thereby exposing margins to the soldering operation. The powder and liquid of the soldering investment should be dispensed accurately.

Solution c. Overheating the investment assembly for a long period can transfer heat to the protected margins, thus causing them to melt. Adequate temperature should be reached in the furnace, after which the reducing flame of the torch should be applied properly. The solder should be fused promptly.

Problem 6. A full crown wax pattern was sprued to the bulkiest portion with a single sprue. After casting, porosity was observed on the pulpal floor of the gold crown. What could have caused the problem, and how can the problem be avoided on the next casting?

Solution. The porosity, commonly known as suckback porosity, resulted from improper freezing of the alloy so that molten alloy could not compensate for shrinkage of the molten to the solid alloy. Several conditions could have caused the problem: (1) The diameter of the sprue may have been too small and/or the length of the sprue was too long, resulting in the alloy's freezing in the sprue before freezing in the crown; a larger diameter and shorter sprue should be used. (2) The single sprue directed the molten alloy to the area of the pulpal floor, and the investment in this area became much hotter than the surrounding investment. This condition, coupled with the poor thermal conductivity of the investment, caused the alloy in this area to stay molten after it had frozen in the sprue; the direction of the sprue should be toward the margin, and a Y-shaped sprue should be used to distribute the flow of the alloy more uniformly. Increasing the temperature of the high-heat investment before casting reduces the differences in temperature of the investment from the impingement of the molten alloy. (3) The amount of alloy forming the sprue button may have been too small in relationship to the size of the pattern; again the sprue and button froze before the alloy in the crown, causing the porosity.

Problem 7. A cobalt-chromium partial denture alloy was melted with an oxygen-acetylene flame. However, problems with adjustment of the torch resulted, and the alloy was heated three times longer than normal. What, if any, problems might be expected with the cast partial denture framework?

Solution. Extended heating of the alloy with such a flame probably will increase the carbon content of the cast alloy. The alloy contains several elements that form carbides under such conditions, and their precipitation increases the brittleness and decreases the elongation. As a result, the clasps of the cast partial denture will be susceptible to fracture during minor adjustments.

Problem 8. A low-fusing nickel-chromium alloy was to be cast to embedded platinum-gold-palladium (PGP) wire in the preparation of a partial denture framework. A gypsum-bonded investment was used but after the investment had been heated to the casting temperature casting of the alloy was delayed for four hours. Later when the PGP wire was bent to form a clasp it was brittle and broke. What caused the embrittlement and how can it be prevented in the next casting?

Solution. Low-fusing nickel-chromium alloy melt at substantially higher temperatures than gold alloys, just under 1300° C compared to 900-1000° C. Therefore, special gypsum-bonded investments are used that contain oxalic acid, oxalates, carbonates, and carbon that release CO_2 at various temperatures during heating of the investment, and keep the mold cavity flushed with CO_2 to remove any sulfur oxides from the calcium sulfate binder. On extended heating these agents are eliminated and the sulfur oxides react with the PGP wire causing embrittlement. Embrittlement will also occur if a gypsum-bonded casting investment designed for gold alloys is used that does not contain these protective chemicals, even if there is no delay in casting procedure.

When casting a low-fusing nickel-chromium alloy to embedded PGP wire the casting should be made promptly after the investment has reached the proper casting temperature.

Problem 9. Why is it necessary to prepare a duplicate investment cast from the master stone model in the preparation of a wax pattern for a partial denture framework?

Solution. The large wax pattern is too fragile to be handled and sprued as a free-standing wax pattern.

Waxing must be done on the investment cast, which becomes part of the investment mold, and unlike the stone model it must be able to withstand the burnout and casting tempertures.

The master stone model must be saved to be used in the processing of the acrylic denture base material to the metal partial denture framework.

■ REFERENCES

Casting Procedures

Allan FC, Asgar K: Reaction of cobalt-chromium casting alloy with investment, *J Dent Res* 45:1516, 1966.

Asgar K: Casting restorations. In Clark, JW, editor: *Clinical dentistry,* vol 4, New York, 1976, Harper & Row.

Asgar K, Arfaei AH: Castability of crown and bridge alloys, *J Prosthet Dent* 54:60, 1985.

Asgar K, Mahler DB, and Peyton FA: Hygroscopic technique for inlay casting using controlled water additions, *J Prosthet Dent* 5:711, 1955.

Asgar K, Peyton FA: Effect of casting conditions on some mechanical properties of cobalt-base alloys, *J Dent Res* 40:73, 1961.

Barreto MT, Goldberg AJ, Nitkin DA, Mumford G: Effect of investing on casting high-fusing alloys, *J Prosthet Dent* 44:504, 1980.

Blackman R, Barghi N, Tran C: Dimensional changes in casting titanium removable partial denture frameworks, *J Prosthet Dent* 65:309, 1991.

Campagni WV, Preston JD, Reisbick MH: Measurement of paint-on-die spacers used for casting relief, *J Prosthet Dent* 47:606, 1982.

Cecconi BT, Asgar K: Modified hygroscopic gold casting technique, *J Prosthet Dent* 33:216, 1975.

Cooney JP, Caputo AA: Type III gold alloy complete crowns cast in phosphate-bonded investment, *J Prosthet Dent* 46:414, 1981.

Craig RG, Anthony DH, Peyton FA: Dimensional changes in duplicated investment casts, *Dent Prog* 2:35, 1961.

Dootz ER, Craig RG, Peyton FA: Influences of investments and duplicating procedures on the accuracy of partial denture castings, *J Prosthet Dent* 15:679, 1965.

Eames WB, MacNamara JF: Evaluation of casting machine for ability to cast sharp margins, *Oper Dent* 3:137, 1978.

Earnshaw R: Casting shrinkage of cobalt chromium alloys, *Aust Dent J* 3:159, 1958.

Earnshaw R: The effect of restrictive stress on the thermal expansion of gypsum-bonded investments. II. Inlay casting investments, "hygroscopic expansion" type, *Aust Dent J* 12:123, 1967.

Earnshaw R: The effect of restrictive stress on the thermal expansion of gypsum-bonded investments. III. Dental casting investments, *Aust Dent J* 12:270, 1967.

Earnshaw R: The effect of restrictive stress on the hygroscopic setting expansion of gypsum-bonded investments, *Aust Dent J* 14:22, 1969.

Eden GT, Franklin OM, Powell JM, Ohta Y, Dickson G: Fit of porcelain-fused-to-metal crown and bridge castings, *J Dent Res* 58:2360, 1979.

Harcourt JH, Cotterill WF: Induction melting of cobalt-chromium alloys, *Br Dent J* 118:325, 1965.

Kasloff Z: Recent advances in casting techniques and their evaluation, *Int Dent J* 13:331, 1963.

Kono A, Hosoda H, Fusayama T: Heating rate of a gypsum investment related to crack formation, *J Dent Res* 45:1419, 1966.

Leinfelder KF, Fairhurst CW, Ryge G: Porosities in dental gold castings. II. *J Am Dent Assoc* 67:816, 1963.

Lewis AJ: The effect of variations in mould temperature, metal temperature and mould size on the development of internal porosity in cast structures, *Aust Dent J* 22:243, 1977.

O'Brien WJ, Nielsen JP: Decomposition of gypsum investment in the presence of carbon, *J Dent Res* 38:541, 1959.

Ryge G, Kozak SF, Fairhurst CW: Porosities in dental gold castings, *J Am Dent Assoc* 54:746, 1957.

Shell JS, Hollenback GM: Physical properties of dental gold castings closely approximating dental dimensions, *J South Calif Dent Assoc* 33:20, 1965.

Smyd ES: Factors which influence casting accuracy: a universal casting technic, *J Am Dent Assoc* 36:160, 1948.

Stevens L: An additional measure to ensure unidirectional solidification in dental casting, *Aust Dent J* 28:33, 1983.

Strandman E: Influence of different types of acetylene-oxygen flames on the carbon content of dental Co-Cr alloy, *Odontol Revy* 27:223, 1976.

Tuccillo JJ, Nielsen JP: Sprue design for cast gold alloys, *Dent Lab Rev* 39:14 (June), 14 (July), 1964.

Wagner AW: Causes and cures for porosities in dental castings, *Quintess Dent Technol* 3:57, 1979.

Webb EL, Murray HV, Holland GA, Taylor DF: Effects of preparation relief and flow channels on seating full coverage castings during cementation, *J Prosthet Dent* 49:777, 1983.

17 Ceramics

The art of fusing dental porcelain has remained, to a great extent, with those persons who have learned the art directly from others. The laboratory portion of porcelain restorations usually is made in commercial dental laboratories by skilled technicians working with specialized equipment and from models and color specifications provided by the dentist. Skilled technicians and artisans also are employed by the manufacturers of artificial teeth to produce the many forms, types, and shades necessary in this application of porcelain.

■ COMPOSITION

The quality of any porcelain depends on the choice of ingredients, the correct proportioning of each ingredient, and the control of the firing procedure. Only the purest ingredients are used in the manufacture of dental porcelains because of the stringent requirements of color, toughness without brittleness, insolubility, and translucency, as well as the desirable characteristics of strength and thermal expansion. In many instances, the result must be a compromise of a number of these properties.

Ceramics from the finest porcelain to china and earthenware are composed of essentially the same materials; the principal difference being in the proportion of the primary ingredients and the firing procedures. The ingredients are feldspar, silica (quartz or flint), and kaolin (clay). Other compounds such as potash, soda, or lime often are added to give special properties. Glass is a fusible combination of silica and potash, whereas porcelain contains infusible elements held together by lower-fusing materials and is less transparent.

In its mineral state, feldspar, the main raw material of dental porcelains, is crystalline and opaque with an indefinite color between gray and pink. Chemically it is designated as potassium aluminum silicate, with a composition of $K_2O \cdot Al_2O_3 \cdot 6SiO_2$. When heated, it fuses at about 1290° C, becomes glassy, and, unless overheated, retains its form without rounding. This last property is desirable because it is necessary to retain the form of porcelain restorations while they are fusing.

Iron and mica are commonly found as impurities in feldspar. It is particularly important to remove the iron, because metallic oxides act as strong coloring agents in porcelain. For removal of iron, each piece of feldspar is broken with a steel hammer, and only the uniformly light-colored pieces are selected for use in the porcelain. These pieces are ground in ball mills until they become a fine powder. The final particle size is carefully controlled by screening to remove the coarser particles, and flotation processes are used to remove the excessively fine particles. The dry powder is then slowly vibrated down inclined planes equipped with a series of narrow ledges formed by induction magnets. In this way the remaining iron contaminants are separated and removed, and the feldspar is made ready for use.

Dental porcelains in recent years are made mainly with potash feldspar. The feldspar is heated with alkali metal carbonates as fluxes to about 1000° C in large crucibles. The feldspar decomposes to form a glass and leucite $KAlSi_2O_6$ (or $K_2O \cdot Al_2O_3 \cdot 4SiO_2$). The thermal expansion of the leucite is high ($>20 \times 10^{-6}/°$ C) and the amount present controls the thermal expansion coefficient of the porcelain. Leucite also contributes strength to the porcelain, and high leucite porcelains are around twice as strong as those containing low concentrations.

Pure quartz crystals (SiO_2) are used in dental porcelain and are ground to the finest grain size possible. Silica contributes stability to the mass during heating by providing a framework for the other ingredients.

Kaolin is a clay represented by the formula $Al_2O_3 \cdot 2SiO_2 \cdot 2H_2O$. Kaolin gives porcelain its properties of opaqueness. When mixed with water, it becomes sticky and aids in forming a workable mass of the porcelain during molding. When subjected to high heat, it adheres to the framework of quartz particles and shrinks considerably.

The coloring pigments added to the porcelain mixture are called "color frits." These powders are added in small quantities to obtain the delicate shades necessary to imitate the color of the natural teeth. They are prepared by grinding together metallic oxides with fine glass and feldspar, fusing the mixture in a furnace, and regrinding it to a powder. The metallic pigments include titanium oxide for yellow-brown shades, manganese oxide for lavender, iron oxide for brown, cobalt oxide for blue, copper or chromium oxides for green, and nickel oxide for brown. In the past, uranium oxide was used to provide fluorescence; however, because of the small amount of radioactivity, lanthanide earths are being substituted for this purpose. Tin oxide is used to increase opacity.

The manufacturers do not publicize the exact formulas for their porcelains. Without the precise preparation and firing technic for each formula, however, the composition would be only a matter of general interest. Of the formulas published in the literature, feldspar constitutes between 75% and 85% of the total; quartz, 12% to 22%; and kaolin, 3% to 5%. Pigments constitute a small percentage of the mixture. A typical formula for tooth body porcelain is given in Table 17-1. In contrast, the formula for the fine porcelain used in figurines and other decorative objects differs in percentage composition, as shown also in Table 17-1. These are two of the many triaxial ceramic products, each of which contains the three primary ingredients—feldspar, quartz, and clay.

The porcelains used for porcelain-fused-to-metal crown and bridgework have lower fusing temperatures. Typical compositions are given in Table 17-2. They are essentially potassium-sodium aluminosilicate glasses with TiO_2, SnO_2, and ZrO_2 added as opacifiers.

TABLE 17-1   Ingredients of Porcelains

Ingredient	Dental Porcelain (weight %)	Decorative Porcelain (weight %)
Feldspar	81	15
Quartz	15	14
Kaolin	4	70
Metallic pigments	<1	1

■ GENERAL APPLICATIONS IN DENTISTRY

The strength, hardness, and range of toothlike colors of porcelain offer advantages as a single tooth restorative material. However, its brittleness, difficulties in matching tooth structure in color and texture, and the problem of compensating for the comparatively large shrinkage that occurs during firing are disadvantages and have somewhat limited the application of porcelain for individual tooth restorations.

Because of its natural appearance and durability, porcelain is widely used for the restoration of individual teeth and for fixed bridgework. Porcelain has been used for jacket crowns since the early 1900s and covers the entire coronal part of the tooth, as shown in Fig. 17-1. Recently, the ordinary jacket crown has been reinforced by strong core ceramics and substituted by castable glass-ceramics.

The porcelain inlay, as shown in Fig. 17-2, has not been used as much in recent years. However, currently there is experimentation with casting inlays with glass-ceramics and machining ceramic inlays.

Porcelains for fusing to high-temperature alloy crowns are widely used. This development was the result of successfully matching the coefficients of thermal expansion of porcelain with alloys and the achievement of a proper bond.

Porcelain is used in the commercial manufacture of artificial teeth. Individual or complete sets of teeth of excellent quality are available in a wide range of molds and shades from a number of manufacturers.

TABLE 17-2   Composition of Dental Ceramics for Fusing to High Temperature Alloys

Compound	Biodent Opaque BG 2 (%)	Ceramco Opaque 60 (%)	V. M. K. Opaque 131 (%)	Biodent Dentin BD 27 (%)	Ceramco Dentin T 69 (%)
SiO_2	52.0	55.0	52.4	56.9	62.2
Al_2O_3	13.55	11.65	15.15	11.80	13.40
CaO	–	–	–	0.61	0.98
K_2O	11.05	9.6	9.9	10.0	11.3
Na_2O	5.28	4.75	6.58	5.42	5.37
TiO_2	3.01	–	2.59	0.61	–
ZrO_2	3.22	0.16	5.16	1.46	0.34
SnO_2	6.4	15.0	4.9	–	0.5
Rb_2O	0.09	0.04	0.08	0.10	0.06
BaO	1.09	–	–	3.52	–
ZnO	–	0.26	–	–	–
UO_3	–	–	–	–	–
B_2O_3, CO_2, and H_2O	4.31	3.54	3.24	9.58	5.85

From Nally JN, Meyer JM: *Schweiz Monatsschr Zahnheilkd* 80:250, 1970.

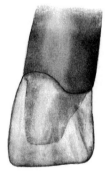

Fig. 17-1 Drawing of a porcelain jacket crown in position.

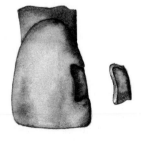

Fig. 17-2 Drawing of a porcelain inlay for an anterior tooth.

■ PORCELAIN AS TOOTH RESTORATIVE MATERIAL

The esthetic appearance of a well-constructed porcelain inlay or jacket crown is generally quite satisfactory. The glazed surface produces a restoration that is color-stable, compatible with the soft tissues, resistant to sudden thermal changes, strong, and relatively easy to place from the standpoint of the patient. Baked porcelain has many favorable qualities to recommend it as a restorative material.

There are certain limitations, however, to the use of porcelain. Matching the exact color and texture of the teeth is complicated because the optical properties of porcelain are different from those of enamel and dentin. Restorations of porcelain are constructed outside the mouth and are cemented into position, which means that they must be free of overhanging margins and undercuts. In some instances, particularly in cavities between the anterior teeth, this may require the removal of additional sound tooth structure. If a cement line should occur at the margin of the restoration, the cement will tend to wash out, and staining will occur. The strength of porcelain is normally adequate but varies with the composition, manipulation, and firing procedure. To avoid breakage, it should preferably be well supported by sound tooth structure or metal.

Porcelain offers considerable resistance to abrasion because of its hardness, but this may be a disadvantage where it contacts opposing natural teeth. Even when the glaze is removed and the surface is roughened, the porcelain surface does not wear as much as the neighboring teeth. This combination may result in excessive wear of the teeth in the opposing arch or excessive forces exerted during biting, which are damaging both to the restoration and to the tissues that support the teeth.

Porcelain Technic

The production of a satisfactory porcelain restoration requires careful attention to the principles and details of the operation. These procedures have been well described in the dental literature, so that they have come to be recognized as conventional practice for crown and inlay technics.

After the tooth has been prepared, an impression of it is made, and a working model or die is formed of a suitable die material. The portion of the die to be contacted with porcelain is carefully covered with a thin layer of platinum foil approximately 0.025 mm thick. Overlapping portions at the margins are either trimmed or soldered to provide a uniform thickness around all of the borders. This platinum form or matrix retains the porcelain mix in the shape of the tooth preparation during firing and determines, to a great extent, the accuracy of fit of the restoration.

The porcelain powder in the color selected for the body or dentin portion is mixed with distilled water to a creamy consistency and is applied in the correct proportion to the platinum matrix, with allowances made for shrinkage. To produce minimum shrinkage and a dense strong porcelain, it is important to achieve a thorough condensation of the particles at this stage. Various means of condensation may be employed. The vibration method is particularly useful in simple inlays, in which flow is restricted. The wet porcelain is applied to the platinum matrix with a spatula and vibrated gently until the particles settle together. The excess water is then removed with a clean towel or an absorbent medium.

Other methods of condensation include both the spatulation and brush technics. The spatulation method consists of smoothing and burnishing the wet porcelain with a suitable spatula until the excess water is brought to the surface, where it is absorbed. The brush or capillary attraction method depends on the action of dry porcelain powder to remove the excess water by capillary attraction. The dry powder is applied with a brush to a small area of the wet porcelain mass, and as the water is withdrawn toward the dry area, the wet particles are pulled closely together. This process is repeated with the dry powder placed on the opposite side from each new addition of the wet mix.

Experienced operators sometimes complete the fusion of a porcelain restoration in only two firing operations, one for the dentin portion and another for the enamel, stain, and glaze. Generally, however, three firings are employed. In the first firing, the dentin portion, which is formed approximately 13% oversize, is heated to the biscuit bake. This temperature is 56° C below the fusing temperature of the porcelain. During this firing, virtually all the shrinkage takes place. After cooling, the enamel portion is added, also oversize, and the second firing is made. If an enamel with a slightly lower fusing temperature than the dentin portion has been used, a lower temperature may be required for the second firing.

After the second firing and cooling, the restoration, with the platinum matrix undisturbed, may be placed on the tooth in the patient's mouth. At this time it may be adjusted to size and the final contouring done by grinding or adjusting to match the restoration with the remaining tooth structure or the adjoining teeth.

After the porcelain is cleaned and any necessary stains are applied, it is returned to the furnace for the final firing. As it is held at the correct fusing temperature, complete fusion takes place, and a thin glaze is formed on the surface. Overglazing is to be avoided, because it gives the restoration an unnatural glassy appearance and may cause slumping, or loss of contour, as well as weaken the porcelain mass.

After being annealed by careful slow cooling, the platinum matrix is removed, and the completed restoration is prepared for cementation. The accuracy of the final fit will be reduced slightly by the thickness of the platinum foil plus a certain amount of shrinkage of the porcelain. These factors tend to produce restorations that are slightly inaccurate and may account for the cement line sometimes found around fused porcelain inlays and jacket restorations.

Types of Tooth Restorative Porcelain

The various components of the porcelain blended together by the manufacturer result in two principal phases. One is the vitreous (or glass) phase, and the other is the crystalline (or mineral) phase. The glass phase formed during the firing process has properties typical of glass, such as brittleness, nondirectional fracture pattern, flow under stress, and high surface tension in the fluid state. The crystalline phase includes leucite and certain metallic oxides added as coloring agents or opacifiers, such as iron, tin, or titanium oxides. The vitreous phase is prominent in dental porcelain powders and contributes to many characteristic properties as well as bonds together the crystalline particles. The high-fusing porcelains have a fusing range from 1315° to 1370° C; the medium-fusing porcelains, from 1090° to 1260° C; and the low-fusing porcelains, from 870° to 1065° C.

The medium-fusing and low-fusing porcelains are usually modified by the manufacturer with chemicals or fluxes of low melting temperature and are prefused and reduced to powder form again. The addition of fluxing agents results in narrower fusing ranges and increases the tendency for the porcelain to slump during repair or when making additions, staining, or glazing. Prefusing and regrinding, however, increase the homogeneity of the powder, which may be an advantage in the handling and fusing operations. Low firing temperatures are a definite asset in the fusion of porcelain to metal, because the differences in the coefficients of expansion of the porcelain and metal can be tolerated better at lower temperature ranges. Porcelain enamels that have a fusion temperature below 1040° C have been developed.

High-fusing porcelains are considered superior in strength, insolubility, translucency, and maintenance of accuracy in form during repeated firings. Recent tests of low-fusing products, however, indicate that they are essentially as strong as the high-fusing types, and their solubility and translucency are adequate. The principal practical advantage of high-fusing porcelain is therefore its ability to be repaired, added to, stained, or glazed without distortion.

Fusion of Porcelain

Porcelain restorations may be fired either by temperature control alone or by controlled temperature and a specified time. In the first method the furnace temperature is raised at a constant rate until a specified temperature is reached. In the second method the temperature is raised at a given rate until certain levels are reached, after which the temperature is maintained for a measured period until the desired reactions are completed.

Either of these methods gives satisfactory results, but the time and temperature method generally is preferred because it is less critical and more likely to produce a uniform product. Porcelain is a poor thermal conductor, and for this reason too rapid heating may overfuse the outer layers before the inner portion is properly fused.

Acceptable technics have been developed that employ either air firing or vacuum firing of the porcelain. Slightly less porosity exists when vacuum firing is used. Some evidence exists to indicate that the surface roughness is less with vacuum-fired specimens than with air-fired specimens.

During firing, the porcelain undergoes several changes. The first change involves the loss of the water, which was added to the powder to form the workable mix. The excess water is partially removed by warming the mix before it is placed into the preheated furnace. This prevents the sudden formation of steam and possible physical damage to the porcelain mass. After the mass is placed in the furnace, both the free and combined water are removed in various stages of heating until a temperature of 480° C is reached.

The second change occurs as the temperature is raised, and the particles of porcelain fuse together by sintering. Sintering is the process responsible for the fusion of the enamel particles to form a continuous mass. During this densification, the volume change, ΔV, in the early stages is related to the surface tension of the enamel, γ; viscosity, η; particle radius, r; and sintering time, t, by the relation

$$\frac{\Delta V}{V_0} = \frac{9\gamma}{4\eta r} t$$

As this equation indicates, the lower the viscosity and the finer the particle size, the greater is the rate of densification. Thoroughly dried porcelain may be placed directly into a moderately hot furnace if it is preheated a few minutes by the open furnace door. After the drying stage, the temperature and time should be controlled carefully during the final fusing and glazing stages.

The glazing stage is reached in the last firing and is held only long enough for a glossy surface to form. The fusion range for porcelain glaze is from about 955° to 1065° C. Overglazing produces too thick a glaze, an increase in porosity, and loss of strength, form, and color.

Slow cooling of the fired mass is preferred to prevent a too-rapid cooling of the outer layers, which may result in surface crazing or cracking. This slow cooling is accomplished by removal of the porcelain from the furnace as soon as the firing is finished and placement of it under a glass cover to protect it from air currents and from possible contamination by dirt.

Properties of Fused Porcelain

From the information available on the properties of fused porcelain, it is obvious that two factors of manipulation have a pronounced effect on the quality of the finished porcelain mass: (1) the manner and degree of condensation or compaction of the porcelain powder in the shaping of the restoration before the firing operation and (2) the degree of firing and procedure followed to fuse the porcelain mass.

The properties that have been most reported include the linear and volumetric shrinkage, the transverse strength, and the specific gravity of the fired porcelain mass. The linear shrinkage of glazed porcelain has been reported to be approximately 14% for low-fusing porcelain and 11.5% for high-fusing porcelain. Overglazed porcelain has a greater percentage of shrinkage for both the low-fusing and high-fusing types, and the volumetric shrinkage shows even greater differences of approximately 8%. Several studies have shown that the low-fusing type has a volumetric shrinkage of from 32% to 37% and the high-fusing porcelain can shrink as much as 28% to 34%. The medium-fusing porcelain has shrinkage values between the high-fusing and low-fusing types. As pointed out earlier in this chapter, a precise control of the condensation and firing technic is required to compensate for such shrinkage values during the construction of the porcelain restoration.

The specific gravity of the fused porcelain mass is less influenced by manipulation technics than other properties are, and little difference exists between the high-fusing and low-fusing types. The apparent specific gravity is 2.2 to 2.3, whereas the true value is approximately 2.4. Little variation in specific gravity appears to exist between different brands of porcelain.

The transverse strength of porcelain is between 62 and 90 MPa. The shear strength value for porcelain is 110 MPa, and the diametral tensile strength is lower at 34 MPa.

The compressive strength is about 172 MPa, the elastic modulus is 69 GPa, and the Knoop hardness is 460 kg/mm^2.

The thermal properties of porcelain include a conductivity of 0.0030 cal/sec/cm^2 (° C/cm), a diffusivity of 0.64 mm^2/sec, and a linear thermal coefficient of expansion of 12.0×10^{-6}/° C.

Porcelain Crowns

The jacket crown is a popular individual tooth restoration constructed of baked porcelain. Anterior teeth that have been fractured, that contain extensive decay involving the incisal angles, and that are malformed or discolored are primary indications for this type of restoration. Sufficient dentin must remain to provide a strong core or to hold a reinforcing casting. In selected patients, teeth slightly out of line, rotated, or with unsightly spaces between them also may be covered with porcelain jackets for esthetic reasons. Porcelain rarely is indicated for crowns on posterior teeth because of the bulk and uniform thickness required to provide adequate strength.

The brittleness of porcelain requires that a layer of nearly equal thickness be placed over the entire tooth to avoid areas of weakness. All outside forces should be directed, if possible, at right angles to a plane of supporting tooth structure. The finished jacket preparation therefore should have the appearance of a miniature tooth, with no undercuts and a shoulder about 0.5-mm wide placed slightly beneath the gingival tissues around the entire tooth. In many instances it is easier to match the color of an entire tooth than only a portion of it with an inlay. Reproducing the exact size and form of a tooth requires considerable skill and experience, because the jacket is formed from several overlapping layers of porcelain, and each layer must be built oversize to allow for shrinkage.

Porcelain Inlays

Perhaps the brittle character of porcelain is the most important factor in determining its application as a restorative material. Because of this quality, porcelain is indicated primarily for restoring gingival cavities in the buccal or labial surfaces of the teeth where the restoration is free from direct force applications. In general, these class 5 cavities are prepared to give a relatively uniform thickness to the inlay, with the outer walls tapered outward only slightly.

Cavities on the proximal surfaces of the anterior teeth occasionally are restored by porcelain inlays. These class 3 preparations must have the entire lingual or labial wall of the cavity removed to provide access for the impression and placement of the inlay. Retention is provided by undercutting the remaining walls or by a dovetail prepared in the lingual surface. Etching the finished inlay with hydrofluoric acid and undercutting the cavity slightly after the impression is taken aid in developing a cement bond for adequate inlay retention.

Incisal angles and edges of the anterior teeth also may be restored with porcelain inlays. Usually a step is prepared in the remaining portion of the tooth, and platinum pins are cemented in the dentin to provide adequate retention. Porcelain rarely is indicated for either occlusal or two-surface inlays in the posterior teeth because of its tendency to fracture under direct force application.

For inlay fabrication, some laboratories use an alternate procedure that permits the fusion of the porcelain directly on a ceramic investment die material. Three types of investment materials have been developed for this purpose, including a silicate, a phosphate, and a calcium sulfate–bonded type, having different physical properties. Although the process eliminates the platinum matrix, it is time-consuming and does not effectively shorten the procedure. Results of one study did not yield an inlay with significantly improved margin accuracy over that obtained with the conventional platinum matrix technic.

The conventional technic for porcelain inlays, with the platinum matrix, has been modified to what recently has been described as the "rapid inlay technic." The use of this modification has increased in popularity. Essential to the procedure is the proper cavity design and the formation of accurate impressions on good dies, as well as careful adaptation of the platinum matrix. In this technic, time is saved in the three firing operations by inserting the porcelain directly into the furnace at 1205° C on a special quick-heating tray, after it has been dried briefly by being placed in front of the furnace door. The firing time at this temperature is about 25 seconds, after which it is air-cooled to room temperature. The second and third applications of porcelain are made with comparable firing time for each. This method has significantly shortened the inlay firing operation.

Color matching is a critical problem in replacing portions of the teeth. Porcelain, being partially amorphous in structure, does not resemble the crystalline enamel completely. As a result, various kinds of light are reflected and absorbed in a different manner by the tooth tissue and porcelain, and restorations viewed from an angle may not appear the same as they do from the front. The cementing medium is also an important factor in the final appearance of the restoration because shrinkage tends to make porcelain inlays undersize and a fine cement line may become visible at the margins. The more translucent glass ionomer rather than the opaque zinc cement is sometimes selected as a cementing medium for porcelain restorations. Special blends and shades of color of zinc phosphate and glass ionomer cements also are used to retain porcelain inlays and crowns, as indicated in Chapter 8. A jacket crown often may be cemented with zinc phosphate cement, but a porcelain inlay surrounded by tooth structure usually requires the use of translucent cements.

Machined Restorations

Equipment is available for milling machinable ceramics to form inlays, onlays, and veneers. Research is also underway for milling ceramics to form crowns. One system uses CAD/CAM (*C*omputer-*A*ssisted *D*esign/*C*omputer *A*ssisted *M*achining) technology to produce restorations in one office visit. After cavity preparation, the restoration is designed with the aid of a monitor screen as

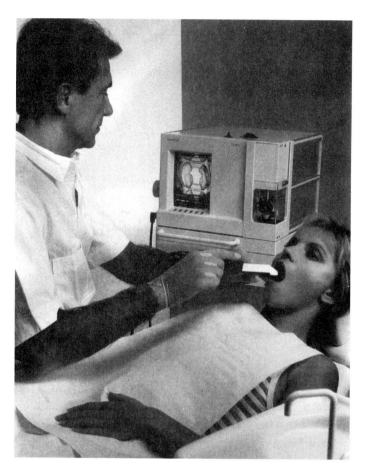

Fig. 17-3 The Cerec chairside CAD/CAM system for porcelain inlay fabrication. (Courtesy Siemens Corp., Munich, Germany, 1995.)

shown in Fig. 17-3. The restoration is then machined to achieve this design using an attached milling machine from ceramic blocks. Although convenient, the CAD/CAM system is very expensive and the marginal accuracy is poor with values of 100 to 150 μm. Bonding of the restorations with resin cements may overcome the problems associated with poor marginal fit. Another system for machining ceramics is to form inlays, onlays, and veneers using copy milling. In this system, a hard-resin pattern is made on a traditional stone die. This handmade pattern is then copied using a device that machines a block of machinable ceramic similar to those for copying house keys. Again, marginal accuracy is a concern and there are high equipment costs.

Porcelain Enamel-Metal Restorations

Porcelain enamels are vitreous ceramic coatings fired on metals. During the manufacturing process, crystalline ingredients such as feldspar and silica are heated with fluxes to form glasses that have a vitreous amorphous structure as illustrated in Fig. 17-4. This vitreous enamel is powdered and supplied in various shades for coating specific alloys. It is essential that the coefficients of thermal expansion of the enamel and alloy be matched to ensure strong bonds.

In practice, the alloy crown is cast and then coated with a veneer of enamel by layers of the powdered ceramic being baked on the surface. In Fig. 17-5 a cast metal crown with a porcelain enamel

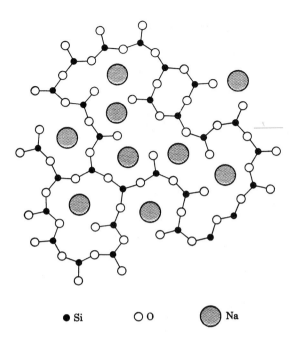

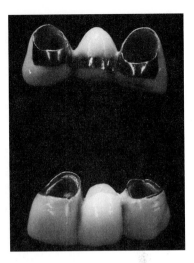

Fig. 17-6 Lingual and labial views of cast metal bridge with Ceramco porcelain fused to surface. (Courtesy Aderer J, Long Island City, NY, 1967.)

● Si   ○ O   ◉ Na

Fig. 17-4 Two-dimensional structure of sodium silicate glass. (After Warren BE, Biscoe J: *J Am Ceram Soc* 21:259, 1938.)

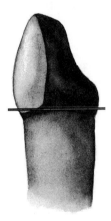

Fig. 17-5 Drawing of a porcelain veneer fused to a cast metal crown.

veneer is illustrated, and Fig. 17-6 shows a three-unit bridge with an enamel veneer. The main advantage of these restorations is the excellent esthetics possible, along with the strength of the alloy structure. The alloys used for casting the substructure are usually gold-platinum alloys containing tin, indium, and iron. Gold-palladium, palladium-silver, and nickel-chromium alloys also have been developed as lower-

cost alternatives. The ceramic-metal systems are described in detail in Chapter 18.

Core Materials

A core porcelain containing 40% to 50% alumina crystals bonded in a low-fusing fritted glass is used. The crown is formed on a platinum matrix with use of this aluminous porcelain. A veneer of the usual glass type is then fired over the crown for esthetics. Strengthening as a result of the alumina component has been claimed with a doubling of the modulus of rupture. It has been proposed that the bonding between the alumina and the glass phase is responsible for this increase in strength. In a related development, an aluminous core was used with a vitreous veneer. This reinforcement is suggested as a replacement for the gold alloy–porcelain jacket crowns currently being used. Aluminous core porcelains have transverse strengths of about 138 MPa and shear strengths of 145 MPa.

Fig. 17-7 illustrates the construction of an aluminous porcelain jacket crown. Less tooth structure needs to be removed because the aluminous porcelain core requires a thinner veneer for good esthetics than a metal crown does. Aluminous porcelain also has application in denture teeth in which brittleness has been a problem. During the firing of these porcelains, a sintering mechanism is responsible for densification.

A new process for preparing aluminous cores involving glass infiltration has been introduced that gives flexure strength values around 500 MPa. The process involves the slip casting of fine grained pure alumina followed by sintering at 1120° C. The sintered alumina core is then infiltrated with a glass at 1100° C for 4 hours. After the excess glass is trimmed off the core, the rest of the crown is built up using compatible body and incisal porcelains. Due to the high strength of the core, small anterior bridges are being made using this process. However, no long-term clinical data are available on the success of these bridges.

A high-expansion magnesia core material has been developed that is compatible with the same body porcelains used with metals. The construction of a crown using this core material is shown in Fig. 17-8. The strength of the high-expansion core material is around 138 MPa with an average coefficient of expansion of $14.5 \times 10^{-6}/°$ C. The main advantage of this core material is that it allows a laboratory to utilize the more widely available porcelains for bonding to metals for reinforced jacket crown construction.

■ CAST GLASS CERAMICS

A glass ceramic is a material fabricated in the vitreous or noncrystalline state and then converted to a crystalline state by heat treatment. Recent research has led to the development of a castable glass for forming crowns by the lost wax process. The most widely used glass ceramic product in dentistry is a silica material that crystallizes to form mica upon heat treatment. A phosphate-bonded investment mold is used in the lost wax process. A two-stage burnout procedure is used with a hold at 250° C and a second hold at 950° C. The mold temperature for casting is 900° C. A motor-driven casting machine with a thermostatically controlled platinum wound muffle is used (Fig. 17-9). The casting temperature of the glass is around 1380° C. Typical castings before and after ceramming and external coloration are shown in Fig. 17-10. After removal of the sprue, the glass crown is invested and heat-treated for several hours at 1075° C to produce crystallization of glass to form a mica ceramic. The recrystallized ceramic has a flexure strength of around 152 MPa and a Knoop hardness of 362 kg/mm². The final shade is achieved by applying a colored glass to the surface and firing.

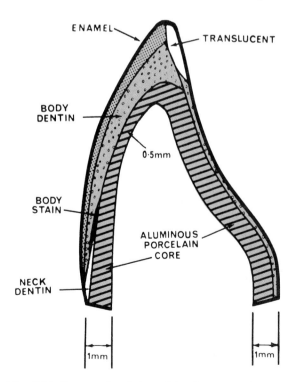

Fig. 17-7 Cross-sectional view of aluminous porcelain jacket crown. (From McLean JW: *J Am Dent Assoc* 75:621, 1967.)

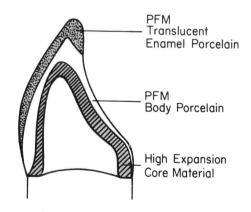

Fig. 17-8 All-ceramic crown made with porcelain-fused to metal-(PFM) type of translucent porcelains over a high-expansion magnesia core material. (From O'Brien WJ, *J Dent Res, IADR Abstract* 410, p 216, March 1984.)

Another glass ceramic based on calcium phosphate also has been developed. This glass is cast at 1050° C in a gypsum-bonded investment and converted to a crystalline ceramic by heat treating at 645° C for 12 hours.

The main concern about these systems is the need for external coloration, which is considered not as natural and durable as porcelain with pigments dispersed throughout the material.

High-Temperature Injection Molding

This system is designed to produce all ceramic crowns, inlays, and onlays by injection molding. The porcelain is a high leucite content glass. The high leucite ($KAlSi_2O_6$) glass ingots are heated to

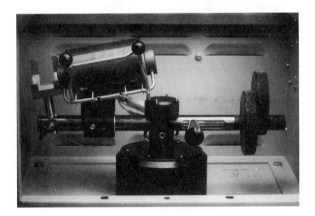

Fig. 17-9 Casting machine used for fabricating glass ceramic restorations.

around 1180° C and injected into an investment mold cavity produced by the lost wax process (Fig. 17-11). The crown produced is then cut back with a handpiece to a dentin porcelain understructure. An outer layer of incisal porcelain is then added and fired by the conventional means to supply color and translucency over the preshaded dentin porcelain. The flexure strength of this porcelain is about 200 MPa, which is about double that of conventional feldspar porcelains. The main disadvantages are the initial cost of the equipment and complexity of the process.

■ OPTICAL PROPERTIES

The colors of commercial premixed dental porcelains are in the yellow to yellow-red range. Because the range of colors of natural teeth is much greater than available in a kit of premixed porcelains, modifier porcelains are also supplied for adjustments. These modifier porcelains are strongly pigmented porcelains usually supplied in blue, yellow, pink, orange, brown, and gray. The dental technician may add the modifier porcelain to the opaque and body porcelains during the building of the crown. Surface staining is another way of changing the color of a dental porcelain crown and involves the application of highly pigmented glazes. The main disadvantages of surface staining are a lowered durability as a result of high solubility and the reduction of translucency.

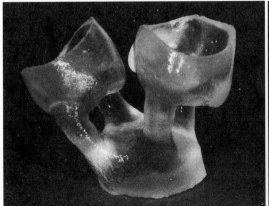
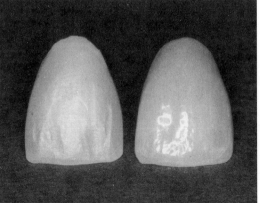

Fig. 17-10 Glass ceramic castings (*left*), a glass ceramic crown after heat treatment or ceramming (*middle*), and a glass ceramic crown after external coloration (*right*). (Courtesy Dootz ER, Ann Arbor, 1987, University of Michigan School of Dentistry.)

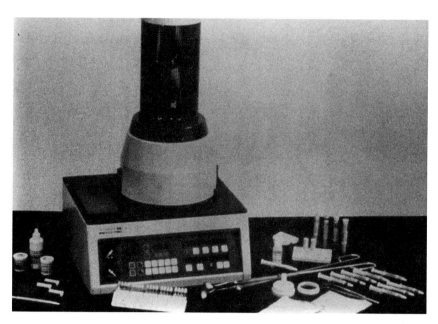

Fig 17-11 The Empress high-temperature injection molding systems for all ceramic restorations. (Courtesy Ivoclar Inc., Amherst, NY, 1995.)

TABLE 17-3   Total Percent Transmission of 1-mm Thick Porcelains

Shade	Ceramco	Vita	Neydium	Will-Ceram	Steeles
59	29.97	22.66	31.93	26.06	27.23
62	27.85	–	–	27.88	–
65	23.31	20.39	35.39	33.50	22.10
67	26.32	18.04	23.58	19.03	23.42
91	31.81	–	38.41	–	–

Adapted from Brodbelt RHW, O'Brien WJ, Fan PL: *J Dent Res* 59:70, 1980.

Translucency is another critical property of dental porcelains. The translucencies of opaque, body, and incisal porcelains differ considerably. Opaque porcelains have very low translucency values to mask metal substructure surfaces. Body porcelain translucency values range between 20% and 35% as seen in Table 17-3. Incisal porcelains have the highest values of translucency ranging between 45% and 50%.

Because dental enamel is fluorescent under ultraviolet light, uranium oxide had been added to produce fluorescence with porcelain. However, because of the low but detectable radioactivity of uranium, newer formulations contain rare earth oxides (such as cerium oxide), which produce fluorescence.

Because the outer layers of a porcelain crown are translucent, the apparent color is affected by reflectance from the inner opaque or core porcelain. Subtractive color mixing results from combining the light reflected from the inner opaque porcelain surface and the light transmitted through the body porcelain. The thickness of the body porcelain layer determines the color obtained with a given opaque porcelain. This thickness effect may be minimized if the body porcelain and the opaque porcelain are the same color as that of some commercial systems.

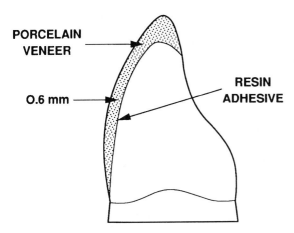

PORCELAIN
VENEER

0.6 mm

RESIN
ADHESIVE

Fig 17-12 Porcelain veneer bonded to facial surface of tooth. (From Craig RG, O'Brien WJ, Powers JM: *Dental materials: properties and manipulation,* ed. 6, St Louis, 1996, Mosby.)

ESTHETIC PORCELAIN VENEERS

A porcelain esthetic veneer is a layer of porcelain that is bonded to the surface of a tooth to cover an unsightly area (Fig. 17-12). Porcelain veneers are custom-made veneers that are fabricated in a dental laboratory. Previously, denture teeth were shaped to fit the area to be covered. Currently, the porcelain veneer is constructed on a die of the tooth from the opaque and body porcelains normally used for porcelain-fused-to-metal crowns and bridges. The porcelain is fired either on a phosphate refractory die material or a platinum matrix. To obtain sufficient adhesion, the tooth enamel is etched with phosphoric acid and the bonding surface of the porcelain is etched with an acid and treated with a silane coupling agent. Composite resins specifically formulated for bonding to porcelain are employed as the adhesive.

PORCELAIN ARTIFICIAL TEETH

Individual porcelain teeth, either air-fired or vacuum-fired, are used generally for both complete and partial dentures. The anterior teeth have one or two gold-covered pins to provide retention to the denture base. Only one brand is available that uses undercut areas in the proximal surfaces instead of pins for retention. The posterior teeth in general use have undercut diatoric holes located centrally in the underside of the teeth.

Manufacture

In the production of porcelain teeth, the powder ingredients are weighed and mixed with water containing starch, gum tragacanth, or other organic materials to form a puttylike mass that can be handled conveniently. Anterior teeth are made of both a body portion, which forms the bulk of the tooth and corresponds roughly to the dentin of the human tooth, and a lighter, more translucent enamel portion, which covers the surface and forms much of the incisal edge of the tooth. To readily distinguish the mix for each portion during molding, a vegetable dye is added to one or both mixes. This burns away at low temperatures and does not affect the final colors.

The molding technic varies with different manufacturers. Generally, the split molds are made of bronze and may be separated so that one portion contains the negative pattern for the lingual surface of 12 teeth and the other portion contains the negative pattern for the labial surface, or face, of the teeth. One technic employs a third portion, which also fits against the labial surface, for the purpose of accurately forming the enamel-colored porcelain separately before the body portion is added.

When the two-piece molds are used, a thin layer of the enamel mix is placed in the labial mold to provide the enamel color, and the body mix, which forms the bulk of the tooth, is placed over this. A thin veneer of enamel mix then is placed in the incisal portion of the lingual mold and covered with body mix. When combined, the two mold halves with the porcelain mixes form a tooth with contours and coloration similar to natural teeth.

The technic for the three-piece molds involves placing the doughlike enamel mix in the labial half first, pressing the third or blender mold into it, and heating the molds until the mix stiffens. They are then opened, the excess mix is trimmed away, and the body mix is added to fill the second and larger lingual half of the mold.

Small noble-metal rings are embedded in the porcelain to provide a base for the gold-plated nickel pins used for the retention of the teeth in the denture base. These rings are made of a metal or alloy with a high melting point and usually are split to allow for the shrinkage of the surrounding porcelain during fusion. Before the molds are filled, the rings are placed over the tips of tapered posts that extend into the tooth from the lingual half of the mold.

The posterior teeth are molded in somewhat the same manner but without provision for pins. Retention of posterior teeth to the denture base is provided by openings (diatorics) in the underside of the finished teeth. A typical set of porcelain teeth is shown in Fig. 17-13.

After the molds are filled by either method, they are placed in a press and heated until the porcelain mix develops sufficient hardness to allow handling. Each anterior tooth at this "biscuit" stage is approximately one-fifth oversize to allow for shrinkage and has one or two tapered openings extending from the lingual surface to the embedded platinum alloy rings.

The biscuited teeth are placed on trays of coarsely ground quartz and are moved slowly through a furnace in which the temperature and time are precisely controlled. Each tooth size and color requires a different firing schedule.

The first stage of the firing operation involves the removal of water and the elimination of the organic binders and coloring matter by burning. This leaves a loosely joined mass of particles in the shape of a tooth, interspersed with approximately 50% by vol-ume of voids. In the second, or densification, stage, the feldspar fuses and unites solidly with the particles of quartz and kaolin, and the particles pull together, resulting in a linear shrinkage of approximately 18%. Thus to produce a tooth 8.5-mm wide, the molds and biscuits must be 10.3 mm in width. The final fusion takes place in the third stage, and a gloss is formed over the entire surface of the tooth.

After the teeth have been cooled slowly to prevent crazing, all that remains is the attachment of the pins. For this operation small bits of solder are stamped to the ends of the gold-clad pins, and they are inserted, solder downward, to contact the metal rings at the base of the tapered openings in the lingual body of the teeth. When heated, either in a furnace or electrically, the solder melts and joins the pins firmly to the embedded rings, as indicated in Fig. 17-14.

Vacuum firing

Gas bubbles have always been a problem in the production of dental porcelain. The extent to which bubbles may exist in air-fired porcelain is shown in Fig. 17-15. The specimen shown was ground and polished, and the round black spots are the cross-sectioned bubbles. It has been calculated that air-fired

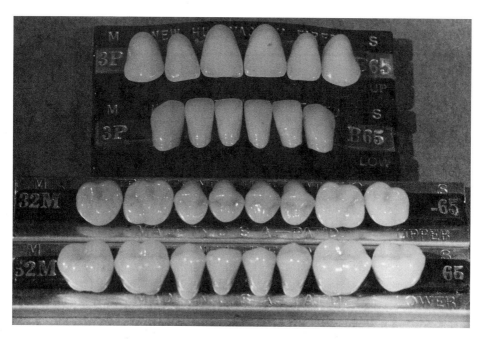

Fig 17-13 A complete set of porcelain artificial teeth as supplied by the manufacturer.

porcelain contains as much as 6.3% voids. This not only results in undesirable roughness when a tooth must be ground, but it also exerts an even more undesirable effect on the optical properties of the porcelain.

It has been determined that the bubbles were caused by the entrapment of air during melting and fusing. Air spaces become spherical under the influence of surface tension and expand with increased temperature. A method was developed for firing porcelain in a vacuum while the shrinkage was taking place. The first stage, when the organic material is burning off, is completed in normal atmosphere, but at about 980° C. Before the fusion begins, the

teeth in loose powder or biscuit form are subjected to a vacuum and held until partial melting takes place and the shrinkage is complete. The vacuum is then broken, and the final gloss is formed at normal atmospheric pressure to prevent boiling or blistering during this last 30° C rise.

Actually, the mechanism of densification under a vacuum is more involved than this. Because the vacuum is not absolute, there are still a number of small spherical air bubbles entrapped in the interstitial spaces of the porcelain mass. When air at atmospheric pressure is allowed to enter the furnace, it has a strong compressive effect on these low-pressure bubbles through the medium of the semimolten porcelain. This results in a dense, relatively pore-free porcelain, as illustrated in Fig. 17-16.

An alternate method may be used in which the principle of diffusion is used to secure improved density in fused porcelain. A diffusible gas such as helium may be introduced to the furnace at low pressure during the second, or densification, stage. The helium gas instead of air is entrapped in the interstitial spaces, and because its molecular diameter is smaller than the porcelain lattice, it diffuses outward under the pressure of the shrinking porcelain.

In another method, known as the pressure-firing process, only the third or gloss stage is involved in the operation. Normal air-fired porcelain is gloss-fired in a furnace completely encased in a pressure shell, and the pressure is held at 1.55 MPa during cooling to about 980° C. This causes the air bubbles

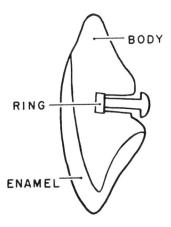

Fig 17-14 Cross-sectional outline of an anterior porcelain tooth showing various layers and pin anchorage.

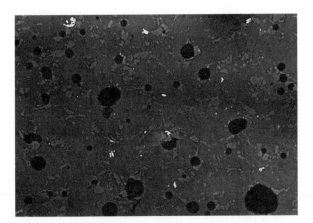

Fig 17-15 Microscopic view of air-fired porcelain, showing porosity. (Courtesy Semmelman JO, York, Pa, 1959, Dentsply International.)

Fig 17-16 Microscopic view of vacuum-fired porcelain showing minimal porosity. (Courtesy Semmelman JO, York, Pa, 1959, Dentsply International.)

to be reduced in size and produces density comparable to vacuum firing or diffusible gas firing. Pressure-fired porcelain may not be refired to self-glazing temperatures under normal atmospheric pressure, however, because the compressed bubbles expand to produce the porosity of air-fired porcelain. Nevertheless, pressure firing is economical and of value in producing teeth for certain uses.

Before the development of these improved firing methods, fine texture and translucency were not possible at the same time. Maximum translucency was obtained only by use of coarse powders that trapped only a few relatively large bubbles of air but at the same time produced an undesirable granular appearance. Fine-grained powders developed a better texture but increased the opacity because of the large number of small bubbles. With vacuum firing it is possible to have both fine texture and translucency, but an entirely new coloring system is necessary. Studies of pigment dispersion soon made it possible to produce teeth that compared favorably with the natural teeth. This quality has long been sought in artificial teeth and is called opalescence. The cross section of a modern anterior vacuum-fired porcelain tooth is shown in Fig. 17-17.

With the improvement in density and color came an increase of approximately 50% in the impact strength. This has always been a critical factor in ceramics. Vacuum-fired porcelain will resist over 300 g cm of impact energy as compared with approximately 200 g cm for the same porcelain that is air-fired. The impact strength of a porcelain tooth is further improved when moderate tempering stresses are pro-

vided in the outer glaze. As the tooth cools, the slightly lower coefficient of expansion of this layer develops a slight compression stress in the porcelain. Because all glasses and glazes are stronger under compression than tension, this property is used to an advantage to provide increased resistance to shattering.

A porcelain tooth is complex from the standpoint of thermal expansion. There is a high-expansion metal core embedded for a retention of pins, a medium-expansion body porcelain, and a low-expansion enamel portion. The various compositions are formulated to balance the thermal stresses of each layer to obtain the maximum strength by the action of compression.

It is often necessary to "spot" grind porcelain teeth or to heat them momentarily in a flame during the waxing of a denture. Overheating during these procedures may cause a small area to expand and become too large to be compatible with the remainder of the tooth. This may result in immediate breakage or perhaps only in cracking the tooth so that failure occurs in service. Therefore it is advisable to keep a porcelain tooth wet during all grinding operations and to avoid rapid heating or cooling.

A low-expanding porcelain tooth that is more resistant to thermal shock is possible, because silica in the vitreous stage has an expansion curve below that of feldspar and may be substituted for it. This new type of porcelain is not thermally compatible with the high-expansion metal inserts in anterior teeth and is better indicated for posterior teeth in which grinding is often necessary. Such posterior porcelain teeth have become available in recent years.

Properties

The physical properties of tooth porcelain perhaps may be best shown when they are compared with the properties of plastic teeth and, when possible, with those of natural teeth. These properties, however, often are so radically different that they cannot be measured with the same equipment or compared quantitatively. The hardness values of porcelain compared with plastic and natural tooth structures are shown in Table 17-4.

It is evident from these values that the two standard tooth replacement materials are quite different in hardness values. Porcelain is harder than enamel, whereas the best plastic teeth are softer than dentin.

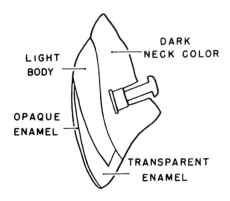

Fig 17-17 Cross-sectional drawing of a modern vacuum-fired porcelain tooth.

In regard to abrasion resistance, dental porcelain has been clinically evaluated as being equal to or slightly more wear resistant than natural tooth structure. At present, clinical data represent the only measure of abrasion believed to be of real significance. On this basis, porcelain has been estimated to have from 10 to 20 times the abrasion resistance of plastic teeth.

Porcelain is resistant to the action of solvents, with only hydrofluoric acid known to have any significant effect on it. The cross-linked plastics are relatively craze resistant and are immune to reasonable amounts of ordinary solvents. They may, however, be softened to some extent by a number of organic solvents.

Water bleaching and sunlight have no effect on porcelain, but repeated cycles of drying and water immersion may cause whitening and loss of color in plastic teeth. Continued exposure to ultraviolet light may cause a slight yellowing. When plastic is softened by solvents, organic dyes may penetrate the outer layer and cause discoloration.

The flexural strength of dental plastics is unquestionably superior to that of the dental porcelains. The pin anchorage and the strength of the porcelain that surrounds it are the determining factors in the basic strength of a porcelain tooth. At present this is adequate for most service conditions.

The high impact strength of plastic gives it a definite advantage. Vacuum firing has improved the fracture resistance of dental porcelain by about 50%, but this does not preclude the possibility of fracture from sudden shock.

In dimensional stability or permanence of form, plastic is less acceptable than porcelain. The superior strength of plastic is indicated by its ability to cushion the impact blow of mastication and avoid fracture because of brittleness. Unfortunately, plastic does not return to its original form each time it

yields, and there is cumulative loss of dimension described as flow. Porcelain, like tooth enamel, is incapable of cold flow.

Both porcelain and plastic withstand heating well enough for the usual dental procedures. Plastic teeth will withstand temperatures of approximately 200° C, and porcelain is unaffected by temperatures in excess of 1100° C if the heat is applied slowly.

A direct and more complete comparison of the characteristic properties of porcelain and plastic teeth is discussed under plastics in Chapter 19.

SELECTED PROBLEMS

Problem 1. A porcelain that normally glazes at 982° C was found to require 1010° C for glazing. Explain.

Solution a. The pyrometer of the porcelain furnace requires periodic calibration, usually with silver disks that are supplied by the furnace manufacturer.

Solution b. If the particle size is changed, the sintering and glazing temperatures change also. It is important to shake up the porcelain before using it to counteract any settling of particles.

Problem 2. A porcelain crown fractured as a result of excessive porosity. What can be done to avoid porosity?

Solution a. The mix of porcelain should not be stirred too much because bubbles may be entrapped.

Solution b. Porcelain should be heated gradually when first fired to evaporate the water holding the particles together without creating steam. Rapid heating results in steam, which can create porosity.

Problem 3. A patient showed considerable wear of enamel on the teeth in occlusion with porcelain crowns. Explain.

Solution. Dental porcelain is harder than tooth enamel and can wear it away. Porcelain fused to metal with metal lingual surfaces on anterior crowns results in less wear. However, because the porcelain crowns are already cemented, the use of a bite splint in the case of bruxism may be indicated.

■ REFERENCES

Asaoka K, Nuwayama N, Tesk JA: Influence of tempering method on residual stress in dental porcelain, *J Dent Res* 71:1623, 1992.

Baran GR, O'Brien WJ, Tien TY: Colored emission of rare earth ions in a potassium feldspar glass, *J Dent Res* 56:1323, 1977.

Brodbelt RHW, O'Brien WJ, Fan PL: Translucency of dental porcelain, *J Dent Res* 59:70, 1980.

TABLE 17-4 Hardness of Natural and Artificial Teeth

Material	KHN (kg/mm^2)
Porcelain	460
Enamel	343
Dentin	68
Plastic	20

Clark EB: Porcelain as a filling material. In Anderson GM, editor: *Proceedings of the Dental Centenary Celebration,* Baltimore, 1940, Maryland State Dental Association, Waverly Press.

Denry IL, Rosenstiel SF: Flexural strength and fracture toughness of Dicor glass-ceramic after embedment modification, *J Dent Res* 72:572, 1993.

Denry IL, Rosenstiel SF, Holloway JA, Niemiec MS: Enhanced chemical strengthening of feldspathic dental porcelain, *J Dent Res* 72:1429, 1993.

Gray HS: The porcelain jacket crown, *NZ Dent J* 59:283, 1963.

Hodson JT: Some physical properties of three dental porcelains, *J Prosthet Dent* 9:235, 1959.

Johnston WM, O'Brien WJ: Color analysis of dental modifying porcelains, *J Dent Res* 60(Spec Issue A):441, 1981.

Kelly JR, Tesk JA, Sorensen JA: Failure of all-ceramic fixed partial dentures *in vitro* and *in vivo:* analysis and modeling, *J Dent Res* 74:1253, 1995.

Kingery WD, editor: *Ceramic fabrication processes,* New York, 1958, John Wiley & Sons.

Kulp PR, Lee PW, Fox JE: Impact test for dental porcelain, *J Dent Res* 40:1136, 1961.

Kurzeja R, O'Brien WJ: The fluorescence of porcelain containing cerium, *J Dent Res* 60(Spec Issue A):435, 1981.

Lehman ML, Hampson EL: A study of strain patterns in jacket crowns on anterior teeth resulting from different tooth patterns, *Br Dent J* 113:337, 1962.

Leone EF, Fairhurst CW: Bond strength and mechanical properties of dental porcelain enamel, *J Prosthet Dent* 18:155, 1967.

Mackert JR Jr, Twiggs SW, Evans-Williams AL: Isothermal anneal effect on leucite content in dental porcelains, *J Dent Res* 74:1259, 1995.

McLean JW: A higher strength porcelain for crown and bridge work, *Br Dent J* 119:268, 1965.

McLean JW: The alumina reinforced porcelain jacket crown, *J Am Dent Assoc* 75:621, 1967.

McLean JW, Hughes TH: The reinforcement of dental porcelain with ceramic oxides, *Br Dent J* 119:251, 1965.

Meyer JM, O'Brien WJ, Yu R: Sintering of dental porcelain enamels, *J Dent Res* 55:696, 1976.

Milleding P, Örtengren V, Karlsson S: Ceramic inlay systems: some clinical aspects, *J Oral Rehabil* 22:571, 1995.

Mora GP, O'Brien WJ: Thermal shock resistance of core reinforced all-ceramic crown systems, *J Biomed Mater Res* 28:189, 1994.

O'Brien WJ: *Ceramics,* Dental Clinics of North America, vol 29, no 4, Philadelphia, Oct 1985, WB Saunders.

O'Brien WJ: Recent developments in materials and processes for ceramic crowns, *J Am Dent Assoc* 110:547, 1985.

O'Brien WJ, Craig RG, editors: Recent developments in dental ceramics, *Ceramic Eng and Sci Proc,* Columbus, Ohio, 1985, American Ceramic Society.

O'Brien WJ, Johnston WJ, Fanian F: Filtering effects of body porcelain on opaque color modifiers, *J Dent Res, IADR Abstracts* 61:330, 1982.

O'Brien WJ, Nelson D, Lorey RE: The assessment of chroma sensitivity to porcelain pigments, *J Prosthet Dent* 49:63, 1983.

Paquet GH: A comparison of surface roughness, hardness, and porosity of air-fired and vacuum-fired porcelain, *Northwestern Univ Bull* 66:14, 1966.

Preston JD, Bergen SF: *Color science and dental art,* St Louis, 1980, Mosby.

Sherrill CA, Jr, O'Brien WJ: The transverse strength of aluminous and feldspathic porcelains, *J Dent Res* 53:683, 1974.

Smith BB: Esthetic restoration of anterior teeth, with emphasis on rapid fabrication of fired porcelain units, *J Am Acad Gold Foil Oper* 6:6, 1963.

Smith BB: *Porcelain inlays for the general practitioner,* Dental Clinics of North America, Philadelphia, March 1967, WB Saunders.

Thompson JY, Anusavice KJ: Effect of surface etching on the flexure strength and fracture toughness of Dicor disks containing controlled flaws, *J Dent Res* 73:505, 1994.

Vines RF, Semmelman JO: Densification of dental porcelain, *J Dent Res* 36:950, 1957.

Wozniak WT, Moore BK, Smith E: Fluorescence spectra of dental porcelain, *J Dent Res* 55(Spec Issue B):B186, 1976.

Yamada HN: *Dental porcelain, the state of the art—1977,* Los Angeles, 1977, University of Southern California.

18 *Ceramic-Metal Systems*

All-ceramic anterior restorations can appear very natural. Unfortunately, the ceramics used in these restorations are brittle and subject to fracture from high tensile stresses. Conversely, all-metal restorations are strong and tough but, from an esthetic viewpoint, acceptable only for posterior restorations. Fortunately the esthetic qualities of ceramic materials can be combined with the strength and toughness of metals to produce restorations that have both a natural toothlike appearance and very good mechanical properties. A cross section of a ceramic-metal anterior crown is shown in Fig. 18-1. The cast metal coping provides a substrate on which a ceramic coating is fused. The ceramics used for these restorations are porcelains, hence the common name, porcelain-fused-to-metal restorations. These ceramic-metal restorations are highly popular and are used for most of the crown and bridge restorations made today.

Ceramic-metal restorations were made possible by the following developments: (1) ceramics and alloys that form a strong bond, (2) ceramics and alloys with matching coefficients of thermal expansion, (3) low-fusing ceramic materials, and (4) alloys that resist deformation at the ceramic fusing temperature. The ceramic must fuse and bond to the alloy without the metal coping deforming, and, on cooling, the ceramic and metal must contract in unison so the ceramic will not crack or separate from the alloy. When these conditions are met, strong restorations with excellent esthetics are produced.

■ CERAMIC-METAL BONDING

Perhaps the most important requirement in the design of ceramic-metal restorations is that the ceramic and metal adhere to each other. In fact, the most common mechanical failure of these restorations is porcelain debonding from the metal. Many factors control metal-ceramic adhesion: the formation of strong chemical bonding, mechanical interlocking between the two materials, and residual stresses. In addition, the ceramic must wet and fuse to the surface to form a uniform interface with no voids. These factors are also important for ceramic coatings on metallic implants (Chapter 15).

An interface between a metal and a ceramic with many strong chemical bonds between them, with the bonds acting as tags that hold the two materials together, would obviously lead to strong bonding. However, methods producing a ceramic-metal interface with strong chemical bonding, or even showing that strong chemical bonding exists, have not been developed. But the formation of oxides on the surface of the metal are proven to contribute to the formation of strong bonding. Noble metals, which are resistant to oxidizing, must have other, more easily oxidized elements, added to form surface oxides. When these elements are added, bonding is improved. The common practice of degassing or preoxidizing the metal coping before porcelain application creates surface oxides that improve bonding.

From both theoretical and practical standpoints, the roughness, or more generally the topography, of a ceramic-metal interface plays a large part in adhesion. The ceramic penetrating into a rough metal surface can mechanically interlock with the metal, like Velcro®, improving adhesion. The increased area associated with a rougher interface also provides more room for chemical bonds to form. However, rough surfaces can reduce adhesion if the ceramic does not penetrate into the surface and voids are present at the interface; this may happen with improperly fired porcelain or metals that are

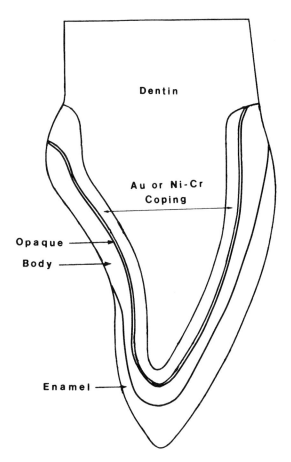

Fig. 18-1 Cross section of a ceramic-metal crown showing the coping and the opaque, body, and enamel porcelain layers.

poorly wetted by the porcelain. Sandblasting is often used to roughen the surface of the metal coping to improve the bonding of the ceramic.

High residual stresses between the metal and ceramic can lead to failure. If the metal and ceramic have different thermal expansion coefficient the two materials will contract at different rates during cooling and strong residual stresses will form across the interface. If these stresses are strong enough the porcelain on porcelain-fused-to-metal restorations will crack or separate from the metal. Even if the stresses are less strong and do not cause immediate failure, they can still weaken the bond. To avoid these problems the porcelains and metal alloys are formulated to have closely matched thermal expansion coefficients. Typically the porcelains have coefficients of

thermal expansion between 13.0 and $14.0 \times 10^{-6}/^{\circ}$ C and the metals have coefficients between 13.5 and $14.5 \times 10^{-6}/^{\circ}$ C. The difference of $0.5 \times 10^{-6}/^{\circ}$ C in thermal expansion between the metal and porcelain causes the metal to contract slightly more than does the ceramic during cooling after firing the porcelain. This condition puts the ceramic under slight residual compression, which makes it less sensitive to applied tensile forces.

Wetting is important for formation of good ceramic-metal bonding. The porcelain during firing must wet and flow over the metal surface. The contact angle between the porcelain and metal is a measure of the wetting and to some extent the quality of the bond that forms. The wetting of the alloy surface by the fused porcelain indicates an interaction between surface atoms in the metal with the porcelain. Low contact angles indicate good wetting. The contact angle of porcelain on a gold type of ceramic alloy is shown in Fig. 18-2; the contact angle is about 60 degrees. The surface of the noble alloys containing tin and indium after heating have these oxides, and they diffuse into and interact with the porcelain, forming an adhesive bond. The oxide surface of a Type 1, 98% noble alloy is shown at high magnification in Fig. 18-3.

Evaluation of Ceramic-Metal Bonding

Many tests have been used to determine the bond strength between ceramics and metals; however, the ideal test currently does not exist. In addition, data obtained from different tests often are not comparable. However, new fracture toughness tests may be an improvement over the more established tests. One of the established bond-strength tests is the planar shear test. A sketch of the test is shown in Fig. 18-4. Other commonly used tests are the flexural tests, which require layers of porcelain to be bonded to a strip or plate of metal. The coated metal plate is flexed in a controlled manner until the porcelain fractures off. A variant of this test is used for the ANSI/ADA Specification No. 38 and the ISO/TC 106/SC2 Specification. In these specification tests opaque and body porcelains are applied and fired to a thickness of approximately 1 mm on 20 mm × 5 mm × 0.5 mm alloy sheets. The specimen is then bent over a 1-cm diameter rod with the porcelain on the outside and then straightened.

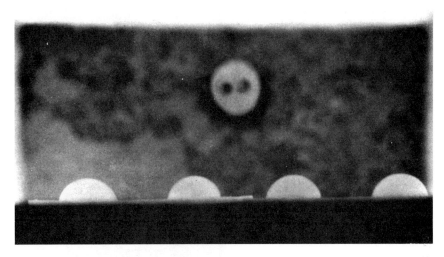

Fig. 18-2 Enamel resting on a high noble ceramic alloy (*left*) and alloy treated with a gold coating agent (*right*), both at 1040° C. (From O'Brien WJ, Ryge G: *J Prosthet Dent* 15:1094, 1965.)

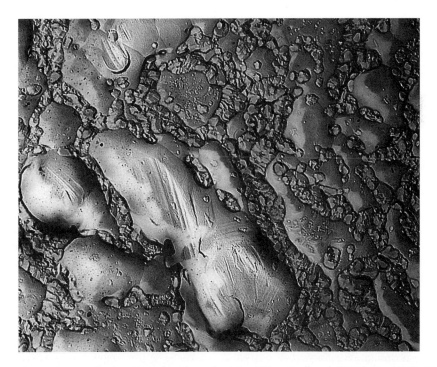

Fig. 18-3 Electron photomicrograph of replicated surface of oxidized Type 1 alloy. (×8000.) (From Kelly M, Asgar K, O'Brien WJ: *J Biomed Mater Res* 3:403, 1969.)

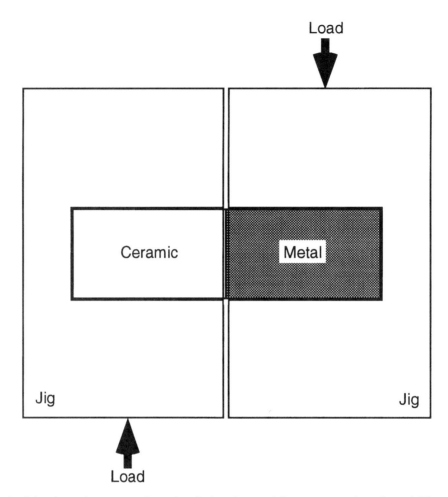

Fig. 18-4 Sketch of the planar shear test to determine the bond strength between ceramic and metal. The ceramic and metal are held in a jig and loaded in opposite directions until shear failure at the interface occurs.

Then the surface is viewed under low magnification and the percent of the surface with retained porcelain is reported. Tests based on tensile and torsional loading schemes have also been used.

The failure of a ceramic-metal bond can occur in six possible locations (Fig. 18-5). Knowing the location of the fracture provides considerable information. The highest strength metal-ceramic specimens will fracture in the porcelain when tested (Fig. 18-5, *III*); this is observed with some alloys that were properly prepared and had porcelain applied and fused. Testing these high-strength specimens using the push-through shear test shows that the maximum strengths are approximately the same as the shear strength of the ceramic. Fractures are rarely observed through the metal; however, fracture through the oxide (Fig. 18-5, *V*) and interfacial fracture (Fig. 18-5, *I*) are commonly observed with poor bonding. Base metal alloys commonly fracture through the oxide (Fig. 18-6) if an excessively thick oxide layer is present. Interfacial fracture is observed with metals that are resistant to forming surface oxides, such as pure gold or platinum.

■ CERAMICS FOR PORCELAIN-FUSED-TO-METAL BONDING

The ceramics used for porcelain-fused-to-metal restorations must fulfill five requirements: (1) they must simulate the appearance of natural teeth,

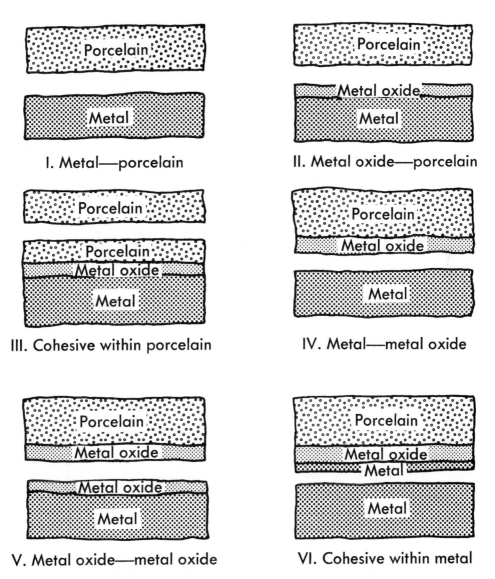

Fig. 18-5 Classification of porcelain enamel failures. (In Valega TM, editor: *Alternatives to gold alloys in dentistry,* HEW Pub No. (NIH) 77–1227, Washington, DC, 1977, US Government Printing Office.)

(2) they must fuse at relatively low temperatures, (3) they must have thermal expansion coefficients compatible with the metals used for ceramic-metal bonding, (4) they must withstand the oral environment, and (5) they must not abrade opposing teeth. The ceramic is carefully formulated to achieve these requirements. These porcelains are composed of crystalline phases in an amorphous and glassy (vitreous) matrix. They comprise primarily SiO_2, B_2O_3, Al_2O_3, and K_2O (see Table 17–2). Opacifiers and

various pigments are also added to the porcelain. Some newer low-fusing porcelains also contain significant quantities of Na_2O and hydroxyl groups. Porcelain is supplied by the manufacturer in the form of a fine powder.

In developing porcelains for ceramic-metal bonding, a major breakthrough was formulating porcelains that had sufficiently high thermal expansion coefficients to match those of dental alloys. This higher expansion was made possible by the addition

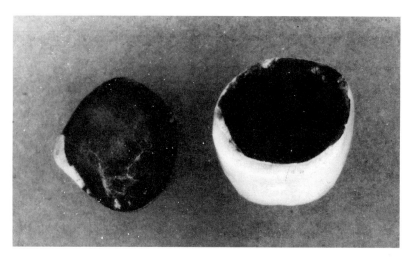

Fig. 18-6 A failure through oxide layer of nickel-chromium alloy. (From O'Brien WJ. In Yamada H, editor: *Dental porcelain: the state of the art—1977,* Los Angeles, 1977, University of Southern California.)

of potassium oxide and the formation of a high-expansion phase called leucite ($KAlSi_2O_6$). This phase increased the thermal expansion of the porcelain so that it could match that of dental alloys.

Very natural-appearing restorations are made using porcelains. The nature of porcelains, with their glassy matrix and crystalline phases, produces a translucency much like that of teeth. Pigments and opacifiers control the color and translucency of the restoration.

Porcelains have other qualities that make them well suited for ceramic-metal restorations. They fuse at lower temperatures than do many other ceramic materials, lessening the potential of distorting the metal coping. Sodium and potassium oxides in the glassy matrix are responsible for lowering the fusing temperatures to the range 930° to 980° C. The new low-fusing porcelains have hydroxyl groups and more Na_2O to lower fusing temperatures to as low as 660° C. Porcelains, because they do not corrode, are also resistant to the fluids present in the oral environment. Porcelain can be abrasive to opposing teeth because of their hardness. This becomes a significant problem if the porcelain surface is rough due to improper processing or becomes rough in the oral environment. New porcelains have been developed that have been shown to be less abrasive to natural teeth. These ceramics are also strong in compression, which permits their use on the occlusal surfaces of the restorations. The porcelains used to bond to met-

als have tensile strengths of 35 MPa, compressive strengths of 860 MPa, shear strengths of 120 MPa, and transverse strengths of 60 MPa.

■ ALLOYS FOR PORCELAIN-FUSED-TO-METAL BONDING

To be suitable for porcelain-fused-to-metal restorations, a metal must meet several qualifications. In processing, the alloy must not deform or change the color of the porcelain. It must form strong bonding with the porcelain. The alloy must have good mechanical properties and must match the thermal expansion of the porcelains. Six types of noble and three types of base metal casting alloys meet these requirements. These are shown in Tables 18-1 and 18-2.

Composition of Noble Metal Alloys

The Type 1 alloy was the first of the gold-based alloys to be introduced for ceramic-metal restorations. It is a very high noble alloy, 96% to 98%, with iron present as a strengthening element. The platinum and palladium increase the melting range and decrease the coefficient of expansion, whereas the indium and tin contribute to form a good ceramic-metal bond. The iron reacts with platinum to form $FePt_3$ precipitates, which strengthen the alloys. The optimum heat treatment is 30 minutes at 550° C,

TABLE 18-1 Range of Compositions of Six Types of Noble Metal Alloys for Ceramic-Metal Restorations

| Type | Description | Elements (in weight percent) | | | | | | Casting Temperature (°C) | Total Noble Metal Content (%) |
		Au (%)	Pd (%)	Pt (%)	Ag (%)	Cu (%)	Other (%)		
1	Very high noble metal alloys	84-86	5-7	4-10	0-2	—	Fe, In, Sn–2-3	1150	96-98
2	High noble metal alloys	45-52	38-45	—	0	—	In–8.5; Ga–1.5	1320-1330	89-90
3	High noble metal alloys with moderate silver content	51-52	26-31	—	14-16	—	In, Sn–5-7	1320-1330	78-83
4	Palladium-silver alloys	—	53-88	—	30-37	—	In–4-7; Sn–4-7	1310-1350	49-62
5	Palladium-copper alloys	0-2	74-79	—	—	10-15	Ga–9	1170-1190	76-81
6	Palladium-cobalt alloys	—	88	—	—	—	Co–4-5	1343	88

TABLE 18-2 Composition of Base Metal Alloys for Ceramic-Metal Restorations

Type	Cr	Mo	W	Be	Al	V	Fe	Sn	Ga	Ru	P	Ni	Co	Ti
							Elements (in weight percent)							
Nickel	11-20	4-6	0-2	0-2	0-5	0	0-1	0-2	0-1	0	0-1	Balance	0	0-2
Cobalt	15-20	0-4	0-4	0	0-2	0	0-1	0	0-5	0-3	0	0	Balance	0
Titanium	0	0	0	0	0-6	0-4	0-0.3	0	0	0	0	0	0	Balance

which results in a 30% to 50% increase in the tensile strength. In practice this hardening is accomplished during the firing of the ceramic.

Type 2 and 3 alloys contain substantially less gold than does Type 1. In Type 2 alloys the decrease is made up by an increase in the palladium concentration to 38% to 45% (with no silver present), whereas in Type 3 alloys the decrease in gold is made up by an increase in the palladium concentration to 26% to 31% plus an increase in the silver to 14% to 16%. Neither of these alloys contain iron or platinum and both are strengthened mainly by a solid solution-hardening mechanism. These alloys may contain some tin, indium, gallium, or cobalt. Even though the total percentage of these additives is less than 20%, their effect on properties is great. These additives increase the strength of the alloys, produce good bond strengths, and lower the fusion temperature. These are the properties that make the alloys suitable for ceramic-metal restorations.

Types 4, 5, and 6 are the palladium alloys. Type 4 is a palladium-silver alloy. The silver in Type 4 alloys can contaminate porcelain and cause a greenish tint; however, most porcelains currently produced no longer show this effect. Type 5 alloys contain palladium, copper, and gallium. Type 6 alloys are the palladium-cobalt alloys. The copper in Type 5, and the cobalt in Type 6, may produce a dark oxide that may be difficult to mask and may cause dark margins on the restorations.

Recently a new type of alloy was introduced and has become popular. This gold alloy has a composition similar to the Type III golds (Chapter 14) with additives for compatibility with a special low-fusing porcelain. Type III golds would soften excessively and sag at normal porcelain firing temperatures; however, with the low-fusing porcelain this is no longer a problem as the porcelain firing temperature is approximately 270° C lower.

Many alloys of the same type are produced by different manufacturers, and although these alloys may have the same noble metal content, they may behave differently because of different additives.

Composition of Base Metal Alloys

Considerable compositional variation is found in the base metal alloys for ceramic-metal restorations; however, they can be divided into three major types: nickel, cobalt, and titanium alloys. The range of compositions of these alloys are given in Table 18-2. It can be seen that some of the base metal alloys have wide compositional ranges, which is reflected in their mechanical properties.

The nickel and cobalt alloys contain large amounts of chromium to prevent the alloy from tarnishing and corroding. Nickel alloys containing aluminum or titanium form Ni_3Al or Ti_3Al, which strengthen the alloy. Beryllium in nickel alloys reduces the melting temperature, but its main contribution is to produce a strong bond between the alloy and the ceramic. Some cobalt alloys contain small amounts (3% to 6%) of ruthenium. Small amounts of ruthenium increase the castability. The main difference between cobalt alloys used for fabricating partial denture prostheses and those used for ceramic-metal restoration is their carbon content. Cobalt alloys formulated for partial denture applications contain some carbon, which strengthens the alloy by carbide formation; however, for crown and bridge purposes such a high strength is not needed, and these alloys are strengthened by a solid solution-hardening mechanism.

Few titanium alloys are used for porcelain-fused-to-metal restorations; they are infrequently used because of processing difficulties. Relatively new technics for processing titanium are being introduced, which should increase the use of these alloys. Crowns and bridges can be cast from titanium alloys (see Chapter 16) or they can be machined using recently developed processes. One process uses both machine duplication and spark erosion to make accurate titanium copings. Commercially pure titanium and the alloy Ti-6Al-4V may become important porcelain-fused-to-metal alloys.

Properties of Alloys for Ceramic-Metal Restorations

The properties of the alloys for ceramic-metal restorations are given in Tables 18-3 and 18-4.

Type 1 alloys have good corrosion resistance; moreover, they are easily cast and reasonably easy to solder. They do have disadvantages; they have lower strengths, lower resistance to distortion on firing the ceramic, higher densities, and higher costs than the other alloys. Type 1 alloys are the only ceramic-metal alloys that have the desirable yellow

TABLE 18-3 Properties of Noble Metal Alloys Used in Ceramic-Metal Restorations

Type	Ultimate Tensile Strength (MPa)	0.2% Yield Strength (MPa)	Elastic Modulus (MPa × 10³)	Elongation (%)	Hardness (DPH, kg/mm²)	Density (g/cm³)
1	480-500	400-420	90-96.5	3-5	175-180	18.6
2	700-730	550-575	116-117	8-12	210-230	13.5
3	650-680	475-525	100-105	8-10	210-230	13.8
4	550-730	400-525	95-117	10-15	185-235	10.7-11.0
5	690-1300	550-1100	94-97	8-10	350-400	10.6
6	793	572	120-125	25	210-235	11.0

TABLE 18-4 Properties of Base Metal Alloys Used in Ceramic-Metal Restorations

Type	Ultimate Tensile Strength (MPa)	0.2% Yield Strength (MPa)	Elastic Modulus (MPa × 10³)	Elongation (%)	Hardness (DPH, kg/mm²)	Density (g/cm³)	Casting Temperature (°C)
Nickel	400-1000	255-730	150-210	8-20	210-380	7.5-7.7	1300-1450
Cobalt	520-820	460-640	145-220	6-15	330-465	7.5-7.6	1350-1450
Titanium	242-896	173-827	103-114	10-20	125-353	4.4-4.5	1760-1860

color. All other alloys have a gray color that is more difficult to mask with porcelain. Type 2 alloys are characterized by excellent mechanical properties, high fusion temperatures, good corrosion resistance, and ease of casting and soldering. Type 3 alloys are noted for their high mechanical properties, high fusion temperature, ease of casting and soldering, high resistance to distortion during firing of ceramic, lower density, and reasonable cost. Type 4 alloys contain no gold and thus are noted for their low density and cost; their other qualities are similar to those of Type 3 alloys. Type 5 alloys are characterized by high strength, moderate elongation, ease of casting and soldering, and low cost; however, the alloys are gray in color, form dark oxides, and do not have a high resistance to distortion on firing. Type 6 alloys have similar mechanical properties to the Type 4 alloys but with higher elongation; they have high resistance to distortion on firing of ceramic, but like Type 5 alloys they form dark oxides that can be difficult to mask. In general the properties of all six types of noble metal alloys improve during the firing of the ceramic.

The properties of the three types of base metal alloys are presented in Table 18-4. The nickel alloys show wide variation in mechanical properties. These are harder than noble metal alloys, but many have lower yield strengths. Variation in strength among cobalt alloys is not as large as among nickel alloys, and cobalt alloys typically show higher strength than noble metal alloys. Like the nickel alloys, the titanium alloys show a wide range of mechanical properties. The higher strength titanium alloys compare favorably with the other alloys.

It is important for the alloy coping to provide rigid support for the ceramic because the ceramic can withstand very little deformation before it fractures. The nickel and cobalt alloys, with their higher elastic moduli, would be expected to provide better support. Calculations using the equation for deformation of a transverse beam (see Chapter 4) show that the modulus plays a relatively minor part. The thickness is much more important because it is present in the equation at the third power. Therefore no practical reduction in thickness of copings is possible with the nickel and cobalt alloys despite their higher moduli.

A general comparison of the properties of noble and base metal ceramic alloys shows that the base metal alloys have higher hardness and elastic moduli and lower densities. Because of the lower melting temperatures and lower hardness of the noble metal alloys, casting and finishing are easier with them than with the base metal alloys. Titanium is particularly difficult to cast because of its high casting temperatures. Good adhesion of porcelain to the alloy can be achieved with all the alloys; however, the bonding with some base metal alloys is more technic sensitive. Although little literature exists on adhesion of porcelain to titanium alloys, it appears successful bonding is achieved if special porcelains are used.

■ PREPARATION OF PORCELAIN-FUSED-TO-METAL RESTORATIONS

The processing of the metal coping for porcelain-fused-to-metal restorations is much like that of all-metal crowns and bridges. One significant difference relates to the reuse of metal. When the metal is melted and cast, certain alloying elements can be lost, especially the elements that readily form oxides. These elements are important for bonding with some noble metal alloys. To conserve metal, portions of the casting are commonly remelted. Each time the metal is remelted, some of these easily oxidized elements are lost. Therefore a certain portion of new alloy should be added each time the metal is reused to replenish the lost alloying elements.

Surface treatment of the metal coping before porcelain application is important for good bonding. These treatments are used to roughen the coping surface and form surface oxides. The surface may be roughened by gritblasting with a fine abrasive (25 to 50 μm alumina); in some cases this results in a large increase in bond strength. In most cases the metal coping is heat treated either in air or under partial vacuum to produce a surface oxide to improve bonding. In some palladium alloys the heat treatment not only forms surface oxides but also forms internal oxides that penetrate into the metal from the surface and effectively roughen the surface, thereby improving bonding. Some base metal alloys tend to form excessively thick interfacial oxides, which weaken the metal-ceramic bond (see Fig. 18-6). With these alloys the coping is heat treated and then gritblasted to achieve highest bonding. If this process is not used, failure through the oxide may occur.

Porcelain application is similar to that described in Chapter 17. However, there are several important considerations. The first layer of porcelain is especially important with porcelain-fused-to-metal restorations because it must hide the metal; special opaque porcelain must be used. The porcelain-alloy compatibility is another important consideration. The thermal expansions must be matched and the porcelain firing temperatures must be low enough that the alloy will not sag; the manufacturer usually supplies compatibility information. The titanium alloys require special porcelains, otherwise processing of the porcelain is similar to that of the other alloys.

SELECTED PROBLEMS

Problem 1. The porcelain of a metal-ceramic crown placed in the mouth fractured from the metallic substructure. What factors might have produced such a failure, and how can it be avoided?

Solution a. Surface contamination of the alloy before placing the porcelain may be a causative factor. Impurities on the metal surface, such as organic powder from the grinding stones or grease and oils from fingers, may prevent a good wetting of the porcelain, and air bubbles will be present at the ceramic-metal interface. To avoid this problem, you should use vitrified grinding stones, protect the metal surface from polishing debris, and not touch the metal with the fingers.

Solution b. Underfired opaquer may be a factor. When the opaque porcelain has not been brought up to its fusing point, a complete fusion into the surface of the metal has not been achieved. Proper firing technic with the opaque material will eliminate this trouble.

Solution c. Another cause for the fracture may be improper metallic thickness. A uniform metal thickness is very important to prevent failures in the metal-ceramic bond. A minimum thickness of 0.4 mm is allowable. Thinner metal substructure will not protect the porcelain from fracture.

Solution d. The reuse of alloys may cause a fracture in the substructure. When sprue buttons are employed to cast a new substructure, zinc, tin, or indium may be decreased or eliminated, and a very weak bonding with the porcelain is the result. The use of fresh alloys for casting the substructure is ideal, but a combination of a 50% (75% is better) fresh alloy and 25% to 50% used alloy may be employed without detrimental effects on the metal-ceramic bond.

Problem 2. When a ceramic-metal restoration was removed from the oven, cracks in the porcelain were observed. What factors may have caused this failure, and how can it be avoided?

Solution a. Improper selection of porcelain and alloy will cause such cracks. Manufacturers frequently produce porcelain with special characteristics to match the thermal properties of a particular alloy. When another metal is tried with the same porcelain, a mismatch in the thermal expansion may be sufficient to cause cracking. Only the alloy and the porcelain suggested by the manufacturer should be used.

Solution b. Another causative factor may be overglazed or overfired porcelain because it no longer matches the alloy properly. Irregularities on porcelain surfaces should be finished before glazing to avoid overglazing.

Solution c. When the ceramic-metal restoration is allowed to cool in the furnace after the porcelain has been baked, cracks in the ceramic material will be produced. The porcelain should never be cooled in the furnace because slow cooling may change some physical properties of the porcelain, creating a mismatch with the alloy.

Solution d. When hot porcelain is touched with a cold instrument, a thermal shock can produce cracks.

Problem 3. When a metal-ceramic fixed appliance was completed, the shades appeared too gray. What could be the cause of such a dark porcelain, and how can it be avoided?

Solution a. When the coating of opaque porcelain is too thin or the coating is incomplete, the transparency of the body porcelain will allow the gray coping to show through. The opaque bake should be examined for gray areas and reopaqued if any are present. Two thin coats of opaque porcelain with separate firings are often recommended.

Solution b. When opaque porcelain has been fired to maturity at the opaque bake, by the time a third or fourth bake is made, the opaque may have become too glazed and lost some of its opacifying qualities, thereby allowing the metal to reflect through the opaque layer, creating a gray shade. The manufacturer's suggested technic to bake the opaque should be carefully followed.

Solution c. When a crucible contaminated by an alloy containing base metals is used, a dark shade may be obtained. To avoid this problem do not use a crucible that has been used to cast any other alloy. Only clean crucibles without ceramic liners or fluxes should be employed to cast the alloys for metal-ceramic restorations.

Solution d. Non-precious alloys may contaminate the oven. Another source of oven contamination is the formation of volatilized impurities when the porcelain furnace has been used frequently for degassing and soldering operations. When the contamination accumulates in the oven, porcelain fired there will be dark. To avoid this problem you should purge the porcelain oven frequently.

Problem 4. A metal-ceramic restoration was cemented in the mouth. After insertion, flaking or chipping of the porcelain was observed. What may have been the cause of this failure?

Solution. The main problem with the porcelain is that this material does not withstand much bending without fracture. When fired on a thin or flexible substructure, deformation of the metal under stresses may deform the porcelain beyond its limit, and flakes or chips in the ceramic material are produced. The alloy selected to prepare ceramic-metal restorations or appliances should be built with enough bulk and have a high enough rigidity to withstand masticatory stresses without excessive deformation.

■ REFERENCES

Anthony DH, Burnett AP, Smith DL, Brooks MS: Shear test for measuring bonding in cast gold alloy-porcelain composites, *J Dent Res* 49:27, 1970.

Anusavice KJ, Dehoff PH, Fairhurst CW: Comparative evaluation of ceramic-metal bond tests using finite element stress analysis, *J Dent Res* 59:608, 1980.

Anusavice KJ, Ringle RD, Fairhurst CW: Bonding mechanism evidence in a ceramic non-precious alloy system, *J Biomed Mater Res* 11:701, 1977.

Anusavice KJ, Ringle RD, Fairhurst CW: Identification of fracture zones in porcelain-veneered-to-metal bond test specimens by ESCA analysis, *J Prosthet Dent* 42:417, 1979.

Anusavice KJ, Ringle RD, Morse PK, Fairhurst CW, King GE: A thermal shock test for porcelain metal systems, *J Dent Res* 60:1686, 1981.

Asgar K, Giday Z: Refinements on testing of porcelain to metal bond, *J Dent Res* 57:292, 1978.

Baran GR: Phase changes in base metal alloys along metal-porcelain interfaces, *J Dent Res* 58:2095, 1979.

Baran GR, Woodland EC: Forming of cast precious metal alloys, *J Dent Res* 60:1767, 1981.

Bartolotti RL, Moffa JP: Creep rate of porcelain-bonding alloys as a function of temperature, *J Dent Res* 59:2062, 1980.

Bergman M, Bergman B, Soremark R: Tissue accumulation of nickel released due to electrochemical corrosion of non-precious dental casting alloys, *J Oral Rehabil* 7:325, 1980.

Civjan S, Huget EF, Dvivedi N, Cosner HJ Jr: Further studies on gold alloys used in fabrication of porcelain-fused-to-metal restorations, *J Am Dent Assoc* 75:659, 1975.

Council on Dental Materials and Devices: How to avoid problems with porcelain-fused-to-metal restorations, *J Am Dent Assoc* 95:818, 1977.

Dent RJ, Preston JD, Moffa JP, Caputo A: Effect of oxidation on ceramometal bond strength, *J Prosthet Dent* 47:59, 1982.

Donachie MJ Jr, editor: *Titanium, a technical guide,* Metals Park, Ohio, 1988, ASM International.

Duncan JD: Casting accuracy of nickel-chromium alloys: marginal discrepancies, *J Dent Res* 59:1164, 1980.

Duncan JD: The casting accuracy of nickel-chromium alloys for fixed prostheses, *J Prosthet Dent* 47:63, 1982.

Duncanson MG Jr: Non-precious metal alloys for fixed restorative dentistry, *Dent Clin North Am* 20:422, 1976.

Eden GT, Franklin OM, Powell JM, Ohta H, Dickson G: Fit of porcelain-fused-to-metal crown and bridge casting, *J Dent Res* 58:2360, 1979.

Fairhurst CW, Anusavice KJ, Hashinger DT, Ringle RD, Twiggs SW: Thermal expansion of dental alloys and porcelains, *J Biomed Mater Res* 14:435, 1980.

Farah JW, Craig RG: Distribution of stresses in porcelain-fused-to-metal and porcelain jacket crowns, *J Dent Res* 54:255, 1975.

Faucher RR, Nicholls JI: Distortion related to margin design in porcelain-fused-to-metal restorations, *J Prosthet Dent* 43:149, 1980.

German RM: Hardening reactions in a high-gold content ceramo-metal alloy, *J Dent Res* 59:1960, 1980.

Huget EF, Dvivedi N, Cosner HE Jr: Characterization of gold-palladium-silver and palladium-silver for ceramic-metal restoration, *J Prosthet Dent* 36:58, 1976.

Huget EF, Dvivedi N, Cosner HE Jr: Properties of two nickel-chromium crown and bridge alloys for porcelain veneering, *J Am Dent Assoc* 94:87, 1977.

Jones DW: Coatings of ceramics on metals. In Ducheyne P, Lemons JE, editors: *Bioceramics: materials characteristics versus in vivo behavior,* vol 523, New York, 1988, New York Academy of Science.

Könönen M, Kivilahti J: Bonding of low-fusing dental porcelain to commercially pure titanium, *J Biomed Mater Res* 28:1027, 1994.

Lautenschlager EP, Greener EH, Elkington WE: Microprobe analysis of gold-porcelain bonding, *J Dent Res* 48:1206, 1969.

Lenz J, Schwarz S, Schwickerath H, Sperner F, Schäfer A: Bond strength of metal-ceramics systems in three-point flexure bond test, *J Appl Biomater* 6:55, 1995.

Lubovich RP, Goodkind RJ: Bond strength studies of precious, semiprecious, and non-precious ceramic-metal alloys with two porcelains, *J Prosthet Dent* 37:288, 1977.

Mackert JR Jr, Twiggs SW, Evans-Williams AL: Isothermal anneal effect on leucite content in dental porcelains, *J Dent Res* 74:1259, 1995.

Malhotra ML, Maickel LB: Shear bond strength of porcelain-fused-to-alloys of varying noble metal contents, *J Prosthet Dent* 44:405, 1980.

Meyer JM, Payan J, Nally JM: Evaluation of alternative alloys to precious ceramic alloys, *J Oral Rehabil* 6:291, 1979.

O'Brien WJ: Ceramics, *Dent Clin North Am* 29:851, October 1985.

Ohno H, Kanzawa I, Kawashima I, Shiokawa N: Structure of high-temperature oxidation zones of gold alloys for metal-porcelain bonding containing small amounts of In and Sn, *J Dent Res* 62:774, 1983.

Ringle RD, Fairhurst CW, Anusavice KJ: Microstructures in non-precious alloys near the porcelain-metal interaction zone, *J Dent Res* 58:1987, 1979.

Sarkar NK, Fuys RA Jr, Stanford JW: The chloride corrosion behavior of silver-base casting alloys, *J Dent Res* 58:1572, 1979.

Saxton PL: Post soldering of non-precious alloys, *J Prosthet Dent* 43:592, 1980.

Shell JS, Nielsen JP: Study of the bond between gold alloys and porcelain, *J Dent Res* 41:1424, 1962.

Smith DL, Burnett AP, Brooks MS, Anthony DH: Iron-platinum hardening in casting golds for use with porcelain, *J Dent Res* 49:283, 1970.

Valega TM, editor: *Alternatives to gold alloys in dentistry,* proceedings of a conference held at NIH, January 1977, Bethesda, Md, DHEW Publication No. (NIH) 77–1227.

Vermilyea SG, Huget EF, Vilca JM: Observations on gold-palladium-silver and gold-palladium alloys, *J Prosthet Dent* 44:294, 1980.

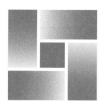

19 Prosthetic Applications of Polymers

Acrylic polymers were introduced as denture base materials in 1937. Previously, materials such as vulcanite, nitrocellulose, phenol formaldehyde, vinyl plastics, and porcelain were used for denture bases. The acrylic resins were so well received by the dental profession that by 1946, 98% of all denture bases were constructed from methyl methacrylate polymers or copolymers. Other polymers that have been developed since that time include vinyl acrylic, polystyrene, epoxy, nylon, vinyl styrene, polycarbonate, polysulfone-unsaturated polyester, polyurethane, polyvinylacetate-ethylene, hydrophilic polyacrylate, silicones, light-activated urethane dimethacrylate, rubber-reinforced acrylics, and butadiene-reinforced acrylic.

In spite of the advances in restorative dentistry in the last few decades, a recent survey of dentists in Great Britain indicated that 57% felt they were treating about the same number of denture patients as previously, 35% noticed a decrease, and 9% indicated an increase. Acrylic plastics have a wide variety of applications in prosthetic dentistry as artificial teeth, denture repair materials, facings in crown and bridge restorations, impression trays, baseplates, temporary crowns, and obturators for cleft palates. The physical and mechanical properties of these polymers should be considered when selecting a material for specific purposes.

■ PROPERTIES OF DENTURE BASE MATERIALS

The following list indicates the requirements for a clinically acceptable denture base material.
1. Adequate strength and durability
2. Satisfactory thermal properties
3. Processing accuracy and dimensional stability
4. Good chemical stability (unprocessed as well as processed material)
5. Insolubility in and low sorption of oral fluids
6. Absence of taste and odor
7. Biocompatibility
8. Natural appearance
9. Color stability
10. Adhesion to plastics, metals, and porcelain
11. Easy to fabricate and repair
12. Moderate cost

There are many commercially available materials that meet these requirements. The majority of dentures made today are heat-cured poly(methyl methacrylate). Fractures of dentures are still common, but they usually are associated with carelessness or unreasonable use by the patient. Considering functional stresses, the oral environment, and expected service life, denture base materials perform remarkably well.

Physical Form and Composition

Denture base plastics commonly are supplied in a powder-liquid or a gel form. The powder-liquid type may contain the materials listed in Table 19-1.

Powder

Most commercial materials contain poly(methyl methacrylate), which may have been modified with small amounts of ethyl, butyl, or other alkyl methacrylates to produce a polymer somewhat more resistant to fracture by impact. The powder also contains an initiator such as benzoyl peroxide (see following formula) or diisobutylazonitrile to initiate the polymerization of the monomer liquid after being added to the powder.

The peroxide initiator may be added to the polymer or be present as a residual from the polymerization reaction and is present in amounts from 0.5% to 1.5%.

Pure polymers, such as poly(methyl methacrylate), are clear and are adaptable to a wide range of pigmentation. The pigments used to obtain the various

TABLE 19-1 Principal Ingredients of Acrylic Denture Base Powder and Liquid

Powder	Liquid
Acrylic polymer (or copolymer) beads	Monomer
Initiator	Inhibitor
Pigments	Accelerator
Dyes	Plasticizer
Opacifiers	Cross-linking agent
Plasticizer	
Dyed organic fibers	
Inorganic particles	

tissuelike shades are compounds such as mercuric sulfide, cadmium sulfide, cadmium selenide, ferric oxide, or carbon black, although the use of cadmium salts is suspect because of demonstrated toxicity. These pigments may be locked into the polymer beads by addition during the commercial polymerization, as shown in Fig. 19-1, *A,* or they may be mechanically mixed with the polymer beads after polymerization, as shown in Fig. 19-1, *B.* Generally, the latter method is used, and the uneven distribution of the pigment in the final denture gives a mottled, natural-appearing denture. Dyes, as well as pigments, occasionally are used, but generally they are not as satisfactory, because they tend to leach out of the plastic by the oral fluids, which results in a gradual lightening of the shade. In addition to coloring agents, zinc or titanium oxides are used as opacifiers, with titanium dioxide being most effective. Dyed synthetic fibers made from nylon or acrylic usually are added to the denture material to simulate the minute blood vessels underlying the oral mucosa.

Plasticizers such as dibutyl phthalate may be incorporated in the powder or the monomer. Inorganic particles such as glass fibers and beads or zirconium silicate have been added to plastics. The particles

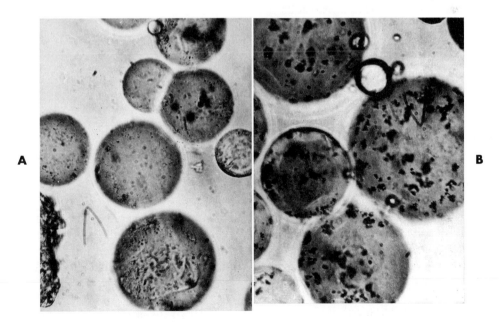

Fig. 19-1 Polymer beads with the pigment locked into the polymer, **A,** and mechanically mixed with the polymer, **B.** (×450.) (Courtesy The LD Caulk Co, Milford, Del, 1959.)

usually are treated with a coupling agent such as an unsaturated triethoxysilane to improve the wetting and bonding of the inorganic particles and the plastic. Studies also have reported on the addition of whiskers of alumina, silicon carbide, boron nitride, and carbon fibers to dental plastics. Addition of glass fibers and alumina (sapphire) whiskers increases the stiffness and decreases the thermal coefficient of expansion. Polyethylene-woven yarn and polyaramid fabric also have been used to reinforce acrylic polymers.

Most denture base materials are transparent on x-ray examination. Pieces of fractured dentures have been aspirated by patients during traumatic injury and these pieces have been difficult if not impossible to locate. A few denture base materials contain heavy metal compounds of elements such as barium or radiopaque glass fillers added to improve the radiopacity. It is necessary to add up to 20% by weight of these compounds to give sufficient radiopacity, and this results in a reduction in the strength of the material and a change in the appearance of the denture. A 3-year clinical study of a commercial radiopaque polymer, however, showed the dentures performed well and remained radiopaque. Other additives that provide radiopacity include bismuth or uranyl salts at concentrations of 10% to 15% and zirconyl dimethacrylate at 35%. It has been shown that esthetically pleasing radiopaque denture plastics can be made that do not demonstrate cytotoxicity or mutagenicity. In the future, efforts must be made to improve the handling properties, transverse deflection, and water sorption of radiopaque denture base materials.

Liquid

The liquid component of the powder-liquid type of acrylic resin is, in most cases, methyl methacrylate, but it may be modified by the addition of other monomers. Because these monomers may be polymerized by heat, light, or traces of oxygen, inhibitors are added to give the liquid adequate shelf life. The inhibitor most commonly used to prevent premature polymerization is hydroquinone, shown below, which may be present in concentrations of 0.003% to 0.1%.

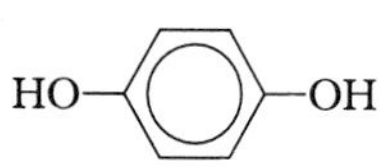

When a chemical accelerator rather than heat is used to speed up the peroxide decomposition and enable the polymerization of the monomer at room temperature, an accelerator is included in the liquid. These accelerators are tertiary amines, sulfinic acids, or the more stable salts of sulfinic acid. Commonly used amines are *N,N*-dimethyl-para-toluidine, and *N,N*-dihydroxyethyl-para-toluidine.

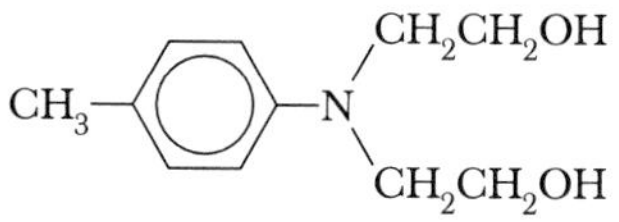

Chemically accelerated plastics also are referred to as self-curing, cold-curing, or autopolymerizing resins. The pour type of denture resin is included in this category.

Plasticizers are sometimes added to produce a softer, more resilient polymer. They are generally relatively low molecular weight esters, such as dibutyl phthalate.

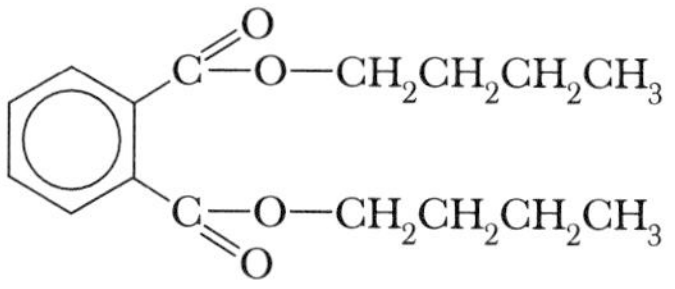

These plasticizer molecules do not enter the polymerization reaction but are distributed throughout the polymerized mass. In this way they interfere with the interaction between polymer molecules. This makes the plasticized polymer considerably softer than the pure polymer. One disadvantage in using plasticizers is that they gradually leach out of the plastic into oral fluids, resulting in hardening of the denture base. A polymer also may be plasticized by the addition of some higher ester such as butyl or octyl methacrylate to methyl methacrylate. The esters polymerize and form a more flexible plastic. This type of internal plasticizing does not leach out in the oral fluids, and the material remains flexible.

If a cross-linked polymer is desired, organic compounds such as glycol dimethacrylate are added to the monomer.

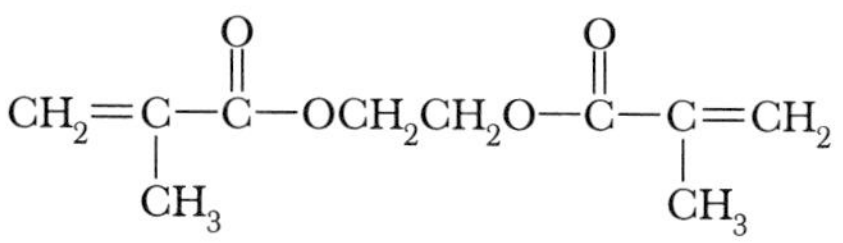

Cross-linking compounds are characterized by the reactive–CR $=$ CH–groups at opposite ends of the molecules and serve to link two long polymer molecules together. The main advantage in using cross-linking agents is that the final polymer has greater resistance to minute surface cracking, termed *crazing*. Cross-linking materials may be present in amounts of 2% to 14%, but up to 25% have little effect on the tensile strength, transverse properties, or hardness of the acrylic plastics, although the recovery from an indentation by a metal ball like a Rockwell Hardness indenter is somewhat improved.

Gel types

It also is possible to supply denture base plastics such as vinyl acrylics in a gel form. These gels have, in general, the same components as the powder-liquid type, except that the liquid and powder have been mixed to form a gel and have been shaped into a thick sheet. Chemical accelerators cannot be used in a gel because the initiator, accelerator, and monomer would be in intimate contact. The storage temperature of a gel and the amount of inhibitor present have a pronounced effect on the shelf life of the material. When stored in a refrigerator, the shelf life is about 2 years. Accuracy of proportioning and thoroughness of mixing are the advantages claimed for the gel type of denture base plastics.

Other Denture Materials

Several modified poly(methyl methacrylate) materials have been used for denture base applications. These include the pour type of denture resins, hydrophilic polyacrylates, high-impact strength resins, rapid heat-polymerized acrylics, and light-activated denture base materials.

Pour type of denture resins

The chemical composition of the pour-type denture resins is similar to poly(methyl methacrylate) materials that are polymerized at room temperature. The principal difference is in the size of the polymer powder or beads. The pour-type denture resins, which are commonly referred to as "fluid resins," have powder particles that are much smaller, and when they are mixed with monomer, the resulting mix is very fluid. The mix is quickly poured into an agar-hydrocolloid or modified plaster mold and allowed to polymerize under pressure at 0.14 MPa. Centrifugal casting also has been used to inject the slurry into the mold.

High-impact strength materials

Denture base materials that have greater impact strength than conventional poly(methyl methacrylate) have been introduced. These polymers are reinforced with butadiene-styrene rubber. The rubber particles are grafted to methyl methacrylate to bond to the acrylic matrix. These materials are supplied in a powder-liquid form and are processed in the same way as other heat-accelerated methyl methacrylate materials.

Rapid heat-polymerized resins

Dentists and technicians are always looking for ways to do things quicker and better. The rapid heat-polymerized materials were introduced with that in mind. These are hybrid acrylics that are polymerized in boiling water immediately after being packed into a denture flask. The initiator is formulated from both chemical and heat-activated initiators to allow rapid polymerization without the porosity that one might expect. After placing in boiling water, the water is brought back to a full boil for 20 minutes. After the usual bench cooling to room temperature, the denture is deflasked, trimmed, and polished in the conventional manner.

Light-activated denture base resins

This denture base material consists of a urethane dimethacrylate matrix with an acrylic copolymer, microfine silica fillers, and a photoinitiator system. It is supplied in premixed sheets having a claylike consistency. The denture base material is adapted to the cast while it is still pliable. The denture base can be polymerized in a light chamber without teeth and used as a baseplate. The teeth are processed to the base with additional material and the anatomy is sculptured while the material is still plastic. The acrylic is polymerized in a light chamber (curing unit) with blue light of 400 to 500 nm. The denture is rotated on a table in the chamber to provide uniform exposure to the light source. This material is now used for many prosthetic applications.

An argon laser also has been used to polymerize composite resins. The results are of interest because the physical/mechanical properties are improved when compared with the same material processed with blue light. This method may find application with light-cured denture base materials.

ANSI/ADA Specification No. 12 for Denture Base Resins

The scope, requirements, and procedures for evaluating denture base plastics are listed in ANSI/ADA Specification No. 12. The specification includes acrylic, vinyl, and styrene polymers, or mixtures of any of these polymers, as well as copolymers. Denture base resins may be heat-curing or self-curing.

The specification lists a number of general requirements for the nonprocessed materials. The liquid should be as clear as water and free of extraneous material, and the powder, plastic cake, or pre-cured blank should be free of impurities such as dirt and lint. The specification further states that (1) a satisfactory denture shall result when the manufacturer's instructions are followed, (2) the denture base should be nonporous and free from surface defects, (3) the cured plastic should take a high gloss when polished, (4) the processed denture should not be toxic to a normal, healthy person, (5) the color should be as specified, (6) the plastic should be translucent, and (7) the cured plastic should not show any bubbles or voids.

The specific requirements are that (1) within 5 minutes after reaching the proper consistency, indicated by clean separation from the walls of a glass mixing jar, the material shall have adequate flow properties so that it will intrude to a depth of at least 0.5 mm into a 0.75-mm diameter hole when a load of 5000 g is placed on a plate 5-mm thick and 50 mm^2 in area (this test is modified for pour type of plastics); (2) the water sorption shall not be more than 0.8 mg/cm^2 after immersion for 7 days at 37° C; (3) the solubility shall not be more than 0.04 mg/cm^2 after the water sorption specimen is dried to constant weight; (4) the plastic shall show no more than a slight color change when exposed 24 hours to a specified ultraviolet lamp test; and (5) the transverse deflection shall be within the limits listed in the discussion on transverse deflection.

The results of several tests listed in ANSI/ADA Specification No. 12 for various types of plastics are shown in Table 19-2. Although the values are typical for each group, they can vary considerably for different commercial products.

■ PROPERTIES OF DENTAL PLASTICS

Strength Properties

Conventional heat-accelerated acrylic resins are still the predominant denture base materials in use. These materials are typically low in strength, soft and fairly flexible, brittle on impact, and fairly resistant to fatigue failure. The properties of poly(methyl methacrylate) and polyvinyl acrylic are shown in Table 19-3. Several properties of newer denture base materials are seen in Table 19-4.

Tensile and compressive strength

Table 19-3 reveals small differences between poly(methyl methacrylate) and polyvinyl acrylic. The two plastics have adequate tensile and compressive strength for complete or partial denture applications. Fractures that occur usually are caused by accidental dropping of a denture or by faulty construction. Fractures also may be caused by flexure fatigue from cyclic stresses of low magnitude in service.

Elongation

Elongation, in combination with the ultimate strength, is an indication of the toughness of the plastic. The larger the area under the stress-strain curve, the tougher the material is. Materials having a combination of reasonable tensile strength and elongation will be tough materials, and those with low elongation will be brittle. Examples of tough materials are polyvinylchloride or polyethylene, whereas poly(methyl methacrylate) is more brittle.

Values for percent elongation of polyvinyl acrylics are considerably higher than for poly(methyl methacrylate) and, as expected, the polyvinyl acrylics are considerably tougher and permit larger deformation before fracture.

Elastic modulus

The higher strain or elastic deformation for a given stress for polyvinyl acrylic is reflected in the lower value for the elastic modulus of 2.8×10^3 MPa.

TABLE 19-2 Properties of Various Types of Denture Acrylics According to ANSI/ADA Specification No. 12

Property	Conventional	Rubber Reinforced	Vinyl	Light-Activated Acrylic*	Pour Type	Rapid Heat Cure
Transverse deflection (mm)						
At 3500 g	2.0	2.4	1.8	1.9	2.2	1.7
At 5000 g	4.1	5.0	3.8	3.6	Fractured	3.5
Water sorption (mg/cm^2)	0.60	0.55	0.50	0.64	0.50	0.64
Water solubility (mg/cm^2)	0.02	0.02	0.02	0.01	0.01	0.02
Color change	None	Slight	Slight	Slight	Slight to moderate	Slight

*Data supplied by Dentsply International, York, Pa.

TABLE 19-3 Strength Characteristics of Denture Base Plastics

Property	Poly(methyl methacrylates)	Polyvinyl Acrylics
Tensile strength (MPa)	48.3-62.1	51.7
Compressive strength (MPa)	75.9	70.0-75.9
Elongation (%)	1-2	7-10
Elastic modulus (GPa)	3.8	2.8
Proportional limit (MPa)	26.2	29.0
Impact strength, Izod (kg m/cm notch)	0.011	0.023
Transverse deflection (mm)		
At 3500 g	2.0	1.9
At 5000 g	4.0	3.9
Fatigue strength (cycles at 17.2 MPa)	1.5×10^6	1×10^6
Recovery after identation (%)		
Dry	89	86
Wet	88	84
KHN (kg/mm^2)		
Dry	17	16
Wet	15	15

This value may be compared with that of 3.8×10^3 MPa for poly(methyl methacrylates). A denture constructed of polyvinyl acrylic will deform elastically to a greater extent under the forces of mastication than a comparable poly(methyl methacrylate) denture. The modulus of elasticity for several newer denture base materials is seen in Table 19-4. In comparison with metals used as denture bases, the elastic moduli of all plastics is quite low.

Proportional limit

There is some question as to whether dental plastics possess a true proportional limit because they may be permanently deformed at low stresses, and, as a result, the proportional limit obtained is a function of the rate of stress application. Despite this characteristic, the proportional limit determined under standard conditions is important. A plastic with a low proportional limit will begin to deform permanently at a low stress. If the percent elongation is relatively high, it may deform permanently to a considerable extent before rupture. If the proportional limit is high, considerable stress is required before permanent deformation will occur. A denture material should have a proportional limit sufficiently high that permanent deformation does not result from the stress applied during mastication. Perm-

anent deformation may result in loss of retention or loosening of the teeth embedded in the denture base. The values reported in Table 19-3 for the proportional limit of poly(methyl methacrylates) and polyvinyl acrylics are approximately the same, and the dimensional stability of dentures made of these materials would be expected to be similar.

Impact strength

Impact strength is a measure of the energy absorbed by a material when it is broken by a sudden blow.

The impact strength for the polyvinyl acrylics is about twice that of poly(methyl methacrylates) (see Table 19-3), which indicates that polyvinyl acrylic absorbs more energy on impact and is more resistant to fracture.

Although the addition of plasticizing ingredients may increase the impact strength of plastics, the increases are accompanied by decreases in hardness, proportional limit, elastic modulus, and compressive strength. Ideally, a denture base plastic should have a sufficiently high impact strength to prevent breakage on accidental dropping, but not at the expense of the other properties.

The impact strength of various types of denture base materials is listed in Table 19-5. There are

TABLE 19-4 Mechanical Properties of New Denture Resins

Material	Processing Condition	Knoop Hardness (kg/mm²)	Rockwell Indentation (μm)	Rockwell Recovery (%)	Transverse Strength (MPa)	Modulus of Elasticity (GPa*)	Izod Impact Strength (J/m)
20 min cure PMMA	100° C 20 min	15-17	70-74	74-78	79-86	1.3-1.6	12-15
Light-cured resins	10 min in light chamber	18	73	72	80	2.1	13
Rubber reinforced PMMA	74° C 9 hr	14	79	73	78	1.1	31
Autopolymerizing PMMA	45° C 0.14 MPa	16	73	76	84	1.6	15
Microwave Cured PMMA	3 min 500 W	17	74	75	92	1.7	14

Adapted with permission from Smith LT, Powers JM, Ladd D: Mechanical properties of new denture resins polymerized by visible light, heat and microwave energy, *Int J Prosthodont* 5:315, 1992.
*1 GPa = 10^3 MPa

TABLE 19-5 Impact Strength of Denture Base Plastics

Material	Charpy Impact* Strength (joules)	Hounsfield Impact† Test ($Nm \times 10^{-4}$)
Conventional heat-cured acrylic	0.26	455
Vinyl acrylic	0.20	578
Rubber-reinforced acrylic	0.58	1063
Hydrophilic acrylic	0.18	NA

*Adapted from Soni PM, Powers JM, Craig RG: *J Mich Dent Assoc* 59:418, 1977.
†Adapted from Stafford GD, Bates JF, Hugget R, Handley RW: *J Dent* 8:292, 1980.
NA, Not applicable.

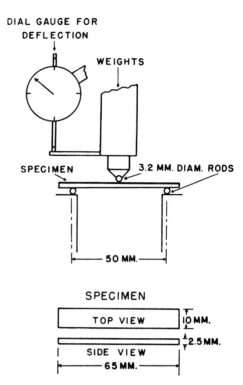

Fig. 19-2 Simplified sketch of equipment for determining transverse deflection and strength.

differences in the relative impact strength using both tests. However, the impact strength of the rubber-reinforced acrylic plastic is considerably higher in both instances. In a recent study of several denture base materials (see Table 19-4), the rubber-reinforced acrylic had a much higher impact strength than any of the other materials. When small surface defects are present, however, this improved impact resistance is significantly reduced.

Transverse strength and deflection

In the evaluation of denture plastics, transverse strength measurements are used to a greater extent than either tensile or compressive strength, because this test more closely represents the type of loading applied to a denture in the mouth. The transverse strength is determined by applying an increasing load until fracture along a line at the center of a plastic strip $65 \times 10 \times 2.5$ mm that is supported on each end by metal rollers spaced 50-mm apart, as shown in Fig. 19-2. In the process of obtaining the transverse strength, the deflection in millimeters at the middle of the plastic specimen is recorded at a load of 3500 and 5000 g. Transverse strength is therefore a combination of tensile and compressive strength and includes some of the elements of proportional limit and elastic modulus. The values listed in Table 19-4 show that the transverse

strength varied from 78 to 92 MPa for various poly(methyl methacrylates) and polyvinyl acrylic.

A transverse deflection test is included in ANSI/ADA Specification No. 12 for denture base resins. The requirements are that the deflection in the center of the specimen shall be no more than 2.5 mm between a load of 1500 and 3500 g and that the deflection between 1500 and 5000 g shall be between 2.0 and 5.5 mm. All specimens are tested in water at 37° C after being allowed to absorb water for 2 days at 37° C.

A comparison of the transverse deflection of several types of materials is seen in Table 19-2. Note that the pour-type resin fractured in this test and the rapid-cure acrylic was slightly less flexible than the other materials.

Fatigue strength

In addition to impact forces, dentures are subjected to a large number of smaller cyclic stresses during mastication. For this reason, the fatigue properties of denture plastics are important. Fatigue strength

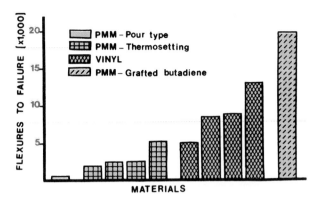

Fig. 19-3 Flexural fatigue of various types of denture base materials. (Adapted from Johnson EP: *J Prosthet Dent* 46:478, 1981.)

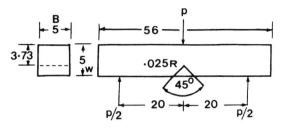

Fig. 19-4 Sketch of specimens for measuring fracture toughness. p, Load; R, radius; w, thickness; **B**, width; dimensions in millimeters. (Adapted from Stafford GD, Bates JF, Huggett R, Handley RW: *J Dent* 8:292, 1980.)

TABLE 19-6   Fracture Toughness of Denture Base Plastics

Material	$MN/m^{-3/2}$
High impact resin	2.0
Rapid heat cure	3.0
Conventional acrylic	2.3
Pour type of acrylic	1.5

Adapted from Stafford GD, Bates JF, Hugget R, Handley RW: *J Dent* 8:292, 1980.

represents the number of cycles before failure at a certain stress. Values of the fatigue strength at a stress of 17.2 MPa for poly(methyl methacrylates) and polyvinyl acrylic plastics are 1.5×10^6 and 1×10^6, respectively. Because the current denture base plastics hold up well in service, a value of 1×10^6 cycles at 17.2 MPa is apparently an adequate fatigue strength value.

There are many flexural fatigue tests reported in the literature for denture base resins. The results from one of these tests are shown in Fig. 19-3. The samples were repeatedly flexed in a fatigue-testing machine under a load of 3650 g at 342 flexures per minute. The flexural fatigue strength of the rubber-reinforced acrylic plastic was superior to the other materials, and the pour type of acrylic plastic had the lowest value.

Fracture toughness

Because the geometry of denture bases is complex and stresses can be concentrated in flaws on the surface or in frenum notches, cracks can occur in the denture base. Several tests are available for estimating fracture toughness. One method for testing the fracture toughness is to bend a notched specimen and record the force required for crack propagation (Fig. 19-4). Several denture base materials are compared in Table 19-6. The fracture toughness of the high-impact resin appears to be no better than the vinyl or conventional acrylic resin. The rapid heat-cured resin had the highest fracture toughness, and the pour type of resin had the lowest toughness. The

fracture toughness of acrylic is much greater when samples are saturated with water rather than dry.

Compressive creep

When denture base resins are placed under a load they will deform (creep) with time. The lowest compressive creep rates are found for the heat-polymerized materials. The chemically accelerated acrylics, both dough and pour type, have higher values for compressive creep. At low stress levels, the type and quantity of cross-linking agents have no major affect on creep. However, at higher stress levels, creep values decrease with increasing quantities of cross-linking agents. For heat-polymerized materials, when the temperature is increased from 37° to 50° C the mode of failure changes from brittle to ductile. For autopolymerizing acrylics, the materials fail in a ductile manner at both temperatures.

Recovery after indentation

Indentation recovery of plastics in equilibrium with water generally is lower than when they are dry. The recovery from indentation of a 1.27-cm diameter steel ball loaded for 10 minutes at 30 kg is given in Table 19-3. The time allowed for recovery was 10 minutes. The recovery on dry specimens was from 86 to 89% and on wet specimens from 84 to 88%. The results for several new products are seen in Table 19-4.

A modified Wallace hardness tester has been used to measure the hardness, creep, and recovery of denture base polymers as well as the effects of cyclic loading. Results demonstrate the viscoelastic nature of denture base polymers. A torsional pendulum also may be used to evaluate the viscoelastic properties of denture base resins. These tests are useful in evaluating the effect of free monomer, plasticizers, and degree of cross-linking.

Hardness

The low Knoop hardness number of the denture base plastics (Tables 19-3 and 19-4) indicates that these materials may be scratched easily and abraded. Cross-linked poly(methyl methacrylate) is only slightly harder than regular poly(methyl methacrylate) (about 1 kg/mm^2). The incorporation of fillers in plastics may alter the resistance to abrasion, but the hardness of the plastic matrix remains unchanged. Polishing, shell blasting, and cleaning denture bases by brushing should be carried out with this in mind.

Abrasion resistance

Abrasion resistance of denture base resins has been evaluated by abrading specimens against 600-grit silicon carbide paper for 1 hour under a stress of 0.26 MPa in water at 37° C and measuring loss of material (Table 19-7). All materials had similar wear characteristics. However, the vinyl acrylic had the best and the pour type of acrylic had the least wear resistance.

Thermal Characteristics

The thermal properties of plastics are important in dentistry, because the plastic materials usually are processed at 74° C and in service they are in contact with hot and cold foods and beverages. If a chemical accelerator is used rather than heat, the material is still subjected to the exothermic heat resulting from the polymerization reaction.

TABLE 19-7 Abrasion Resistance of Denture Base Plastics

Material	Material Loss (mm × 10^{-3})
Conventional acrylic	595
Rubber reinforced acrylic	588
Vinyl acrylic	499
Rapid heat cured	530
Pour type of acrylic	611

Thermal conductivity

Dental plastics are poor thermal and electrical conductors. Compared with gold, cobalt alloys, or even human dentin, which have thermal conductivities of 0.7, 0.16, and 1.3 × 10^{-3} cal/sec/cm^2 (° C/cm), respectively, the values for the various types of plastics listed in Table 19-8 are low. Low thermal conductivity results in plastic denture bases serving as an insulator between the oral tissues and hot or cold materials placed in the mouth.

Specific heat

Specific heat, or the heat required to raise the temperature of a gram of plastic 1 degree Celsius is a thermal property closely related to thermal conductivity. Although it is not obvious, it may be shown that the ratio of thermal conductivity to the product of specific heat and density is a constant for a particular material and represents the velocity of temperature disturbance in a plastic. The higher this ratio, termed *diffusivity,* the greater the velocity of heat transfer through a material. The specific heats for poly(methyl methacrylates) and polyvinyl acrylics are similar, and the respective thermal conductivities are not greatly different; therefore the diffusivity of plastics will be roughly equivalent, 0.123 mm^2/sec.

Thermal coefficient of expansion

The temperature differences from processing temperature to room temperature or to mouth temperature indicate the importance of the thermal coefficient of expansion. These plastics have relatively high thermal coefficients of expansion (71 to 81 × 10^{-6}/° C) compared with other dental materials. Gold, amalgam, and tooth structure have values of 14.4 × 10^{-6}/° C, 22 to 28 × 10^{-6}/° C, and 11.4

TABLE 19-8   Thermal Characteristics of Denture Base Plastics

Property	Poly(methyl methacrylates)	Polyvinyl Acrylics
Thermal conductivity (cal/sec/cm^2) (° C/cm)	5.7×10^{-4}	2.2×10^{-4}
Specific heat (cal/° C/g)	0.35	0.2-0.28
Thermal coefficient of expansion (/° C)	81×10^{-6}	71×10^{-6}
Heat distortion temperature (° C)	71-91	54-77

$\times 10^{-6}$/° C, respectively. The addition of fillers such as glass reduces the thermal coefficient of expansion, although the reduction is not a linear function of the amount of the filler present. Thermal expansion is important in the fit of denture bases, because it is apparent that a denture that fits a cast accurately at room temperature will not fit the same at mouth temperature.

Heat distortion temperature

A measure of the ability of a plastic to resist dimensional distortion by heat is the temperature at which a specimen loaded in a transverse manner at 1.8 MPa stress deflects the distance of 0.25 mm. These temperatures are generally sufficiently high that they are of little concern except in the repair of dentures. The heat distortion temperature for polyvinyl acrylic is 54° to 77° C and for poly(methyl methacrylates) it is 71° to 91° C. These values suggest the need for keeping repair temperatures low and indicate the use of chemically or light polymerized materials for this purpose.

Plastics or polymers, when heated, are transformed from a glassy or brittle condition to a rubbery condition. The temperature of this transition is called the glass transition, T_g. Molecular motions are allowed above this temperature that are not permitted at lower temperatures and thus plastics are easier to deform above T_g.

Other Properties of Denture Plastics

Density

The density, or the weight in grams of a cubic centimeter (g/cc) of material, varies in plastics because of variations in molecular weight. Denture base plastics have densities ranging from 1.16 to 1.36 g/cc (Table 19-9), or slightly greater than the density for water.

Polymerization shrinkage

The density of methyl methacrylate monomer is only 0.945 g/cc at 20° C, compared with 1.16 to 1.18 g/cc for poly(methyl methacrylate). This increase in density is mainly accounted for by an approximate 21% decrease in volume of monomer during polymerization. Because the ratio of polymer to monomer used in the preparation of dental poly(methyl methacrylates) and polyvinyl acrylics is usually 3:1, the free volumetric shrinkage amounts to approximately 6%.

The light-activated denture base material has low polymerization shrinkage of 3% because higher molecular weight oligomers are used compared with acrylic monomer. It should be pointed out that the linear shrinkage values reported in the literature are generally much less than would be expected (Table 19-10) on the basis of the free volumetric shrinkage because a portion of the polymerization takes place after the plastic has attained a solid condition, resulting in residual stresses in the plastic rather than additional shrinkage. An ideal plastic would be one that had no polymerization shrinkage, but even if this requirement was attained, thermal dimensional change would still result from cooling the plastic from molding temperature to room temperature.

Dimensional stability and accuracy

The dimensional stability of the denture during processing and in service is important in the fit of the denture and the satisfaction of the patient. In general, if the denture is properly processed, the original fit and the dimensional stability of the various denture base plastics are good. However, excess heat generated during finishing of the denture can easily distort a denture base by releasing residual stresses.

It has been shown that chemically activated denture bases processed by dough molding with a

TABLE 19-9   Miscellaneous Properties of Denture Base Plastics

Property	Poly(methyl methacrylates)	Polyvinyl Acrylics
Density (g/cc)	1.16-1.18	1.21-1.36
Polymerization shrinkage (% by volume)	6*	6*
Dimensional stability	Good	Good
Water sorption (mg/cm^2; ADA Test)	0.69	0.26
Water solubility (mg/cm^2)	0.02	0.01
Resistance to weak acids	Good	Excellent
Resistance to weak bases	Good	Excellent
Effect of organic solvents	Soluble in ketones, esters, and aromatic and chlorinated hydrocarbons	Soluble in ketones and esters and swells in aromatic hydrocarbons
Processing ease	Good	Good
Adhesion to metal and porcelain	Poor	Poor
Adhesion to acrylics	Good	Good
Colorability	Good	Good
Color stability	Yellows very slightly	Yellows slightly
Taste or odor	None	None
Tissue compatibility	Good	Good
Shelf life	Powder and liquid, good; gel, fair	Gel, fair

*Monomer shrinkage in mixes with polymer/monomer ratios of approximately 3:1.

TABLE 19-10   Polymerization Shrinkage of Posterior of Maxillary Denture Bases

Material	Shrinkage (%)
Conventional acrylic	0.43
High impact acrylic	0.12
Vinyl acrylic	0.33
Rapid heat-cured acrylic	0.97
Pour type of acrylic	0.48

Adapted from Stafford GD, Bates JF, Huggett R, Handley RW: *J Dent* 8:292, 1980.

dimensional accuracy of –0.1% were more accurate than heat-activated denture bases at –0.4%. The most accurate dentures were produced using either a chemically activated pour resin processed under pressure at 45° C or a microwave-activated resin. A visible light-activated resin was more accurate than a conventional heat-activated resin. In the past, injection-molded dentures were less accurate than compression-molded materials. Two recent studies demonstrated that an acrylic processed by a new injection molding process was significantly more accurate than a standard compression-molded material. The increase in vertical dimension of occlusion was very small for the injection-molded acrylic when compared with the conventional compression-molded acrylic.

In another report, six different denture base materials were processed by heat, light, or microwave energy. The denture bases were removed from the casts, finished, and polished. After storage in distilled water for 42 days to allow for water sorption, the dentures were placed back on the stone casts on which they were made and ranked for accuracy of fit by five evaluators. Denture bases processed by microwave energy, low heat at 45° C (autopolymerizing resins), or visible light fit better than those resins processed at either 74° C (conventional resins) or 100° C (quick heat-cured resins).

When evaluated in two dimensions, the dimensional stability of denture bases is usually reported at <1%. In one study the accuracy of maxillary dentures was measured at six locations from anterior to posterior. For all materials studied, the accuracy was better from the anterior of the denture to the middle of the palate (generally <100 μm) and became worse toward the posterior of the denture. In a recent study of three-dimensional stability of several products, changes ranged from 0.2% to 8.1% in the frontal dimension, and 0.2% to 9% in the lateral dimension. Changes were greatest in the cross-arch dimension.

There are numerous articles in the literature that report conflicting results for accuracy of denture base resins. However, it is encouraging that emphasis is being placed on dimensional accuracy and some of the newer materials appear superior to older products.

Water sorption and solubility

The sorption of water also alters the dimensions of acrylic dentures. This change in dimension is, for the most part, reversible and the plastic may go through numerous expansions and contractions when alternately soaked in water and dried. However, repeated wetting and drying of finished dentures should be avoided by the patient because irreversible warpage of the denture bases may result. Denture plastics of the same type may vary considerably in water sorption because of the presence of additives. Poly(methyl methacrylates) have relatively high water sorption values of 0.69 mg/cm^2. Polyvinyl acrylics have lower values of 0.26 mg/cm^2. The thickness of the plastic specimen and the type of polymer influence whether equilibrium water sorption will be attained in 24 hours.

Temperature also affects the rate at which water is absorbed because the diffusion coefficient is increased by a factor of two between room and oral temperature and the equilibrium absorption value does not change.

ANSI/ADA Specification No. 12 for denture plastics includes a water sorption test, in which a dried plastic disk 50 mm in diameter and 0.5-mm thick is stored in distilled water at 37° C for 7 days, after which the increase in water is determined and the sorption is recorded in milligrams per square centimeter. In addition, the solubility of the plastic is measured on the same specimen by re-drying to constant weight in a desiccator and reweighing to determine the loss in weight in milligrams per square centimeter. For a plastic to meet the specification, it should have a water sorption value of not more than 0.8 mg/cm^2 and a solubility not greater than 0.04 mg/cm^2 (see Table 19-2).

Resistance to acids, bases, and organic solvents

The resistance of denture plastics to water solutions containing weak acids or bases is good to excellent. Denture plastics are quite resistant to organic solvents, with poly(methyl methacrylate) being more resistant than polyvinyl acrylic. Both are soluble in aromatic hydrocarbons, ketones, and esters. Alcohol will cause crazing in certain denture plastics. Ethanol also functions as a plasticizer and can reduce the glass transition temperature. Therefore solutions containing alcohol should not be used for cleaning or storing dentures. Incorporating ethylene glycol dimethacrylate as a cross-linking agent in denture base resins has little effect on water sorption, but significantly improves solvent resistance.

Processing ease

A comparison of the processing ease of the various types of denture plastics is difficult. In general, with the proper equipment and facilities all of the denture plastics have satisfactory processing properties.

Adhesion properties

The adhesion of denture plastics to untreated porcelain or metals is generally poor. As a result, porcelain teeth or combined metal and plastic bases should be designed so that the porcelain or metal is held by mechanical retention. It has been shown that the lack of adhesion between a plastic base and porcelain teeth provides an area in which microorganisms present in the oral fluids may incubate, and this makes maintenance of a clean denture more difficult. This problem can be avoided by the use of plastic teeth, which form a bond with denture base materials or by organosilane treatment of porcelain teeth (although this treatment is not routinely used). The silane coupling agent, γ-methacryloxypropyl-trimethoxysilane, provides a bond between the porcelain and the plastic surface. The use of 4-META has been shown to provide a bond to metal.

Esthetics

The esthetic qualities of the denture base plastics include such properties as colorability, color stability, taste, and odor. The ability of the plastics to be colored and their compatibility with dyed synthetic fibers for characterization are both good. Color-measuring systems have been used to compare the actual color of denture base resins with the color of gingival tissues. Results indicate that few commercial products actually match the color of the tissue they are replacing. The color stability of denture base materials must conform to the ANSI/ADA Specification No. 12. The specification requires that a specimen exposed for 24 hours to an ultraviolet light source shall not show more than a slight change in color when compared with an original specimen. One study questioned the stain resistance of the light-activated denture acrylic. The current denture products have no taste or odor when properly processed.

Tissue compatibility

The tissue compatibility or allergic sensitization of the skin to the components of denture plastics or to the processed plastics has been a subject of considerable contention. It may be concluded that completely polymerized poly(methyl methacrylate) or polyvinyl acrylics do not cause allergic reactions but that methyl methacrylate monomer or other trace components in the monomer may produce a contact type of allergic reaction of the skin or oral tissues. Dentures prepared by polymerization of methyl methacrylate with a chemical accelerator may have sufficient residual methyl methacrylate monomer present in the finished denture to cause an allergic reaction in patients who are sensitive to methyl methacrylate. This reaction diminishes as the residual monomer is leached out of the plastic. Allergic reactions to heat-processed denture base plastics also occur but less frequently than with chemically accelerated plastics. Again, residual monomer is considered to be the allergen, and strict adherence to processing instructions recommended by the manufacturer can keep the residual monomer to a minimum. When patients are known to have suffered from an allergic reaction, processing the denture for extended periods (such as 24 versus 8 hours) may be helpful. Residual monomer levels can also be reduced dramatically by processing heat-polymerized poly(methyl methacrylate) in a water bath for 7 hours at 70° C, followed by boiling for 1 hour. Boiling has only a slight effect on the dimensional accuracy of the processed dentures.

The light-activated denture base materials are an alternative choice for those patients who are sensitive to methyl methacrylate monomer because none is present in the formulation.

In one study, 53 patients wearing dentures and suffering from "burning-mouth syndrome" were evaluated for allergies related to various components of denture base plastics. Epicutaneous patch tests were used. Fifteen patients demonstrated a positive skin test to one or more of the following: *N,N*-dimethyl-para-toluidine, hydroquinone, formaldehyde, methyl methacrylate, and *p*-phenylenediamine, as well as several metallic compounds. Pigments also may be toxic.

Plasticizers are used to lower the glass transition temperature of poly(methyl methacrylate), which in turn produces a tougher, less brittle material. Additionally, the use of plasticizers decreases water sorption because they are hydrophobic. There is evidence that plasticizers fill microvoids within acrylic. This "microvoid concept" is also related to water sorption where water may replace the plasticizer in the microvoids over time or is absorbed directly into the polymer. Plasticizers are commonly used in fairly high concentrations in soft denture liners. Unfortunately, some plasticizers, particularly phthalates, are known toxins, and products that contain these materials should be evaluated for biocompatibility. With the demand for safety from health-related products, greater attention will be focused on the tissue compatibility of denture base materials.

The growth of *Candida albicans* on the surfaces of dentures is a concern for many denture patients. This organism often is associated with denture stomatitis. An *in vitro* study has demonstrated the effectiveness of chlorhexidine gluconate in eliminating this organism. The chlorhexidine apparently can bind to acrylic surfaces for at least 2 weeks. Treating acrylic with Nystatin, followed by drying, produces similar results. *In vivo* studies are planned to evaluate the effectiveness of these antimicrobial agents with denture patients who suffer from this condition.

In addition to *Candida albicans,* many other microorganisms can adhere to denture base acrylics, such as *Streptococcus oralis, Bacteroides gingivalis, B. intermedius,* and *S. sanguis.* It is not surprising that many organisms adhere more strongly to rougher surfaces than to those that are highly polished. Future studies will probably evaluate the effectiveness of antimicrobial agents to control this problem.

Shelf life

The shelf life, or useful storage time at room temperature, for denture base plastics varies considerably. Acrylic plastics packaged in the powder-liquid form have excellent shelf life because the powder is almost indefinitely stable and the liquid usually is adequately protected from polymerization during storage by a hydroquinone inhibitor. The vinyl acrylic plastics, packaged as a gel in which the monomer is in contact with the polymer, must be stored at refrigerator temperature (about 2° C) to have a reasonable storage life of 1 to 2 years. The shelf life of light-activated denture base materials has not been reported.

Summary

It is fortunate that many types of denture base materials are available that will produce satisfactory dentures. The requirements may vary for different patients, and the processing facilities can dictate which material to use. There are also significant differences between products in each category, and it is wise to choose materials that have passed the ANSI/ADA specification.

■ MANIPULATION AND PROCESSING OF DENTURE BASE PLASTICS

As mentioned previously, denture base plastics are supplied in several forms. The technics used to process these materials into a finished complete or partial denture are briefly described, and the justifications for the various procedures are presented.

Texts on prosthetic dentistry describe impression technics, pouring master stone casts, setting denture teeth, preparing the waxed denture, investing in a denture flask, removing the wax, and coating the stone mold to prevent adhesion of the plastic. A set of waxed dentures on stone casts with the teeth in position is shown in Fig. 19-5, and a flask that contains maxillary porcelain teeth ready for packing the plastic dough is shown in Fig. 19-6.

Heat-Accelerated Acrylic Denture Plastics

The general method for processing a heat-accelerated acrylic denture base material consists of proportioning and mixing the polymer powder and the liquid monomer and allowing the monomer to react physically with the polymer in a sealed jar until a doughy consistency is reached. Before packing, all stone surfaces of the mold are coated with an alginate separator and allowed to dry. Metal foil separators may also be used. The dough is then packed into the treated denture mold containing the artificial teeth and "trial packed" by repeated application of slow pressure with a flask press until no excess flash remains and the material has a glossy surface. Polymerization is accomplished by applying heat and pressure, which are maintained until polymerization is complete. The flask is then bench cooled to room temperature, and the denture is deflasked, finished, and polished.

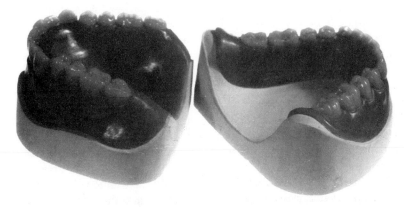

Fig. 19-5 Waxed maxillary and mandibular dentures on the stone casts.

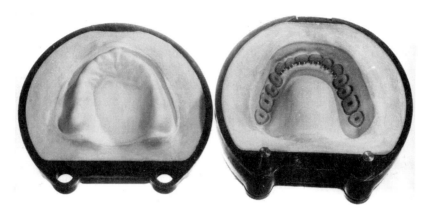

Fig. 19-6 Flask containing maxillary porcelain teeth, ready for packing the plastic dough.

$$\underbrace{Polymer + Peroxide\ initiator}_{Powder} + \underbrace{Monomer + Inhibitor}_{Liquid} + \underset{(external)}{Heat} \longrightarrow Polymer + \underset{(reaction)}{Heat}$$

The reaction involved in the heat-accelerated powder-liquid type is outlined in a simplified equation above.

The powder, consisting of the polymer plus the initiator, and the liquid monomer, containing the inhibitor, are proportioned in the ratio of approximately 3:1 by volume.

Proportioning

The main requirement for the quantity of liquid used is that it completely wet the polymer powder. The powder and liquid are mixed with a stainless steel spatula and then kept in the sealed jar during the initial stages of reaction to avoid loss of monomer by evaporation. Incompletely wetted portions can result in a streaked or blanched appearance in the denture because of incomplete polymerization of the plastic during processing. Care should be taken to avoid breathing the monomer vapor. Animal studies have shown that the monomer can affect respiration, cardiac function, and blood pressure.

The polymer-monomer mixture, on standing, goes through several distinct consistencies, which may be qualitatively described as (1) sandy, (2) stringy or sticky, (3) doughy or puttylike, (4) rubbery or elastic, and (5) stiff. When the mixture is in the doughy consistency, it has desirable qualities for packing into a denture flask. Different products vary considerably in the time required to reach the doughy condition and the length of time they remain at the packing consis-

tency. These stages or consistencies are represented by a model of the viscosity of the polymer/monomer mix (Fig. 19-7). Nf represents the final viscosity and $nf/2$ is one-half of this value. ANSI/ADA Specification No. 12 for denture base plastics requires that the powder-liquid mixture be at the packing consistency when the mixture separates cleanly from the walls of the glass mixing jar and that this consistency be attained in less than 40 minutes from the start of mixing. The consistency, determined 5 minutes after the packing consistency is reached, should be such that when 6 to 10 g of the material are placed over 0.75-mm diameter holes in a brass plate and loaded with a 5000-g weight, the dough intrudes into the holes to a depth of not less than 0.5 mm. If the material passes this test, adequate time should be available for trial packing of the denture mold and for final closure. During the various consistency stages, little polymerization is taking place and the reaction occurring is physical in nature. This reaction includes some solution of the polymer in the monomer and some absorption of the monomer by the polymer, as well as wetting of the polymer particles. For conventional acrylic plastics, no substantial polymerization occurs until the denture flask is heated to above 70° C. If too much monomer is used in the mixture, polymerization shrinkage will be greater than necessary, additional time will be required to reach the packing consistency, and there will be a tendency for porosity to occur in the denture. If too little monomer is used,

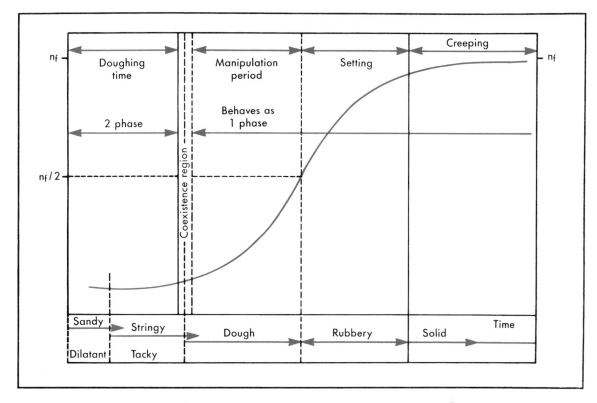

Fig. 19-7 Rheology stages of prepolymerized denture acrylic after mixing of powder and liquid: nf is the final viscosity and nf/2 is half of the final value. (From Mutlu G, Huggett R, Harrison P, Goodwin JW, Hughes RW: *Dent Mater* 6:288, 1990.)

the polymer will be insufficiently wetted, the dough will be difficult to manage, and in extreme cases the mass may not fuse into a continuous unit of plastic during processing.

Packing

The powder-liquid mixture should be packed into the flask at the doughy stage (Fig. 19-8, *A*) for several reasons. If it is packed at the sandy or stringy stages, too much monomer will be present between the polymer particles, the material will be of too low a viscosity to pack well, and will flow out of the flask too easily. Packing too early may also result in porosity in the final denture base. If packed at the rubbery-to-stiff stage, the material will be too viscous to flow well under the pressure of the flask press, and metal-to-metal contact of the flask halves will not be obtained. Delayed packing will result in loss of detail in the denture, movement or fracture of the teeth, and an increase in the contact vertical dimension of the den-

ture. Some plastics now have increased working time and remain in the dough stage for periods approaching 1 hour. This permits the packing of several dentures at the same time. Other products, particularly the rubber-reinforced materials, have shorter working times, and in some instances only one or two dentures should be packed with one mix. The plastic dough should not be manipulated excessively with bare hands. The monomer is a good solvent for body oils and may pick up dirt from the hands, resulting in a nonesthetic denture. Monomer may also enter the bloodstream through the skin.

The acrylic dough is packed into the flask in slight excess by use of a hydraulic, pneumatic, or mechanical press (Fig. 19-8, *B*), and this excess is removed by trial-packing procedures, with a damp cellophane or polyethylene film used as a separator for the upper half of the flask. The film separator allows easy separation of the flask halves during trial-packing procedures. The closing force of the press is applied slowly

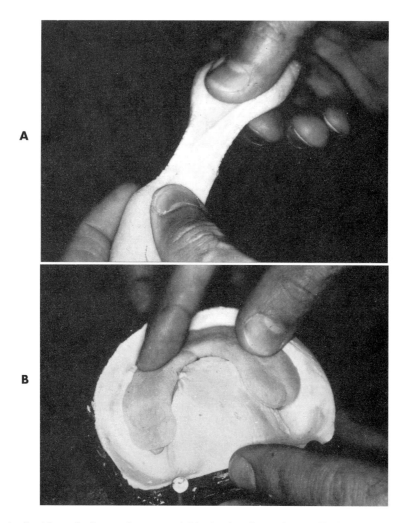

Fig. 19-8 A, Powder-liquid acrylic denture base material in the dough consistency. **B,** An excess being placed in the mold. (Adapted from Craig RG, O'Brien WJ, Powers JM: *Dental materials: properties and manipulation,* ed 6, St Louis, 1996, Mosby.)

during the trial packing to allow the excess or flash to flow out between the halves of the flask (Fig. 19-8, *C*). The flask is opened at intervals and the flash trimmed away (Fig. 19-8, *D*). Before final closure, the separating film is removed and discarded. During final closure of the flask metal-to-metal contact of the flask halves is completed in the press, the flasks are placed in a flask press that maintains pressure, and the denture is processed.

Processing

For heat-polymerized plastics the curing temperature must be maintained close to 74° C because the polymerization reaction is strongly exothermic. The heat of reaction will be added to the heat used to raise the material to the polymerization temperature. The temperature rise at various positions in a denture flask during a curing cycle is illustrated in Fig. 19-9. The initial temperature increases are in the following order: flask, plaster or stone, tinfoil, and plastic because the outside of the flask is in contact with the water bath. The temperatures in the different areas increase at approximately the same rate until the temperature of the plastic dough reaches about 70° C. At this point the material becomes quite fluid, and the decomposition rate of the ben-

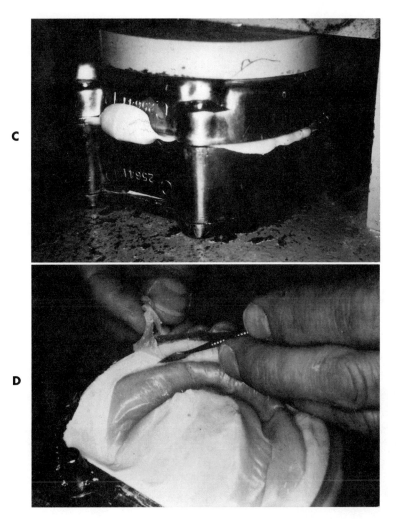

Fig. 19-8, cont'd. C, The excess being forced out between the two portions of the flask. **D,** The flash being trimmed away. (Adapted from Craig RG, O'Brien WJ, Powers JM: *Dental materials: properties and manipulation,* ed 6, St Louis, 1996, Mosby.)

zoyl peroxide initiator is rapid enough for a substantial amount of polymerization to take place. As the polymerization reaction proceeds, the exothermic heat of reaction increases the temperature of the plastic to values considerably above the surrounding materials and above the boiling point of the methyl methacrylate monomer. This occurs because both the plastic and stone are poor thermal conductors and the heat of reaction is dissipated slowly. Also the larger the mass or bulk of material, the higher the peak temperature attained in the plastic. In thick sections of a denture the temperature rise will be greater than in thin sections. It has been demon-strated that the strength of thin sections of a denture may be less than that of the thick sections because of a lower degree of polymerization. Because of the excessive temperature rise, porosity will more likely occur in thick sections of the denture.

The porosity that developed in two plastics cured at 74°, 82°, and 100° C is shown in Fig. 19-10. Product A showed no porosity at 74° C, a negligible amount at 82° C, and moderate porosity at 100° C. Product B, however, evidenced no porosity at 74° C, a moderate amount at 82° C, and severe porosity at 100° C. On the basis of a large number of studies, a satisfactory processing temperature for most products

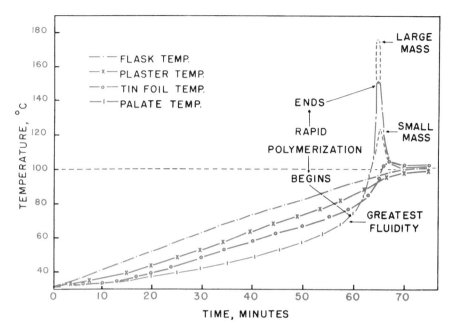

Fig. 19-9 Temperature observed at various positions in a denture flask during processing. (Adapted from Tylman SD: *J Am Dent Assoc* 29:1845, 1942.)

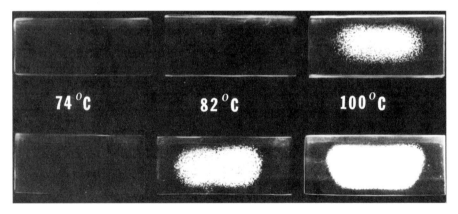

Fig. 19-10 Effect of the processing temperature on the porosity of two acrylic dental plastics. (From Peyton FA: *J Am Dent Assoc* 40:525, 1950.)

is between 71° and 77° C, although as indicated in Fig. 19-10 some products can be processed at higher temperatures without serious difficulty. A satisfactory processing procedure is to cure the plastic in a constant temperature water bath at 74° C for 8 hours or longer. Longer curing times, such as overnight, will not result in any degradation of properties. Another satisfactory processing method, which permits curing in a shorter time, is to heat at 74° C for 1.5 hours and then increasing the temperature of the water bath to boiling for an additional hour.

The porosity shown in the specimens in Fig. 19-10 is in the center. The absence of porosity in the periphery of the specimens results from lower temperatures in these areas because the heat can be dissipated to the surrounding dental stone. The center of the specimens experience higher temperatures because poor thermal conductivity of the plastic prevents the dissipation of heat. Porosity in thick sections of dentures therefore may exist below the surface of the plastic, and in pigmented materials it may not be noticed until grinding or polishing exposes the deeper layers.

Porosity also results when insufficient pressure is maintained on the flask during processing, but the distribution of the porosity is different from that shown in Fig. 19-10. Porosity resulting from insufficient pressure is distributed uniformly throughout the material, rather than concentrated in the center.

Other problems associated with rapid initial heating of the acrylic dough above 74° C are production of internal stresses, warpage of the denture after deflasking, and checking or crazing around the necks of the artificial teeth. High internal stresses resulting from rapid heating combined with the heat of polymerization may be released later and cause distortion and misfit of the denture base.

A variety of other methods of supplying the necessary heat to accelerate the polymerization reaction have been used. They include steam, dry heat supplied by electric platens, dry-air oven, infrared heating, induction or dielectric heating, and microwave radiation. The results of various processing studies have shown that equally satisfactory clinical results may be obtained with any of these methods compared with the water bath method if adequate temperature control and pressure are maintained.

Deflasking and finishing

After polymerization, the flask is removed from the water bath and allowed to cool to room temperature. If the flask is opened prematurely while the plastic is still warm, warpage is likely to occur. Rapid cooling also tends to increase stresses in the denture, which may be released at a later time. During the cooling process, thermal shrinkage occurs due to the relatively high thermal coefficient of expansion of the plastic. The magnitude of this thermal shrinkage will depend on the difference between the temperature at which the plastic hardens and room or mouth temperature, whichever is the final reference point. It is apparent that as long as the plastic is soft, it will shrink with the stone cast, which has a different thermal coefficient. When the plastic hardens, stresses are induced as cooling continues because the plastic is forced to follow the shape of the cast despite the dif-

ferences in thermal coefficients. Deflasking of the denture after cooling, however, allows some of the stresses in the denture to be released, and warpage occurs. Numerous studies dealing with the linear shrinkage of denture bases, measured across the posterior region, have shown that for normal processing conditions, the linear shrinkage is 0.3% to 0.5%. Usually more shrinkage is observed in mandibular than in maxillary dentures because of their shape.

A change in the contact vertical dimension of a denture during processing, as measured on an articulator, is also important. These changes are caused by variations in flask pressure, flask temperature, consistency of the dough, and strength of the stone mold. The pressure developed during closure of the flask is possibly the most important factor. If proper precautions are taken, the vertical opening may be held to 0.5 mm rather than reported variations of 2 to 5 mm.

After cooling, the denture is ejected from the flask and the stone is removed. Stone adhering to the plastic may be removed by shell blasting, a process where ground-up walnut shells are used to abrade the stone with little or no effect on the plastic. After deflasking, the denture is trimmed with an arbor band and acrylic burs and polished. A wet polishing wheel and a slurry of pumice and water should be used to avoid heating the acrylic, which can cause measurable warpage. Tin oxide has been used to produce the final polish. However, tin oxide recently has been identified as a biological hazard and should not be used for polishing dentures. After finishing, the denture should be stored in water.

Residual monomer

During the polymerization process the amount of residual monomer decreases rapidly at first and, later, more slowly. The amount of residual monomer in a denture plastic processed at 70° C and at 100° C is shown as a function of the time and processing in Fig. 19-11. At zero time the monomer content was 26.2%. After 1 hour at 70° C it decreased to 6.6%, and at 100° C it decreases to 0.31%. After 4 hours the residual monomer was 4.0% and 0.29%, respectively. It required 168 hours at 70° C for the residual monomer to approximate the value obtained after 1 hour at 100° C. These data support the use of a 1-hour terminal boil for processing dentures as described earlier. However,

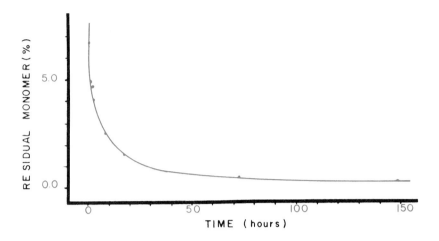

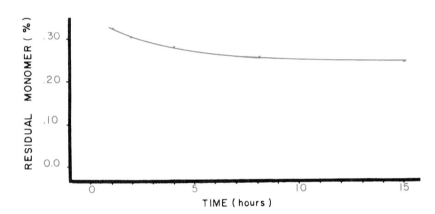

Fig. 19-11 Residual monomer concentration in the polymerization of methyl methacrylate in dental plastics at 70° C, **A,** and 100° C, **B,** as a function of the time of processing. (Adapted from Smith DC: *Br Dent J* 105:86, 1958.)

the processing temperature should not be raised to boiling until most of the polymerization is completed, or porosity may result.

The highest residual monomer level is observed with chemically accelerated denture base plastics at 1% to 4% shortly after processing. Storing the denture for several days at elevated temperatures (up to 50° C) and excluding oxygen can significantly reduce the monomer level. However, this may be impractical. The rapid heat-cured denture base materials have significant residual monomer levels from 1% to 3% when they are processed in less than 1 hour in boiling water. If they are processed for 7 hours at 70° C and then boiled for 3 hours, the residual monomer content may be less than 0.4%.

If heat-processed materials are to be used for patients sensitive to residual monomer, processing for longer times in boiling water should reduce the monomer to an acceptable level. Because there is evidence that poly(methyl methacrylate) monomer has poor biocompatibility, every effort should be made to eliminate residual monomer or reduce it to very low levels.

Dimensional changes

Dimensional changes take place when dentures are stored in water or are in contact with oral fluids. A considerable number of studies have reported on dimensional changes occurring during processing and storage of dentures. The area described with

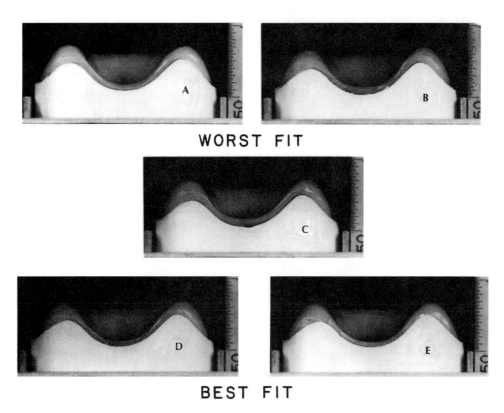

WORST FIT

BEST FIT

Fig. 19-12 Fit of denture bases after finishing and storage in water at 37° C for 42 days. **A,** Conventional acrylic. **B** and **C,** Rubber-modified acrylic. **D,** Vinyl-modified acrylic. **E,** Hydroxyethyl-modified acrylic. (From Soni PM, Powers JM, Craig RG: *J Oral Rehabil* 6:35, 1979.)

the most uniform results has been the posterior region. In general, heat-cured dentures stored in water show a linear expansion in this region of 0.1% to 0.2%, which partially but not completely compensates for the processing shrinkage of 0.3% to 0.5%. The net linear change can vary from a shrinkage of 0.1% to 0.4%. The major portion of the expansion in water takes place during the first month, and changes are insignificant after 2 months.

The results of a study comparing the fit of maxillary dentures made from five different commercial products are seen in Fig. 19-12. The denture bases were placed on their respective casts after being stored in water at 37° C for 42 days to ensure equilibrium. The materials were ranked from best fit to worst fit by a panel of trained observers. The relative fit is determined by the space between the base and the cast in the palatal region. One rubber-modified material, *C,* had the worst fit, whereas another, *B,* had a fit that was similar to the conventional acrylic. The best fit was observed with the vinyl-modified, *D,* and the hydroxethyl, *E,* acrylics. There was no correlation with water sorption values, and therefore the fit of the denture bases may be related more to the glass transition temperature (glassy to brittle transition) than to water sorption for these materials.

There is always concern regarding what a net shrinkage of 0.1% to 0.4% represents clinically. A number of other steps in the preparation of a complete denture may cause dimensional inaccuracies, such as making the impression, pouring the stone cast, and preparing and investing the waxed denture. The oral tissues apparently compensate for small dimensional changes in the dentures, and a dimensional change of 0.1% to 0.4% is tolerated by most patients.

Chemically Accelerated Acrylic Denture Plastics–Compression Molding

Chemically accelerated dental plastics, often called chemically curing resins, self-curing resins, cold-curing resins, or autopolymerizing resins, are similar to the heat-accelerated dental plastics. The principal difference is that the polymerization reaction is accelerated by a chemical, such as *N,N*-dihydroxyethyl-para-toluidine, rather than by heat, as indicated by the simplified equation below (compare with the equation given in the earlier section on heat-accelerated acrylic denture plastics).

The amine accelerator reacts with the peroxide initiator at room temperature, and sufficient free radicals are produced to initiate the polymerization reaction. Except for the initiation step, the remainder of the polymerization reaction is the same as for the heat-accelerated type. The reaction is exothermic, and polymerization still results in volumetric shrinkage, but the plastic does not reach as high a peak temperature.

Manipulation and processing

The general procedure for compression molding a chemically accelerated plastic is much the same as for the heat-accelerated type, except that after final flask closure the dough is allowed to polymerize at room temperature or in a warm water bath in a pressure vessel.

The denture mold is packed when the polymer-monomer mixture reaches the doughy stage. Several trial closures are made and the flash is removed. Care must be taken to make both the trial closures and final closure before the dough becomes so stiff that final closure is not possible. The chemically accelerated materials start to polymerize soon after the powder and liquid are mixed and proceed more rapidly through the various consistency stages than the heat-accelerated types. The average time needed to reach packing consistency is only 5 minutes for the chemically accelerated type, compared with 15 minutes for the heat-polymerized acrylic. Therefore it is more difficult to pack a number of denture flasks from one mix and still obtain complete flask closure. Additional working time may be obtained when the ingredients and the mixing jar are cooled in a refrigerator.

Properties

After the flask is packed it should remain closed and under clamp pressure for a minimum of 2.5 hours to ensure polymerization. Compared with the heat-cured plastics, the chemically cured types do not reach the same degree of polymerization. The higher residual monomer acts as a plasticizer, which results in higher transverse deflection values and lower transverse strengths. After 15 days in water, however, the chemically cured acrylics are nearly as hard as the heat-cured type. If, after 2.5 hours of curing at room temperature, the flask is boiled for 0.5 to 1 hour, properties comparable to the heat-cured type are obtained, and the residual monomer content is considerably reduced.

Peak temperatures observed at various positions in a denture cured by chemical acceleration are not as high as for heat-polymerized types. The linear shrinkage across the posterior region of a chemically cured maxillary denture after deflasking is about 0.3% compared with 0.5% for a heat-cured maxillary denture. As in the case of heat-cured dentures, mandibular dentures prepared with chemically accelerated denture plastics show more dimensional change than corresponding maxillary dentures. The lower dimensional change of the chemically cured type results because less residual stress is produced in the denture during the processing cycle. This is substantiated by the fact that the chemically accelerated denture plastics produce less shrinkage when processed at 20° to 25° C rather than at 37° C. When chemically cured dentures are placed in water, an increase in the molar-to-molar distance is observed, and after 1 month this expansion amounts to about 0.3%, which approximately compensates for the processing shrinkage of 0.3%. Additional storage up to 9 months results in a total expansion of 0.4%, and the net dimensional change at this time is +0.1%, compared with the master model. It should be noted that the water sorption of the chemically cured acrylics is between 0.5 and 0.7 mg/cm^2, or about the same as the heat-cured

$$\underbrace{\text{Polymer + Peroxide initiator}}_{\text{Powder}} + \underbrace{\text{Monomer + Inhibitor + Amine accelerator}}_{\text{Liquid}} \longrightarrow \text{Polymer} + \underset{\text{(reaction)}}{\text{Heat}}$$

type. However, the solubility is 0.05 mg/cm^2 for the chemically cured type compared with 0.02 mg/cm^2 for the heat-cured type. This larger value for solubility is caused by the loss of residual monomer from the chemically cured acrylic.

On the basis of these observations, it can be concluded that chemically cured acrylic dentures are generally about 0.1% oversize after several months of service and heat-cured acrylic dentures are 0.3% to 0.4% undersize.

In addition to strength, water sorption, solubility, and dimensional changes, the color stability of the chemically cured denture base should be considered. The presence of some amine accelerators causes problems in color stability. These amines produce colored products on oxidation, and therefore the color stability of the chemically cured acrylics may not be as good as for heat-cured acrylics, although definite improvements in the color stability of chemically cured acrylics have taken place since their introduction. Several products are now available that comply with the ANSI/ADA Specification No. 12 color stability test. Activators such as organic sulfinic acids can be used to improve color stability, but these compounds have certain disadvantages, such as chemical instability.

Fluid Resin Acrylic Denture Plastics

The fluid resin technic takes advantage of the flow properties of polymer-monomer mixtures in the early consistency stage and a smaller size of the polymer powder particles. A very fluid mix also results from a much higher monomer-polymer ratio of about 1:2.5. The polymer and monomer are mixed and then poured into the mold in the denture flask, and no trial packing is required. This procedure is advantageous in the preparation of the saddles for partial dentures in which trial packing is difficult and flow of plastic around the metal framework is required. It also requires less expensive equipment than the heat-accelerated acrylic. Manufacturers claim that a denture can be produced in much less time using this procedure. However, this was not substantiated in a laboratory survey.

This technic involves the use of agar or alginate hydrocolloid or, less commonly, a soft stone or silicone mold. The presence of water in the hydrocolloid does not interfere with the polymerization of the slurry of polymer and monomer. The technic involves preparation of an hydrocolloid gel mold of the waxed-up model, as shown in Fig. 19-13, *A*. After the gel is formed, the model, including the waxed denture, is removed. The wax is removed from the model and teeth, and the teeth are reinserted into the mold (Fig. 19-13, *B*). The model is repositioned in the mold after an alginate separator has been applied and allowed to dry. The denture flask is constructed so that two or three circular holes can be cut from the side of the flask through the gel to the posterior portion of the model. A slurry of chemically activated acrylic is poured through one of these holes into the mold space provided by the loss of the wax (Fig. 19-13, *C*). The remaining hole or holes provide vents for the excess acrylic slurry, thus ensuring adequate filling of the mold space. After pouring of the acrylic the flask is placed in a pressure vessel containing warm water, and air pressure of 0.1 to 0.2 MPa is applied. Only 30 to 45 minutes are necessary for polymerization. After processing, the gel is easily broken away from the denture and the denture looks as clean as the one shown in Fig. 19-13, *D*. Dentures fabricated by this technic are slightly less accurate than heat-activated dentures processed in a stone mold because of higher polymerization shrinkage. When compared with heat-cured resins, pour-type acrylics are characterized by lower impact and fatigue strengths, higher creep values, lower transverse bend strength, lower water sorption values, and higher solubility. The technic is interesting because the hydrocolloid mold is easy to prepare, processing time is shortened considerably, the agar hydrocolloid may be reused, problems of broken teeth are eliminated, and deflasking is simplified.

Commercially available fluid resins may vary considerably in apparent viscosity. Fig. 19-14 demonstrates the dramatic increase in apparent viscosity of six different fluid resins as a function of time and at a constant shear rate (rotational speed). It illustrates the importance of pouring the fluid resins into the mold soon after the powder and liquid phases are mixed if lower viscosities are to be obtained. The apparent viscosity of fluid resins appears to be an important factor when fluid resin denture materials are evaluated.

Light-Cured Denture Plastic

Light curing of a denture is a novel method compared with other processing methods. After the try-in of the waxed-up trial denture is completed, a roll of light-activated acrylic is placed over the occlusal

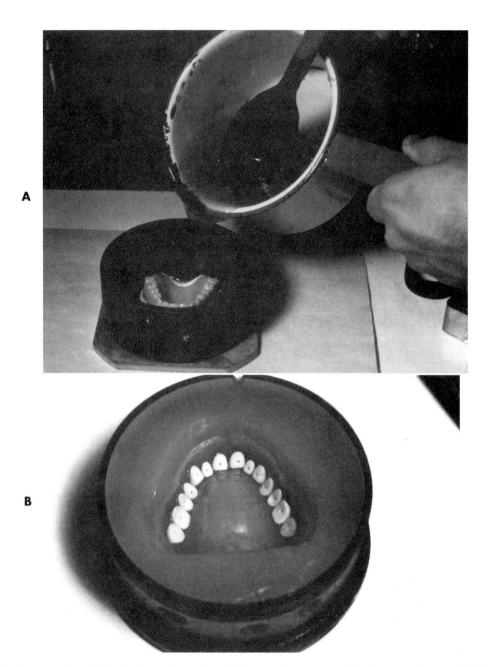

Fig. 19-13 Slurry casting of chemically accelerated acrylic denture base material. **A,** Pouring of agar mold. **B,** Agar mold with denture teeth in position.

surfaces of the teeth to form a template having three reference areas on the master cast (Fig. 19-15, *A*). The template is cured in the light chamber for 10 minutes, and then the teeth are removed from the trial denture.

Removal is simple because the wax softens under the heat of the high-intensity light bulbs. The teeth, the attached template, and the cast are placed in boiling water to remove all traces of wax (Fig. 19-15, *B*).

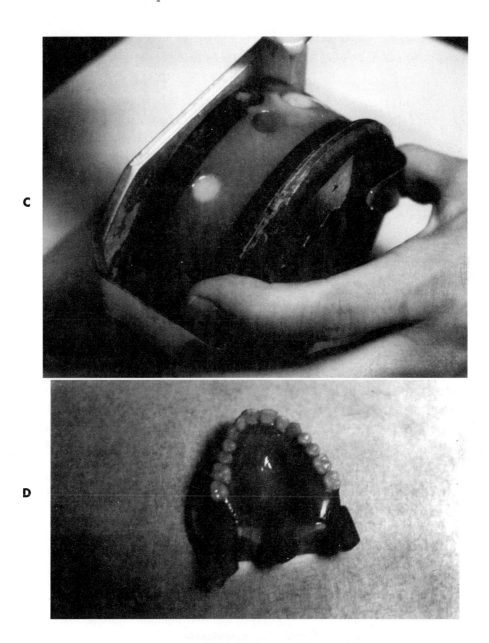

Fig. 19-13, cont'd. C, Pouring of powder-liquid slurry into the agar mold. **D,** Appearance of denture after processing.

After coating the master cast with a release agent, a sheet of the light-activated denture base material is adapted to the cast and trimmed to the boxing edge (Fig. 19-15, *C*). The base is then polymerized in the light chamber.

A strip of the light-activated acrylic is placed on the underside of the teeth after they have been coated with a bonding agent. The teeth are then repositioned on the denture base using the template to place them in the original location (Fig. 19-15, *D*).

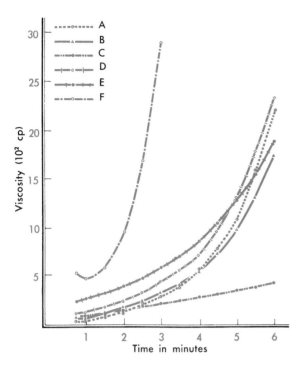

Fig. 19-14 Viscosity of six fluid resins as a function of time at 10 rpm. (From Vermilyea SG, Powers JM, Koran A: *J Dent Res* 57:227, 1978.)

The teeth are fixed in position by polymerization in the light chamber.

The anatomical portion of the denture is completed using more of the base material to sculpt the surface and develop the final shape of the denture (Fig. 19-15, *E*). After contouring, final polymerization is accomplished in the light chamber. After processing and removal from the cast, the denture is finished in a conventional manner.

Forces Involved in Denture Retention

The accuracy of fit of a denture has been cited as one of the important factors in the retention of denture bases but no explanations have been given. Other factors are (1) capillary forces involving the liquid film between the oral tissues and the denture base, (2) surface forces controlling the wetting of the plastic denture base by the saliva, (3) the thickness of the saliva film between the denture and the oral tissues, (4) the surface tension of the saliva, (5) the viscosity of the saliva, and (6) atmospheric pressure. High surface tension, area, and wetting increase retention, as does a thin film of saliva (see Chapter 2). A technical discussion of all factors involved in the retention of dentures is not within the scope of this text.

Effect of Auxiliary Materials on Denture Plastics

A number of materials are used in making a denture. These materials may affect the final properties and function of the denture. Examples of such materials are (1) dental plaster and stone, (2) impression materials, (3) wax, (4) mold separators, (5) artificial teeth, (6) characterization materials, (7) metal inserts, (8) repair and reline materials, and (9) denture cleansers.

Plaster and stone

The strength of the plaster or stone used to invest the wax denture is of concern because a weak investment resulting from a thin mix or incomplete mixing will not adequately support the artificial teeth during packing of the denture mold. As a result of teeth shifting, the finished dentures may have faulty occlusion. Another problem involved in the use of a stone mold is that the thermal coefficient of expansion, or contraction, is different from the thermal coefficients of the teeth and the plastic used to form the denture. After the polymerization reaction, the plastic and investment cool to room temperature and attempt to contract according to their individual thermal coefficients. The stone cast with a different thermal coefficient creates residual stresses in the acrylic as it cools. These stresses may be released after the processed denture is deflasked and deformation or crazing (numerous small cracks) may result.

Impression materials

When agar or alginate materials are used to make the original impression, it is important that the cast be poured as soon as possible. If dimensional changes occur in the impression, these inaccuracies will be reflected in the final fit of the denture base. The presence of any residual zinc oxide–eugenol on the cast from the impression will function as an inhibitor in the polymerization of the plastic.

Waxes

Baseplate wax that is not removed from the crown portion of the teeth before the denture is

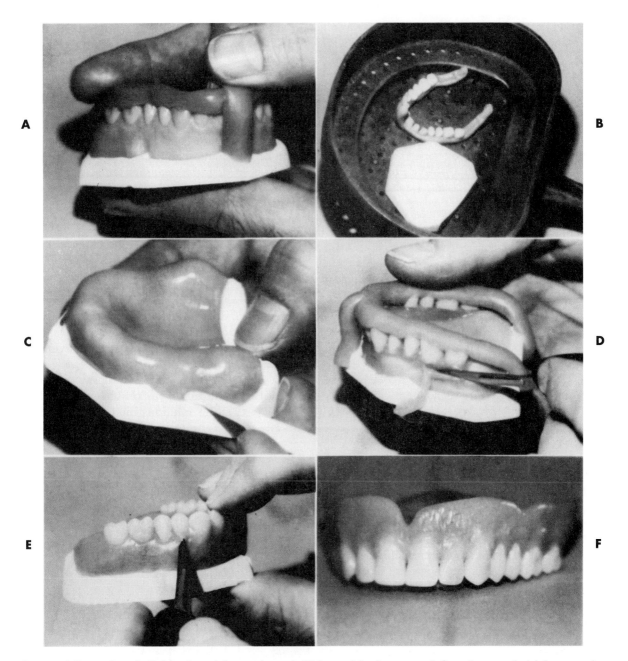

Fig. 19-15 Processing of a light-activated denture base. **A,** Pick-up of the denture teeth from the waxed trial denture using a rope of the light-activated acrylic. **B,** Removal of all traces of wax from the teeth and master cast. **C,** Adaptation of light-activated denture base material to the master cast. **D,** Reseating the teeth on the master cast and beginning the shaping of the anatomical portion of the denture. **E,** Final adaptation of the anatomical portion of the denture just before polymerization in the light chamber. **F,** Completed light-activated acrylic denture. (Courtesy Dentsply International, York, Pa, 1987.)

flasked will cause problems. During the removal of the wax by boiling in water, the wax on the teeth is also removed and will result in shifting of the teeth, poor articulation, or broken teeth when the denture is packed. A more common problem is the presence of a residual wax film on the gingival portions of the artificial teeth after the boilout of the wax, which prevents the adherence of the plastic base to the teeth. This may be avoided by the addition of detergents to the water used in the boilout procedure, followed by rinsing with clear boiling water.

Mold separators

For many years tinfoil was the most acceptable separating medium. Tinfoil, however, is difficult to apply and as a result a number of tinfoil substitutes have been developed. Materials such as aqueous solutions of sodium silicate, calcium oleate, or sodium or ammonium alginate have been used. The common alginate separators contain about 2% sodium alginate in water with small amounts of glycerin, alcohol, sodium phosphate, and preservatives. Care must be exercised to avoid coating plastic teeth with these release agents because this will interfere with the bond between the denture base and the teeth.

Characterization materials

A variety of materials are used for the characterization of dentures, including dyed synthetic fibers, pigments, dyes, and clear plastic powder. These materials improve the esthetics of the dentures and have no substantial effects on the strength or other properties of dental plastics. For example, the addition of dyed acrylic fibers to simulate the blood vessels of the oral mucosa does not alter the water sorption or strength of the dental plastic significantly. There is a justified concern regarding the toxicity of some of the pigments used to color denture base materials.

Denture cleansers

Denture cleansers and cleaning methods may have pronounced effects, including causing scratches and wear, on plastic dentures. For this reason, denture acrylic has been tested for wear using various commercially available denture cleaning pastes, an experimental paste, soap and water, and

water against a reciprocating soft toothbrush. The results shown in Fig. 19-16 are dramatic. The use of water, or soap and water, produced little or no wear compared with the commercial denture cleansers and toothpaste. Daily brushing with a very soft brush (similar to the toothbrushes used in periodontal therapy) is very effective in keeping dentures clean and will not abrade the denture or teeth appreciably if abrasive cleansers are not used. Most immersion denture cleansers are effective in the removal of mucin, stains, and loosely attached food debris. Some immersion cleaners have been demonstrated to be effective sanitizing agents. A water solution containing a hypochlorite and a glassy phosphate (Calgon) is an effective denture cleanser that does not cause discoloration of the dental plastic or the metal retainer pins used in porcelain artificial teeth when used occasionally. A solution consisting of 1 tsp of a hypochlorite, such as Clorox, and 2 tsp of Calgon in half a glass of water has been recommended for occasional overnight immersion of plastic dentures. This cleanser is not recommended for use on prostheses containing cobalt-chromium or nickel-chromium alloys because chlorine solutions tend to darken these metals.

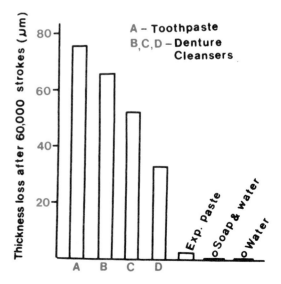

Fig. 19-16 Wear of denture base acrylic in various media. (Adapted from Heath JR, Davenport JC, Jones PA: *J Oral Rehabil* 10:159, 1983.)

Repair Materials

An important application of plastics in prosthetic dentistry is in the repair of broken dentures. The repair materials are usually acrylic plastics of the powder-liquid type, similar to those used for denture bases, and are either heat-accelerated or chemically accelerated. Recently, light-activated acrylic has been shown to be a fast and effective repair material. The material of choice will depend on the following factors: (1) length of time required for making the repair, (2) transverse strength obtainable with the repair material, and (3) degree to which dimensional accuracy is maintained during repair.

One technic for making a repair requires holding, or luting, the broken pieces together with sticky wax, pouring a stone model on the inside of the denture, and investing the model and denture in a flask. Then the wax is removed, the fracture line is opened with a bur to allow for a reasonable amount of repair plastic, and the ground surfaces are painted with monomer or a 4:1 mixture of monomer and polymer. Acrylic dough is packed into the area being repaired, and the material is cured, cooled, deflasked, and finished.

If a heat-accelerated acrylic is used, the denture should be completely flasked, and curing of the repair material preferably should be carried out at temperatures no greater than 74° to 77° C for 8 hours or longer. This procedure minimizes the dimensional change of the denture base.

In a similar manner, the repair may be done without flasking, by use of a chemically accelerated acrylic. After a cast is poured, the fracture line is opened and the acrylic is painted into the defect. The denture is then placed in a pressure vessel under air pressure until polymerization is complete. Repairs using light-activated acrylic are done in a similar manner. After the acrylic dough is packed into the defect, curing is done in the light chamber. A bonding agent is used to increase the strength of the repair.

The use of chemically accelerated and light-activated acrylic resins for making repairs has the advantage of not requiring flasking of the denture. The procedure is rapid and may be done while the patient waits. The dimensional accuracy is maintained because not enough heat is present during polymerization to cause warpage from the release of stresses. The chemically accelerated acrylic resins, however, have the disadvantage of lower transverse strength in the repaired area than a heat-cured acrylic. In general, the transverse strength of a heat-cured repair is about 80% of that of the original plastic, and the transverse strength of a chemically cured repair is approximately 60% of the original material. Regardless of the type of plastic used for repair, the edges in the repair area should be tapered and all corners should be rounded to avoid areas of high stress concentration. These ground edges are painted with monomer to soften the plastic before the flask is packed to obtain a chemical bond between the repair material and the denture.

The use of chemically accelerated repair material without flasking, at room temperature and pressure, may result in a repair area containing porosity. The polymerization in the center of the repair proceeds rapidly, but the polymerization at the surface is slowed by the inhibiting effect of the oxygen. When the repair is done in water, under air pressure of 0.2 MPa and a temperature of 30° C, the porosity is greatly reduced. The residual monomer content of specimens processed either in air or under pressure is approximately 3%.

The reported net dimensional change across the molar region of a maxillary denture for a heat-cured repair conducted at 73.5° C is –0.3%, whereas for a chemically cured repair it is +0.2%. It also has been reported that a denture repaired with chemically accelerated plastic will fit the model better. This may be the result of less warpage or because the denture is slightly oversized. Studies have been done on the contour of denture bases before they were broken and after repair. The results indicate that better reproduction of dimensions results when chemically accelerated repair materials are used to repair dentures originally prepared from heat-cured or self-cured acrylic plastics. Superior results also are obtained when a heat-curing acrylic repair material is used to repair a denture prepared from a chemically accelerated acrylic plastic. Less satisfactory reproduction of dimensions is obtained when a heat-curing repair material is used to repair a heat-cured denture. If the cause of breakage is not corrected, such as faulty occlusion, fit, or both, repairs usually will fail regardless of what repair material is used.

ANSI/ADA Specification No. 13 for denture self-curing repair resins

The requirements of the chemically accelerated repair plastics or the self-curing repair resins are listed in ANSI/ADA Specification No. 13. The specification includes self-curing powder-liquid plastics, which may be either pink or clear. These materials must satisfy the requirements of the previously described ANSI/ADA Specification No. 12 for denture base plastics with the following exceptions. The plasticity test shall be conducted as in the denture base specification, except that the test should be started 3 minutes, rather than 5 minutes, after the proper plasticity is reached. This change allows for the faster setting of the repair materials.

The transverse deflection between a 1500- and 2500-g load shall be not more than 1.5 mm, and the deflection between a 1500- and 4000-g load shall be not less than 1 mm and not more than 4.5 mm. This transverse deflection requirement is difficult to compare with the test for chemically accelerated denture base plastics because the loads used are different and therefore the deflection limits are not the same. It does appear, however, that the deflection limits for the repair materials are somewhat more lenient.

In general, the color stability test (ANSI/ADA Specification No. 12) is difficult for chemically accelerated repair materials to pass.

Relining and Rebasing Dentures

The fit of a denture may be satisfactory when it is first delivered to the patient. However, because of changes in the contour of the soft tissues and resorption of underlying bone, the denture may gradually lose retention. If the occlusion and vertical dimension of the dentures have not been greatly altered, the retention may be regained by either relining or rebasing.

Relining

Relining is a process in which a film of plastic is added to the inside of the denture to obtain an improved fit with the denture-bearing mucosa. This is accomplished by (1) making an impression of the denture-bearing mucosa using the denture as a tray, reflasking the denture, removing the impression material, and packing and curing the new liner, or (2) making a chairside reline where the reline material is used to make the impression.

Two different types of reline materials may be used. One is designed as a permanent reline, and the other is used only as a temporary reline. The former may be either a heat-accelerated, chemically accelerated, or light-activated acrylic. The relining process is carried out either by a flasking procedure or curing in a light chamber depending on the type of material. Permanent reline materials may be identical to those from which permanent denture bases are made.

The problems involved in relining a denture are much the same as in repairing a denture: (1) a good chemical bond is desired between the reline plastic and the denture plastic, (2) satisfactory strength of the relined denture is necessary, (3) no warpage or dimensional change should result in the denture because of the relining procedure, and (4) the relining should take as short a time as possible for patient convenience. Precautions should be taken to reline the denture with a compatible repair material. The area to be relined is softened by monomer and the acrylic is packed soon after reaching the doughy consistency to achieve a chemical bond between the two materials. The polymerization of the reline material should be done at temperatures between 74° to 77° C to prevent warpage. Chemically accelerated reline materials have an advantage because lower peak temperatures during polymerization may minimize warpage.

The light-activated material is used directly in the denture to record the tissue surface. A bonding agent is used before placing the material in the denture. The light-activated acrylic allows the entire reline procedure to be completed in 30 to 45 minutes.

Temporary relining plastics are used directly in the mouth, and a chemically accelerated curing system is used. These materials are considered temporary because they are porous and stain easily or foul. In addition, most of these products are not color stable. These temporary reline materials polymerize at mouth temperature, with peak polymerization temperatures of 59° to 79° C and peak temperature times of 6 to 11 minutes, with the lower temperatures generally corresponding to the longer times. Peak temperatures of 79° C are certainly uncomfortable. To avoid burning of the tissues, the denture is usually taken from the mouth after a few minutes, chilled in cool water, and returned to the mouth. In addition to the heat, direct contact of monomer and the oral tissues may elicit a burning sensation. Temporary reline plastics, however, do not cause any clinically significant warpage of the denture.

ANSI/ADA Specification No. 17 for denture base temporary relining resin

The ANSI/ADA Specification No. 17 for temporary relining resin is for hard-setting, self-curing plastics of the powder-liquid type. This specification contains requirements for the consistency, temperature rise, hardening time, ease of polishing, translucency, porosity, hardness, water sorption and solubility, and color stability. The peak temperature reached during processing should not be more than 75° C, and the time of hardening should be between 6 and 15 minutes. The processed plastic should have a smooth glossy surface when polished by usual methods and should be translucent and free of large numbers or sizes of bubbles. The surface hardness shall be not less than 10 Knoop hardness numbers (kg/mm^2). The water solubility and sorption shall be less than 0.07 and 0.7 mg/cm^2, respectively, when stored for 24 hours at 37° C. The requirements for hardness and solubility in water therefore are less demanding for the temporary relining materials than for the denture base plastics. The temporary relining plastics, however, must pass the color stability test listed in the ANSI/ADA Specification No. 12, which requires that the specimen show no more than a slight color change after an exposure of 24 hours. This requirement may be difficult to satisfy because many products show noticeable color changes when exposed to ultraviolet light.

Rebasing

Rebasing refers to a technic in which the dimensional relations of the teeth are maintained and the entire denture base is replaced. A cast is prepared from an impression made in the denture. After flasking, the old plastic is removed except perhaps for that around the teeth. The denture is then rewaxed and processed according to standard procedures with new acrylic. The discussion presented for permanent reline materials also applies for rebasing.

Tissue conditioners

Tissue conditioners are soft elastomers used to treat an irritated mucosa supporting a denture. They are mixed at chairside, placed in the denture, and seated in the patient's mouth. These materials will conform to the anatomy of the residual ridge, gel in that position, and continue to flow slowly after application. They are used only for short-term applications and should be replaced every 3 days. Inhibition of the growth of oral bacterial flora is associated with some materials, and this should promote healing of inflamed tissues.

Tissue conditioners are composed of a powder containing poly(ethyl methacrylate) and a liquid containing an aromatic ester-ethyl alcohol (up to 30%) mixture. Tissue conditioners are very soft elastomers with a hardness of from 13 to 49 Shore A hardness units 24 hours after mixing. They also will show a weight loss of from 4.9% to 9.3% after 24 hours as a result of the loss of alcohol. These materials deform easily, and with a stress of 200 g/cm^2 applied 15 minutes after the set of the material, the compression will range from 60% to 83% of the original length. When the stress is removed, there will be a recovery of from 22% to 48%. When unstrained samples are left in a humidifier for 24 hours, they will tend to "slump" or shorten under their own weight. Within a few days the tissue conditioners become stiffer as a result of the loss of alcohol.

Tissue conditioners are formulated to have specific viscoelastic properties. The viscosity of a number of tissue conditioners is listed in Table 19-11. The values were obtained 2 hours after mixing and under prolonged static loads. Under cyclic loading, which parallels cyclic masticatory forces, the materials demonstrated elastic behavior, particularly when the frequency was more than 1 Hz.

The properties that make tissue conditioners effective are (1) viscous behavior, which allows adaptation to the irritated denture-bearing mucosa over a period of several days and (2) viscoelastic and elastic behavior, which cushions the cyclic forces of mastication and bruxism.

It has been suggested that the initial flow depends on the time of loading, volume of the material, and the load applied when seating the denture. A rheologic study has shown that different products must be seated in the mouth at different times from the start of mixing because they may differ both in viscosity and/or gelation time.

An evaluation of the viscoelastic properties of tissue conditioners consisting of poly(ethyl methacrylate) powders and butyl phthalate/butyl glycolate-ethanol liquids demonstrated that the elastic modulus, relaxation time, and instantaneous modulus increased as a function of time. The rate of increase in the coefficient of viscosity was greater than the elastic modulus in all cases. This confirms that compliance measurements and the Maxwell model are the most useful when describing the viscoelastic properties of tissue conditioners.

Viscoelastic finite element analysis has been used to evaluate the stress concentrations caused by simulated dentures with soft liners during function. The results indicate that viscous flow of both soft liners and tissue are affected by the load and the duration of the load placed on the denture. This of course affects the stress distribution in the supporting tissues.

Soft or resilient denture liners

Soft or plasticized acrylic, vinyl polymers copolymers, as well as natural and silicone rubber products, have been used as denture liners. As mentioned previously, these soft liners are suggested for use in patients having irritation of the denture-bearing mucosa, areas of severe undercuts, or con-

genital or acquired defects of the palate. Some products reportedly have an inhibitory effect on the growth of *Candida albicans* whereas others appear to support the growth of microorganisms. Desirable properties are (1) high bond strength to the denture base, (2) dimensional stability of the liner during and after processing, (3) permanent softness or resilience, (4) low water sorption, (5) color stability, (6) ease of processing, and (7) biocompatibility. Soft liners may be mouth-cured or processed in the laboratory.

Mouth-cured soft liners

Mouth-cured soft liners are used for short periods (up to several weeks) to improve the comfort and fit of an old denture until it can be remade or permanently relined. After several weeks they may begin to foul and debond from the denture. They are mixed chairside, placed in the denture, and seated in the patient's mouth until polymerized, which generally takes a few minutes. Two types of materials are generally used:

1. Powder—poly(ethyl methacrylate) and peroxide initiator; liquid—aromatic esters, ethanol, and tertiary amines.
2. Powder—poly(ethyl methacrylate), plasticizers such as ethyl glycolate, and a peroxide initiator; liquid—methyl methacrylate and tertiary amines.

TABLE 19-11 Viscosity of Tissue Conditioners 2 Hours after Mixing

Material	Liquid/Powder Ratio	Viscosity (10^6 poise)	
		(20° C)	(37.4° C)
A	1.03	2.00	1.20
B	0.98	7.40	4.90
C	0.97	2.73	1.30
D	0.98	5.75	1.87
E	0.89	6.75	3.78
F	1.03	2.70	1.23
	0.8	5.80	2.455
G	1.04	0.187	0.029
	0.77	3.98	–
H	1.15	0.78	–
I	1.01	1.16	2.66
J	0.92	1.47	–

Adapted from Braden M: *J Dent Res* 49:496, 1970.

Biocompatibility of these materials is of interest because it has been demonstrated both *in vitro* and *in vivo* that both tissue conditioners and chairside soft liners leach out significant amounts of alcohol and phthalate esters.

Processed soft liners

Processed soft liners are used with denture patients who experience chronic soreness with their dentures because of heavy bruxism or poor health. Although these materials fulfill a need, they will not last long in use. A year is considered good service. These materials tend to pull away from the denture base or become porous and foul smelling. They are processed in the laboratory in a manner similar to processing of a denture base. Finishing of soft denture liners is often difficult as a result of the resilient nature of the material. Several types of processed soft liners are available and include plasticized acrylics, plasticized vinyl acrylics, heat- and room temperature–cured silicones, hydrophilic acrylates, and more recently a polyphosphazine. The compositions of various commercial products of plasticized acrylic and silicones are shown in Tables 19-12 and 19-13.

Several physical properties determined 24 hours after processing are seen in Table 19-14 for four categories of laboratory-processed soft liners. For all materials there is a wide range of properties. This variability is difficult to interpret because there is no ANSI/ADA specification for laboratory processed soft liners. For example, a plasticized acrylic may have very high tear resistance but at the same time also may have a high Shore A hardness value. Because softer materials are generally considered kinder to the tissues, the gain in tear resistance is offset by hardness. Conversely, a silicone soft liner may have a low Shore A hardness value and low tear resistance. Many of these materials tend to increase in hardness with time, and the physical and mechanical properties also are affected by prolonged storage in water or in the oral environment.

Water solubility and sorption of soft liners is complex. When placed in water, plasticizers and other components may leach out over extended periods while water is absorbed until equilibrium is reached. Absorbed water can have a detrimental effect on the adhesion of soft liners to acrylic denture bases, particularly if the rate of diffusion is rapid. At 1 week, water sorption will range from 0.2 to 5.6 mg/cm^2 and solubility will range from 0.03 to 0.40 mg/cm^2 for various commercial products. An ideal processed soft liner would have no soluble components and would have low water sorption.

Processed soft liners are intended to be used for extended periods. In some patients it has been observed that a yeast, *Candida albicans,* and other microorganisms may grow on and within the liner, resulting in a rough and hardened surface. Antimicrobial agents have been proposed to eliminate this problem. Color changes have also been demonstrated for some liners subjected to accelerated aging.

Silicone liners do not adhere as well to denture bases as plasticized acrylic resin. When a peel test is used, the adhesion of silicone liners (0.6×10^2 Nm^{-2}) may be less than 25% of plasticized acrylic (2.3×10^2 Nm^{-2}). Some silicone liners also have poor tear resistance, particularly after storage in water for extended periods.

TABLE 19-12   Composition of Plasticized Acrylic Soft Lining Materials

Material	Polymer	Monomer	Plasticizer	Percentage of Plasticizer
A	Poly(ethyl methacrylate)	Methyl methacrylate	Butyl phthalyl butyl glycollate	31.2
B	Poly(ethyl methacrylate)	*n*-Butyl methacrylate	Butyl phthalyl butyl glycollate	24.9
C	Poly(methyl methacrylate)	Methyl methacrylate	Butyl phthalyl butyl glycollate	58.8
D	Poly(ethyl methacrylate)	Methyl methacrylate + Ethyl acetate	Di-*n*-butyl phthalate	36.2
E	Poly(ethyl methacrylate)	Ethyl methacrylate	2-Ethylhexyl diphenyl phosphate	39.0

Adapted from Wright RS: *J Dent* 9:210, 1981.

TABLE 19-13 Composition of Silicone Soft Lining Materials

Material	Polymer	Cross-Linking Agent	Catalyst	Percentage of Filler	Adhesive
A	α-ω-dihydroxy end-blocked poly(dimethyl siloxane)	Triethoxy silanol	Dibutyltin dilaurate	34.5	Silicone polymer in solvent
B	α-ω-dihydroxy end-blocked poly(dimethyl siloxane)	Ethyl polysilicate	Dibutyltin dilaurate	16.5	Silicone polymer in solvent
C	α-ω-dihydroxy end-blocked poly(dimethyl siloxane)	Tetraethoxy silane	Stannous octoate	42.6	Silicone polymer in solvent
D	α-ω-dihydroxy end-blocked poly(dimethyl siloxane)	Methyltriacetoxy silane	Moisture	11.35	Silicone polymer in solvent
E	α-ω-dihydroxy end-blocked poly(dimethyl siloxane)	Acryloxyalkyl silane	Heat + Benzoyl peroxide	21.5	γ-Methacryloxypropyl trimethoxysilane

Adapted from Wright RS: *J Dent* 9:210, 1981.

TABLE 19-14 Properties of Laboratory-Processed Soft Liners

Materials	Tensile Strength (kg/cm^2)	Percent Elongation	Hardness Shore A	Tear Resistance (kg/cm)
Plasticized poly(methyl methacrylate)	8.1–84.9	150–300	30–95	3–26
Plasticized vinyl acrylics	20–37	250–280	35–55	5–11
Silicones	25–44	325–340	25–45	5–7
Polyphosphazine	37	240	50	9

Adapted from Dootz ER, Koran A, Craig RG: *J Prosthet Dent* 67:707, 1992.

The bond strength for the materials listed in Table 19-14 are seen in Table 19-15. The materials were tested in a two-phase tensile test. Two test conditions were used. The soft liners were processed against both polymerized and unpolymerized acrylic resin. Again the results were variable. For both test conditions the polyphosphazine material demonstrated higher bond strength. It also was surprising that for three of the four groups, the bond strength was higher to polymerized acrylic than to unpolymerized acrylic. Most manufacturers recommend processing the soft liner and the denture base acrylic at the same time to improve the bond strength. Only the plasticized vinyl acrylic had a higher bond strength when processed against unpolymerized acrylic.

Unfortunately, many of the short- and long-term resilient denture liners contain significant amounts of plasticizers, many of which have questionable biocompatibility. The phthalate esters have caused epithelial changes when polymer disks containing these esters have been implanted in the hampster cheek pouch. The potentially premalignant changes are a cause for concern because the amount of this plasticizer leached from a typical soft liner may be between 10 and 40 times greater than environmental and food uptake. Although even this amount of plasticizer is low, demonstrated biocompatibility of soft denture liners should be considered.

Recently, a rather unique concept in soft denture liners has been introduced. In this technique a soft

TABLE 19-15   Bond Strength of Laboratory Processed Soft Denture Liners

Materials	Processed to Unpolymerized PMMA (kg/cm^2)	Processed to Polymerized PMMA (kg/cm^2)
Plasticized poly(methyl methacrylate)	5–13	11–17
Plasticized vinyl acrylics	27	11
Silicones	8.6–14	10–18
Polyphosphazine	20	26

Adapted from Kawano F, Dootz ER, Koran A, Craig RG: *J Prosthet Dent* 68:367, 1992.

denture liner is made from an envelope covered with a polyethylene film and filled with a viscous silicone liquid. This soft liner is designed to allow continuous adaptation of the denture base. The method is interesting and warrants further evaluation.

It appears that soft liners will have a place in denture prosthetics in the future, but improved strength, adhesion to the denture base, and the growth of microorganisms are problems that need to be solved before these materials will be considered permanent.

■ DENTURE TEETH

Plastic teeth are prepared from acrylic and modified acrylic materials similar to denture plastics. Different pigments are used to produce the various tooth shades, and usually a cross-linking is used to improve strength and prevent crazing. Plastic teeth are prepared in layers of different colors so that the shade is gradually lightened toward the incisal and occlusal portions to give these areas a translucent appearance. The gingival or body portion may not be as highly cross-linked as the incisal or occlusal portion. This is done to improve the chemical bond between the teeth and the denture base. Fillers also may be added to increase resistance to wear. Recently, composite materials have received some interest as denture tooth materials.

As indicated in the discussion on physical properties of dental plastics, poly(methyl methacrylate) has satisfactory chemical properties for use as plastic teeth. It is nontoxic and insoluble in oral fluids but is soluble to some extent in ketones and aromatic hydrocarbons. The mechanical properties of com-

pressive strength (76 MPa), abrasion resistance, elastic modulus (2700 MPa), elastic limit (55 MPa), and hardness (18 to 20 kg/mm^2) are low when compared with other restorative materials or with human enamel and dentin.

Of necessity, a discussion of the merits of plastic teeth includes a general comparison of the properties of plastic and porcelain teeth, a number of which are listed in Table 19-16. Certain properties may be listed as a disadvantage or an advantage depending on the particular purpose and point of view involved. For example, the softness and low abrasion resistance of plastic teeth may be cited as a disadvantage because the teeth are more easily abraded and the occlusion and vertical dimension of the denture may be altered. The low wear resistance also has been quoted as an advantage, however because plastic teeth are easy to grind and polish, and they tend to be self-adjusting in service. The hardness of porcelain teeth compared with plastic teeth is an advantage, whereas the resulting brittleness of porcelain compared with the toughness of plastic teeth is a disadvantage.

One may summarize the main difference between porcelain and plastic teeth by stating that plastic teeth are softer but tougher than porcelain teeth. This difference also is reflected in the low elastic modulus, low resistance to cold flow, low abrasion resistance, and high impact strength of plastic teeth. Both plastic and porcelain teeth are insoluble in oral fluids; in addition, porcelain teeth are resistant to organic solvents such as ketones and aromatic hydrocarbons, which will attack non-cross-linked plastic teeth. This advantage is slight because the

TABLE 19-16   Comparison of Properties of Plastic and Porcelain Teeth

Plastic Teeth	Porcelain Teeth
High resilience	Very brittle
Tough	Friable
Soft–low abrasion resistance	Hard–high abrasion resistance
Insoluble in mouth fluids–some dimensional change	Inert in mouth fluids–no dimensional change
Low heat-distortion temperature, cold flow under pressure	High heat-distortion temperature; no permanent deformation under forces of mastication
Bond to denture base plastic	Poor bond-to-denture base plastic*; mechanical retention provided in tooth design
Natural appearance	Natural appearance
Natural feel–silent	Possible clicking sound in use
Easy to grind and polish	Grinding removes surface glaze
Crazing and blanching–if non-cross-linked	Occasional cracking

*Does not apply if silane-treated.

denture base is plastic and also is attacked by these organic solvents. The plastic teeth composed of poly(methyl methacrylate) change dimensions, as all acrylic teeth do when placed in water. As expected, vinyl acrylic teeth do not show as much dimensional change as the totally acrylic teeth. Porcelain teeth show no dimensional change when stored in water and exhibit no permanent deformation from forces exerted on them in the mouth.

The coefficient of friction of acrylic against acrylic in the presence of water or saliva is lower than the coefficient for porcelain against porcelain. The lowest coefficients of friction, however, are obtained when porcelain and acrylic specimens oppose each other.

In Fig. 19-17 the frictional behavior of acrylic denture teeth is shown for central incisors from two manufacturers. The tangential force on a diamond slider being drawn across the teeth was measured under various loads in distilled water. The width of the wear track was also measured. In general, low values of track width occurred with low tangential force values, and higher track widths and more severe surface failure were associated with higher values of tangential force. The "enamel" surfaces, which were the labial surfaces of the teeth, were more resistant to penetration and surface damage than the "dentin" surfaces, which were prepared by removal of 1 mm of acrylic from the ridge lap area of the tooth.

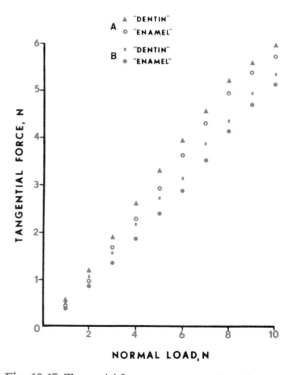

Fig. 19-17 Tangential force versus normal load for a diamond slider on "enamel" and "dentin" surfaces of two manufacturers' acrylic teeth (*A* and *B*) in water. (Adapted from Raptis CM, Powers JM, Fan PL: *J Dent Res* 60:908, 1981.)

Plastic teeth possess low heat-distortion temperatures, although the use of cross-linked plastics has improved this property considerably. Care should be taken not to flame plastic teeth during the preparation of a waxed denture. Porcelain teeth have high heat-distortion temperatures; however, sudden temperature changes may cause crazing or cracking. As indicated previously, plastic teeth exhibit cold flow, or permanent deformation, under stresses below their elastic limit, and their dimensions may be altered slightly during use. Plastic teeth are of a similar material to the denture base and may be chemically bonded to the base. The bond strength between chemically accelerated acrylics and plastic teeth is lower, and the use of mechanical retention on the underside of the teeth may prove useful. Highly cross-linked acrylic denture teeth also may be treated with 4-methacryloxyethyl trimellitic anhydride to improve the bond strength to denture base resins. An adhesive containing this compound also is available for bonding acrylic to nickel-chromium and cobalt-chromium metal denture bases. This allows for adding acrylic posterior palatal seals to metal bases or relining metal base dentures when necessary.

Porcelain teeth usually are constructed so that mechanical retention in the denture base occurs. It has been shown that treatment of porcelain teeth with a silane coupling agent, such as γ-methacryloxypropyltrimethoxy silane, provides a surface treatment that allows the teeth to be chemically bonded to the denture base material. When the bond was tested in tension, the porcelain, rather than the bond, ruptured. The use of cross-linked acrylic teeth has made the chemical bonding to the denture base more difficult, and therefore mechanical retention is often provided for plastic teeth. The chemical bond produced between the plastic and porcelain teeth and the denture base has the distinct advantage of preventing capillary spaces around the teeth, which are difficult to clean and are prone to microorganism growth.

Both types of artificial teeth have a realistic appearance, but the noise or clicking of porcelain teeth rubbing against each other is about three times greater than plastic against porcelain or plastic against plastic. The processing of a single tooth replacement and the characterization of plastic teeth are considerably easier than for porcelain teeth. In addition, plastic teeth may be ground and polished with ease, whereas grinding of porcelain teeth removes the surface glaze, making repolishing more difficult. Porcelain teeth should not be used opposing natural teeth or gold restorations because excessive wear will occur.

The choice between plastic and porcelain teeth depends to a great extent on the preferences of the dentist and the patient. Plastic teeth are used opposite natural teeth or gold restorations and in patients poor ridge conditions or limited space. Porcelain teeth are indicated for patients who have good ridge support, adequate space, and both maxillary and mandibular dentures. There is no ANSI/ADA specification available for porcelain teeth, although one is available for plastic teeth.

ANSI/ADA Specification No. 15 for Plastic Teeth

On the basis of the desired properties available for plastic teeth, ANSI/ADA Specification No. 15 has been developed. Only an abstract of this specification is included here because a large number of requirements are listed.

Types of teeth: anatomical anterior teeth and anatomical and nonanatomical posterior teeth

Materials: polyacrylates, substituted polyacrylates, polyvinyl esters, polystyrenes, and copolymers or mixtures of these plastics

Size and shape: as specified by the purchaser

Blend: teeth shall consist of a gingival or body portion and a more translucent incisal or occlusal portion, with gradual shading between portions

Color: as specified by the purchaser; natural shades ranging from light to dark that shall match the shade guide

Porosity: none on or 2 mm below the surface at $10\times$

Surface finish: retained on processing or reprocessing with slight buffing; also certified that no stain will occur in service and that any deposit can be removed with slight buffing

Bonding: chemically bonds to base; bond strength or tooth strength of 31 MPa

Hardness: KHN not less than 15 kg/mm^2

Indentation resistance: gingival portion; not less than 0.11 mm by 12.7 mm steel ball at 30 kg load for 10 minutes; recovery at least 80% in 10 minutes after load release

Blushing: none, and no color change when heated in 100° C water for 3 hours

Distortion: no distortion when heated in 100° C water for 3 hours

Craze resistance: shall be resistant before and after curing cycle in water bath

Color stability: not more than slight color change by using ANSI/ADA Specification No. 12 ultraviolet lamp test

Most of the requirements for plastic teeth are self-explanatory or have been discussed previously. The requirement of indentation resistance involves several physical properties, which may not be evident. The indentation resistance of the plastic to a 12.7-mm steel ball loaded to 30 kg is a measure of the hardness of the material. The size of the indentation depends on the amount of permanent deformation and the retarded elastic deformation of the plastic. This retarded elastic deformation gradually recovers with time, and the indentation decreases until it represents the permanent deformation. The specification requires that the recovery be at least 80% after 10 minutes or that the permanent deformation be only 20% of the initial value.

■ MAXILLOFACIAL MATERIALS

Maxillofacial materials are used to correct facial defects resulting from cancer surgery, accidents, or even congenital deformities. Noses, ears, eyes and orbits, or any other part of the head and neck may be replaced by these prostheses (Fig. 19-18).

Maxillofacial prostheses are difficult to construct and have a relatively short life of 6 months to several years in service. They fail because of inherent problems with static and dynamic properties over varying periods and because of color degradation. The prostheses are expensive to fabricate, and many patients cannot afford frequent replacement.

Several types of materials are available for maxillofacial prostheses, and they vary considerably in ease of preparation and physical properties.

Poly(methyl methacrylate)

Poly(methyl methacrylate) was once commonly used for maxillofacial prostheses, and it is still used occasionally to make artificial facial parts. When properly pigmented, these prostheses can look quite realistic. The main disadvantages are that the acrylic is hard and heavy, does not flex when the face moves, and does not have the feel of skin. Stone molds are generally used with poly(methyl methacrylate), and these are sacrificed when the prosthesis is deflasked after processing.

Plasticized polyvinylchloride

Polyvinylchloride has been used widely for maxillofacial applications, but it has been replaced by newer materials with superior properties. Polyvinylchloride is a rigid plastic with a glass tran-

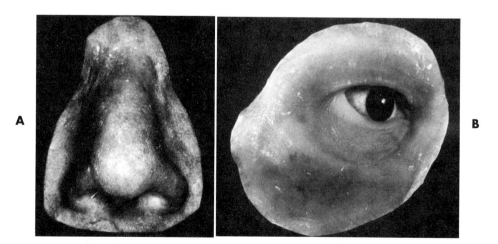

Fig. 19-18 Maxillofacial appliances. **A,** Nose. **B,** Eye and orbit. (From Craig RG, editor: *Dental materials: a problem-oriented approach,* St Louis, 1978, Mosby.)

sition temperature higher than room temperature. For maxillofacial applications, plasticizers are added to produce an elastomer at room temperature. Other ingredients added to polyvinylchloride include cross-linking agents for added strength and ultraviolet stabilizers for color stability. There is no chemical reaction involved when the material is processed. The product is supplied as finely divided polyvinylchloride particles suspended in a solvent. When the fluid is heated above a critical temperature, the polyvinylchloride will dissolve in the solvent. When the mix is cooled, an elastic solid is formed. Plasticized polyvinylchloride is processed at 150° C, and metal molds are generally used.

Polyurethane

Polyurethanes are used as maxillofacial materials. The formation of polyurethane is the result of the direct addition of diisocyanate to a polyol in the presence of an initiator, as shown below. An isophorone polyurethane has also been used as a maxillofacial material.

$$O=C=N-R-N=C=O + OH\sim OH \xrightarrow{\text{Initiator}}$$

Diisocyanate   **Polyol**

$$O=C=N-R-\overset{H}{\underset{|}{N}}-\overset{O}{\underset{\|}{C}}-O\sim O-\overset{O}{\underset{\|}{C}}-\overset{H}{\underset{|}{N}}-R-\overset{H}{\underset{|}{N}}-\overset{O}{\underset{\|}{C}}-O-$$

Polyurethane

The reaction must be carried out in a dry atmosphere, or carbon dioxide will be produced and a porous elastomer will result. The diisocyanates are very toxic and must be handled with extreme care. The processing temperature of 100° C is reasonable, and stone molds can be used.

Heat-vulcanized silicone

The heat-vulcanized silicones are used occasionally for maxillofacial prostheses. The vulcanization mechanism is achieved by an addition reaction. The components of heat-vulcanized silicones are a polydimethylvinyl siloxane copolymer with approximately 0.5% vinyl side chains, 2,4-dichlorobenzoyl peroxide as an initiator, and a silica filler obtained from burning methyl silanes (see following). Vulcanization results from thermal decomposition of the initiator to form free radicals that cross-link the copolymer into a three-

Polydimethylvinyl siloxane

2,4-Dichlorobenzoyl peroxide

dimensional structure. The processing temperature is 220° C, and metal molds are used. The copolymer is supplied as a rubbery solid with a high viscosity. The pigments are incorporated into the polymer with roller mills. Although this material is more difficult to pigment and process, excellent results can be obtained.

Room temperature–vulcanized silicones

Room temperature–vulcanized (RTV) silicones have become popular as maxillofacial materials not only because of good physical properties but also because they are easy materials to process. Currently, they are used more often than any other material. They have good physical and mechanical properties, are easy to color and process, and allow the use of stone molds. There has been a steady improvement in the physical and mechanical properties of these materials. They are affected by accelerated aging, but not to a degree that would compromise usefullness as maxillofacial materials. These RTV silicones are similar to addition silicone impression materials in that they consist of vinyl- and hydride-containing siloxanes and are polymerized with a chloroplatinic acid catalyst.

Experimental elastomers

Several elastomers have been investigated for use as maxillofacial materials: aliphatic polyurethanes, chlorinated polyethylene, silphenylene polymers, organophosphazenes, butadiene-styrene butadiene-acrylonitrile, and silicone-PMMA block copolymers.

Fabrication of the prostheses

The method for fabricating a prosthesis is similar for most materials. An impression is made of the affected area with alginate. A master cast is poured that is a duplicate of the defect on the patient. The artificial part (such as a nose) is then carved in wax or clay on the master cast and tried on the patient to see if it fulfills the esthetic requirements for form.

The pattern is then invested in a manner similar to that used for complete dentures. In fact, denture flasks often are used for this purpose. When the prosthesis is quite complex (such as an eye and orbit), three- or four-part molds are made. With some materials, metal models and molds are required because of high processing temperatures. After the pattern is invested, it is removed from the mold by use of a boiling water bath.

The mold is now ready to make the prosthesis. At this time, the patient should be present so that pigments may be added to the elastomer to give a realistic appearance and match the patient's skin color. Generally, dry mineral earth pigments or artist's oil-base pigments are used. Color matching is done by mixing small amounts of the pigments into the elastomer. Some clinicians use color tabs and predetermined pigment formulations to match skin color. When a color match is achieved, the elastomer is compression molded and processed according to the manufacturer's instructions.

After processing, the prosthesis is removed from the mold and the excess flash is removed. The prosthesis is then delivered to the patient. Surface pigmentation is generally done to give the prosthesis a more lifelike appearance. When mechanical undercuts are not present for retention, the patient may use adhesives to keep the prosthesis in place.

Physical properties

The static and dynamic properties of the more popular maxillofacial materials are shown in Table 19-17. Values are representative of the best commercial products in each category.

Heat-vulcanized silicone has the highest tensile strength at 59.8 kg/cm^2 and polyurethane has the lowest at 8.52 kg/cm^2. The remaining materials have tensile strengths about 30% lower than the heat-vulcanized material. Tensile strength is important because when the patient removes the prosthesis, high tensile forces are applied, particularly in thin areas.

Three of the materials are similar in maximum percent elongation with values from 422% to 445%. Plasticized polyvinylchloride has a lower percent elongation at 215%. Knowing the percent elongation is helpful because different parts of the face have different requirements in terms of how far the elastomer must stretch to accommodate facial movement.

Tear resistance is important for maxillofacial materials because prostheses may be torn when patients remove them. In the pants tear test, a thin sheet of the elastomer is made in the shape of a pair of pants. The "legs" of the pants are then pulled slowly apart, and the energy required to propagate a tear is measured. The heat-vulcanized silicone and RTV silicone have excellent tear resistance because the samples did not tear but stretched, as in tensile elongation. The plasticized polyvinylchloride and polyurethane have good tear resistance at 4.3×10^6 and 6.7×10^6 dynes/cm, respectively.

TABLE 19-17 Static and Dynamic Properties of Maxillofacial Materials

Material	Ultimate Tensile Strength (kg/cm^2)	Maximum Elongation (%)	Pants Tear Energy (dynes/cm × 10^6)	Dynamic Modulus (kg/cm^2)
Plasticized polyvinylchloride	40.7	215	4.3	44.0
Polyurethane	8.5	422	6.7	35.3
Heat-vulcanized silicone	59.8	441	Does not tear but stretches, as in tensile elongation	47.5
RTV silicone	42.8	445	Does not tear but stretches, as in tensile elongation	21.6

The evaluation of maxillofacial materials should involve not only the static but also the dynamic physical properties because the stress-strain curves for elastomers are nonlinear, which causes them to function differently at high and low rates of loading. The dynamic modulus is the ratio of stress to strain applied for small cyclic deformations at a given frequency at a specified point on the normal stress-strain curve, or it is the slope of the stress-strain curve at a given point corresponding to a given frequency.

In practical terms, elastomers with a high dynamic modulus are rather rigid materials, whereas materials with a low dynamic modulus are more flexible. In Table 19-17 the heat-vulcanized silicone has the highest dynamic modulus at 47.5 kg/cm^2, and the RTV silicone has the lowest dynamic modulus at 21.6 kg/cm^2.

Efforts have been made to modify the stress-strain properties of maxillofacial materials to match living facial tissues. Medical-grade silicone adhesive has been combined with an RTV silicone base in various ratios to control the elastic properties. The stress-strain profiles of human facial tissues and various ratios of the silicone elastomers are shown in Fig. 19-19. The curves demonstrate that it is possible to formulate silicones that will match the elastic properties of facial tissues.

Major advances have been made in the last few years in the area of maxillofacial materials. It seems likely that in the not-too-distant future it may be possible to make very lifelike maxillofacial prostheses that will last longer in a service environment.

■ PLASTIC FACINGS FOR CROWN AND BRIDGE APPLICATIONS

Before the introduction of porcelain-fused-to-metal crowns, acrylic facings were the only type available for crown facings. Currently, porcelain facings have replaced acrylic in all but a few applications. When used for facings, the acrylic materials are similar in composition and properties to the best available denture teeth.

■ TEMPORARY CROWN AND BRIDGE RESTORATIONS

Chemically accelerated plastics have become popular as temporary restorations. They have decreased the use of aluminum shell and polycarbonate temporary crowns because they are easy to fabricate and are esthetic. They are similar to chemically accelerated denture base plastics and are available in several shades to approximate the color of the patient's

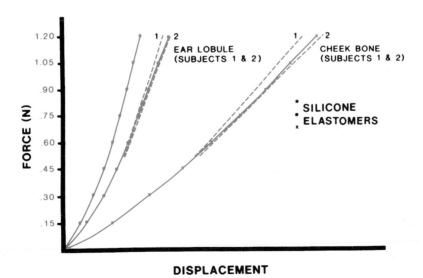

Fig. 19-19 Stress-strain properties of human facial tissues and various silicone elastomers. (Adapted from Farah JW, Robinson JC, Hood JAA, Koran A, Craig RG: *J Oral Rehabil* 15:277, 1988.)

teeth. In one widely accepted technic, a thin polystyrene sheet is heated and then vacuum-formed over a wet gypsum model of the patient's teeth taken before tooth preparation. The thin template is then trimmed to include the teeth to be prepared and the teeth on either side. In the case of a bridge, a denture tooth can be waxed to the model before vacuum-forming, and this allows space in the template for the pontic of the temporary bridge. After the teeth are prepared for crowns and the final impression has been made, the thin polystyrene template is used to make the temporary restoration. The tooth preparations are lubricated, and the chemically accelerated plastic powder and liquid are mixed and placed into the template in the area of the restorations. Chemically activated temporary resins are now also available in automixing syringes and can be directly injected into the matrix. When the acrylic approaches the doughy stage, the template and acrylic are placed over the prepared teeth and seated. The patient is then asked to bring the teeth into occlusion. The temporary restoration may be removed and cooled in water several times during polymerization to control the heat and then reinserted into the mouth. When the restoration is still slightly elastic, it is removed from the mouth and allowed to continue polymerization at room temperature. The restoration is then trimmed, polished, and cemented to the prepared teeth with a temporary cement. The resulting restoration simulates the teeth as they were before preparation and has acceptable esthetics. There is generally little trouble with the occlusion because the teeth are in contact during polymerization. In the dental literature there are reports of some allergic reactions to the temporary crown and bridge plastics, and they are believed to be caused by monomer or the amine accelerator. Heat generation from polymerization also can be harmful to the teeth. Using thermocouples and extracted teeth prepared for crowns, temperatures of 40° to 84° C have been recorded in the pulp chambers during polymerization. With external cooling of a restoration, the temperature rise is minimal.

Accuracy of various products should be considered when selecting a material. Marginal opening can be caused by the polymerization shrinkage.

Light-activated polymers used to make temporary restorations are available in several tooth shades. The method used is similar to that used for chemically activated acrylics but with several advantages. The material can be removed from the mouth in the template, the flash can be removed before curing, and the restoration can be reinserted several times to ensure easy seating after processing. The final polymerization is done in a light chamber identical to that used for processing light-activated denture bases. The light-activated material allows fast and accurate fabrication of temporary restorations, and it has the added advantage of no methyl methacrylate monomer in the formulation, thus reducing the potential for allergic reactions.

Light-activated and chemically activated composites are also gaining popularity for use as temporary restorations. A review of these materials is found in Chapter 10.

■ OCCLUSAL SPLINTS

The use of occlusal splints in the treatment of patients with temporomandibular joint syndrome has become a routine procedure. These splints are made by the same technique used for processing dentures. The splint is waxed on a model of the patient's teeth, usually the maxillary arch. The model and wax pattern are invested in a denture flask, and the wax is boiled out. After cooling, alginate separator is painted onto the mold and allowed to dry. A clear, heat-accelerated acrylic resin is packed into the mold and processed. The acrylic resin is mixed and packed when it has reached the doughy stage. Chemically accelerated acrylic resin also may be used, but less often. The properties of acrylic splints are similar to those of heat-accelerated denture materials. Recently, a clear light-activated acrylic has been introduced that simplifies the construction of occlusal splints. A major advantage is that the splint can be made quickly and without flasking.

■ ATHLETIC MOUTH PROTECTORS

The use of custom-made rather than stock tray athletic mouth protectors has been increasing rapidly. Materials used for this application include plasticized acrylic polymers, vinyl acetate–ethylene copolymers, silicone rubber, rubber latex, and polyurethane, with the vinyl acetate–ethylene copolymer type becoming the most popular. The plasticized acrylic material is formed into a mouth protector by a method similar to processing a denture.

The vinyl acetate–ethylene copolymers are supplied in 3.2-mm thick sheets that are softened by heating and adapted to the cast by a variety of methods such as hand pressure, vacuum, or pressure forming. Polyurethane polymers also are supplied in the form of sheets, but because of the high softening temperature, pressure forming is necessary for proper adaptation to the cast. The latex products are painted on the model, and then the moisture is driven off by heating in an oven. Chemically accelerated silicones have been used for mouth protectors by actually forming the material around the teeth after mixing and allowing it to polymerize in the mouth.

Evaluation of the physical properties of poly-vinylacetate–polyethylene (PVAC-PE) products have a wide range of values, as indicated in Table 19-18. This variation results from the use of various copolymers and the selection or use of fillers. The polyurethane materials are characterized by high water sorption and high energy absorption when struck by an 18.8-mm diameter steel ball. The latex material has low strength, hardness, and energy absorption. It also has been demonstrated that the static and dynamic properties of various mouthguard materials are altered in time by saliva, as seen in Table 19-19. The data represent the properties of two commercial mouth-guard materials before and after they were worn by 280 football players 9 to 12 years of age. Significant changes are seen in

dynamic modulus (23° and 37° C), tensile strength, and tear strength for both materials.

Numerous studies have shown the advantage of wearing athletic mouth protectors in contact sports, and it appears that almost any type of protector worn by the player is better than not wearing one. Such factors as comfort, ease of speaking or breathing, and esthetics may control the selection of material. Studies of the stress transferred to models through mouth protectors show that the thickness is critical and that most of the thicker stock mouth protectors transfer less stress than the thinner, custom-made varieties. For example, increasing the thickness of the latex protector from 1.5 to 2 mm produces a significant decrease in the stress transferred. The polyurethane protector, which has the highest energy absorption, also transfers the most stress to the teeth on the model. Therefore energy absorption alone should not be used to select a material for a mouth protector.

■ INLAY PATTERNS

Chemically accelerated acrylic is used to fabricate inlay patterns and direct posts and cores. Commercial products have good dimensional stability and are convenient to use. The pattern is made by painting the powder-liquid onto the die or tooth in layers and allowing it to polymerize. After polymerization, the pattern can be modified with stones and burs. If necessary, inlay wax may be added to complete the pattern. Considerably longer burnout times must be used with acrylic patterns.

TABLE 19-18   Physical Properties of Materials Used for Custom-Made Mouth Protectors

Property	Polyvinylacetate-Polyethylene	Polyurethane	Latex
Tensile strength (MPa)	6.9–13.8	18.6	5.0
Elongation (%)	700–1000	450	780
Tear strength (N/cm)	244–454	646	279
Hardness, Shore A	67–90	80	35
Water sorption, equilibrium (mg/cm^2)	0.1–0.4	2.8	—
Water solubility, equilibrium (mg/cm^2)	0.01–0.02	0.06	—
Energy absorption (cm-N)	30.4	46.2	20.2
Energy absorption (%)	56	84	37

TABLE 19-19   Properties of Mouth Protector Materials Before and After Use

Material	Dynamic Modulus (MPa)		Dynamic Resilience (%)		Tensile Strength (MPa)	Tear Strength (N/cm)	Shore A Hardness
	23° C	37° C	23° C	37° C			
Sta-Guard							
Before use	13.7	9.4	27.7	23.4	3.0	240	71
After use	11.8	7.2	25.8	20.2	2.1	250	66
Proform							
Before use	22.5	15.7	34.7	30.7	4.4	320	82
After use	21.1	14.0	34.9	30.1	3.0	380	82

Adapted from Godwin WC, Craig RG, Koran A, Lang BR, Powers JM: *Physician and Sportsmedicine* 10:47, 1982.

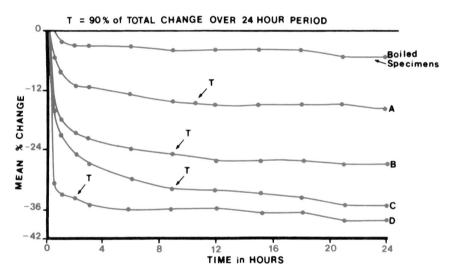

Fig. 19-20 Dimensional change of various tray materials. *A* to *D,* During 24 hours. (Adapted from Pagniano RP, Schied RC, Clowson RL, Dagefoerde RO, Zardiackas LD: *J Prosthet Dent* 47:280, 1982.)

■ IMPRESSION TRAYS AND RECORD BASES

Chemically accelerated acrylic is used to produce impression trays. These trays provide a nearly constant distance between the tray and the tissues. This results in a more even distribution of the impression material during the impression procedure, resulting in improved accuracy. The same material also may be used to make record bases for prosthetic applications. The principal change in the composition of the plastics for this purpose is the addition of substantial quantities of fillers, which decrease the warpage of the material during setting. Shrinkage of chemically accelerated acrylic trays can occur for up to 7 days, although the greatest shrinkage takes place during the first 24 hours. The dimensional changes of five commercially available tray materials are shown in Fig. 19-20. Significant shrinkage occurs after the initial polymerization. The products differ considerably in the length of time required to reach 90% of the total dimensional change. Although the maximum shrinkage is less than 0.4%, chemically accelerated acrylic impression trays should be allowed to stand from 2 to 9 hours, depending on the product, if dimensional changes are to be minimized. In practice, many dentists have a dental laboratory fabricate the impression trays, and the time between fabrication and use will be adequate. If trays are to be used soon after fabrication, the tray should be boiled for 5 minutes and then cooled to room temperature before use.

Vacuum-formed polystyrene also is used to make impression trays and baseplates. This material is popular with commercial laboratories because the trays and record bases can be made rapidly. These trays must be handled carefully because they are more flexible than acrylic trays and can be deformed easily by the application of heat.

Light-activated tray materials have become quite popular and have many advantages over chemically accelerated acrylic. They are similar to light-activated denture base materials but are of a different color. The trays are easy to make, contain no methyl methacrylate, and have negligible polymerization shrinkage in the light chamber. They can be used soon after processing because there is no clinically significant dimensional change after polymerization.

SELECTED PROBLEMS

Problem 1. A denture is to be made for a patient who has previously fractured a denture several times. How will this influence your choice of a denture base material?

Solution. A rubber-reinforced acrylic is the material of choice because this type of denture base material exhibits superior impact resistance and flexural fatigue strength. A metal base also might be used in cases where maximum strength is desired.

Problem 2. A denture is delivered from a dental laboratory with obvious porosity in the denture base. Why might this have occurred? Where is the porosity most likely to occur, and why?

Solution. Several conditions may have caused the porosity. Most commonly, the processing temperature exceeded 74° C. Other causes may be insufficient flask pressure, excessive monomer in the mix, and packing of the material before it reached the doughy consistency. Porosity almost always will occur in the thicker sections of acrylic because the polymerization reaction is exothermic and the heat cannot be dissipated as quickly from the larger mass.

Problem 3. A patient is having a maxillary denture made that opposes a natural dentition in the mandible. Should acrylic or porcelain teeth be used, and why?

Solution. Acrylic teeth always should be used when opposing natural teeth or restored teeth. Porcelain teeth

are abrasive against these surfaces, and excessive wear will quickly occur.

Problem 4. A patient has a history of sensitivity to denture base materials. In making a new denture for this patient, what might decrease the potential for an allergic reaction?

Solution. Residual monomer is almost always the cause of an allergic or toxic reaction to a denture base material. To reduce the residual monomer content to a very low level, the denture should be boiled for at least 1 hour at the end of the processing cycle. Another choice might include the selection of a light-activated denture base material.

Problem 5. A new set of dentures is delivered to a patient, and there is no retention on the maxillary denture. At the trial-denture stage, there was good retention of the baseplate. What are the probable causes?

Solution. Assuming that a denture base material had passed the ANSI/ADA Specification test, the most probable causes are improper processing variables such as processing too rapidly and at elevated temperatures during the early stages, deflasking before the flask has bench-cooled to near room temperature, quenching the hot flask in cold water, and overheating the denture during trimming and polishing. These processing variables can affect the accuracy of even the best denture base materials.

Problem 6. A finished denture is returned from the laboratory, and in several areas there is insufficient material in the interproximal areas. What is the probable cause?

Solution. The probable cause is packing the denture acrylic when it is not in the doughy consistency. Because of the lower viscosity, even with adequate packing pressure the material will squeeze out of the flask before it is forced into all areas of the mold cavity. Conversely, if the acrylic dough has reached the rubbery consistency, it may be too viscous to fill all areas of the mold.

Problem 7. A patient has fractured a lingual cusp and comes to the office for emergency care. You would like to prepare the tooth for a gold crown, and you would like to have your dental assistant make a custom tray for the final impression while you are preparing the tooth. In terms of the dimensional accuracy of the tray, what must be considered?

Solution. Autopolymerizing tray materials continue to change dimensionally during the first few hours after they are made. Use of a tray before this polymerization is complete can affect the accuracy of the impression. Two things can be done to eliminate this problem: (1) have the dental assistant boil the tray for a short time to force the polymerization reaction to completion or (2) use a light-activated tray material because after processing there is no significant dimensional change.

Problem 8. A patient has excessive wear on the anatomical areas of a denture caused by aggressive cleaning with an abrasive cleaner and a toothbrush. What instructions might you give the patient for cleaning the new denture that you will be making?

Solution. Use a soft toothbrush and soap and water (a nonabrasive hand soap) to regularly clean the denture. The patient may also soak the denture occasionally in a commercial cleanser or a solution of 1 tsp of a hypochlorite, such as Clorox, and 2 tsp of Calgon in half a glass of water. Some immersion cleansers have also been demonstrated to be effective sanitizing agents.

Problem 9. A patient needs a soft denture liner for an extended period. (a) What material would you choose, and what would you tell the patient? (b) What problems are associated with these materials?

Solution a. Both the silicone and plasticized acrylics will work, although the silicones generally are softer with a lower Shore A hardness value. More recently, a polyphosphazine product has received favorable clinical acceptance and has demonstrated excellent bond strength to denture base materials. The patient should be told that any soft liner will have to be replaced occasionally because they are not as long-lasting as the denture base material.

Solution b. Growth of microorganisms, *Candida albicans* in particular; poor adhesion to the denture base; and poor tear strength are deficiencies normally associated with these materials.

Problem 10. A patient requires a maxillofacial prosthesis that includes an area of movable tissue near the mouth. How might a silicone maxillofacial material be modified to be more elastic in this instance?

Solution. Medical-grade silicone adhesive can be combined at various ratios with an RTV silicone base to control the elastic properties. By selecting the proper ratio, the stress-strain profiles of the silicone elastomer can be matched to that of human facial tissues. This is most important when the prosthesis rests on movable tissue.

■ REFERENCES

General

Anthony DH, Gibbons P: The nature and behavior of denture cleansers, *J Prosthet Dent* 8:796, 1958.

Berg E, Gjerdet NR: The effects of pressure and curing temperature on porosity of two chemically activated acrylics, *Dent Mater* 1:204, 1985.

Berzins G: How to bond acrylic to metal, *Trends Tech Contemp Dent Lab* 6:45, 1989.

Craig RG: Denture materials and acrylic base materials, *Curr Opin Dent* 1:235, 1991.

Craig RG, Godwin WC: Physical properties of materials for custom-made mouth protectors, *Mich Dent Assoc J* 49:34, 1967.

Davidson CL, Boere G: Liquid-supported dentures. I. Theoretical and technical considerations, *J Prosthet Dent* 63:303, 1990.

Donovan TE, Hurst RG, Campagni WV: Physical properties of acrylic resin polymerized by four different techniques, *J Prosthet Dent* 54:522, 1985.

Godwin WC, Craig RG, Koran A, Lang BR, Powers JM: Mouth protectors in junior football players, *Physician and Sportsmedicine* 10:41, 1982.

Godwin WC, Koran A, Craig RG: Evaluation of the dynamic and static physical properties of mouth protectors, IADR Abst, *J Dent Res* 53:67, 1974.

Harrison A, Huggett R, Murphy WM: Complete denture construction in general dental practice: an update of the 1970 survey, *Br Dent J* 169:159, 1990.

Moore TC, Smith DE, Kenny GE: Sanitization of dentures by several denture hygiene methods, *J Prosthet Dent* 52:158, 1984.

Pagniano RP, Scheid RC, Clowson RL, Dagefoerde RO, Zardiackas FD: Linear dimensional change of acrylic resins used in the fabrication of custom trays, *J Prosthet Dent* 47:279, 1982.

Powers JM, Fan PL, Dootz ER, Litvin SB: Properties of plastic facing materials, *Mich Dent Assoc J* 63:625, 1981.

Roberts BJ: A study of the viscosity of saliva at different shear rates in dentate and edentulous patients, *J Dent* 5:303, 1977.

Tarbet WJ, Grossman E: Observations of denture-supporting tissue during six months of denture adhesive wearing, *J Am Dent Assoc* 101:789, 1980.

Denture Base Materials

Andreopoulos AG, Polyzois GL, Demetriou PP: Repairs with visible light-curing denture base materials, *Quintess Int* 22:703, 1991.

Anthony DH, Peyton FA: Dimensional accuracy of various denture-base materials, *J Prosthet Dent* 12:67, 1962.

Arab J, Newton JP, Lloyd CH: The effect of an elevated level of residual monomer on the whitening of a denture base and its physical properties, *J Dent* 17:189, 1989.

Blanchet LJ, Bowman DC, McReynolds HD: Effects of methyl methacrylate monomer vapors on respiration and circulation in unanesthetized rats, *J Prosthet Dent* 48:344, 1982.

Braden M: The absorption of water by acrylic resins and other materials, *J Prosthet Dent* 14:307, 1964.

Braden M, Stafford GD: Viscoelastic properties of some denture base materials, *J Dent Res* 47:519, 1968.

Chandler HH, Bowen RL, Paffenbarger GC: Physical properties of a radiopaque denture base material, *J Biomed Mater Res* 5:335, 1971.

Clark RL: Dynamic mechanical thermal analysis of dental polymers. I. Heat cured poly(methyl methacrylate)-based materials, *Biomaterials* 10:494, 1989.

Ellsworth K: Fatigue failure in denture base polymers, *J Prosthet Dent* 21:257, 1969.

Firtell DN, Harman LC: Porosity in boilable acrylic resin, *J Prosthet Dent* 49:133, 1983.

Fletcher AM, Purnaveja S, Amin WM, Ritchie GM, Moradians S, Wood AW: The level of residual monomer in self-curing denture-base materials, *J Dent Res* 62:118, 1983.

Grant AA, Atkinson HF: Comparison between dimensional accuracy of dentures produced with pour-type resin and with heat-processed materials, *J Prosthet Dent* 26:296, 1971.

Hargreaves AS: Equilibrium water uptake and denture base resin behavior, *J Dent* 6:342, 1978.

Hargreaves AS: The effects of cyclic stress on dental polymethylmethacrylate, *J Oral Rehabil* 10:137, 1983.

Harrison WM, Stansbury BE: The effect of joint surface contours on the transverse strength of repaired acrylic resin, *J Prosthet Dent* 23:464, 1970.

Heath JR, Davenport JC, Jones PA: The abrasion of acrylic resin by cleaning pastes, *J Oral Rehabil* 10:159, 1983.

Hill RG: The crosslinking agent ethylene glycol dimethacrylate content of the currently available denture base resins, *J Dent Res* 60:725, 1981.

Hill RG, Bates JF, Lewis TT, Rees N: Fracture toughness of acrylic denture base, *Biomaterials* 4:112, 1983.

Huggett R, Brooks SC, Bates JF: The effect of different curing cycles on the dimensional accuracy of acrylic resin denture base materials, *Quintess Dent Technol* 8:81, 1984.

Jagger RG, Huggett R: The effect of crosslinking on sorption properties of a denture base material, *Dent Mater* 6:276, 1990.

Kaaber S, Cramers M, Jepsen FL: The role of cadmium as a skin sensitizing agent in denture and non-denture wearers, *Contact Dermatitis* 8:308, 1982.

Kaaber S, Thulin H, Nielsen E: Skin sensitivity to denture base materials in the burning mouth syndrome, *Contact Dermatitis* 5:90, 1979.

Kalachandra S, Turner DT: Water sorption of poly(methyl methacrylate). III. Effects of plasticizers, *Polymer* 28:1749, 1987.

Kalachandra S, Turner DT: Water sorption of plasticized denture acrylic lining materials, *Dent Mater* 5:161, 1989.

Kelsey WP, III, Blankenau RJ, Powell GL, Barkmeier WW, Cavel WT, Whisenant BK: Enhancement of physical properties of resin restorative materials by laser polymerization, *Laser Surg Med* 9:623, 1989.

Khan Z, von-Fraunhofer JA, Razavi R: The staining characteristics, transverse strength, and microhardness of a visible light-cured denture base material, *J Prosthet Dent* 57:384, 1987.

Koda T, Tsuchiya H, Yamauchi M, Hoshino Y, Takagi N, Kawano J: High-performance liquid chromatographic estimation of eluates from denture base polymers, *J Dent* 17:84, 1989.

Lamb DJ, Ellis B, Priestly D: The effects of processing variables on levels of residual monomer in auto-polymerizing dental acrylic resin, *J Dent* 11:80, 1983.

Latta GH Jr, Bowles WF, Conkin JE: Three-dimensional stability of new denture base resin systems, *J Prosthet Dent* 63:654, 1990.

Lorton L, Phillips RW: Heat-released stress in acrylic dentures, *J Prosthet Dent* 42:23, 1979.

Mutlu G, Huggett R, Harrison A, Goodwin JW, Hughes RW: Rheology of acrylic denture base polymers, *Dent Mater* 6:288, 1990.

Oysaed H, Ruyter IE: Creep studies of multiphase acrylic systems, *J Biomed Mat Res* 23:719, 1989.

Polyzois GL, Karkazis HC, Zissis AJ: Dimensional stability of dentures processed in boilable acrylic resins: a comparative study, *J Prosthet Dent* 57:639, 1987.

Powers JM, Koran A: Color of denture resins, *J Dent Res* 56:754, 1977.

Powers JM, Lepeak PJ: Parameters that affect the color of denture resins, *J Dent Res* 56:1332, 1977.

Rawls HR, Starr J, Kasten FH, Murray M, Smid J, Cabasso J: I. Radiopaque acrylic resins containing miscible heavy-metal compounds, *Dent Mater* 6:250, 1990.

Robinson JG, McCabe JF: Impact strength of acrylic resin denture base materials with surface defects, *Dent Mater* 9:355, 1993.

Rodford RA: Further development and evaluation of high-impact-strength denture base materials, *J Dent* 18:151, 1990.

Ruyter IE, Espevik S: Compressive creep of denture base polymers, *Acta Odont Scand* 38:169, 1980.

Ruyter IE, Svendsen SA: Flexural properties of denture base polymers, *J Prosthet Dent* 43:95, 1980.

Smith LT, Powers JM: Relative fit of new denture resins polymerized by heat, light and microwave energy, *Am J Dent* 5:140, 1992.

Smith LT, Powers JM, Ladd D: Mechanical properties of new denture resins polymerized by visible light, heat and microwave energy, *Int J Prosthodont* 5:315, 1992.

Soni PM, Powers JM, Craig RG: Physical and mechanical properties of acrylic and modified acrylic denture resins, *Mich Dent Assoc J* 59:418, 1977.

Spiechowicz E, Santarpia RP, Pollock JJ, Renner RP: *In vitro* study on the inhibiting effect of different agents on the growth of *Candida albicans* on acrylic resin surfaces, *Quintess Int* 21:35, 1990.

Stafford GD, Huggett R, Causton BE: Fracture toughness of denture base acrylics, *J Biomed Mater Res* 14:359, 1980.

Strohaver RA: Comparison of changes in vertical dimension between compression and injection molded complete dentures, *J Prosthet Dent* 62:716, 1989.

Sykora O, Sutow EJ: Comparison of the dimensional stability of two waxes and two acrylic resin processing techniques in the production of complete dentures, *J Oral Rehabil* 17:219, 1990.

Takamata T, Setcos JC: Resin denture bases: review of accuracy and methods of polymerization, *Int J Prosthodont* 2:555, 1989.

Tsao DH, Guilford HJ, Kazanoglu A, Bell DH: Clinical evaluation of a radiopaque denture base resin, *J Prosthet Dent* 51:456, 1984.

Vermilyea SG, Powers JM, Koran A: The rheological properties of fluid denture base resins, *J Dent Res* 57:227, 1978.

Wollff EM: The effect of cross-linking agents on acrylic resins, *Aust Dent J* 7:439, 1962.

Yamauchi M, Yamamoto K, Wakabayashi M, Kawano J: *In vitro* adherence of microorganisms to denture base resin with different surface texture, *Dent Mater J* 9:19, 1990.

Denture Liners

Amin WM, Fletcher AM, Ritchie GM: The nature of the interface between polymethylmethacrylate denture base materials and soft lining materials, *J Dent* 9:336, 1981.

Braden M: Tissue conditioners. I. Composition and structure, *J Dent Res* 49:145, 1970.

Braden M: Tissue conditioners. II. Rheologic properties, *J Dent Res* 49:496, 1970.

Braden M, Wright PS: Water sorption and water solubility of soft lining materials for acrylic dentures, *J Dent Res* 62:764, 1983.

Cornish HH, Block WD: The toxicology of uncured epoxy resins and amine curing agents, *Arch Ind Health* 20:390, 1959.

Council on Dental Research: Resilient liners, *J Am Dent Assoc* 67:558, 1963.

Dootz ER, Koran A, Craig RG: Comparison of the physical properties of eleven soft dental liners, *J Prosthet Dent* 67:707, 1992.

Duran RL, Powers JM, Craig RG: Viscoelastic and dynamic properties of soft liners and tissue conditioners, *J Dent Res* 58:1801, 1979.

Eick JD, Craig RG, Peyton FA: Properties of resilient denture liners in simulated mouth conditions, *J Prosthet Dent* 12:1043, 1962.

Graham BS, Jones DW, Sutow EJ: An *in vivo* and *in vitro* study of the loss of plasticizer from soft polymer-gel materials, *J Dent Res* 70:870, 1991.

Graham BS, Jones DW, Sutow EJ: Clinical implications of resilient denture lining material research. II. Gelation and flow properties of tissue conditioners, *J Prosthet Dent* 65:413, 1991.

Harsanyi BB, Foong WC, Howell RE, Hidi P, Jones DW: Hamster cheek-pouch testing of dental soft polymers, *J Dent Res* 70:991, 1991.

Hayakawa I, Hirano S, Kobayashi S, Nagao M, Masuhara E: The creep behavior of denture-supporting tissues and soft lining materials, *Int J Prosthodont* 7:339, 1994.

Hayakawa I, Kawae M, Tsuji Y, Masuhara E: Soft denture liner of a fluoroethylene copolymer and its clinical significance, *J Prosthet Dent* 51:310, 1984.

Jones DW, Sutow EJ, Graham BS: Rheology and strength of denture soft lining materials, *J Dent Res* 62(abstr): 661, 1983.

Jones DW, Sutow EJ, Hall GC, Tobin WM, Graham BS: Dental soft polymers: plasticizer composition and leachability, *Dent Mater* 4:1, 1988.

Kawano F, Asaoka K, Nagao K, Matsumoto N: Effect of viscoelastic deformation of soft tissue on stresses in the structure under complete dentures, *Dent Mater J* 9:70, 1990.

Kawano F, Dootz ER, Koran A, Craig RG: Bond strength of soft denture liners to denture base resin, *J Prosthet Dent* 68:368, 1992.

Kawano F, Dootz ER, Koran A, Craig RG: Sorption and solubility of 12 soft denture liners, *J Prosthet Dent* 72:393, 1994.

Kawano F, Koran A, Asaoka K, Matsumoto N: Effect of soft denture liner on stress distribution in supporting structures under a denture, *Int J Prosthodont* 6:43, 1993.

Murata H, Shigeto N, Hamada T: Viscoelastic properties of tissue conditioners: stress relaxation test Maxwell model analogy, *J Oral Rehabil* 17:365, 1990.

Razavi R, Kahn Z, von Fraunhoffer JA: The bond strength of a visible light-cured reline resin to acrylic resin denture base material, *J Prosthet Dent* 63:485, 1990.

Razek MKA, Mohamed ZM: Influence of tissue-conditioning materials on the oral bacteriologic status of complete denture wearers, *J Prosthet Dent* 44:137, 1980.

Shotwell JL, Razzoog ME, Koran A: Color stability of long-term soft denture liners, *J Prosthet Dent* 68:836, 1992.

Wright PS: Characterization of the rupture properties of denture soft lining materials, *J Dent Res* 59:614, 1980.

Wright PS: The effect of soft lining materials on the growth of *Candida albicans*, *J Dent* 8:144, 1980.

Wright PS: Composition and properties of soft lining materials for acrylic dentures, *J Dent* 9:210, 1981.

Wright PS: Characterization of the adhesion of soft lining materials to poly(methyl methacrylate), *J Dent Res* 61:1002, 1982.

Denture Teeth

Cornell JA: Composite tooth and veneer gel composite formed of non-volatile dimethacrylate as the sole polymerizable constituent, US Patent 3,265,202, Aug 9, 1966.

Ekfeldt A: Incisal and occlusal tooth wear and wear of some prosthodontic materials, *Swed Dent J* 65(suppl):1, 1989.

Ekfeldt WA, Ivanhoe JR, Adrian ED: Wear mechanism of resin and porcelain denture teeth, *Acta Odontol Scand* 47:391, 1989.

Huggett R, John G, Jagger RG, Bates JF: Strength of the acrylic denture base tooth bond, *Br Dent J* 153:187, 1982.

Koran A, Craig RG, Tillitson EW: Coefficient of friction of prosthetic tooth materials, *J Prosthet Dent* 27:269, 1972.

Raptis CM, Powers JM, Fan PL: Frictional behavior and surface failure of acrylic denture teeth, *J Dent Res* 60:908, 1981.

Rupp NW, Bowen RL, Paffenbarger GC: Bonding to cold-curing denture base acrylic resin to acrylic resin teeth, *J Am Dent Assoc* 83:601, 1971.

Suzuki S, Sakoh M, Shiba A: Adhesive bonding of denture base to plastic denture teeth, *J Biomed Mater Res* 24:1094, 1990.

Maxillofacial Materials

Chalian VA, Drane JB, Standish SM: *Maxillofacial prosthetics,* Baltimore, 1971, Williams & Wilkins.

Craig RG, Koran A, Yu R: Color stability of elastomers for maxillofacial appliances, *J Dent Res* 57:866, 1978.

Craig RG, Koran A, Yu R: Elastomers for maxillofacial applications, *Biomaterials* 1:112, 1980.

Dootz ER, Koran A, Craig RG: Physical properties of three maxillofacial materials as a function of accelerated aging, *J Prosthet Dent* 71:379, 1994.

Hill RG, Bates JF, Lewis TT, Rees N: The fracture of acrylic polymers in water, *J Mater Sci* 19:1904, 1984.

Koran A, Craig RG: Dynamic properties of maxillofacial prostheses, *J Dent Res* 54:1216, 1975.

Kouyoumdjian J, Chalian VA, Moore BK: A comparison of the physical properties of a room temperature vulcanizing silicone modified and unmodified, *J Prosthet Dent* 53:388, 1985.

Ogle RE, Sorensen SE, Lewis EA: A new visible light-cured resin system applied to removable prosthodontics, *J Prosthet Dent* 56:497, 1986.

Ouellette J: Spray coloring of silicone elastomers for maxillofacial prostheses, *J Prosthet Dent* 22:271, 1969.

Parker S, Braden M: Soft prosthesis materials based on powdered elastomers, *Biomaterials* 11:482, 1990.

Price CA, Earnshaw R: Impact testing of a polysulphone denture base polymer, *Aust Dent J* 29:398, 1984.

Schaaf NG: Color characterizing silicone rubber facial prostheses, *J Prosthet Dent* 24:198, 1970.

Sweeney WT, Fisher TE, Castleberry DJ, Cowperthwaite GF: Evaluation of improved maxillofacial prosthetic materials, *J Prosthet Dent* 27:297, 1972.

Turner GE, Fisher TE, Castleberry DJ, Lemons JE: Intrinsic color of isophorone polyurethane for maxillofacial prosthetics, *J Prosthet Dent* 51:673, 1984.

Temporary Crown and Bridge Materials

Grajower R, Shaharbani S, Kaufman E: Temperature rise in pulp chamber during fabrication of temporary self-curing resin crowns, *J Prosthet Dent* 41:535, 1979.

Lui JL: Hypersensitivity to a temporary crown and bridge material, *J Dent* 7:22, 1979.

Robinson FB, Hovijitra S: Marginal fit of direct temporary crowns, *J Prosthet Dent* 47:390, 1982.

Acrylic Tray Materials

Goldfogel M, Harvey WL, Winter D: Dimensional change of acrylic resin tray materials, *J Prosthet Dent* 54:284, 1985.

Appendix

Table of weights and measures

Lengths

1 millimeter (mm)	=	0.001 meter	=	0.03937 inch
1 centimeter (cm)	=	0.01 meter	=	0.3937 inch
1 meter (m)			=	39.37 inches
1 yard (yd)	= 0.9144 meter		=	36 inches
1 inch (in)	=	2.54 centimeters	=	25.4 millimeters
1 micrometer (μm)	=	0.001 millimeter	= 0.00003937 inch	
1 micrometer (μm)	= 10,000 Angstrom units			
1 Angstrom unit (Å) =		0.1 nanometer	= 3.937×10^{-9} inch	
1 nanometer (nm)	=	0.001 micrometer	=	10 Angstrom units

Weights

1 milligram (mg)	= 0.001 gram	= 0.015 grain
1 gram (g)	= 0.0022 pound	= 15.432 grains
1 gram (g)	= 0.035 ounce	
1 kilogram (kg)	= 1000 grams	= 2.2046 pounds
1 ounce (oz)	= 28.35 grams	
1 pound (lb)	= 453.59 grams	= 16 ounces
1 pennyweight (dwt) (troy)	= 1.555 grams	= 24 grains
1 grain	= 0.0648 gram	
1 Newton (N)	= 0.2248 pound = 0.102 kilogram	= 100,000 dynes
1 dyne	= 0.00102 gram	

Capacity (liquid)

1 milliliter (ml)	=	1 cubic centimeter	= 0.0021 pint
1 liter (l)	=	1000 cubic centimeters	= 1.057 quarts
1 quart (qt)	= 0.946 liter		= 32 ounces
1 ounce (oz)	=	29.6 milliliters	
1 cubic foot (cu ft)	= 28.32 liters		

Area

sq in (in²)	*sq ft (ft²)*	*sq mm (mm²)*	*sq cm (cm²)*
1	0.00694	645.16	6.4516
144	1	92,903	929.03
0.00155	0.000011	1	0.01
0.155	0.0011	100	1

Volume

cu in (in³)	cu mm (mm³)	cc (cm³)
1	16,387	16.387
0.0000610	1	0.001
0.0610	1000	1

Note: 1 ml (or cc) of distilled water at 4° C weighs 1 g

Conversion tables

Conversion factors (linear)

	mm	cm	in
1 Angstrom unit (Å)	0.0000001	0.00000001	0.000000003937
1 nanometer (nm)	0.000001	0.0000001	0.00000003937
1 micrometer (µm)	0.001	0.0001	0.00003937

Conversion factors (force per area)

To change kilograms per square centimeter (kg/cm^2) to pounds per square inch (lb/in^2), multiply by 14.223 (1 kg/cm^2 = 14.223 lb/in^2).

To change kilograms per square centimeter (kg/cm^2) to megapascals (MPa), multiply by 0.0981 (1 kg/cm^2 = 0.0981 MPa). Note 1 MN/m^2 =1 MPa.

To change pounds per square inch (lb/in^2) to kilograms per square centimeter (kg/cm^2), multiply by 0.070307 (1 lb/in^2 =0.0703 kg/cm^2).

To change meganewtons per square meter (MN/m^2) to pounds per square inch (lb/in^2), multiply by 145 ($1MN/m^2$ =145 lb/in^2).

To change meganewtons per square meter (MN/m^2) to giganewtons per square meter (GN/m^2), divide by 1000.

Conversion of thermometer scales

Temperature Fahrenheit (° F) = ⅞ Temperature Celsius + 32°
Temperature Celsuis (° C) = ⅝ Temperature Fahrenheit – 32°

or

$$(°\ C \times 1.8) + 32 = °\ F$$

$$\frac{°\ F - 32°}{1.8} = °\ C$$

Conversion factors (miscellaneous)

1 foot-pound (ft-lb) = 13,826 gram-centimeters = 1.356 Newton-meters
1 radian = 57.3 degrees
1 watt = 14.3 calories/minute

Conversion of exponentials to decimals

Exponential no.	Decimal no.
1×10^{-5} (or 10^{-5})	0.00001
1×10^{-3}	0.001
1×10^{-1}	0.1
1×10^{0} (or 10^{0})	1
1×10^{1}	10
1×10^{4}	10,000
1×10^{7} (or 10^{7})	10,000,000

Comparative table of troy, avoirdupois, and metric weights

Grain	Troy dwt	Troy oz	Avoirdupois oz	Avoirdupois lb	G
1	1.042	0.002	0.00228	0.00014	0.065
24	1	0.05	0.0548	0.0034	1.555
480	20	1	1.097	0.0686	31.10
437.5	18.23	0.91	1	0.063	28.35
7000	291.67	14.58	16	1	453.59
15.43	0.64	0.032	0.035	0.0022	1

Index

A

Abrasion resistance, gypsum products and, 342-343
Absorption coefficient, vs. wavelength, for shades of
 composite, *37*
Acid etching, tooth structure, effect of, 14
Acrylic; *see also* Resin
 abrasion resistance of, 510
 athletic mouth protectors and, 544-545
 bond strength of, 536
 chemically accelerated, 523-525
  athletic mouth protectors and, 545
  characteristics of, 523-525
  impression trays and baseplates and, 546
  inlay wax patterns and, 545
  for repairing, 531
  as temporary crown and bridge restorations,
   543-544
 contact angle of water on, 22
 elastic modulus of, 66
 as facings for crowns and bridges, 541
 fluid resin, 525
 hardness of, 88, 510
 heat-accelerated, 515-523
 indentation depth of, 90
 light-cured, 525-528
 packing of, 517-518
 percent recovery of, 90
 Poisson's ratio of, 66
 polymerization shrinkage of, 511
 polyvinyl; *see* Polyvinyl acrylic
 pour type of, 503
  abrasion resistance of, 510
  fracture toughness of, 509
  polymerization shrinkage of, 511
  transverse deflection of, 508
 prosthetic applications of, 500; *see also* Polymers,
  prosthetic applications of
 rapid heat-polymerized; *see* Rapid heat-polymerized
  acrylic

Acrylic–cont'd
 rubber-reinforced
  abrasion resistance of, 510
  impact strength of, 506
 shear strength of, 72
 specific heat of, 44
 thermal conductivity of, 43
 thermal diffusivity or expansion of, 44
 transverse deflection of, 508
 two-body abrasion of, 92
 unfilled, 196-198
  biocompatibility of, 260
  history of, 244
Acrylics
 denture base, powder, liquid, principal ingredients
  of, 501t
 properties of, ANSI/ADA specification No. 12,
  505t
 soft lining materials, plasticized, composition of,
  535t
Admixed alloys
 composition of, 210
 compressive strength of, 217
 creep of, 217
 dimensional stability of, 218
 mercury and, 213-214
 tensile strength of, 217
Adsorption, 20
Agar
 alginate combination impressions, 293-295, *294-295*,
  295t
 hydrocolloids, 289-296
 impression material, composition of, 290t
Agar overlay test 149, 150
Air firing of artificial teeth, 471, 480, 481
Air pressure casting machines, 450
Albumin diffusion, 142
Alcohol
 heat of fusion of, 42
 specific heat of, 44
 surface tension of, 21

Alginate
    hydrocolloids, 283-289, *284*
    impression powder, ingredients in, 285t
    properties of, 286t
Allen, Charles, 8
Alloys
    amalgam, 209-212
    cast microstructures, *119*, 120-121, *121*
    casting and, 404
    for ceramic-metal restorations, properties of, 493-496,
        494-495t
    classification of systems, 110-111, *111*
    cold-worked microstructures, 121-122, *122*
    eutectic, 111, 113-115, *114-116*, 116t, 117
    general requirements of, 408-409
    grain growth, 122-123, *123*
    hardening of, 389-390
    intermetallic compounds, 111, 115, 117
    melting, methods of, 449-450
    metallic bonding and, 104
    metallic elements used in, 383-395
        base metals, 386
        binary combinations of metals, 387
        composition, 387-389
        copper, 386-387
        gallium, 387
        gold, 383-385
        indium, 387
        iridium, 386
        nickel, 387
        palladium, 385-386
        platinum, 385
        rhodium, 386
        ruthenium, 386
        silver, 386
        tin, 387
        zinc, 387
    nature of, 109-111
    in partial dentures, mechanical properties of, 413t
    phase diagrams, *112*, 112-117
        construction of, 116-117, *117*
        types of, 113-115
    for porcelain-fused-to-metal bonding, 490-496, 491-492t
    properties of, 104, 117-123
    recrystallization, 122-123, *123*
    selection of, 223-224
    solid solution, 111, 113, 113t, *113-114*, 117
    solidification of, *116*, *119*, 119-120
    strengthening techniques, *123-125*, 124-125
    temperature of, 387-389
    ternary phase diagrams, 115-116, *117*
Aluminous core porcelain, 475

Aluminum, 410
    ductility of, 85
    heat of fusion of, 42
    malleability of, 85
    oxidation-reduction potential of, 48
    specific heat of, 44
Alveolar bone, 144
Amalgam, 209-243
    alloys, 209-212
    amalgamation processes, 212-214
    ANSI/ADA specification No. 1 for amalgam alloy, 215
    blood, mercury in, 234
    bonding of, 231-232
    composition, 209-211, 210t, *211*
    compressive strength, 215-218, 217t, 227
    condensation, 228
        delay in, 228-229
        hand, 228
        mechanical, 228
    copper amalgam alloys, composition, 210t
    corrosion, 221-222, *223*
        products, release of, 234
    creep, 217t, 219-220, *220*, 227-228
    dimensional change, 218t, 220-221, *221*, 227
    elastic modulus, 219
    finishing amalgam restorations, 230, 231t
    high-copper alloys, 213-214
    irregular particles, *211*, 211-212
    local reactions, 235
    low-copper alloys, 212-213
    manipulation of, 223-232
    mechanical properties, 215-222
    mercury
        concentration of, 233-234
        content, 229
        daily intake of, 233t
        forms of, 232-233
        properties of, 222-223
        proportions, of alloy to, 224, *224-225*
        reaction of
            in admixed high-copper alloy, 213-214
            in unicompositional alloy, 214
        sources of, 232, 233t
        toxicity, 232-237
    microstructure of, 214, *215-216*
    mix, 224-228, *226*, 226-228, *227*
    moisture contamination, during insertion, 229-230
    morphology, 209-211, 210t, *211*
    office personnel, risks to, 236-237
    overmix, 226-228, *227*
    physical properties, 215-222
    poisoning, 234-236

Amalgam—cont'd
  production, 211-212
  properties of, 214-223
  risks to dentists, 236-237
  selection of alloy, 223-224
  silver-tin alloy, 212, *213*
  size of mix, 224
  spherical particles, *211*, 212
  strength, various phases, 218-219, *219*
  surface roughness, various methods of
      instrumentation, 231t
  systemic reactions, 235-236, *236*
  tensile strength, 218, 218t, 227
  transverse strength, 218
  undermix, 226-228, *227*
  urine, mercury in, 233-234
  working time, 227
Amalgamation processes, 212-214
American Dental Association, 13
  acceptance program, 13, 95
  Council on Dental Materials, Instruments, and
      Equipment, 11
  specifications of, 95, 96-97t
American Journal of Dental Science, establishment of, 8
American National Standards, 13
American National Standards Institute/American Dental
      Association specifications, 95-98
  on agar hydrocolloids, 292
  on alginate hydrocolloids, 285-87
  on amalgam alloys, 215
  on casting investments, 347-351
  on cobalt-chromium casting alloys, 409
  on denture base resins, 504
      and temporary relining, 533
      and transverse deflection test and, 508
  on denture plastics
      and color stability, 513
      and powder-liquid mixture, 516
      and water sorption test, 513
  on duplicating materials, 296
  on gold alloys
      and classification, 391
      and composition and mechanical properties,
          391-392
  on gypsum products, 337, 338
  on impression materials, 311, 319
  on nickel-chromium alloys and, 409
  on oxidation of base metals, 455
  on plastic teeth, 539-540
  research fellowship and, 13
  on self-curing repair resins, 532
  on tray compound, 320

American National Standards Institute/American Dental
      Association specifications—cont'd
  on wax
      and baseplate, 372-378
      and inlay pattern, 372, 373
      and properties, 439-340
  on zinc oxide–eugenol cement, 184, 187, 316-320
  on zinc phosphate cement, 175, 178, 181
  on zinc polyacrylate cement, 190
American Society of Dental Surgeons, 9
  establishment of, 8
American Textbook of Operative Dentistry, 12
Ames' test, 151, 152
Amine-accelerated sealant, 271
Amine-cured cement, 196
Ammonium diacid phosphate, 355
Ancient history of dentistry, 4
Animal waxes, 362, 364
Ankylosis, 143
Anodic polarization curves, amalgam in synthetic saliva,
      50
Anterior veneers, 264-265
Appliances, construction of, 4
Applied technics and, clinical dentistry, relationship, 2
Arthur, Robert, 10
Artificial teeth, from bone, ivory, 6
Ash tube tooth, 8
Assyrians, history, restorative metals, 4
Auxiliary materials, effect, on denture plastics, 528-530

B

Babylonians, history, restorative metals, 4
Baltimore College of Dental Surgery, establishment of, 8
Barnum, Phineas Taylor, 10
Base metal
  alloys, 386
      composition of, 492t, 493
  crowns, prefabricated, 427-428, 430t
      mechanical properties of, 430t
Baseplate wax, 376-378
  requirements for, 378t
Basic sciences, applied to restorative materials, 2, *2*
Beeswax, 362, 364
  elastic modulus of, 367-368
  ester in, 362
  flow of, 368, 369
  heat of fusion of, 42
  thermal conductivity of, 43
  thermal expansion of, 366-367
Bending, *72*, 72-73
Beta-titanium alloy, wrought, 431-432
Binary combinations of metals, in alloys, 387

Biocompatibility, 137-171
   bone, 143-144
      alloys, reactions to, 166
      formation
         endochondral, 144
         membranous, 143-144
      implant materials
         other materials, 166-167
         overview, 167
         reaction to, 165-167
            ceramic implant materials, 165-166
      metals, pure, reactions to, 166
   cell response after injury, stages of, 138t
   cytotoxicity assays, 147-151, *148-149*
   dentin
      permeability, 142-143
      pulp and, 140-142, *140-143*
   enamel, 140
   gingiva, mucosa and, 145-146
   host tissue morphological changes, after injury,
         138t
   implants into bone, 154-155
   initial tests, 147-153
   intermediate tests, 153
   mucosa, gingival usage tests and, 155
   mutagenesis assays, 151-152, 152t
   oral tissue, 143-144
      alloys, reactions to, 166
      biology, 140-146
      implant materials
         other materials, 166-167
         overview, 167
         reaction to, 165-167
            ceramic implant materials, 165-166
            reactions to, ceramic implant materials, 165-166
      inflammatory response, to injury, 140-146
      metals, pure, reactions to, 166
      reaction to implant materials, 165-167
      restorative materials, reaction to, 163
   overview, 146, 156
   periodontium, 144-145
   pulp, 156-163
      amalgams, 159-161
      bleaching agents, 163
      cast alloys, 159-161
      dentin bonding, *141*, 157-159
      glass ionomers, 161
      irritation tests, 154
      liners, 161-163, *162*
      microleakage, 156-157
      nonresin cements, 161-163, *162*
      resin-based materials, 159, *160*

Biocompatibility—cont'd
   pulp—cont'd
      varnishes, and nonresin cements, 161-163, *162*
   reactions of materials, comparison of
         screening, usage tests, 155t
   restorative materials, esthetic, direct, 260
   screening tests, correlation among, 138-139t, 155t,
         155-156
   secondary tests, 153
   tests, types of, 146-156
   tooth and, 140-143
   usage tests
      in animals, 154-155
      correlation, 138-139t, 155t, 155-156
   in vitro mutagenesis tests, comparison of, 152t
Biological technics, clinical dentistry, relationship, 2
Bis-GMA-amine-accelerated sealant, 271
Bis-GMA-light-accelerated sealant, 271
Bis-GMA resin, 268-270
   sealants, restorative materials, esthetic, direct, physical
         properties of, 269t
Bite registration
   rubber impression materials, 314, 314t
   wax, 380
Black, G.V., 11, 12
Blandy, Alfred A., 10
Blood, mercury in, 234
Bond formation, to tooth structure, restorative materials,
         esthetic, direct, 256-260
Bond strengths, 72
   of ceramic and metal, 485-488
   of dentin-bonding systems, 258-260
   of glass ionomer cement, 193
   of processed soft liners, 536-537
   of resin cement, 196
   of zinc polyacrylate cement, 191
Bonding
   ceramic-metal, 485-488
   penetration coefficient in, 24
   porcelain, 265
   pulp reactions and, 157-158
   to tooth structure, 256-258
Bonding, amalgam, 231-232
Bone
   alloys, reactions to, 166
   biocompatibility, 143-144
   implant materials
      other materials, 166-167
      overview, 167
      reaction to, 165-167
         ceramic implant materials, 165-166
   metals, pure, reactions to, 166

Bone formation
    endochondral, 144
    membranous, 143-144
Bourdet, Etienne, 7
Boxing wax, *361*, 378-379, 379t
    federal specifications for, summary of requirements,
        379t
Boyle, Robert, 7
Branched polymer, 129-130
Brazilian test, 70
Brazing, 397
Bridge
    biting force and, 56
    casting alloys for, 414
    dental plastics and, 543-544
    plastic facings for, 543
    porcelain and, 468
    resin cement and, 195
    stress distribution of, 59
Bridge, casting alloys, 413t, 414
Bridge restorations, polymer, 543-544
Bridgework, history of, 4
Brinell hardness test, 87-88, *88*, 88t
Brittle materials, tensile properties, 69-70, 70t
Bull, Marcus, 8
Burning-mouth syndrome, 514
Burnishing
    of amalgam, 230
    of gold alloys, 450
Burnout time of wax, 448
Byram, J.Q., 10

C

Calcium hydroxide bases, 200-201, 201t
Calcium sulfate-bonded investment, 347, 352t
    gypsum products, 351-354, 352t
    hygroscopic expansion of, 351-354, 352t
    properties of, 347-350, 348-349t
Calcium sulfate dihydrate, solubility of, 336t
Calcium sulfate hemihydrate, solubility of, 336t
Calculus, 51
Calorimetry, differential scanning, 40
Candelilla waxes, 362, 363
Candida albicans
    dentures and, 514
    soft liners and, 534, 535
Capillary
    around teeth, formature of, 26
    penetration, depression, 25
    rise, 24-26, *25*
        curves, for water, between plates of dissimilar
            materials, 25

Capillary—cont'd
    rise—cont'd
        isolated capillaries, 24-26, *26*
        penetration coefficient, 24, *26*
    systems, two classes of, 26
Capsules for amalgamation, 224, 225, 226
Carat of gold, 391
    in solder, 400
Carbide burs, 38
Carbon
    bone and soft tissue reactions to, 166
    in cast base metal alloys, 409
Carcinogen assay, 151-152
Carding wax, 377-378
Carious teeth. *See also* Filling
Carnauba wax, 362-363
    differential thermal analysis of, 40-41, 365-366
    elastic modulus of, 367-368
    flow of, 368
    proportional limit of, 367, 368
    thermal expansion of, 366
Carving of amalgam, 230
Cast base metal alloys, 408-436, 414-415
    composition of, 409t
    microstructure of, 410-411, *411*
Cast glass ceramics, 476-477, *477*
Cast microstructures, alloys, *119*, 120-121, *121*
Casting
    alloys, 404
        crown, bridge, 413t, 414
        melting, methods of, 449-450
    cobalt-chromium alloys, casting of, 456-463, *457-459*,
        461-463
    compensation, means of, 438-439
    dimensional changes, 438-439
    direct wax patterns, 439
    distortion, 442
    embedded metals, 404
    facilities, 449-450
    glass, 464
    gold alloys
        cleaning, "pickling," 455-456
        low-fusing, casting practices for, 437
    hand-investing procedure, 442-444, *443-444*
    heating mold, 445-446, *446*
    hygroscopic, high-heat technics, differences between, 448
    indirect wax patterns, 439-440, *440*
    inlay patterns, formation of, 439-442
    investing patterns, for water-added technic, 445
    investing procedure, for wax patterns, 442-448
    investments, gypsum, 346-347
    machines, 450

Casting—cont'd
  oven temperature, 448
  porcelain veneer metal structures, 454-455, *455*
  problems, *451*, 451-453
  procedures, 437-466
  soldering, casting, fluxes, 453-454
  spring pattern, 440-441, *441*
  titanium, 463-464
  vacuum-investing procedure, 444-445, *445*
  wax, *361*, *374*, 374-376
    elimination, 446-448, *447*
    federal specifications, summary of requirements
      of, 375t
  wettability, 441-442, *442*
Cavity liners, cement, 199-200
Cavity varnishes, cement, 198-199
Cell response after injury, stages of, 138t
Cellini, Benvenuto, 6
Celsus, 5
Cements, 172-208
  acidity, 182, *182*, 191
  adhesive resin cements, 195-198
  ANSI/ADA specification No. 57 (ISO 6876),
      187-189, 188t
  ANSI/ADA specification No. 96, 176t, 190
  ANSI/ADA specification No. 96 for water-based
      cements, 175, 176-177t
  base, 186
    low- and high-strength, mechanical properties of, 201t
  biological properties, 189, 193-194
  bond strength, 191, 193
  bonding
    esthetic restorations, 196
    orthodontic brackets, 196-198
  bridges
    conventional, cementation of, 195-196
    resin-bonded, cementation of, 195-196
  calcium fluoroaluminosilicate glass, nominal
      composition of, 192t
  calcium hydroxide bases, 200-201, 201t
  care of liquid, 174
  cavity liners, 199-200
  cavity varnishes, 198-199
  cementation of orthodontic bands, 183
  characteristic properties, 175-183, 177t, 184-186,
      185t, 194
  chemistry of setting, 174, 184, 194, 200
  composite, 195-198
  compressive strength, 177t, 186, 189
  consistency, film thickness, 175-179, *178*
  crowns, cementation of, 195-196
  dimensional change, 189

Cements—cont'd
  dimensional stability, 182, 191
  disintegration, 176-177t, 191, 193
  dispensing, 184
  effect of powder/liquid ratio, 179-180
  electrical conductivity, 182-183
  endodontic filling materials, types II and III,
      specification requirements for, 188t
  endodontic sealers, 187
  film thickness, 175-179, 177t, *178*, 184, 189, 191,
      193
  frozen slab method, 175
  glass ionomer cement, 192-194
  high-strength bases, 201t, 202
  hybrid ionomer cement, 194-195
  liquid, 173, 173t
  low-strength bases, 200-201
  luting cements
    mechanical properties of, 177t
    physical properties of, 177t
  mixing procedure, 174-175, 184
  mixing slab, 174
  non-eugenol cements, 183-189
  permanent cementation, 177t, 187
  powder, 173, 173t
  powder/liquid ratio, 174
  radiopacity, 189
  resin, 195-198
  resin-bonded bridge cements, to various substrates,
      bond strengths, 195t
  resin-metal bonding, 196
  solubility, 176-177t, 181-182, 186, 189, 191, 193
  strength, 181, 191, 193
  temperature, mixing slab, 180
  temporary cementation, 186-187
  temporary restorations, 187
    cementation of, 195-196
  thermal conductivity, 182-183
  tissue management, 189
  types of, bracket base, effect of, 198t
  viscosity, 179, *180*, 189, 190
  water-based cements, specification requirements for,
      176t
  water content of mix, 181
  zinc oxide-eugenol, 183-189, 185t, 200, 201, 201t
    endodontic sealers, composition of, 187t
    temporary filling cement, formula for, 183t
  zinc phosphate cement, 173-183
    manipulative variables, effects of, 181t
    rate of set of, factors governing, 180t
    typical composition of, 173t
  zinc polyacrylate cement, 189-192

Centrifugal casting machine, 450
    bar sprue and, 454
    glass casting and, 464
Ceramic-metal restorations, 485-488, *487*
    evaluation of, 486-488, *488-490*
    noble metal alloys, 491t, 494t
Ceramic-metal systems, *485*, 485-499
    alloys
        for ceramic-metal restorations, properties of, 493-496, 494-495t
        for porcelain-fused-to-metal bonding, 490-496, 491-492t
    base metal alloys, composition of, 492t, 493
    ceramic-metal restorations, 485-488, *487*
        base metal alloys for, composition of, 492t
        evaluation of, 486-488, *488-490*
        noble metal alloys, 491t, 494t
    ceramic-metal systems, ceramic-metal restorations, base metal alloys for, composition of, 492t
    ceramics, for porcelain-fused-to-metal bonding, 488-490
    noble metal alloys, composition of, 490-493
    porcelain-fused-to-metal restorations, preparation of, *490*, 496-497
Ceramics, 467-484
    applications, 468, *469*
    cast glass ceramics, 476-477, *477*
    composition, 467-468, 468t
    core materials, 475-476, *476*
    esthetic porcelain veneers, 479, *479*
    fusion
        to high temperature alloys, composition of, 469t
        of porcelain, 471-472
    hardness, of natural, artificial teeth, 482t
    high-temperature injection molding, 477, *478*
    machined restorations, 473-474, *474*
    manufacture, 479-482, *480-481*
    optical properties, 477-478, 478t
    porcelain artificial teeth, 479-483
    porcelain crowns, 472-473
    porcelain enamel-metal restorations, 474-475, *475*
    for porcelain-fused-to-metal bonding, 488-490
    porcelain ingredients, 468t
    porcelain inlays, 473
    porcelain technic, 470-471
    porcelain tooth restorative, 469-476
    porcelains total percent transmission of, 478t
    properties, of fused porcelain, 472
Ceresin, 362-363
Certification programs, 95
Charpy impact strength, 84
Chemical acceleration, acrylic denture plastics, compression molding, 524-525

Chemical reaction
    gypsum, 334-337
    restorative materials, esthetic, direct, 244-249
Chemical technics, clinical dentistry, relationship, 2
Chemistry, impression materials, 283-285, 285t
Chewing force, 56-57
    new restorations and, 230
Chlorhexidine, 515
Chloropercha, 10
Christensen, W.E., 10
Chroma, 32-34
    direct esthetic resins and, 260, 261
Chromaticity diagram, 33
Chromium
    in cobalt-chromium alloys; *see* Cobalt-chromium cast alloys
    in cobalt-chromium-molybdenum alloys, 166
    elastic modulus of, 66
    electrode potential of, 48
    flux and, 467
    heat of fusion of, 42
    Knoop hardness of, 89
    in nickel-chromium alloys, 409
    oxidation-reduction potential of, 48
    percent elongation of, 64
    yield strength of, 63
Chromium release assay, 148
Classification, alloy systems, 110-111, *111*
Clinical Products in Dentistry—A Desktop Reference, 13
Cloves, oil of, 6
Cobalt-chromium alloys, casting of, 456-463, *457-459*, *461-463*
Cobalt-chromium casting alloys, 409-415
Cobalt-chromium-nickel alloy, wrought, 428-429
Cobalt-chromium-nickel wires, cold bending of, 430t
Cocoa butter, 362, 363
Coefficient
    of friction, 538
    of thermal expansion, 44-45; *see also* Thermal expansion
Coherent precipitate formation, 124
Cohesion of gold, 385
Cold-worked microstructures, alloys, 121-122, *122*
Coleman, R.L., 13
Colloid systems, 19
    emulsions, 20
    gels, 19
    syneresis, 20
Colloidal state, 18-20
Colloids, nature of, 18-19

Color, 30-31, 31t
    measurement of, 31-34, *33*
        chromaticity diagram, 33
        instrumental technic, 31t, 31-32, *32-33*
        Munsell scales, 34
        surface finish, thickness, 34
        visual technic, 32-34, *34*
    quantities for, in reflected daylight, 31
    restorative materials, esthetic, direct, 260-261, *261*, 261t
    solders, 400
    spectral reflectance, vs. wavelength, for composite
        resin, 32
Composite, dentin, shear bond strengths, 258t
Composite resin
    color characteristics, variation in, 261t
    posterior, critical physical properties for, 266t
Composite restorative resins, 244-252
Composites, 85-86, *86*, 195-198, 244-252
    anterior veneers and, 264-265
    biocompatibility of, 260
    bonding and, 256
    composition of, 244-249
    compressive strength of, 71, 253-254
    depth of cure of, 255-256
    elastic modulus of, 253
    extended applications for, restorative materials,
        esthetic, 264-267
    fine, properties of, 253t
    indentation depth of, 90
    inorganic phase in, 244
    Knoop hardness of, 253, 254
    manipulation and handling of, 262-264
    mechanical properties of, 85-86
    microfine; *see* Microfine composite resin
    organic phase in, 244
    percent recovery of, 89
    Poisson's ratio of, 66
    polymerization shrinkage in, 253
    posterior resins and, 265-267
    properties of, 177
    radiopacity in, 255
    restorative materials, esthetic, direct, 262
    screening and usage tests of, 155, 156
    selection of, 261-262
    solubility of, 253, 254
    tensile strength of, 70, 253
    thermal conductivity of, 43, 253-254
    thermal diffusivity of, 44
    thermal expansion of, 45, 253-254
    transverse strength of, 73
    two-body abrasion of, 92
    water sorption of, 253, 254
    wear rate of, 255

Composition, impression materials, 283-285, 285t,
        300-303, 319t
Compressive properties, 70-71, *71*, 71t
Compressive strength
    of agar hydrocolloids, 292
    of alginate hydrocolloids, 287
    amalgam, 215-218, 217t, 227
    of Bis-GMA resin sealants, 269
    of composite resins, 254-255
    of dental plastics, 506
    of fused porcelain, 472
    of glass ionomer cement, 193
    gypsum, 340t, 341-342, *342*, 342t
    of low- and high-strength cement bases,
        201
    of plastic teeth, 537
    of resin cement, 195, 196
    restorative materials, 71t
    of waxes, 367, 368
    of zinc oxide–eugenol cement, 183-185
    of zinc polyacrylate cement, 191
Condensation, amalgam, 228
    delay in, 228-229
    hand, 228
    mechanical, 228
Condensation polymerization, 133-135
Conduction, faulty, impression materials, 324
Conductivity, electrical, 45-47, 47t
        of zinc phosphate cement, 182-183
        of fused porcelain, 481
        in silver-formed dies, 324
        thermal; *see* Thermal conductivity
Consistency
    of mix, impression materials, 316
    of gypsum products, 340-341
    of zinc oxide–eugenol cement, 184
    of zinc phosphate cement, 175-179
Contact angle
    spreading, wetting, relationship, 22
    water
        on solids, 23
        wax, acrylic plastic, 23
Contact single, formed by balance of energies, between
        liquid, solid, 23
Contraction
    in casting process, 437
    of gypsum products, 335-336
    of impression compound, 320
Contrast ratio, measurement of, *32*, 36
Convection, fluid, 142
Conversion, 132
Conversion tables, 552
Coolants, 38

Cooling, 116-117
  of impression compound, 320
Copal, 363, 366
Copolymers, 127
Copper
  alloys of
    amalgamation and, 212-214
    in ceramic-metal restorations, 491
    electroforming of, 323
    high; see High-copper alloys
    low; see Low-copper alloys
  in amalgam alloys, 10, 210
  characteristics of, 386-387
  creep curves for, 80
  crystals of, 106
  ductility of, 67
  and gold, 110, 387-389
  heat of fusion of, 42
  with lead, 110, 111
  malleability of, 85
  oxidation-reduction potential of, 48
  specific heat of, 44
  surface tension of, 23
  thermal conductivity of, 43
  thermal expansion of, 45
Copper, in alloys, 386-387
Copper amalgam alloys, composition, 210t
Copper-formed dies, 323t, 323-324
Copper-forming bath, composition of solution for, 323t
Core build-up, restorative materials, esthetic, direct, 265, 265
Core materials, ceramics, 475-476, 476
Corrective impression wax, 379-380, 380
Corrosion
  amalgam, 221-222, 223
  electrochemical, 48t, 49-50, 50
Corrosion products, amalgam, release of, 234
Council on Dental Materials and Devices, 14
Council on Scientific Affairs, 11
Coupling agents, restorative materials, esthetic, direct, 247-248
Crawcour brothers, 8
Creep, amalgam, 217t, 219-220, 220, 227-228
Creep compliance, 81-83, 82
  impression materials, 311-312, 312
Crowell, W.S., 12
Crown
  base metal, prefabricated, mechanical properties of, 430t
  casting alloys, bridge, 413t, 414
Crowns
  alloys and, 396
    casting, 414
  aluminous core, 475-476

Crowns—cont'd
  aluminous core, 475-476
  dental plastics and, 543-544
  history of, 10
  plastic facings for, 543-544
  porcelain and, 468, 472
  resin cement and, 195
  zinc oxide–eugenol cement and, 186
Crystal structure, metals, 104-109, 105-107
  physical properties, 105-106, 107
Cubic crystal system, 105
Curing
  of denture plastics, 518-521
  of direct esthetic resins, 255-256
Custer, Levitt Ellsworth, 10
Cytotoxicity assays, 147-151, 148-149

D
Darcet, Jean, 7
Davis crown, 10
De Chemant, Nicholas Dubois, 7
De Saran, Aguilhon, 11
De Vigo, Giovanni, 5
Dean, J.C., 10
Deformation
  metals, 106-108, 107-109
  permanent, impression materials, 286, 286t, 286-287, 292, 310
Dendrites, 118-119
Density
  of dental plastics, 511
  of fused porcelain, 481
  of gold foil, 384, 385
  of low-carat gold alloys, 394, 395
  of metal alloys, 494-495
Density, noble alloys, 394
Dental Device Classification Panel, 13
Dental material testing; see Biocompatibility
Dental plaster; see Impression materials
Dental plastic; see Plastic
Dental societies, 9
Dental stone
  for casts and dies, 321-322
  compressive strength of, 341-342
  consistency of, 340-341
  denture plastics and, 528
  high-strength; see High-strength dental stone
  manufacture of, 333-334
  setting of, 344
  surface hardness of, 342-343
  tensile strength of, 343
  water/powder ratio of, 334
Dental wax, 371-380; see also Wax

Dentifrices
  abrasion and, 92
  denture plastics and, 530
Dentin
  composite
    marginal gap sizes between, 258t
    shear bond strengths, 258t
  compressive strength of, 71
  cytotoxicity assays and, 149, 150-151
  dielectric constant of, 47
  direct esthetic resin bonding to, 258-259
  injury of, 140-143
  Knoop hardness of, 89
  osmotic pressure and, 20
  permeability, 142-143
  pulp and, 140-142, *140-143*
    biocompatibility, 140-142, *140-143*
  restorative materials, esthetic, direct, 253t, 256-260,
      259t
  shear strength of, 72
  specific heat of, 44
  tensile strength of, 70
  thermal conductivity of, 43
  thermal diffusivity of, 44
  usage tests and, 154
  zeta-potential of, 51
Dentin barrier, 155-156
Dentoenamel junction, 140
Denture, 469, 479-483, 537-540.
  complete
    baseplate wax and, 376-378
    biting force and, 56
    historical use of, 7-8
    waxes and, 361-362
  partial, removable, 361-362, 374, 375
    biting force and, 56
    casting wax and, 374, 375
  rebasing, 532-537
  relining, 532-537
  retention of, 528
    surface phenomena in, 26-27
Denture base materials, properties of, polymer, 500-504
Denture retention, forces involved in, 26-27, 528
Denture teeth, polymer, 537-540, *538*, 538t
Depth of cure, photoinitiated resins, restorative materials,
      esthetic, direct, 255-256
Detail, reproduction
  gypsum, 338t, 343-344, *343-344*
  impression materials, 311, 311t
Deviations, of models prepared with various impression
      materials, master die, 295t

Dextran, 142
Diacrylate resin
  filled, 196, 198; *see also* Resin
  two-body abrasion of, 92
Diametral compression test, 70
Diametral tensile strength of fused porcelain, 472
Diamond pyramid indentation test, 89
Dibutyl phthalate, 502
2,4-Dichlorobenzoyl peroxide, 541
Die, 321-325
Dielectric constant, 47, 47t
Dies formed by electrodeposition of metal, 322-325
Differential scanning calorimetry, 40
Differential thermal analysis, 39-41
  for baseplate wax, 377
  for corrective impression wax, 379, 380
  for sticky wax, 377
Diffusion, through membranes, 20
Diffusivity, thermal, 44, 44t
  various materials, 44t
Dimensional change
  amalgam, 218t, 220-221, *221*, 227
  casting, 438-439
  of impressions, impression materials, 316-317
  on setting, impression materials, 306t, 308-309,
      309
Dimensional stability
  cement, 182, 191
  impression materials, 289, *289*, 292-293, *293*, 320
Direct esthetic restorative materials, 244-280
  composite resins and, 244-252
  extended applications of, 264-267
  glass ionomers and, 272-274
  manipulation and handling of, 262-264
  pit and fissure sealants and, 267-271
  properties of, 252-262
    biocompatibility and, 260
    bond formation and, 256-260
    color and, 260-261
    depth of cure and, 255-256
    material selection and, 261-262
    mechanical, 254-255
    polymerization shrinkage and, 252-253
    radiopacity and, 255
    setting time and, 252
    solubility and, 254
    thermal, 253-254
    water sorption and, 254
    working time and, 252
Direct inlay wax patterns, 440; *see also* Inlay
      wax patterns

Discoloration, 51
Disinfection
    impression materials, 289
    of rubber impressions, 312-313
Disintegration, 51
    cement, 181-182, 191
Distortion, casting, 442
Ductility, 66, 67t
    wax, 371
Duplicating impression materials, 294-296
Dynamic modulus, 83t, 83-84

E

Egyptians, history, restorative metals, 4
1840 to 1900, history, restorative metals, 9-11
Elastic limits, 61-62, *62*
Elastic modulus, *61-62*, 65, *65*, 66t
    amalgam, 219
    of bending, 73
    of Bis-GMS resin sealants, 269
    of cement bases, 201
    of composite resins, 253
    of compression material, 71
    of dental plastics, 504, 506
    of glass ionomer cement, 272
    of metal alloys, 494-495
    of plastic teeth, 537
    of waxes, 367-368
    of zinc polyacrylate cement, 272
    values of, 66t
Elastomeric impression materials, 310t
Electrical conductivity, 45-47, 47t
    cement, 182-183
Electrical properties, 45-50
Electrochemical corrosion, 48t, 49-50, *50*
Electroforming impressions, 322-323
Electromotive force, 47-48, 48t
Elongation, *61*, 64, 64t
    of noble alloys, 395
    values of, 64t
Embedded metals, casting and, 404
Emulsions, colloid systems, 20
Enamel, 140
    biocompatibility, 140
    bonding of
        to direct esthetic resin, 256
        penetration coefficient in, 24
    compressive strength of, 71
    elastic modulus of, 66
    etching of, 28
    index of refraction of, 36

Enamel—cont'd
    injury of, 140
    Knoop hardness of, 89
    Poisson's ratio of, 66
    resistivity of, 56
    restorative materials, esthetic, direct, 256, *257*
    shear strength of, 72
    specific heat of, 44
    stress-strain curve for, 70
    surface preparation, restorative materials, esthetic,
        direct, 270, *270*
    tensile strength of, 70
    thermal conductivity of, 43
    thermal diffusivity of, 44
    zeta-potential of, 51
Endodontic instruments, stainless steel, 425-427,
    427
Endodontic sealers, 187
Endosteum, 144
Engineering stress-strain curve, 60; *see also* Stress-strain
    curve
Epoxy die materials, 325, *326*
ESGA spectrum, from surface of hydroxyapatite, 17
Essay upon Various Arts, 6
Essig, C.J., 12
Esters, 361-364
Esthetic restorative materials, direct; *see* Direct esthetic
    restorative materials
Esthetics of dental plastics, 513-514; *see also* Color
Ethanol; *see* Alcohol
Ether, 21
Ethyl, 44
Ethylene imine reaction, 132
Etruria, 4
Eutectic alloy, 113-115, *114-116*, 116t, 117
Eutectic mixture, alloys, 111
Exhausted solution, impression materials,
    324-325
Expansion, thermal, coefficient, 44-45, 45t, *46*
Extra hard gold casting alloys; *see also* Gold alloy
    applications of, 389-390
    properties of, 389-390
    temperature and, 388-389
Extracellular matrix, 140, 143-144
    of bone, 143
Eye protection during photoinitiation, 252

F

Fatigue strength, *76*, 76-77
Fats, 362t, 362-365
Fauchard, Pierre, 7

Federal specifications, standards, 95-98
   on boxing wax, 378
   on casting wax, 374
   on sticky wax, 379
   on utility wax, 379
Federation Dentaire Internationale, 95
Feldspar, 467, 468
Feldspathic porcelain
   compressive strength of, 71
   elastic modulus of, 66
   index of refraction of, 36
   Knoop hardness of, 89
   tensile strength of, 70
   transverse strength of, 73
Ferric oxalate, 256, 258
Fibrinogen, 144
Filler, restorative materials, esthetic, direct, 245-247,
      246-247
Filling
   of carious teeth, 6
   materials, 5, 7
Film thickness, cement, 177t, 184, 191, 193
Finishing
   amalgam restorations, 230, 231t
   restorative materials, esthetic, direct, 263t,
      263-264
Finite element analysis, 93
Fissure sealants, 267-271, *268*
Firing
   of artificial teeth, 480-483
   of porcelain, 471, 472, 480
Flagg, J. F., 10
Flexibility, impression materials, 287, 292
Flow
   impression materials, 310t, 310-311, 319-320
   wax, 368-369, *368-370*
Flow values for compounds, impression materials,
      ANSI/ADA specification No. 3, 320t
Fluid behavior, 77t, 77-79, *78-79*
Fluid resin acrylic, denture plastics, 525, *526-528*
Fluorescence, 35
Fluoride, 200
Flux, 453-454
   porcelains and, 471
Fonzi, Guiseppangelo, 7
Force, on restorations, 56-57
Fracture, of solids, 108-109, *110*
Fracture strength, *61*, 64
Fracture toughness, 67-69, *68*
Free-flowing solders, 399-400
Free-radical polymerization, 130-132
Friable metal deposit, impression materials, 325

Friction, *90*, 90-91
Frozen slab method, cement, 175
Fusion, heat of, 41-42, 42t
   of ceramics, 488
   of gold alloys, 388-389
   of porcelain, 470, 471-472

G

Galileo, 7
Gallium, in alloys, 387
Galvanic series, alloys, in artificial saliva, 48t
Galvanism, 48-49, *49*
Gamma globulin, 137
Gamma phases, 213
   corrosion of, 221-222
   microstructure of, 214, 215
   strength of, 219
Gaylor, M.L.V., 12
Gelatin temperature, impression materials, 292
Gels, surface phenomena, 19
Germany, history, restorative metals, 8
Gingiva, mucosa and, 145-146
Glass, casting, 464
Glass ionomer, 272-274
   cement, 192-194
   bonding and, 157
   compressive strength of, 201
   dielectric constant of, 47
   elastic modulus of, 201
   properties of, 177
   pulp and, 156-157
   resistivity of, 47
   soft tissue and, 163-164
   tensile strength of, 201
   thermal diffusivity or expansion of, 44
   use of, 172
   physical properties of, 272t
Glaze
   penetration coefficient of, 24
   porcelain and, 471-472
Gloves, 303
Glucose, diffusion of, 142
Glycerin, 42, 44
Glyceryl tristearate, 362, 365
Glycol dimethacrylate, 503
Gold
   alloys of; *see* Gold alloys
   characteristics of, 383-385
   copper and, 111
   ductility of, 67
   elastic modulus of, 66
   electrode potential of, 49

Gold–cont'd
    grains of, 122
    hardness of, 89
    heat of fusion of, 42
    historical use of, 4-5
    malleability of, 67
    oxidation-reduction potential of, 48
    percent elongation of, 64
    pulp and, 163
    specific heat of, 44
    surface tension of, 23
    tensile strength of, 70
    thermal conductivity of, 43
    thermal diffusivity or expansion of, 44
    thermal expansion of, 45
    transverse strength of, 73
    weight percentage of, 391
    yield strength of, 63
Gold alloy, 383-385
    cleaning, "pickling," 455-456
    history, restorative metals, 4
    low-fusing, casting practices for, 437
    property requirements for, gypsum-bonded casting
        investment, 349t
Gold crowns, 4
Gold leaf, history, restorative metals, 5-6
Goodyear
    Charles, 8, 10
    Nelson, 10
Grain size, noble alloys, 393-394
Gray, A.W., 12
Great Britain, history, restorative metals, 8
Guillemeau, Jacques, 6
Gums, 362t, 362-365
Gutta-percha, discovery of, 10
Gypsum, impression materials, compatibility
        with, 287-289, 288, 292
Gypsum-bonded casting investment, gold alloy, 348t, 349t
Gypsum products, 333-360
    abrasion resistance, 342-343
    calcium sulfate-bonded investment, 347, 351-354, 352t
        hygroscopic expansion of, 351-354, 352t
        properties of, 347-350, 348-349t
    calcium sulfate hemihydrate, solubility of, 336t
    casting investments, 346-347
    ceramic restorations, investments for, 357
    chemical nature, 333-337
    chemical reaction, 334-337
    composition, 347
    compressive strength, 340t, 341-342, 342, 342t
    consistency, 338t, 340-341, 341
    detail, reproduction of, 338t, 343-344, 343-344

Gypsum products–cont'd
    gypsum-bonded casting investments, for gold alloy,
        expansion requirements for, 348t
    high-melting alloys, investment for casting, 354-357
    hygroscopic-thermal gold casting investment, 354,
        354-355
    investment, properties required of, 346-347
    manipulation, 345, 345-346, 346t
    physical nature of, 333-337
    plaster, manufacture of, 333-334, 334
    properties, 337-345, 338t
    property requirements for, 338t
    setting expansion, 340t, 344, 345
    setting time, 337-340
    soldering investment, 357
    spatulation, effect on setting time, 340t
    stone
        high-strength, manufacture of, 333-334, 334
        and high-strength stones, manufacture of,
            333-334, 334
        properties of, 340t
        viscosity, 341t
    surface hardness, 342-343
    temperature, 350-351
    tensile strength, 343
    viscosity, 341, 341t
    water/powder ratio
        compressive strength, 342t
        effect on setting time, 340t

H

Hand-investing procedure, casting, 442-444, 443-444
Hardening, of alloys, 389-390
Harder, O.E., 12
Hardness
    of dental plastics, 506, 509, 510
    of gypsum products, 342-343
    impression materials, 311, 317
    of indentation, 86-90
    of metal alloys, 395, 494-495
    of natural, artificial teeth, 482t
    of noble alloys, 395
    of plastic teeth, 537, 539
    of soft denture liners, 536
    of solder, 398
    of zinc oxide–eugenol impression pastes, 318
Harris, C.A., 9
Hayden, H.H., 9
Heat, specific, 42-43, 44t
    various materials, 44t
Heat-acceleration, acrylic denture plastics, 515-523
Heat treatment, of base metal alloys, 411-412

Heating
    of dental plastics, 511, 512
    equipment for, 449-450
    of gold casting alloys, 394
    of investment mold, 445-446
    for wax elimination, 446-447
Heating mold, casting, 445-446, *446*
Heister, Lorenz, 7
High-copper alloys, 213-214
    admixed; *see* Admixed alloys
    amalgamation and, 212-214
    composition of, 210
    compressive strength of, 215, 217
    creep of, 217
    dimensional stability of, 218
    finishing of, 230
    microstructure of, 214, 215
    production of, 211-212
    tensile strength of, 218
    unicompositional, 210
        compressive strength of, 215, 217
        creep of, 217
        dimensional stability of, 218
        mercury and, 214
        microstructure of, 214, 215
        tensile strength of, 218
High-heat technic for investing, 449
High impact strength resin, 503, 509, 512
High-melting alloys, investment for casting, 354-357
High-strength bases, cement, 201t, 202
High-strength dental stone
    compressive strength of, 341-342
    consistency of, 340-341
    manufacture of, 333-334
    properties of, 340
    setting of, 344-345
    surface hardness of, 342-343
    viscosity of, 341
    water/powder ratio of, 335
High-temperature injection molding, ceramics, 477, *478*
Hill, Asa, 10
History, restorative materials, 1-15
    acid etching, tooth structure, effect of, 14
    Allen, Charles, 8
    American Dental Association, 13
        acceptance program for dental materials, 13
    American Dental Association Council on Dental
        Materials, Instruments, and Equipment, 11
    American Journal of Dental Science, establishment of, 8
    American National Standards, 13
    American National Standards Institute, 13
    American Society of Dental Surgeons, 9
        establishment of, 8

History, restorative materials–cont'd
    American Textbook of Operative Dentistry, 12
    appliances, construction of, 4
    Arthur, Robert, 10
    artificial teeth, from bone, ivory, 6
    Ash tube tooth, 8
    Assyrians, 4
    Babylonians, 4
    Baltimore College of Dental Surgery, establishment of, 8
    Barnum, Phineas Taylor, 10
    Black, G.V., 11, 12
    Blandy, Alfred A., 10
    Bourdet, Etienne, 7
    Boyle, Robert, 7
    bridgework, 4
    Bull, Marcus, 8
    Byram, J.Q., 10
    Cellini, Benvenuto, 6
    Celsus, 5
    Christensen, W.E., 10
    Clinical Products in Dentistry—A Desktop Reference, 13
    cloves, oil of, 6
    Coleman, R.L., 13
    Council on Dental Materials and Devices, 14
    Council on Scientific Affairs, 11
    Crawcour brothers, 8
    Crowell, W.S., 12
    Custer, Levitt Ellsworth, 10
    Darcet, Jean, 7
    Davis crown, 10
    de Chemant, Nicholas Dubois, 7
    de Saran, Aguilhon, 11
    de Vigo, Giovanni, 5
    Dean, J.C., 10
    Dental Device Classification Panel, 13
    dental metallurgy, usage of term, 12
    early history, 4-5
    Egyptians, 4
    1840 to 1900, 9-11
    Essay upon Various Arts, 6
    Essig, C.J., 12
    Etruria, 4
    Fauchard, Pierre, 7
    filling, 6
        materials, 5, 7
    Fonzi, Guiseppangelo, 7
    Galileo, 7
    Gaylor, M.L.V., 12
    Germany, 8
    gold, 4
    gold crowns, 4
    gold leaf, 5-6
    Goodyear

History, restorative materials—cont'd
    Charles, 8, 10
    Nelson, 10
  Gray, A.W., 12
  Great Britain, 8
  Guillemeau, Jacques, 6
  gutta-percha, discovery of, 10
  Harder, O.E., 12
  Heister, Lorenz, 7
  Hill, Asa, 10
  Hodgen, J.D., 12
  Hudson, Edward, 8
  Hyatt, J. Smith, 10
  International Organization for
    Standardization, 13
  J.M. Ney Company, 8
  Johannes, Arculanus, 5
  Knapp, J.R., 11
  Koenig, Augustus, 12
  Land, Charles, 10
  literature, dental, 7
  McBain, James, 12
  Medical Devices Amendments, 13
  medieval period, 5-7
  Merry, Charles, 10
  Middle Ages, 5
    contemporary arts of, 6-7
  Millberry, G.S., 12
  modern period, early, 5-7
  Montpellier, 5
  Mouton, Claude, 7
  National Bureau of Standards, 11, 12-13
  National Institute for Standards
    and Technology, 11
  Natural History, 6
  Newton, Sir Isaac, 7
  Pare, Ambroise, 6
  Pesso, F.A., 12
  Pfaff, Philip, 8
  Philbrook, B.F., 11
  Phoenician, 5
  Phoenicians, 4
  pivot crown, 10
  plaster models, 8
  Pliny, 6
  Poetske, Paul, 12
  Poppe, W.A., 13
  porcelain, introduction of, 7
  prostheses, 4
  Purmann, Matthaeus Gottfried, 7
  quality, of restorative materials, improving, 12
  Ray, K.W., 12
  Richmond crown, 10

History, restorative materials—cont'd
  Rome, 4
  Ryff, Walter Herman, 5
  Shell, J.S., 12
  silver amalgam, ban on use of, 9
  "silver paste" amalgam, silver, mercury, combination
    of, 8
  silver-tin-mercury alloy, introduction of, 10
  1600 to 1840, 7-9
  Skinner
    E.W., 12
    R.C., 8
  Snell, James, 8
  Souder, Wilmer, 13
  Spalding, E.B., 10
  S.S. White Dental Manufacturing Company, 9
  Swanger, W.L., 13
  Taggart, W.H., 11
  Taveau, O., 8
  Theophilus, 6
  Townsend, Elisha, 10
  twentieth century, 11-14
  United States, 8-9
  van Soolingen, Hornelis, 7
  vulcanite
    development of, 10
    introduction of, 8
  Ward, M.L., 12
  wax models, 7
  Weinstein Research Laboratories, 13
  White, S.S., 9
  Williams, R.V., 12
  wire, to hold teeth, 5
Hodgen, J.D., 12
Host tissue morphological changes, after injury, 138t
Hudson, Edward, 8
Hue, 31, 32; *see also* Color
  direct esthetic resins and, 261
Humidity
  agar hydrocolloids and, 292
  alginate hydrocolloids and, 289
  gypsum products and, 337
  impression plaster and, 318
  zinc oxide–eugenol impression pastes and, 316
Hyatt, J. Smith, 10
Hybrid ionomer cement, 194-195
Hydrocarbons
  in oils, 365
  in waxes, 362, 363, 364
Hydrocolloid heater, 294
Hydrocolloids
  agar, 289-296
  alginate, 283-289

Hydrocolloids—cont'd
   denture plastics and, 525
Hydrogen, 48
Hydrogenated waxes, 364
Hydrophilic acrylic resins, 508, 509
Hydroquinone, 502
   polymerization and, 131
Hydroxyapatite
   in bone, 143
   index of refraction of, 36
   zeta-potential of, 51
Hydroxyethyl methacrylate plus glutaraldehyde, 258, 259
Hygroscopic, high-heat technics, differences between, casting, 448
Hygroscopic-thermal gold casting investment, 354, *354-355*
Hyperalgesia in pulp, 141
Hypersensitivity
   gingiva and, 146
   to glass ionomer cement, 193-194
   mucosa and, 146
   to plastics, 514-515
   skin test and, 153
   to zinc oxide–eugenol cement, 189

I

Ice, 42
Immersion for hygroscopic expansion, 353
Impact resistance, 84
Impact strength, 84, *84*
Implants into bone, 154-155
   biocompatibility, 154-155
Impression, die materials, compared, 325-326
Impression compound, 318-321, *319*
Impression materials, 281-332, 311t, 315, 316, 317, *317*, 321
   accuracy, 320
   agar-alginate combination impressions, 293-295, *294-295*, 295t
   agar hydrocolloids, 289-296
   agar impression material, composition of, 290t
   alginate, properties of, 286t
   alginate hydrocolloids, 283-289, *284*
   alginate impression powder, ingredients in, 285t
   ANSI/ADA specification No. 3 for modeling compound, 320t, 321
   ANSI/ADA specification No. 16 for impression paste–zinc oxide–eugenol type, 317, 318t
   bite registrations, rubber impression materials, 314, 314t
   cast, and model materials, 321-325
   characteristic properties, 316-317
   chemical ingredients, 290t, 290-291

Impression materials—cont'd
   chemistry, 283-285, 285t
   clinical application, relationship of, 313-314
   composition, 283-285, 285t, 300-303, 318-319, 319t
   conduction, faulty, 324
   consistency of mix, 316
   cooling, 320
   copper-formed dies, 323t, 323-324
   copper-forming bath, composition of solution for, 323t
   creep compliance, 311-312, *312*
   detail reproduction, 311, 311t
   deviations, of models prepared with various impression materials, master die, 295t
   die, 321-325
      cast, and model materials, 321-325
      formed by electrodeposition of metal, 322-325
   dimensional change, 316-317
      on setting, 306t, 308-309, *309*
   dimensional stability, 289, *289*, 292-293, *293*, 320
   disinfection, 289
      rubber impressions, 312-313
   duplicating impression materials, 294-296
   effect of wet kneading, 320, 320t
   elastomeric impression materials, 310t
   electroforming impressions, 322-323
   epoxy die materials, 325, *326*
   exhausted solution, 324-325
   flexibility, 287, 292
   flow, 310t, 310-311, 319-320
   flow values for compounds, ANSI/ADA specification No. 3, 320t
   friable metal deposit, 325
   gelatin temperature, 292
   gypsum, compatibility with, 287-289, *288*, 292
   hardness, 311, 317
   impression, die materials, compared, 325-326
   impression compound, 318-321, *319*
   impression plaster, 317-318
   manipulation, critical factors of, *291*, 291-292
   mechanical properties, 309-312, 310-311t
   metal anode, small, 325
   metal-forming, problems in, 324-325
   mixing, 285, 318
   model materials, 321-325
   modification of setting time, 316
   overconcentrated solution, 325
   permanent deformation, *286*, 286t, 286-287, 292, 310
   plaster, 321-322
   polyethers, 303, *305*
   polysulfide, *300*, 300-301, 301t
      rubber impression material, ingredients of, 301t

Impression materials—cont'd
  pouring casts, 317
  proportioning, 285, 318
  purpose of, 281-282, *281-282*
  qualities of, 282-283
  reactions, 300-303
  rubber impression materials, 296-315, *298-300*
    advances in, 314-315
    mechanical properties of, 310t
    setting properties of, 306t
    wettability of, 313t
  separating cast, 317
  setting
    mechanism of, 335
    properties, 303-309, 306t
    reaction, 315
  setting time, 285-286, 306t, 308, *308*
  silicones, 301-303, *303-305*
  silver-formed dies, 324t, 324-325, *325*
  silver-forming bath, composition of solution for, 324t
  softening, 319-320
  specification requirements, duplicating materials, 297t
  stone, 321-322
  storage problems, 318
  strain, 310, 310t
  strength, 287, 292
  tear strength, 311
  thermal conductivity, 319
  thermal contraction, 320
  tray compounds, 320t, 320-321
  types, 283-321
  viscosity, 306t, 306-308, *307*
  wax, as impression material, 318
  wettability of rubber impression materials, 312, 313t
  working time, 285, 306t, 308, *308*
  zinc oxide–eugenol impression paste, 315-317, 318t
Impression plaster, 317-318
Impression trays, polymer, *546*, 546-547
Impurities
  in feldspar, 467
  in gold, 384
  in metals, 120
  in silica, 468
Incisal porcelain, 478
In vitro mutagenesis tests, comparison of, 152t
Indentation hardness, 86-90, *87*
Index of Federal Specifications and Standards, 96
Index of refraction, 36
Indirect inlay wax patterns, 441-442; *see also* Inlay wax patterns
Indirect tensile test, 69-70

Indium, in alloys, 387
Infrared soldering, 403-404
Initial tests, 147-153
Inlay casting, wax, flow requirements for, 372t
Inlay pattern
  formation of, 439-442
  polymer, 545
  wax, 371-374
Inlay wax patterns, 371-374
  acrylic plastics and, 545
  compressive strength of, 367, 368
  direct, 439
  elastic modulus of, 367-368
  flow of, 368-369
  formation of, 439-443
  investment materials and, 442-449
  proportional limit of, 368
  thermal expansion of, 45
  warpage of, 373-374
Inlays, porcelain, 469, 473
Insect wax, 361, 362, 364-368; *see also* Beeswax
Instruments
  for amalgam
    in condensation, 228
    in finishing, 234, 235
    in mixing, 228
    in polishing, 234, 235
  for casting, 450
  for dispensing mercury and alloys, 227
  for finishing composite resins, 263
  for gypsum products, 339
  for hand mechanical spatulation, 443
  historical use of, 5
  for investing wax patterns, 444
  for measurement or test
    of bending, 72
    of cold bending, 74
    of color, 31-33
    of creep, 220
    of dimensional change, 221
    of hardness, 90
    of impact, 84
    of setting time, 308
    of stress, 59
Instrumental technic, color measurement, 31t, 31-32, *32-33*
Interface, sealant, and enamel, scanning electron micrograph, 26
Intermediate tests, 153
Intermetallic compounds, alloys, 111, 115, 117
International Organization for Standardization, 13
Investing patterns, for water-added technic, 445

Investing procedure, for wax patterns, 442-448
Ionic polymerization, 133
Iridium, in alloys, 386
Iron
    in cast base metal alloys, 409
    in ceramic-metal restorations, 491
    crystals of, 106
    ductility of, 67
    malleability of, 67
    oxidation-reduction potential of, 48
    percent elongation of, 64
Irritation test, 153, 154
Ischemia, 137-138
Isochromatic fringe
    transverse bending and, 74
    in two-dimensional photoelasticity, 92-93
Isolated capillaries, 24-26

J

Jacket crowns, 468-469, 472, 473; *see also* Crowns
    aluminous core, 474-475
Japan wax, 362, 363
J.M. Ney Company, 8
Johannes, Arculanus, 5
Journal history, 9
Justi, H.D., 10

K

Kaolin, 467-468
Kauri, 365
Kelvin model, 81
Kerr inlay wax, 366, 367; *see also* Inlay wax patterns
Knapp, J.R., 11
Knoop hardness test, 88-89, *89*, 89t
    of Bis-GMA resin sealants, 269
    of dental plastics, 507, 510
    of direct esthetic resins, 253, 254
Koenig, Augustus, 12

L

Land, Charles, 10
Latex rubber, 544-545
    gloves of, 303
Lathe-cut alloys
    composition of, 210
    creep of, 217
    dimensional stability of, 218, 220
    microstructure of, 214, 215
    production of, 211-212
    selection of, 218, 223
    strength of

Lathe-cut alloys—cont'd
      compressive, 217
      tensile, 218
      trituration time of, 227
Lattice, 105, 107
LD_{50} test, 153
Le Châfatelier, H.L., 335-336
Lead, 67
    copper with, 110
    surface tension of, 23
    zinc with, 110
Life value tests, 76-78
Light, color and, 31
Light-accelerated sealant, 271
Light-activated acrylic resin
    characteristics of, 503-504
    impression trays and, 546
    for repairing, 531
    as temporary crown and bridge restorations, 544
    transverse deflection of, 508
Light-cured cement, 197, 199
Light-cured denture plastic, 525-528, *529*
Light radiation, 249-251
Light reflectivity, 37-38
Linear coefficient of thermal expansion, 45; *see also*
        Thermal expansion
Linear polymer, 129-130
Liners
    cavity, 199-200
    ceramic paper, 443
    reactions of pulp to, 161-163
    soft, 534, 544
      processed, 535-537
Liquid cement, 173, 173t
Literature, history, restorative metals, 7
Local reactions, amalgam, 235
Low-copper alloys, 212-213
    amalgamation and, 212
    composition of, 210
    compressive strength of, 217
    creep of, 217
    dimensional stability of, 218, 220
    lathe-cut; *see* Lathe-cut alloys
    microstructure of, 214, 215
    production of, 211-212
    selection of, 223
    spherical; *see* Spherical alloys
    tensile strength of, 218
Low-strength bases, cement, 200-201
Lubricant for wax release, 440
Luminous reflectance, 31
    direct esthetic resins and, 260, 261

Luting cements; *see* Cements

M

Machined restorations, ceramics, 473-474, *474*
Malleability, 66, 67t
Manipulation
    cement, 196, 197
    critical factors of, *291*, 291-292
    polymer, *515-516*, 515-537
    restorative materials, esthetic, direct, 270-271
Manufacture, ceramics, 479-482, *480-481*
Material selection, restorative materials, esthetic, direct,
        261-262
Materials science, in dentistry, relations of, 2
Maxillary denture bases, polymerization shrinkage,
        posterior of, 512t
Maxillofacial materials, polymer, *540*, 540-543
    static, dynamic properties of, 542t
McBain, James, 12
Mechanical properties
    amalgam, 215-222
    American Dental Association
        acceptance program, 95
        specifications, 95, 96-97t
    bending, *72*, 72-73
    bond strengths, 72
    Brinell hardness test, 87-88, *88*, 88t
    brittle materials, tensile properties, 69-70, 70t
    composites, 85-86, *86*
    compressive properties, 70-71, *71*, 71t
    compressive strength, restorative materials, 71t
    creep compliance, 81-83, *82*
    ductility, 66, 67t
    dynamic modulus, 83t, 83-84
    elastic modulus, *61-62*, 65, *65*, 66t
        values of, 66t
    elongation, *61*, 64, 64t
        values of, 64t
    fatigue strength, *76*, 76-77
    federal specifications, standards, 95-98
    finite element analysis, 93
    fluid behavior, 77t, 77-79, *78-79*
    force, 56-57
        on restorations, 56-57
    fracture, *61*, 64, 67-69, *68*
    friction, *90*, 90-91
    impact strength, 84, *84*
    indentation hardness, 86-90, *87*
    Knoop hardness test, 88-89, *89*, 89t
    malleability, 66, 67t
    occlusal forces, 56
        summary of, 57

Mechanical properties—cont'd
    overview, 93-94
    permanent bending, 74, *75*
    Poisson's ratio, 65-66, 66t
        values of, 66t
    proportional, elastic limits, 61-62, *62*
    resilience, *61*, 66-67, *67*
    restorative materials, esthetic, direct, 253t, 254-255
    Rockwell hardness test, 89-90, 90t
    shear strength, 71-72, 72t
        values of, 72t
    shore A hardness, 90, 90t
    specifications, for restorative materials, 94-98
    strain, 58-59
    stress, 57-59
        analysis, 92-94
        types of, 58, *58-59*
    stress-strain curves, 59-69, *60-61*, *69*
    surface mechanical properties, 86
    tear
        energy, 84-85, 84-85t
            materials, 85t
        strength, 84-85, 84-85t
            materials, 84t
    tensile strength, restorative materials, values of, 70t
    torsion, *75*, 75-76
    toughness, 67, *67*
    transverse strength, 73t, 73-74, *73-74*
        restorative materials, 73t
    two-dimensional photoelasticity, 92-93, *93*
    ultimate strength, *61*, 63-64
    Vickers hardness test, 89, *89*
    viscoelastic materials, 79-80, *80*
    viscoelasticity, 77-83
        mechanical models of, 80-81, *81-82*
    viscosity, 77t, 77-79, *78-79*
        materials, soon after mixing, 77t
    wear, 91-92, 92t
    yield strength, *61*, 62-63, 63t
        values of, 63t
Medical Devices Amendments, 13
Medieval period, history, restorative metals, 5-7
Melting range
    noble alloys, 394
    wax, 365-366, *365-366*
Membrane diffusion, 20
Membrane permeability, 148, 149
Membranous bone formation, 143-144
Mercaptan, 133
Mercury
    concentration of, 233-234
    contact angle of, on various materials, 24

Mercury—cont'd
   content, amalgam, 229
   daily intake of, 233t
   forms of, 232-233
   properties of, 222-223
   proportions of alloy to, 224, *224-225*
   reaction of
      in admixed high-copper alloy, 213-214
      in unicompositional alloy, 214
   sources of, 232, 233t
   toxicity, 232-237
Merry, Charles, 10
Metal anode, small, impression materials, 325
Metal-forming, impression materials, problems in,
      324-325
Metallic bonding, and properties of alloys, 104
Metallic elements, in alloys, 383-395
   base metals, 386
   binary combinations of metals, 387
   composition, 387-389
   copper, 386-387
   gallium, 387
   gold, 383-385
   indium, 387
   iridium, 386
   nickel, 387
   palladium, 385-386
   platinum, 385
   rhodium, 386
   ruthenium, 386
   silver, 386
   temperature, 387-389
   tin, 387
   zinc, 387
Metallurgy, usage of term, 12
Metals, 104-109
   crystal structure, 104-109, *105-107*
      physical properties, 105-106, *107*
   deformation of, 106-108, *107-109*
   fracture of solids, 108-109, *110*
   general characteristics of, 104
   metallic bonding, and properties of alloys, 104
   noble, 383-407
   physical properties, 105-106, *107*
   strengthening techniques, *123-125*, 124-125
   surface tension of, 23
Metamerism, 35
Methacryloxypropyltrimethoxy siloxane, 539
Methyl methacrylate, 127
Metric weights, 553
Microcrystalline wax, 362, 363
Microfine composite resin
   as anterior veneers, 264

Microfine composite resin—cont'd
   compressive strength of, 254
   depth of cure of, 255–256
   elastic modulus of, 253
   Knoop hardness of, 253, 254
   polymerization shrinkage in, 253
   as posterior resins, 265
   radiopacity of, 255
   selection of, 261-262
   solubility of, 254
   tensile strength of, 254
   thermal conductivity of, 254
   thermal expansion of, 253
   water sorption of, 253
   wear rate of, 255
Microleakage, 154
   pulp reactions and, 156-157
Micrometer, 12
Microscopy, 120-121
Microstructure
   amalgam, 214, *215-216*
   wrought alloys, 396
Middle Ages, history, restorative metals, 5
   contemporary arts of, 6-7
Millberry, G.S., 12
Millipore filter assay, 150
Mineral wax
   characteristics of, 361-363
   flow of, 369
   thermal expansion of, 366, 367
Mix, normal, amalgam, 226-228, *227*
Mixing, impression materials, 285, 318
Mixing procedure, cement, 174-175, 184
Mixing slab, cement, 174
Model materials, 321-325
Model plaster
   chemical reaction of, 334-337
   compressive strength of, 341
   consistency of, 340
   manufacture of, 333-334
   setting of, 344
   surface hardness of, 342
   tensile strength of, 343
   water/powder ratio of, 335
Modulus
   dynamic, 83, 84
      of mouth protector materials, 545
   elastic; *see* Elastic modulus
   rupture, 73
Moisture contamination, during insertion, amalgam,
      229-230
Molecular weight, polymers, 128
Molten metals, 23

Molybdenum
    in cast base metal alloys, 409
    in cobalt-chromium-molybdenum alloys, 166
Monel Metal, 432
Monoclinic crystal system, 105
Monomers, 127
    residual, 521-522
Montan wax, 362, 363
    flow of, 369
    thermal expansion of, 366-367
Montpellier, 5
Morphology, amalgam, 209-211, 210t, *211*
Mouth protectors
    athletic, 544-545, 545-546t
    custom-made, physical properties of materials,
        545t
    materials, before, after use, properties of, 546t
Mouton, Claude, 7
Mucosa, gingival usage tests and, 155
Mucositis, contact, 146
Mucous membrane irritation test, 153
Munsell scales, 34
Munsell system, color, for clinical restorations using,
        change in, 261t
Mutagenesis assays, 151-152, 152t
Mutagenesis tests, *in vitro*, comparison of, 152t

N

National Bureau of Standards, 11, 12-13
National Institute for Standards and Technology, 11
Natural History, 6
Natural wax, 362-364
Newton, Sir Isaac, 7
Nickel, in alloys, 387
    in cast base metal alloys, 409
        for ceramic-metal restorations, 493-495
    ductility of, 67
    electrode potential of, 48
    malleability of, 67
    oxidation-reduction potential of, 48
    percent elongation of, 64
    yield strength of, 63
Nickel-chromium alloy, casting, 409-415, 456-463,
        457-459, 461-463
Nickel-titanium alloy, wrought, 430-431
Noble alloys, 383-407
    composition of, 490-493
    density, 394
    elongation of, 395
    formulation of, 390-393
    grain size, 393-394
    hardness, 395

Noble alloys—cont'd
    melting range, 394
    strength, 394-395
Non-eugenol cement, 183-189

O

Occlusal forces, 56
    summary of, 57
Occlusal splints, polymer, 544
Office personnel, risks to, amalgam, 236-237
Oligomers, restorative materials, esthetic, direct, 247
Opacity, 35-36
Optical constants, 36-38
    scattering coefficient, 37, *37*
Optical properties, 30-38
    ceramics, 477-478, 478t
Optical thickness, infinite, *vs.* wavelength, for shades of
        composite, *39*
Oral tissue, 143-144
    alloys, reactions to, 166
    biocompatibility, 143-144
    biology, 140-146
    implant materials
        biocompatibility, 165-167
        other materials, 166-167
        overview, 167
        reaction to, 165-167
            ceramic implant materials, 165-166
        reactions to, ceramic implant materials, 165-166
    inflammatory response, to injury, 140-146
    metals, pure, reactions to, 166
    restorative materials
        biocompatibility, 163
        reaction to, 163
Orthodontic wires
    experimental, 432
    no precious metals requirements, ANSI/ADA
        specification No. 32, 424t
    properties of, in tension, bending, and torsion, 424t
    stainless steel, 423-425
    summary of, 424t, 432
Orthodontics, restorative materials, esthetic, direct, 267
Orthorhombic crystal system, 105
Osmium, 383
Osmotic pressure, 20
Osseointegration, 419-420
Osteoblasts, 143
Osteoclasts, 143
Osteoid, 143
Osteomyelitis, 144
Ouricury waxes, 362-363
Oven temperature, casting, 448

Overconcentrated solution, impression materials, 325
Overmix, amalgam, 226-228, *227*
Oxidation-reduction potentials, corrosion reactions, 48t
Oxygen, polymerization and, 131
Ozokerite, 362-363

P

Packaging, of composites, restorative materials, esthetic, direct, 249-252
Palladium, in alloys, 385-386
Paper mixing pad, 184
Paraffin wax, 362-363
    differential thermal analysis of, 40-41, 365-366
    elastic modulus of, 367-368
    flow of, 368-369
    specific heat of, 44
    thermal expansion of, 366-367
Paraffin-carnauba wax mixture, thermograms, *40*
Pare, Ambroise, 6
Particles, irregular, amalgam, *211*, 211-212
Paste, 27
Pattern wax; *see* Inlay wax pattern
PDL; *see* Periodontal ligament
Penetration coefficient, 24
Penetration curve, 377
Percent elongation, 64; *see also* Elongation
Percent recovery, 90
Periodic table, 384
Periodontal disease, 145
Periodontal ligament, 144
Periodontium, 144-145
Permanent cementation, 177t, 187
Pesso, F.A., 12
Pfaff, Philip, 8
Phase diagrams
    alloys, *112*, 112-117
        types of, 113-115
    construction of, 116-117, *117*
    ternary, 115-116, *117*
Philbrook, B.F., 11
Phoenicians, history, restorative metals, 4, 5
Phosphate-bonded investments
    for high-melting alloys, 354-357
    for porcelain veneers, 454-455
Phosphonates, 258
Photoelasticity
    transverse bending and, 74
    two-dimensional, 92-93
Photoinitiated resins, restorative materials, esthetic, direct, 255-256
Physical techniques, clinical dentistry, relationship, 2

Pigmentation, 34-35
Pigments, restorative materials, esthetic, direct, 248-249
Pit sealants, 267-271, *268*
    indentation depth of, 90
    percent recovery of, 90
    thermal expansion of, 45
    two-body abrasion of, 92
Pitted solder joints, 400
Pivot crown, 10
Plaster, 321-322
    gypsum, manufacture of, 333-334, *334*
Plaster models, 8
Plastic facings, crown, bridge applications, 543
Plastic teeth, porcelain teeth, comparison of properties of, 539t
Plastics
    abrasion resistance of, 510t
    denture base, strength characteristics of, 506t
    fracture toughness, 509t
    impact strength of, 508t
    properties of, 504, 511-515, 512t
    strength characteristics of, 506t
    thermal characteristics of, 511t
Platinum, in alloys, 385
    ductility of, 67
    heat of fusion of, 42
    malleability of, 67
    oxidation-reduction potential of, 48
    specific heat of, 44
    thermal conductivity of, 43
Platinum foil, 385
Platinum-gold alloys, 10
Platinum matrix, 470, 473
Pliny, 6
Poetske, Paul, 12
Poisoning, amalgam, 234-236
Poisson's ratio, 65-66, 66t
        values of, 66t
Polishing; *see also* Finishing
    of amalgam restorations, 230
    of denture plastics, 521
Poly-vinylacetate-poly-ethylene, 545
Polyacrylic acids, 256, 257
Polycarboxylate cement; *see* Zinc polyacrylate
Polycrystalline, 107
Polydimethylvinyl siloxane, 541
Polyether impression materials
    accuracy of, 313
    classification of, 296
    composition and reactions of, 133, 303, 306
    creep compliance of, 311-312
    dimensional stability of, 310

Polyether impression materials—cont'd
    disinfection of, 312-313
    flow of, 310, 311
    hardness of, 311
    permanent deformation of, 310
    setting time of, 306, 308
    silver-formed dies and, 324
    strain of, 310
    tear energy of, 84
    tear strength of, 311
    viscosity of, 306-308
    wettability of, 312, 313
    working time of, 306, 308
Polyethers, 303, *305*
Polyethylene
    resins and, 365
    stress-strain curve for, 69
    waxes and, 362, 364
Polyisoprene, 139
Polymerization, 127-136, 135
    addition, 130-133
    condensation, 133-135
    free-radical, 130-132
    ionic, 133
    ring-opening, 132-133
    shrinkage, restorative materials, esthetic, direct,
        252-253, 253t
Polymers, 127-136, 500-551
    acrylic denture base, powder, liquid, principal
        ingredients of, 501t
    acrylic soft lining materials, plasticized, composition
        of, 535t
    acrylics, properties of, ANSI/ADA specification
        No. 12, 505t
    ANSI/ADA specification No. 12, denture base resins,
        504, 505t
    ANSI/ADA specification No. 15, plastic teeth, 539
    auxiliary materials, effect, on denture plastics, 528-530
    bridge restorations, 543-544
    chemical composition, 127-128
    chemically accelerated acrylic denture plastics,
        compression molding, 524-525
    composition, 500-503, 501t
    denture base materials, properties of, 500-504
    denture materials, 503-504
    denture retention, forces involved in, 528
    denture teeth, 537-540, *538*, 538t
    fluid resin acrylic denture plastics, 525, *526-528*
    heat-accelerated acrylic denture plastics, 515-523
    impression trays, *546*, 546-547
    inlay patterns, 545
    light-cured denture plastic, 525-528, *529*

manipulation, *515-516*, 515-537
maxillary denture bases, polymerization shrinkage,
        posterior of, 512t
maxillofacial materials, *540*, 540-543
    static, dynamic properties of, 542t
molecular weight, 128
mouth protectors
    athletic, 544-545, 545-546t
    custom-made, physical properties of materials,
        545t
    materials, before, after use, properties of, 546t
nature of, 127-130
occlusal splints, 544
physical form, 500-503, 501t
plastic facings, crown, bridge applications, 543
plastics
    abrasion resistance of, 510t
    fracture toughness, 509t
    impact strength of, 508t
    properties of, 504, 511-515, 512t
    strength characteristics of, 506t
    thermal characteristics of, 511t
porcelain teeth, plastic teeth, comparison of properties
        of, 539t
preparation of, 130-135
processing, 513, *515-516*, 515-537
rebasing dentures, 532-537
record bases, *546*, 546-547
relining dentures, 532-537
repair materials, 531-532
resins, mechanical properties of, 507t
silicone soft lining materials, composition of, 536t
soft denture liners, laboratory processed, bond
        strength of, 537t
soft liners, laboratory-processed, properties of,
        536t
spatial structure, 128-130, *129*
strength properties, 504-510, 506-507t
temporary crown, 543-544
thermal characteristics, 510-511
Poly(methyl methacrylate), 127, 195
    bond strength of, 537
    bone and, 167
    in denture base, 500
    hypersensitivity to, 514
    maxillofacial materials and, 540
    properties of, 512
        strength, 506, 508
        thermal, 511
    pulp and, 162-163
    soft tissue and, 167
    water sorption of, 513

Polyoxyethylene wax, 362, 364
Polyphosphazine, 536, 537
Polysiloxanes; *see* Silicone impression materials
Polystyrene, 365
Polysulfide rubber impression material, ingredients
      of, 301t
Polysulfides, *300*, 300-301, 301t
Polysulfide impression materials
    accuracy of, 313, 314
    classificaion of, 296
    composition and reactions of, 300-301
    creep compliance of, 311-312
    disinfection of, 312-313
    flow of, 310, 311
    hardness of, 311
    permanent deformation of, 310
    setting time of, 306, 308
    silver-formed dies and, 324
    strain of, 310
    tear energy or strength of, 84
    thermal expansion of, 45
    viscosity of, 77
    working time of, 306, 308
Polyurethane, 541
    athletic mouth protectors and, 544-545
    for dentin-bonding, 258
    dynamic modulus and resilience of, 83
    physical properties of, 545
    properties of, 541, 542
    tear energy of, 84
Polyvinyl acrylic
    heat distortion of, 511
    hypersensitivity to, 514
    properties of, 512
        strength, 506, 509
        thermal, 510
Polyvinylacetate-polyethylene, 545
    dynamic modulus and resilience of, 83
    Shore A hardness of, 90
    tear strength of, 84
Polyvinylchloride
    dynamic modulus and resilience of, 83
    plasticized, 540-541, 542
    tear energy of, 84
Poppe, W.A., 13
Porcelain
    artificial teeth, 479-483
    bonding, restorative materials, esthetic, direct,
        265, *265*
    crowns, 472-473
    enamel-metal restorations, 474-475, *475*
    fusion, 471-472, *472*

    ingredients of, 468t
    inlays, 473
    introduction of, 7
    technic, 470-471
    teeth, plastic teeth, comparison of properties
        of, 539t
    tooth restorative
        material, 469-476
        types of, 471
    total percent transmission of, 478t
    veneer
        esthetic, 479, *479*
        metal structures, 454-455, *455*
Porcelain-fused-to-metal restorations, preparation of, *490*,
        496-497
Posterior restorations, restorative materials, esthetic,
        direct, 265-267, 266t, *266-267*
Pouring casts, 317
Powder, cement, 173, 173t
Powder/liquid ratio, cement, 174
Precious metals; *see* Gold; Metals; *specific metals*
Precipitation hardening, 124
Pressure firing of artificial teeth, 481
Primary colors, 31
Processing wax, 371
Proportional limit, 61-62
    of dental plastics, 506
    of waxes, 368
Proportioning, impression materials, 285, 318
Prostheses, history, restorative metals, 4
Protein, bone morphogenic, 144
Pseudoplastic liquid, 78
Pulp, 156-163
    amalgams, 159-161
    biocompatibility, 156-163
    bleaching agents, 163
    cast alloys, 159-161
    dentin bonding, *141*, 157-159
    glass ionomers, 161
    irritation tests, 154
    liners, 161-163, *162*
    microleakage, 156-157
    nonresin cements, 161-163, *162*
    resin-based materials, 159, *160*
    varnishes, 161-163, *162*
        and nonresin cements, 161-163, *162*
Purmann, Matthaeus Gottfried, 7

Q

Quality
    impression materials, 282-283
    restorative materials, improving, 12

Quartz
    index of refraction of, 36
    specific heat of, 44
    temperature and, 350

R

Radiopacity
    cement, 189
    restorative materials, esthetic, direct, 255, *255*
Radiopaque polymer, 502
Rapid heat-polymerized acrylic, 503
    abrasion resistance of, 510
    fracture toughness of, 509
    polymerization shrinkage of, 511
    transverse deflection of, 508
Rapid inlay technic, 473
Ray, K.W., 12
Reactions, of materials
    comparison of, screening and usage tests,
            155t
    impression, 300-303
Rebasing dentures, polymer, 532-537
Record bases, polymer, *546*, 546-547
Recrystallization, alloys, 122-123, *123*
Refraction, index of, 36, 36t
Relining dentures, polymer, 532-537
Repair materials, polymer, 531-532
Residual stress, wax, *370*, 370-371
Resilience, *61*, 66-67, *67*
Resin, 362t, 362-365, *365*
    mechanical properties of, 507t
    modeling material, *376*, *376*, 376t
Resistivity
    electrical, 45-47, 47t
    of human tooth structure, cements, 47t
Restorative materials
    esthetic, direct, 244-280
        accelerators, 248, *248-249*
        anterior veneers, 264-265
        biocompatibility, 260
        bis-GMA-amine-accelerated sealant, 271
        bis-GMA-light-accelerated sealant, 271
        bis-GMA resin, 268-270
            sealants, physical properties of, 269t
        bond formation to tooth structure, 256-260
        chemical reaction, 244-249
        clinical application, 272-274, *273*
        clinical studies of sealants, 271
        color, 260-261, *261*, 261t
        composite, 244-252, 262
            color characteristics, variation in, 261t
            microfine, properties of, 253t

Restorative materials—cont'd
    esthetic, direct—cont'd
        composite—cont'd
            posterior, critical physical properties for, 266t
            properties of, 252-262
        composition, 244-249, 272
        core build-up, 265, *265*
        coupling agents, 247-248
        dentin, 253t, 256-260, 259t
            composite, shear bond strengths, 258t
        depth of cure (photoinitiated resins), 255-256
        enamel, 256, *257*
            surface preparation, 270, *270*
        extended applications for composites, 264-267
        filler, 245-247, *246-247*
        finishing, 263t, 263-264
        fissure sealants, 267-271, *268*
        glass ionomer, 272-274
            physical properties of, 272t
        handling characteristics, 262-264
        initiators, 248, *248-249*
        insertion, 262-263
        manipulation, 262-264, 270-271
        material selection, 261-262
        mechanical properties, 253t, 254-255
        Munsell system, color, for clinical restorations
            using, change in, 261t
        oligomers, 247
        orthodontics, 267
        packaging of composites, 249-252
        pigments, 248-249
        pit sealants, 267-271, *268*
        polymerization shrinkage, 252-253, 253t
        porcelain bonding, 265, *265*
        posterior restorations, 265-267, 266t, 266-267
        properties, 269t, 269-270, 272, 272t
        radiopacity, 255, *255*
        reaction, 272
        setting, 252
        single-paste system, 262-263
            for photoinitiation, 249-252, *250-252*
        solubility, 253
        surface roughness, composites finished with various
            abrasives, 263t
        thermal properties, 253t, 253-254
        tooth bleaching agents, effects of, 264
        two-paste system, 249, 262
        water sorption, 253t, 254
        working times, 252
    specifications for, 94-98
Retention, denture, 528
    surface phenomena in, 26-27

Revere, P., 8
Rhazes, 6
Rhodium, in alloys, 386
Richmond crown, 10
Rickert's formula, 187
Ring
    casting, 443
    rubber, 445
Ring-opening polymerization, 132-133
Risks to dentists, amalgam, 236-237
Rockwell hardness test, 89-90, 90t
Rome, history, restorative metals, 4
Room temperature–vulcanized silicone, 541, 542
Root dentin, 142
Rosin, 315
Rotation speed, 38
Rounded margins on castings, 453
Rubber dam, 10
Rubber gloves, 303
Rubber impression materials, 296-315, *298-300*
    advances in, 314-315
    mechanical properties of, 310t
    setting properties of, 306t
    wettability of, 313t
Rubber latex, 544-545
Rubber-reinforced acrylic
    abrasion resistance of, 510
    impact strength of, 508
    transverse deflection of, 508
Rubber ring, 445
Ruthenium, in alloys, 386
Ryff, Water Herman, 5

S

Saliva
    amalgam contamination from, 229
    denture retention and, 27, 528
    gypsum and, 287
    plastic and, 22
Salmonella typhimurium, 151
Salt water, 48
Scanning calorimetry, differential, 40
Scattering coefficient
    absorption coefficient, 37, *37*
    contrast ratio, 38
    light reflectivity, 37-38, *39*
    vs. wavelength, for shades of composite, *37*
Sciences
    application of, to dentistry, 2-3
    basic, applied to restorative materials, 2, *2*
Scope, restorative materials, 1-3

Screening tests, correlation among, 138-139t, 155t,
    155-156
Secondary tests, 153
Setting expansion, gypsum, 340t, 344, 345
Setting properties, impression materials, 303-309, 306t
Setting reaction, impression materials, 315
Setting time, 51-52
    cement, 190-191
    gypsum, 337-340
    impression materials, 285-286, 306t, 308, *308*
    modification of, impression materials, 316
Shear strength, 71-72, 72t
    values of, 72t
Shell, J.S., 12
Shore A hardness, 90, 90t
    of mouth protector materials, 545, 546
    of rubber impression materials, 310
Short-term test, 152
Shrinkage; *see also* Dimensional changes; Dimensional
    stability
    in casting process, 438
    of direct esthetic resins, 252-253
    of plastics, 511-512
    of porcelain, 472
    thermal, 521
    of zinc oxide–eugenol cement, 189
    of zinc phosphate cement, 182
Silica
    ceramics and, 467, 471
    in composite resins, 245, 246
    hygroscopic expansion and, 353
    temperature and, 350-351
    thermal expansion of, 45
Silicate, 10
Silicate cements
    history of, 244
    screening and usage tests of, 155-160
Silicate glass, 474, 475
Silicon, 409
Silicon carbide abrasive, 89
Silicone, 301-303, *303-305*
    addition
        classification of, 296-298
        composition and reactions of, 302-303
        copper-formed dies and, 323
        creep compliance of, 311
        deformation of, 310
        dimensional stability of, 308
        disinfection of, 312
        flow of, 310
        hardness of, 311
        strain of, 310

Silicone—cont'd
  addition—cont'd
    viscosity of, 306
    wettability of, 312
  condensation
    accuracy of, 313
    classification of, 296
    composition and reactions of, 301-303
    creep compliance of, 311
    deformation of, 310
    dimensional stability of, 308
    flow of, 310
    hardness of, 311
    strain of, 310
    viscosity of, 306
    wettability of, 312
  dynamic modulus and resilience of, 83
  in liners, 535, 536
  oils and, 364
  polymerization of, 134
  room temperature—vulcanized, 541, 542
  Shore A hardness of, 90
  soft lining materials, composition of, 536t
Silver, in alloys, 386
Silver amalgam, ban on use of, 9
Silver-formed dies, 324t, 324-325, *325*
Silver-forming bath, composition of solution for, 324t
"Silver paste" amalgam, silver, mercury, combination of, 8
Silver solder, 402
Silver-tin alloy, 212, *213*
Silver-tin-mercury alloy, introduction of, 10
Single-paste system, restorative materials, esthetic, direct, 262-263
Single-paste systems, for photoinitiation, 249-252, *250-252*
1600 to 1840, history, restorative metals, 7-9
Skinner
  E.W., 12
  R.C., 8
Snell, James, 8
Sodium oleate, in water, 21
Soft denture liners, laboratory processed
  bond strength of, 537t
  properties of, 536t
Softening, impression materials, 319-320
Solder, 397-404
  color, 400
  composition of, 398-399
  easy-flowing, 399-400
  joints, microstructure, 400-402
  mechanical properties, 400
  noble metal, 383-407

Solder—cont'd
  pitted solder joints, 400
  selection of, 398
  silver, 402
  tarnish resistance, 400
  types of, 397-398
Soldering, 397-404, *402*
  casting, fluxes, 453-454
  gypsum, 357
  infrared, 403-404
Solid solution, alloys, 111, 113, 113t, *113-114*, 117
Solid surfaces, characterization of, 17-18, *17-18*
Solidification, alloys, *116*, *119*, 119-120
Solubility, 51
  cement, 176-177, 177t, 181-182, 186, 189, 193
  restorative materials, esthetic, direct, 253
Solubility, cement, 191
Souder, Wilmer, 13
Spalding, E.B., 10
Spatial structure, polymers, 128-130, *129*
Spatulation, gypsum, effect on setting time, 340t
Specific heat, 42-43, 44t
  various materials, 44t
Specification requirements, duplicating materials, 297t
Spherical particles, amalgam, *211*, 212
Spring pattern, 440-441, *441*
S.S. White Dental Manufacturing Company, 9
Stainless steel alloys, wrought, 421-428
Stainless steel wires, mechanical properties of, 425t
Sticky wax, *361*, *377*, 379
  federal specifications for, summary of requirements, 379t
Stone, 321-322
  high-strength, manufacture of, 333-334, *334*
  manufacture of, 333-334, *334*
  properties of, 340t
  viscosity, 341t
Storage problems, impression materials, 318
Strain, 58-59
  impression materials, 310, 310t
Strength
  impression materials, 287, 292
  of noble alloys, 394-395
  various phases, amalgam, 218-219, *219*
Strength properties, polymer, 504-510, 506-507t
Strengthening techniques, metals, *123-125*, 124-125
Stress, 57-59
  analysis of, 92-94
  types of, 58, *58-59*
Stress-strain curves, 59-69, *60-61*, *69*
Surface finish, thickness, 34
Surface hardness, gypsum, 342-343

Surface mechanical properties, 86
Surface phenomena, 16-29
    absorption, and sorption, 20-21
    adhesion, 27-28
    adsorption, 20-21
    AES depth profile, for titanium implant surface, 18
    capillaries, around teeth, formature of, 26
    capillary penetration, depression, 25
    capillary rise, 24-26, *25*
        curves, for water, between plates of dissimilar
            materials, 25
        isolated capillaries, 24-26, *26*
        penetration coefficient, 24, *26*
    capillary systems, two classes of, 26
    colloid systems, 19
        emulsions, 20
        gels, 19
        syneresis, 20
    colloidal state, 18-20
    colloids, nature of, 18-19
    contact angle
        spreading, wetting, relationship, 22
        water
            on solids, 23
            wax, acrylic plastic, 23
    contact single, formed by balance of energies, between
            liquid, solid, 23
    denture retention, forces involved in, 26-27
    diffusion, through membranes, 20
    ESGA spectrum, from surface of hydroxyapatite,
            17
    interface, sealant
        and enamel, scanning electron micrograph, 26
        scanning electron micrograph, 26
    mercury, contact angle of, on various materials, 24
    metals, surface tension of, 23
    osmotic pressure, 20
    soap molecules, on wax, water containing, 22
    sodium oleate, in water, 21
    solid surfaces, characterization of, 17-18, *17-18*
    sorption, 20-21
    surface tension, 21t, 21-24, *22-23*, 23-24t
    water, pure, spreading of, 22
    wetting, 21t, 21-24, *22-23*, 23-24t
    XPS spectrum, for Ti implant, 17
Surface roughness
    amalgam, various methods of instrumentation,
            231t
    composites finished with various abrasives, 263t
Surface tension, 21t, 21-24, *22-23*, 23-24t
    metals, 23
Swanger, W.L., 13

Syneresis, surface phenomena, 20
Synthetic waxes, 364
Systemic reactions, amalgam, 235-236, *236*

T

Taggart, W.H., 11
Tarnish, 51
    resistance, solders, 400
Taveau, O., 8
Tear energy, 84-85, 84-85t
    materials, 85t
Tear strength, 84-85, 84-85t
    impression materials, 311
    materials, 84t
Temperature, 38-39, *39*
    of alloys, 387-389
    gypsum, 350-351
    on oral surface, tissue surface, acrylic,
            cobalt-chromium palate, eating, *43*
Temporary cementation, 186-187
Temporary crown, polymer, 543-544
Temporary restorations, 187
Tensile strength
    amalgam, 218, 218t, 227
    gypsum, 343
    restorative materials, values of, 70t
Tests, biocompatibility
    initial, 147-153
    intermediate, 153
Theophilus, 6
Thermal characteristics, polymer, 510-511
Thermal conductivity, 42, *43*, 43t
    cement, 182-183
    impression materials, 319
    various materials, 43t
Thermal contraction, impression materials, 320
Thermal diffusivity, 44, 44t
    various materials, 44t
Thermal expansion
    coefficient, 44-45, 45t, *46*
        of various materials, 45t
    curves, silica, *46*
    wax, *366*, 366-367, 367t
Thermal properties, 38-45
    restorative materials, esthetic, direct, 253t,
            253-254
Ti-6A1-4V, 415-416, *416*
Tin, in alloys, 387
Titanium, 415-421
    alloys, 415-421
    cast, 416-418, *417-418*, 463-464

Titanium—cont'd
   commercially pure, 415
   implants, 418-421
   Ti-6A1-4V, 415-416, *416*
   wrought, applications, 421
Tooth bleaching agents, effects of, 264
Torsion, *75*, 75-76
Townsend, Elisha, 10
Transition temperatures, 40-41, *40-41*
Transverse strength, 73t, 73-74, *73-74*
   amalgam, 218
   restorative materials, 73t
Tray compounds, impression materials, 320t,
     320-321
Twentieth century, history, restorative metals, 11-14
Two-dimensional photoelasticity, 92-93, *93*
Two-paste system, restorative materials, esthetic, direct,
     249, 262

U

Ultimate strength, *61*, 63-64
Undermix, amalgam, 226-228, *227*
United States, history, restorative metals, 8-9
Urine, mercury in, 233-234
Usage tests
   in animals, 154-155
   correlation, 138-139t, 155t, 155-156
Utility wax, 379, 379t
   federal specifications for, summary of
     requirements, 379t

V

Vacuum-investing procedure, 444-445, *445*
Van Soolingen, Hornelis, 7
Vickers hardness test, 89, *89*
Viscoelastic materials, 79-80, *80*
Viscoelasticity, 77-83
   mechanical models of, 80-81, *81-82*
Viscosity, 77t, 77-79, *78-79*
   cement, 179, *180*, 189, 190
   gypsum, 341, 341t
   impression materials, 306t, 306-308, *307*
   materials, soon after mixing, 77t
Visual technic, color measurement, 32-34, *34*
Vulcanite
   development of, 10
   introduction of, 8

W

Ward, M.L., 12
Water, pure, spreading of, 22

Water/powder ratio
   compressive strength, gypsum, 342t
   effect on setting time, gypsum, 340t
Water sorption, 51
   restorative materials, esthetic, direct,
     253t, 254
Wax, *361*, 361-382, 371t, 371-380
   baseplate, 376-378
     requirements for, 378t
   bite registration wax, 380
   boxing, *361*, 378-379, 379t
     federal specifications for, summary of
       requirements, 379t
   casting, *361*, *374*, 374-376
     federal specifications, summary of requirements
       of, 375t
   classification of, 367t
   components of, 362t
   corrective impression wax, 379-380, *380*
   ductility, 371
   elimination, 446-448, *447*
   fats, 364
   flow, 368-369, *368-370*
   gums, 364
   as impression material, 318
   inlay casting, flow requirements for, 372t
   inlay pattern, 371-374
   mechanical properties, *367*, 367-368
   melting range, 365-366, *365-366*
   models, 7
   natural, 362-364
   properties, 365-371
   residual stress, *370*, 370-371
   resin, 365
     modeling material, 376, *376*, 376t
   sticky, *361*, *377*, 379
     federal specifications for, summary of
       requirements, 379t
   synthetic waxes, 364
   thermal expansion, *366*, 366-367, 367t
   utility, 379, 379t
     federal specifications for, summary of
       requirements, 379t
Wax patterns
   direct, casting, 439
   indirect, casting, 439-440, *440*
Weinstein Research Laboratories, 13
Wettability
   casting and, 441-442, *442*
   of rubber impression materials, 312, 313t
White, S.S., 9
Williams, R.V., 12

Wire, 5
  not containing precious metals requirements,
       ANSI/ADA specification No. 32, 424t
  properties of, in tension, bending, and torsion, 424t
Working time
  amalgam, 227
  impression materials, 285, 306t, 308, *308*
Wrought alloys, 395-397
  base metal, 408-436
  composition, 396
  microstructure, 396
  properties, 396-397

X

XPS spectrum, for Ti implant, 17

Y

Yield strength, *61*, 62-63, 63t
  values of, 63t

Z

Zeta-potential, 50, 51t
Zinc, in alloys, 387
Zinc oxide–eugenol bases, cement, 183-189, 185t, 200,
       201, 201t
  specification requirements for, 185t
Zinc oxide–eugenol endodontic sealers, composition
       of, 187t
Zinc oxide–eugenol impression paste, 315-317
  physical properties, 318t
Zinc oxide–eugenol temporary filling cement,
       formula for, 183t
Zinc oxide–non-eugenol cement, specification
       requirements for, 185t
Zinc phosphate cement, 173-183
  manipulative variables, effects of, 181t
  rate of set of, factors governing, 180t
  typical composition of, 173t
Zinc polyacrylate, 189-192, 272t